Nuclear Medicine

THE REQUISITES IN RADIOLOGY

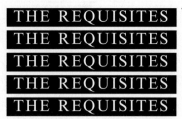

THE REQUISITES ™
THE REQUISITES
THE REQUISITES
THE REQUISITES
THE REQUISITES

THE REQUISITES is a propieary trademark
of Mosby, Inc.

SERIES EDITOR **James H. Thrall,** MD
Radiologist-in-Chief
Massachusetts General Hospital
Juan M. Taveras Professor of Radiology
Harvard Medical School Department of Radiology
Boston, Massachusetts

OTHER VOLUMES IN THE REQUISITES
IN RADIOLOGY SERIES

Breast Imaging

Cardiac Imaging

Gastrointestinal Imaging

Genitourinary Imaging

Musculoskeletal Imaging

Neuroradiology

Nuclear Medicine

Pediatric Imaging

Ultrasound

Thoracic Imaging

Vascular & Interventional Imaging

Nuclear Medicine

THE REQUISITES IN RADIOLOGY

Harvey A. Ziessman, MD
Professor of Radiology
Director of Nuclear Medicine Imaging
The Johns Hopkins University
Baltimore, Maryland

Janis P. O'Malley, MD
Director of Nuclear Medicine & Clinical PET
Assistant Professor Radiology
University of Alabama at Birmingham Medical Center
Birmingham, Alabama

James H. Thrall, MD
Radiologist-in-Chief
Massachusetts General Hospital
Juan M. Taveras Professor of Radiology
Harvard Medical School Department of Radiology
Massachusetts General Hospital
Boston, Massachusetts

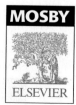

MOSBY

ELSEVIER

ELSEVIER
MOSBY

1600 John F. Kennedy Boulevard, Suite 1800
Philadelphia, PA 19103-2899

NUCLEAR MEDICINE: THE REQUISITES IN RADIOLOGY

ISBN: 978-0-323-02946-9
ISBN: 0-323-02946-9

Notice

Knowledge and best practice in this field are constantly changing. As new research and experience broaden our knowledge, changes in practice, treatment and drug therapy may become necessary or appropriate. Readers are advised to check the most current information provided (i) on procedures featured or (ii) by the manufacturer of each product to be administered, to verify the recommended dose or formula, the method and duration of administration, and contraindications. It is the responsibility of the practitioner, relying on his or her own experience and knowledge of the patient, to make diagnoses, to determine dosages and the best treatment for each individual patient, and to take all appropriate safety precautions. To the fullest extent of the law, neither the Publisher nor the Editor assumes any liability for any injury and/or damage to persons or property arising out or related to any use of the material contained in this book.

Third Edition

Library of Congress Cataloging-in-Publication Data

Ziessman, Harvey A.
Nuclear medicine : the requisites / Harvey A. Ziessman, Janis P. O'Malley, James H. Thrall. – 3rd ed.
   p. ; cm. – (Requisites in radiology)
   Thrall's name appears first on the earlier ed.
   Includes bibliographical references and index.
   ISBN 0-323-02946-9
      1. Nuclear medicine. I. O'Malley, Janis P. II. Thrall, James H. III. Title. IV. Series.
   [DNLM: 1. Radionuclide Imaging. 2. Diagnostic Techniques, Radioisotope. 3. Nuclear Medicine-meth ods. WN 203 Z67n 2006]
   R895.T498 2006
   616.07'575–dc22   2005050503

Acquisitions Editor: Meghan McAteer
Developmental Editor: Karen Lynn Carter
Publishing Services Manager: Joan Sinclair
Project Manager: Mary Stermel
Marketing Manager: Emily Christie

Printed in the United States

Last digit is the print number: 9 8 7 6 5 4 3 2 1

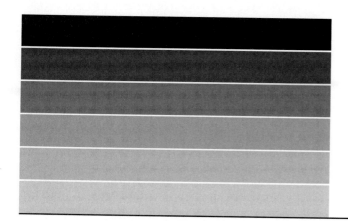

Preface

The 2006 third edition of *Nuclear Medicine: The Requisites in Radiology* closely follows the philosophy and format that has been successful in two prior editions. Our principal aim has been to provide a concise introduction and review of the field of nuclear medicine. Although the textbook has been directed specifically toward radiology and nuclear medicine residents, it has found a much wider audience of practicing physicians, basic scientists, technologists, and medical students.

Dramatic changes have occurred in the field of nuclear medicine since the publication of the second edition in 2001. New radiotracers have been developed and many have become clinically important. Radiopharmaceuticals that depict various aspects of physiology and function continue to be the cornerstone and unique advantage of nuclear medicine. Rapid advances in instrumentation have also powered recent growth in our field.

The use of a radiolabeled glucose analog, F-18 fluorodeoxyglucose (FDG), in conjunction with positron emission tomography (PET) for tumor imaging, has dramatically changed the practice of nuclear medicine. The acceptance and enthusiasm for PET by oncologists, surgeons, and radiation therapists has made FDG PET imaging mandatory for state-of-the-art oncologic care of many cancers.

Medicare and insurance reimbursement for FDG PET scanning resulted in an exponential sales growth of PET scanners in the late 1990s and early 2000s. However, we have now seen a dramatic shift from dedicated PET cameras to hybrid PET/CT systems that allow acquisition of both in a single study. In the second edition, we added a basic science chapter on SPECT and PET because of its growing importance. In the third edition we have added a new clinical chapter dedicated to the subject of oncologic F-18 FDG PET and PET/CT.

PET is also beginning to show growth in areas other than oncology, notably, nuclear cardiology, and neurology. For example, the use of Rb-82 myocardial perfusion imaging is in an early growth phase. F-18 FDG has become the gold standard for the diagnosis of myocardial viability. Neurologic PET, long important for the investigation of pathophysiologic mechanisms, is becoming increasingly important clinically with awareness and concern for the diagnosis and therapy of dementias.

Although single-photon nuclear cardiology is now a mature methodology, SPECT myocardial perfusion imaging continues to grow at a very rapid rate, exceeded only by FDG PET. A complete cardiac study now routinely includes analysis of myocardial perfusion using SPECT, gated wall motion and thickening, left ventricular ejection fraction, attenuation correction, and various two- and three-dimensional quantitative displays.

Single-photon oncologic nuclear medicine is also an important area of growth and change. Peptide imaging with radiolabeled somatostatin receptor imaging agents has become a routine study in many nuclear medicine practices, requested for the evaluation and follow-up of patients with neuroendocrine tumors. Radiolabeled monoclonal antibodies have matured and are used clinically for both diagnosis and therapy. Radioimmunotherapy is coming into its own with growing clinical demand for I-131– and Y-90–labeled monoclonal antibodies for therapy of B-cell lymphoma. A new infection-seeking antibody radiopharmaceutical has recently become available that does not require in vitro labeling, which likely will become a valuable diagnostic imaging agent without the potential dangers of blood handling.

Nuclear Medicine: The Requisites has always emphasized basic principles and concepts of radiopharmaceuticals and instrumentation. An appreciation of the pharmacokinetics, distribution, and clearance of radiopharmaceuticals and the power and limitations of modern single- and dual-photon cameras, in conjunction with an understanding of pathophysiology, provides the tools necessary for choosing optimal imaging protocols and for image interpretation.

Many chapters have been completely rewritten, most notably, Nuclear Cardiology, Neurology, Endocrine, and Genitourinary. Others have been significantly revised and updated (e.g., Skeletal, Single-Photon Oncology, Pulmonary, Infection and Inflammation, Hepatobiliary, and Gastro-enterology). The popular Pearls, Pitfalls, and Frequently Asked Questions has been expanded and updated.

Important principles continue to be highlighted in the boxes and tables in each chapter. Typical protocols are presented for each study type. Schematic diagrams illustrate basic concepts and innumerable scintigraphic examples are provided. Many new figures, tables, and boxes have been added in this edition.

A new co-author, Janis P. O'Malley, MD, has given the textbook new energy and a fresh perspective. We hope that you find the third edition of the *Nuclear Medicine: The Requisites* to be even better than the two previous editions and that it is a continual source of knowledge and ideas, presented is an easy to read and understandable manner.

Harvey A. Ziessman
Janis P. O'Malley
James H. Thrall

Acknowledgments

We would like to thank those persons that have contributed to the preparation of *Nuclear Medicine: The Requisites*, third edition. First and foremost, our gratitude goes out to our many trainees, who over the years who have taught us at least as much as we have taught them. Some have helped in the preparation and review of this third edition. We thank: William Lavely, MD, Heather A. Jacene, MD, Alex Dibona, MD, Matt Larrison, MD, Joel Mixon, MD, Carl Merrow, MD, Robert Morris, MD, Ashok Muthukrishnan, MD, and Jubal Watts, MD. Many colleagues have contributed in direct and indirect ways. We particularly wish to thank Frederic H. Fahey, D.Sc, Jon Baldwin, DO, Honggang Liu, MS, Eva V. Dubovsky, MD, Sharon White, PhD, Douglas F. Eggli, MD, Massoud Madj, MD, James M. Mountz, MD, PhD, and Christopher J. Palestro, MD.

New high-quality original diagrams and illustrations have been provided by Tim Phelps and Kate Weaver in the Johns Hopkins Department of Art as Applied to Medicine, Rick Tracy in the Department of Pathology at Johns Hopkins, and David Fisher in the UAB Medical Education and Design Services.

We would also like to thank our families for supporting us in this endeavor and enduring the many hours of our absences from them to complete this edition. We have been stimulated and taught by our past mentors, our present colleagues, and many trainees. Thus we dedicate the third edition to all of them.

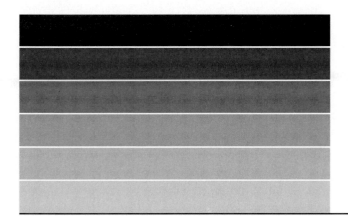

Foreword

The third edition of *Nuclear Medicine: The Requisites* continues to follow the philosophy and format of the first two editions. The basic science chapters are designed to present important principles of physics, instrumentation, and nuclear pharmacy in the context of how they help shape clinical practice. The clinical chapters continue to follow a logical progression from basic principles of tracer distribution and localization to practical clinical applications. The authors believe that understanding tracer mechanisms is fundamental to nuclear medicine practice and that knowledge of how radiopharmaceuticals localize temporally and spatially is the best deductive tool available for analyzing images rather than simply memorizing representative illustrations.

Both the basic science and the clinical chapters have been extensively revised and rewritten to reflect the changing nature of nuclear medicine practice. At the time the first edition of *Nuclear Medicine: The Requisites* was published, single photon computed emission computed tomography (SPECT) was not in ubiquitous use and positron emission computed tomography (PET) was restricted to a small number of research centers. Today, barely a decade later, the use of SPECT is widespread especially for cardiac applications and PET has moved well beyond the halls of academia. SPECT and PET applications now dominate nuclear medicine practice. These methods are fully described and richly illustrated throughout the book.

The basic chapter describing SPECT and PET now also includes material on PET-CT, which is rapidly becoming an important and even dominant new approach to correlative imaging. PET-CT brings the functional and metabolic information available from nuclear medicine studies together with the exquisite anatomical detail available from computed tomography. New pharmaceuticals have been added to the nuclear medicine armamentarium and are included as appropriate in the organ system chapters. Keeping up with the manifold changes occurring in the specialty is challenging to practitioners of nuclear medicine and presented formidable challenges to the authors of *Nuclear Medicine: The Requisites* in making sure that each chapter reflects current state-of-the-art practices.

The Requisites in Radiology have now become old friends to a generation of radiologists. The original intent of the series was to provide the resident or fellow with a text that might be reasonably read within several days at the beginning of each subspecialty rotation and perhaps reread several times during subsequent rotations or during board preparation. The series is not intended to be exhaustive but to provide the basic conceptual, factual, and interpretive material required for clinical practice.

Each book in The Requisites series is written by nationally recognized authorities in their respective subspecialty areas. Each author is challenged to present material in the context of today's practice of radiology rather than grafting information about new imaging modalities onto old out-of-date material. It is our hope in adopting this strategy that readers will find The Requisites to be a very efficient way of accessing the most important material.

The first two editions of *Nuclear Medicine: The Requisites* were well received in the radiology and nuclear medicine community, and we are hopeful that the third edition will be regarded as equally outstanding. We hope that *Nuclear Medicine: The Requisites* will serve residents in radiology as a concise and useful introduction to the subject and will also serve as a very manageable text for review by fellows and practicing nuclear medicine specialists and radiologists.

James H. Thrall, M.D.
Radiologist-in-Chief
Massachusetts General Hospital
Juan M. Taveras Professor of Radiology
Harvard Medical School
Boston, Massachusetts

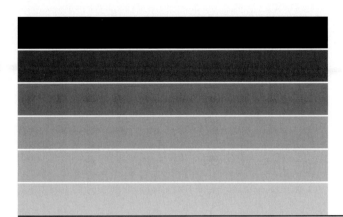

Contents

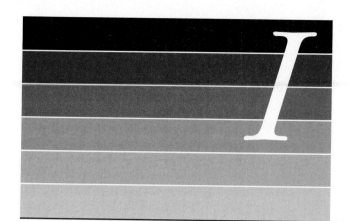

BASIC PRINCIPLES

Radiopharmaceuticals

Radiopharmaceuticals portray the physiology, biochemistry, or pathology of a body system without causing any perturbation of function. They are referred to as *radiotracers* because they are given in subpharmacologic doses that "trace" a particular physiological or pathologic process in the body.

Most radiopharmaceuticals are a combination of a radioactive molecule that permits external detection and a biologically active molecule or drug that acts as a carrier and determines localization and biodistribution. For a few radiotracers, the radioactive atoms themselves confer the desired localization properties and an attached larger pharmaceutical component is not required, such as I-131 or I-123 sodium iodide, gallium-67 citrate (Ga-67), and thallium-201 chloride (Tl-201).

Table 1-1 summarizes some of the localization mechanisms of radiopharmaceuticals important to clinical practice. Understanding the mechanism or rationale for the use of each agent is critical to understanding the normal and pathological findings demonstrated scintigraphically. Because both naturally occurring and synthetic molecules can potentially be radiolabeled, great flexibility exists in designing and developing radiopharmaceuticals.

Radiopharmaceuticals for each major clinical application are considered in detail in chapters on the respective organ systems. This chapter presents some of the general principles of radiopharmaceutical production, radiolabeling, quality assurance, and dispensing.

RADIOPHARMACEUTICALS, RADIOCHEMICALS, AND RADIONUCLIDES

The term *radionuclide* refers only to radioactive atoms. When a radionuclide is combined with a chemical molecule to confer desired localization properties, the combination is referred to as a *radiochemical*. The term

Table 1-1 Mechanisms of Radiopharmaceutical Localization

Mechanism	Applications or examples
Compartmental localization	Blood pool imaging, direct cystography
Passive diffusion (concentration dependent)	Blood-brain barrier breakdown, glomerular filtration, cisternography
Capillary blockade (physical entrapment)	Perfusion imaging of lungs
Physical leakage from a luminal compartment	Gastrointestinal bleeding, detection of urinary tract or biliary system leakage
Metabolism	Glucose, fatty acids
Active transport (active cellular uptake)	Hepatobiliary imaging, renal tubular function, thyroid and adrenal imaging
Chemical bonding and adsorption	Skeletal imaging
Cell sequestration	Splenic imaging (heat-damaged red blood cells), white blood cells
Receptor binding and storage	Adrenal medullary imaging, somatostatin receptor imaging
Phagocytosis	Reticuloendothelial system imaging
Antigen-antibody	Tumor imaging
Multiple mechanisms	
Perfusion and active transport	Myocardial imaging
Active transport and metabolism	Thyroid uptake and imaging
Active transport and secretion	Hepatobiliary imaging, salivary gland imaging

radiopharmaceutical is reserved for radioactive materials that have met legal requirements for administration to patients or subjects. In the United States, this approval must be given by the Food and Drug Administration (FDA) before these substances can be commercially produced and used for clinical purposes.

The term *carrier-free* implies that a radionuclide is not contaminated by either stable or radioactive nuclides of the same element. The presence of carrier material can influence biodistribution and efficiency of radiolabeling. The term *specific activity* refers to the radioactivity per unit weight (mCi/mg). Carrier-free samples of a radionuclide have the highest specific activity.

Design Characteristics of Radiopharmaceuticals

Certain characteristics are desirable in the design of radiopharmaceuticals. The radionuclide decay should result in gamma emissions of suitable energy (100–200 keV is ideal for gamma cameras) and sufficient abundance of emissions for external detection. It should not contain particulate radiation (e.g., beta emissions), which increases the patient's radiation dose without adding diagnostic information. Beta emissions are suitable for therapeutic radiopharmaceuticals. The effective half-life should only be long enough for the intended application, usually a few hours. The specific activity should be high. Technetium-99m (Tc-99m) closely matches these desirable features.

The pharmaceutical component should be free of any toxicity or secondary effects. The radiopharmaceutical should not disassociate in vitro or in vivo, should be readily available or easily compounded, and should have a reasonable cost. The agent should rapidly and specifically localize according to the intended application. Background clearance should be rapid, leading to good target-to-background ratios.

PRODUCTION OF RADIONUCLIDES

Naturally occurring radionuclides have long half-lives (>1000 years) and are heavy, toxic elements (e.g., uranium, actinium, thorium, radium, and radon). They have no clinical role in diagnostic nuclear medicine. The radionuclides most commonly used clinically are artificially produced.

Bombardment of medium atomic-weight nuclides with low-energy neutrons in nuclear reactors (neutron activation) results in neutron-rich radionuclides that undergo beta-minus decay. Neutron bombardment of enriched uranium-235 (U-235) results in fission products in the middle of the atomic chart (Fig. 1-1). The uncontrolled release of radioactive iodines in atomic bomb explosions and during accidents at nuclear power plants is a well-known phenomenon that can also be used for production purposes under controlled conditions in a nuclear reactor. *Proton bombardment* of a wide variety of target nuclides in cyclotrons or other special accelerators produces proton-rich radionuclides that undergo positron decay or electron capture.

Radionuclides produced in nuclear reactors include I-131, Xe-133, Cr-51, and molybdenum-99; those produced in cyclotrons or particle accelerators include F-18, I-123, Ga-67, Tl-201, and In-111. Tables 1-2 and 1-3 summarize the production source and physical characteristics of commonly used radionuclides in clinical nuclear medicine practice.

RADIONUCLIDE GENERATORS

One of the practical issues faced in nuclear medicine is the desirability of using relatively short-lived agents

Periodic Table of Elements

Period	I A																	VIII A
1	1 H	II A											III A	IV A	V A	VI A	VII A	2 He
2	3 Li	4 Be												5 B	6 C	7 N	8 O	9 F	10 Ne
3	11 Na	12 Mg	III B	IV B	V B	VI B	VII B	———	VIII	———	I B	II B	13 Al	14 Si	15 P	16 S	17 Cl	18 Ar
4	19 K	20 Ca	21 Sc	22 Ti	23 V	24 Cr	25 Mn	26 Fe	27 Co	28 Ni	29 Cu	30 Zn	31 Ga	32 Ge	33 As	34 Se	35 Br	36 Kr
5	37 Rb	38 Sr	39 Y	40 Zr	41 Nb	42 Mo	43 Tc	44 Ru	45 Rh	46 Pd	47 Ag	48 Cd	49 In	50 Sn	51 Sb	52 Te	53 I	54 Xe
6	55 Cs	56 Ba	*	71 Lu	72 Hf	73 Ta	74 W	75 Re	76 Os	77 Ir	78 Pt	79 Au	80 Hg	81 Tl	82 Pb	83 Bi	84 Po	85 At	86 Rn
7	87 Fr	88 Ra	**	103 Lr	104 Rf	105 Db	106 Sg	107 Bh	108 Hs	109 Mt	110 Ds	111 Rg	112 Uub	113 Uut	114 Uuq	115 Uup	116 Uuh	117 Uus	118 Uuo

*Lanthanoids	*	57 La	58 Ce	59 Pr	60 Nd	61 Pm	62 Sm	63 Eu	64 Gd	65 Tb	66 Dy	67 Ho	68 Er	69 Tm	70 Yb
**Actinoids	**	89 Ac	90 Th	91 Pa	92 U	93 Np	94 Pu	95 Am	96 Cm	97 Bk	98 Cf	99 Es	100 Fm	101 Md	102 No

Figure 1-1   Periodic table.

Table 1-2   Physical Characteristics of Single-Photon Radionuclides Used in Clinical Nuclear Medicine

Radionuclide	Principal mode of decay	Physical half-life	Principal photon energy in keV (abundance)	Production method
Molybdenum-99	Beta minus	2.8 d	740 (12%), 780 (4%)	Reactor
Technetium-99m	Isomeric transition	6 hr	140 (89%)	Generator (molybdenum-99)
Iodine-131	Beta minus	8 d	364 (81%)	Reactor
Iodine-123	Electron capture	13.2 hr	159 (83%)	Cyclotron
Gallium-67	Electron capture	78.3 hr	93 (37%), 185 (20%), 300 (17%), 395 (5%)	Cyclotron
Thallium-201	Electron capture	73.1 hr	69-83 (Hg x-rays), 135 (2.5%), 167 (10%)	Cyclotron
Indium-111	Electron capture	2.8 d	171 (90%), 245 (94%)	Cyclotron
Xenon-127	Electron capture	36 d	172 (26%), 203 (7%), 375 (17%)	Cyclotron
Xenon-133	Beta minus	5.2 d	81 (37%)	Reactor
Cobalt-57	Electron capture	272 d	122 (86%)	Cyclotron

Table 1-3   Physical Characteristics of Positron-Emitting Radionuclides Used in Nuclear Medicine

Radionuclide	Physical half-life (min)	Positron energy (MeV)	Range in soft tissue (mm)	Production method
Carbon-11	20	0.96	4.1	Cyclotron
Nitrogen-13	10	1.19	5.4	Cyclotron
Oxygen-15	2	1.73	7.3	Cyclotron
Fluorine-18	110	0.635	2.4	Cyclotron
Gallium-68	68	1.9	8.1	Generator (germanium-68)
Rubidium-82	1.3	3.15	15.0	Generator (strontium-82)

<table>
<tr><td colspan="5">**Table 1-4   Radionuclide Generator Systems and Parent and Daughter Half-Lives**</td></tr>
<tr><th>Parent</th><th>Parent's half-life</th><th>Daughter</th><th>Daughter's half-life</th></tr>
<tr><td>Molybdenum-99</td><td>66 hr</td><td>Technetium-99m</td><td>6 hr</td></tr>
<tr><td>Rubidium-81</td><td>4.5 hr</td><td>Krypton-81m</td><td>13 sec</td></tr>
<tr><td>Germanium-68</td><td>270 d</td><td>Gallium-68</td><td>68 min</td></tr>
<tr><td>Strontium-82</td><td>25 d</td><td>Rubidium-82</td><td>1.3 min</td></tr>
<tr><td>Tin-113</td><td>115 d</td><td>Indium-113m</td><td>1.7 hr</td></tr>
<tr><td>Yttrium-87</td><td>3.3 d</td><td>Strontium-87m</td><td>2.8 hr</td></tr>
<tr><td>Tellurium-132</td><td>3.2 d</td><td>Iodine-132</td><td>2.3 hr</td></tr>
</table>

(hours rather than days or weeks) and at the same time the need to have radiopharmaceuticals delivered to hospitals or clinics from commercial sources. One way around this dilemma is the use of radionuclide generator systems. These systems consist of a longer-lived parent and a shorter-lived daughter. With this combination of half-lives, the generator can be shipped from a commercial vendor and the daughter product will still have a useful half-life for clinical applications. Although a number of generator systems have been developed over the years (Table 1-4), the most important one has been the Mo-99/Tc-99m system (Table 1-4).

MOLYBDENUM-99/TECHNETIUM-99M GENERATOR SYSTEMS

The historical production method for Mo-99 was a neutron activation reaction of Mo-98:

$$Mo\text{-}98\ (n,\gamma) \rightarrow Mo\text{-}99$$

This older production method resulted in low specific activity, requiring a large ion exchange column to hold both the desired Mo-99 and the carrier Mo-98 left over from the target material. This process resulted in low specific concentrations of Tc-99m pertechnetate from generator elution because of the large volume of eluant needed for complete removal of the Tc-99m activity.

Mo-99 is now produced by the fission of U-235. The product is often referred to as "fission moly." The reaction is:

$$U\text{-}235\ (n, \text{fission}) \rightarrow Mo\text{-}99$$

After Mo-99 is produced in the fission reaction, it is chemically purified and passed on to an anion exchange column composed of alumina (Al_2O_3) (Table 1-5). The column is typically adjusted to an acid pH to promote binding. The positive charge of the alumina binds the molybdate ions firmly.

<table>
<tr><td colspan="3">**Table 1-5   Molybdenum-99 (Mo-99)/Technetium-99m (Tc-99m) Generator Systems**</td></tr>
<tr><th>Radionuclides</th><th>Parent (Mo-99)</th><th>Daughter (Tc-99m)</th></tr>
<tr><td>Half-life</td><td>66 hr</td><td>6 hr</td></tr>
<tr><td>Mode of decay</td><td>Beta minus</td><td>Isomeric transition</td></tr>
<tr><td>Daughter products</td><td>Tc-99m, Tc-99</td><td>Tc-99</td></tr>
<tr><td>Principal photon energies*</td><td>740 keV, 780 keV</td><td>140 keV (89%)</td></tr>
<tr><td colspan="3">**GENERATOR FUNCTION**</td></tr>
<tr><td>Composition of ion exchange column</td><td>Al_2O_3</td><td></td></tr>
<tr><td>Eluant</td><td>Normal saline (0.9%)</td><td></td></tr>
<tr><td>Time from elution to maximum daughter yield</td><td>23 hr</td><td></td></tr>
</table>

*The decay scheme for Mo-99 is complex, with over 35 gamma rays of different energies given off. The listed energies are those used in clinical practice for radionuclidic purity checks.

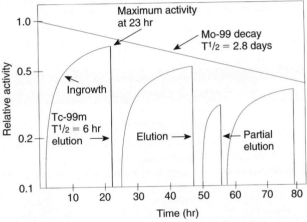

Figure 1-2   Decay curve for molybdenum-99 and ingrowth curves for Tc-99m. Successive elutions, including a partial elution are illustrated. Relative activity is plotted on a logarithmic scale, accounting for the straight line of Mo-99 decay.

The loaded column is placed in a lead container with tubing attached at each end to permit column elution. Commercial generator systems are autoclaved and the elution dynamics are quality controlled before shipment. Alternatively, systems may be aseptically assembled from previously sterilized components.

Generator Operation and Yield

Figure 1-2 illustrates the relationship between Mo-99 decay and the ingrowth of Tc-99m. Maximum buildup of Tc-99m activity occurs at 23 hours after elution. This time point is convenient, especially if sufficient Tc-99m activity is available to accomplish each day's work.

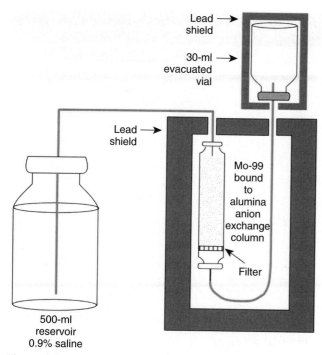

Figure 1-3   "Wet" radionuclide generator system.

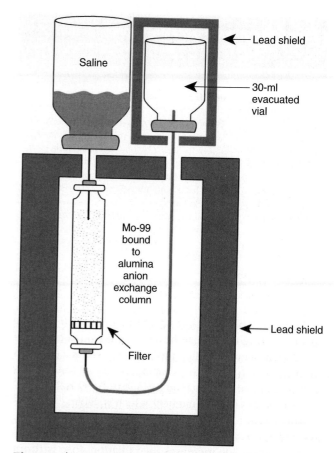

Figure 1-4   "Dry" radionuclide generator system.

Otherwise, the generator can be eluted, or "milked," more than once a day. Partial elution is also illustrated in Fig. 1-2. Fifty percent of maximum is reached in approximately 4.5 hours and 75% of maximum is available at 8.5 hours.

Although greatest attention is paid to the rate of Tc-99m buildup, it should also be remembered that Tc-99m is constantly decaying, with buildup of stable Tc-99 (or "carrier" Tc-99) in the generator. Generators received after commercial shipment or generators that have not been eluted for several days have significant carrier Tc-99 in the eluate. Because the carrier Tc-99 chemically behaves in an identical fashion to Tc-99m, it can compete and adversely affect radiopharmaceutical labeling efficiency. Many labeling procedures require the reduction of Tc-99m from a +7 valence state to a lower valence state. If the eluate contains sufficient carrier Tc-99, complete reduction may not occur, with resultant poor labeling and undesired radiochemical contaminants in the final preparation.

There are two basic types of generator systems with respect to elution. "Wet" systems are provided with a reservoir of normal saline (0.9%) (Fig. 1-3). Elution is accomplished by placing a special sterile vacuum vial on the exit or collection port. The vacuum vial is designed to draw the appropriate amount of saline across the column. In "dry" systems, a volume-calibrated saline charge is placed on the entry port and a vacuum vial is placed on the collection port (Fig. 1-4). The vacuum draws the saline eluant out of the original vial, across the column, and into the elution vial. Elution volumes are typically in the range of 5–20 ml. Elutions can be performed for add-on or emergency studies that come up in the course of a day (Fig. 1-2).

From Figure 1-2, it is obvious that the amount of Tc-99m activity available from a generator decreases each day as a result of decay of the Mo-99 parent. In practice, the 2.8-day half-life of Mo-99 allows generators to be used for 2 weeks, although many larger nuclear medicine operations require two generator deliveries per week.

Quality Control

Although rigorous quality control is performed prior to commercial generator shipment, it is important that each laboratory perform quality control steps each time the generator is eluted (Table 1-6). These quality control steps are good medical practice and are necessary to meet various federal and state regulatory guidelines.

Radionuclidic Purity

The only desired radionuclide in the Mo-99/Tc-99m generator eluate is Tc-99m. Any other radionuclide in the sample is considered a radionuclidic impurity and is undesirable because it will result in additional radiation exposure to the patient without clinical benefit.

The most common radionuclidic contaminant in the generator eluate is the parent radionuclide, Mo-99. Tc-99, the daughter product of the isomeric transition of Tc-99m,

Table 1-6	Purity Checks: Molybdenum-99 (Mo-99)/Technetium-99m (Tc-99m) Generator Systems		
	Problem	**Standard**	
Radionuclidic purity	Excessive Mo-99 in eluant	<0.15 μCi Mo-99/mCi Tc-99m at time of administration	
Chemical purity	Al_2O_3 from generator ion exchange column in elution	<10 μg/ml (fission generator) (aurin tricarboxylic acid spot test)	
Radiochemical purity	Reduced oxidation states of Tc-99m (i.e., +4, +5, or +6 instead of +7)	95% of Tc-99m activity should be in +7 oxidation state	

Table 1-7	Physical Decay of Technetium-99m
Time (hr)	**Fraction remaining**
0	1.000
1	0.891
2	0.794
3	0.708
4	0.631
5	0.532
6	0.501
7	0.447
8	0.398
9	0.355
10	0.316
11	0.282
12	0.251

Tc-99m physical half-life = 6.02 hours.

is also present but is not considered an impurity or contaminant. Although Tc-99 can be a problem from a chemical standpoint in radiolabeling procedures, it is not a problem from a radiation or health standpoint and is not tested for as a radionuclide impurity. The half-life of Tc-99 is 2.1×10^5 years. It decays to ruthenium-99, which is stable.

The amount of parent Mo-99m in the eluate should be as small as possible because any contamination by a long-lived radionuclide increases the radiation dose without providing any benefit to the patient. The Nuclear Regulatory Commission (NRC) sets limits on the amount of Mo-99 in the eluate and this must be tested on each elution. Perhaps the easiest and most widely used approach is to take advantage of the energetic 740- and 780-keV gamma rays of Mo-99 with dual counting of the specimen. The generator eluate is placed in a lead container carefully designed so that all of the 140-keV photons of technetium are absorbed but approximately 50% of the more energetic Mo-99 gamma rays can penetrate. Adjusting the dose calibrator to the Mo-99 setting provides an estimate of the number of microcuries of Mo-99 in the sample. The unshielded sample is then measured on the Tc-99m setting and a ratio of Mo-99 to Tc-99m activity can be calculated.

The NRC limit is 0.15 μCi of Mo-99 activity per 1 mCi of Tc-99m activity in the administered dose (Table 1-5). Because the half-life of Mo-99 is longer than that of Tc-99m, the ratio actually increases with time, which is rarely a problem. However, if the initial reading shows near maximum Mo-99 levels, either the actual dose to be given to the patient should be restudied before administration or the buildup factor should be computed mathematically. From a practical standpoint, the Mo-99 activity may be taken as unchanged and the Tc-99m decay calculated (Table 1-7). Breakthrough is rare but unpredictable.

When it does occur, Mo-99 levels can be far higher than the legal limit.

Chemical Purity

Another routine quality assurance step is to measure the generator eluate for the presence of the column packing material, Al_2O_3. For fission generators, the maximum alumina concentration is 10 μg/ml. Aurin tricarboxylic acid is used for colorimetric spot testing. The color reaction for a standard 10 μg/ml sample of alumina is compared with a corresponding sample from the generator eluate. Acceptable levels are present if the color is less intense than the color of the standard. The comparison is made visually and qualitatively. No attempt is made to measure the alumina concentration quantitatively. Aluminum levels in excess of this limit have been shown to interfere with the normal distribution of certain radiopharmaceuticals, resulting in increased lung activity with Tc-99m sulfur colloid and increased liver activity with Tc-99m–methylene diphosphonate (Tc-MDP).

Radiochemical Purity

When eluted from the generator, the expected valence state of Tc-99m is +7, in the chemical form of pertechnetate (TcO_4^-). The clinical use of sodium pertechnetate as a radiopharmaceutical and the preparation of Tc-99m-labeled pharmaceuticals from commercial kits are based on the +7 oxidation state. The U.S. Pharmacopeia (USP) standard for the generator eluate is that 95% or more of Tc-99m activity be in this +7 state. Reduction states at +4, +5, or +6 result in impurities. However, these reduction states can be detected by thin-layer chromatography. Problems with radiochemical purity of the generator eluate are infrequently encountered but should be considered if

Table 1-8   Measures of Pharmaceutical Purity

Parameter	Definition	Example issues
Chemical purity	Fraction of wanted vs. unwanted chemical in preparation	Amount of alumina breakthrough in Mo-99/Tc-99m generator eluate
Radiochemical purity	Fraction of total radioactivity in desired chemical form	Amount of bound vs. unbound Tc-99m in Tc-99m diphosphonate
Radionuclidic purity	Fraction of total radioactivity in the form of desired radionuclide	Ratio of Tc-99m vs. Mo-99 in generator eluate; I-124 in an I-123 preparation
Physical purity	Fraction of total pharmaceutical in desired physical form	Correct particle size distribution in Tc-99m MAA preparation; absence of particulate contaminates in any agent that is a true solution
Biological purity	Absence of microorganisms and pyrogens	Sterile, pyrogen-free preparations

kit labeling is poor. Measures of pharmaceutical purity are summarized in Table 1-8.

TECHNETIUM CHEMISTRY AND RADIOPHARMACEUTICAL PREPARATION

Tc-99m is the most commonly used radionuclide because of its ready availability, the favorable energy of its principal gamma photon (140 keV), its favorable dosimetry with lack of primary particulate radiations, and its nearly ideal half-life (6 hours) for many clinical imaging studies. However, technetium chemistry is challenging. In most labeling procedures, technetium must be reduced from the +7 valence state. The reduction is usually accomplished with stannous ion. One exception is the labeling of Tc-99m sulfur colloid, which requires heating.

The actual final oxidation state of technetium in many radiopharmaceuticals is either unknown or subject to debate. A number of technetium compounds are chelates, which involve a complex bond at two or more sites on the ligand. Others are used on the basis of their empirical efficacy without complete knowledge of how technetium is being complexed in the final molecule. One exception to the need to reduce technetium from the +7 oxidation state is in the preparation of Tc-99m sulfur colloid (Tc_2S_7).

The details of individual technetium radiopharmaceuticals are discussed in the chapters on individual organ systems and include key points in preparation and the recognition of in vivo markers of radiopharmaceutical impurities. Table 1-9 summarizes the major Tc-99m-labeled agents that are used clinically.

Commercial kits contain a reaction vial with the appropriate amount of stannous ion (tin), the nonradioactive pharmaceutical to be labeled, and other buffering and stabilizing agents. The vials are flushed with nitrogen to prevent atmospheric oxygen from interrupting the reaction. Figure 1-5 illustrates the sequence of steps in a sample labeling process. Sodium pertechnetate is drawn into a syringe and assayed in the dose calibrator. After the proper Tc-99m activity is confirmed, the sample is added to the reaction vial. The amount of Tc-99m activity added for each respective product is determined by the number of patient doses desired in the case of a multidose vial, an estimate of the decrease in radioactivity caused by decay between the time of preparation and the estimated time of dosage administration, and the in vitro stability of the product. The completed product is labeled and kept in a special lead-shielded container until it is time to withdraw a sample for administration to a patient. Each patient dose is individually assayed before being dispensed.

Excessive oxygen can react directly with the stannous ion, leaving too little reducing power in the kit, which can result in unwanted free Tc-99m pertechnetate in the preparation. A less common problem is radiolysis after kit preparation, also resulting in free pertechnetate. The phenomenon is seen when high amounts of Tc-99m activity are used. The kit preparations are usually designed so that multiple doses can be prepared from one reaction vial.

QUALITY ASSURANCE OF TECHNETIUM-99M–LABELED RADIOPHARMACEUTICALS

The difficult nature of technetium chemistry highlights the importance of checking the final product for *radiochemical purity*. This term is defined as the percentage of the total radioactivity in a specimen that is in the specified or desired radiochemical form (Table 1-8). For example, if 5% of the Tc-99m activity remains as free pertechnetate in a radiolabeling procedure, the radiochemical purity would be stated as 95%, assuming no other impurities. Each radiopharmaceutical has a specific radiochemical purity to meet USP standards or FDA requirements, typically 90%. Causes of radiochemical impurities include poor initial labeling, radiolysis, decomposition, pH changes, light exposure, or presence of oxidizing or reducing agents.

Table 1-9   Technetium-99m Radiopharmaceuticals

Agent	Application
Tc-99m sodium pertechnetate	Meckel's diverticulum detection, salivary and thyroid gland scintigraphy
Tc-99m sulfur colloid (filtered)	Lymphoscintigraphy
Tc-99m sulfur colloid	Liver/spleen scintigraphy, bone marrow scintigraphy
Tc-99m pyrophosphate	Acute myocardial infarction detection
Tc-99m diphosphonate	Skeletal scintigraphy
Tc-99m macroaggregated albumin (MAA)	Pulmonary perfusion scintigraphy, liver intra-arterial perfusion scintigraphy
Tc-99m red blood cells	Radionuclide ventriculography, gastrointestinal bleeding, hepatic hemangioma
Tc-99m diethylenetriamine-pentaacetic acid (DTPA)	Renal scintigraphy, lung ventilation (aerosol), glomerular filtration rate
Tc-99m mercaptoacetyltriglycine (MAG$_3$)	Renal dynamic scintigraphy
Tc-99m dimercaptosuccinic acid (DMSA)	Renal cortical scintigraphy
Tc-99m iminodiacetic acid (HIDA) derivatives	Hepatobiliary scintigraphy
Tc-99m sestamibi (Cardiolite, Miraluma)	Myocardial perfusion scintigraphy, breast imaging
Tc-99m tetrofosmin (Myoview)	Myocardial perfusion scintigraphy
Tc-99m teboroxime (CardioTec)	Myocardial perfusion scintigraphy
Tc-99m exametazime (HMPAO)	Cerebral perfusion scintigraphy, white blood cell labeling
Tc-99m bicisate (ECD)	Cerebral perfusion scintigraphy
Tc-99m arcitumomab (CEA)	Monoclonal antibody for colorectal cancer evaluation
Tc-99m apcitide (AcuTect)	Acute venous thrombosis imaging
Tc-99m depreotide (NeoTect)	Tumor imaging
Tc-99m fanolesomab (NeutroSpec)	Infection imaging

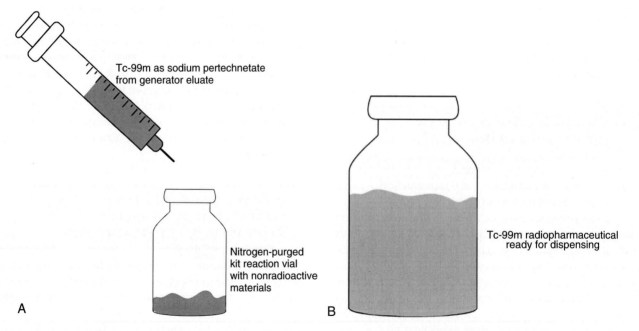

Figure 1-5   Preparation of a technetium-99m-labeled radiopharmaceutical. **A,** Tc-99m as sodium pertechnetate is added to the reaction vial. **B,** Tc-99m radiopharmaceutical is ready for dispensing.

In vivo, radiochemical impurities contribute to background activity or other unwanted localization and degrade image quality. For many agents, the presence of a radiochemical impurity can be recognized by altered in vivo biodistribution. However, intercepting the offending preparation before administration to a patient is desirable. A number of systems have been developed to assay radiochemical purity. The basic approach is to use thin-layer chromatography. Radiochromatography is performed in the same manner as conventional chromatography, by spotting a sample of the test material at one end of a strip. A solvent is then selected for which the desired radiochemical and the potential contaminants have known migration patterns, so the strip can be placed in

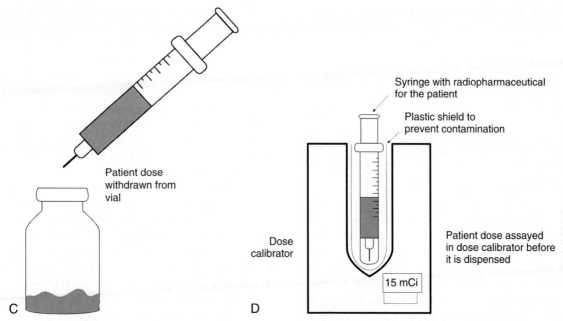

Figure 1-5, cont'd   **C,** The patient dose is withdrawn from the vial. **D,** Each dose is measured in the dose calibrator before it is dispensed.

a dose calibrator for counting. The presence of the radio-label provides an easy means of quantitatively measuring the migration patterns.

For technetium radiopharmaceuticals, the presence of free pertechnetate and insoluble, hydrolyzed reduced technetium moieties are tested using instant thin-layer chromatography techniques. For example, using acetone as the solvent, free pertechnetate migrates with the solvent front in a paper and thin-layer chromatography system, whereas Tc-99m diphosphonate and hydrolyzed reduced technetium remain at the origin (Fig. 1-6). For selective testing of hydrolyzed reduced technetium, a silica gel strip is used with saline as the solvent. In this system, both free pertechnetate and Tc-99m diphosphonate move with the solvent front and hydrolyzed reduced technetium again stays at the origin (Fig. 1-6). This combination of procedures allows measurement of each of the three components. Chromatography systems have been worked out for each major technetium-labeled radiopharmaceutical.

Elaborate systems are available to "read" the chromatography strips. Chromatographic scanners provide detailed strip chart recording of radioactivity distribution. In practice, the easiest way to perform chromatography is simply to cut the chromatography strip into two pieces that can be counted separately.

Chromatography is something of an art form and a number of common pitfalls must be avoided. Inadvertently immersing the chromatography strip into the solvent past the location of the sample spot results in less migration

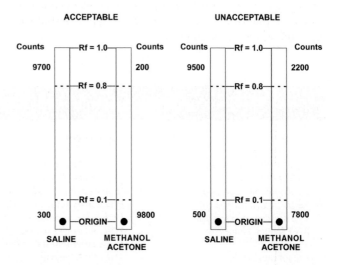

Figure 1-6   Radiochromatography for quality control of Tc-99m diphosphonate. The count-activities on the strips are indicated by the numbers beside the strip diagram. Black dot at the bottom of each strip represents the origin. *Acceptable* (left): 3% of the activity does not migrate with Tc-99m diphosphonate in saline and 2% migrates as Tc-99m pertechnetate with the solvent front using methanol:acetone. Thus, 5% of the radioactivity is not present at Tc-99m diphosphonate. *Unacceptable* (right), 5% of the activity is present as impurities (saline chromatogram) and 22% as free pertechnetate (methanol:acetone chromatogram). This radiopharmaceutical is of unacceptable quality and should not be used clinically. The *Rf* of a compound is the distance from the center of its activity on the strip to the origin (site of application) divided by the distance from the solvent front to the origin. An *Rf* of 1.0 means that the compound moves with the solvent front, whereas an *Rf* of 0 means that the component remains at the origin.

than expected. Also, if spots are not allowed to dry before being used with organic solvents, spurious migration patterns will occur. On the other hand, excessive delay before starting the chromatogram can result in reoxidation of the technetium in the sample; again, spurious results will be encountered.

OTHER SINGLE-PHOTON AGENTS

Radioiodines I-131 and I-123

Radioiodine-131 as sodium iodide was the first radiopharmaceutical of importance in clinical nuclear medicine. It was used for routine studies of the thyroid gland for several years in the late 1940s (Table 1-10). Subsequently I-131 was used as the radiolabel for a variety of radiopharmaceuticals, including human serum albumin, macroaggregated albumin, hippuran for renal studies, and adrenal scintigraphy (metaiodobenzylguanidine and iodocholesterol derivatives).

The disadvantages of I-131 include relatively high principal photon energy (364 keV), long half-life (8 days), and the presence of beta particle emissions. Radioiodine-131 remains an important radiopharmaceutical in nuclear medicine practice for the treatment of hyperthyroidism and differentiated thyroid cancer.

The quality control of radioiodinated pharmaceuticals is important to reduce unwanted radiation exposure to the thyroid gland. In nonthyroid imaging applications of I-131 as a radiolabel, it is common practice to block the thyroid gland with oral iodine (e.g., usually supersaturated potassium iodine; occasionally, potassium perchlorate) to prevent thyroid accumulation of any iodine ion present as a radiochemical impurity or metabolite.

Whenever possible, I-123 is substituted for I-131 for diagnostic purposes. It has a shorter half-life (Table 1-2) and its principal photon energy of 159 keV is better suited to imaging with the gamma scintillation camera. I-123 decays by electron capture, and the dosimetry is favorable compared with that of I-131. Even in applications where imaging over a period of several days allows for improved target-to-background ratio and thus I-131 would seem advantageous, I-123 is now increasingly replacing I-131 (e.g., for whole body thyroid cancer scans and meta-iodo-benzyl-guanidine [MIBG] imaging for neuroblastoma and pheochromocytoma).

Indium-111

Another versatile label that has found applications in clinical nuclear medicine is indium-111 (Table 1-10). Its principal photon energies of 172 keV and 245 keV

Table 1-10 Radiopharmaceuticals for Single-Photon Imaging (Non-Tc-99m labeled agents)

Agent	Application
Tl-201 thallium chloride	Myocardial perfusion scintigraphy
Ga-67 gallium citrate	Inflammatory disease detection, tumor imaging
Xe-133 xenon (inert gas)	Pulmonary ventilation scintigraphy
Xe-127 xenon (inert gas)	Pulmonary ventilation scintigraphy
Kr-81m krypton (inert gas)	Pulmonary ventilation scintigraphy
I-131 sodium iodide	Thyroid cancer scintigraphy; thyroid uptake function studies; treatment of Graves' disease, toxic nodule, and thyroid cancer
I-123 sodium iodide	Thyroid scintigraphy, thyroid uptake function studies
I-131 hippuran	Renal imaging and function studies
I-123 hippuran	Renal imaging and function studies
In-111 oxine leukocytes	Inflammatory disease/infection detection
I-131, I-123 metaiodobenzyl guanidine (MIBG)	Adrenal medullary imaging, neural crest tumor detection
I-131 NP-59 (6β iodomethyl-19 norcholesterol)	Adrenal cortical scintigraphy
In-111 pentetreotide (OctreoScan)	Somatostatin receptor tumor imaging
In-111 capromab pendetide (ProstaScint)	Monoclonal antibody for prostate Ca imaging
Sm-153 lexidronam (Quadramet)	Bone pain palliation
Sr-89 chloride	Bone pain palliation
In-111 satumomab pentetretide (OncoScint)	Monoclonal antibody for colorectal cancer
I-131 tositumomab (Bexxar)	B-cell lymphoma imaging and therapy
In-111 ibritumomab (Zevalin)	B-cell lymphoma scintigraphy prior to therapy

are favorable compared with I-131. The 2.8-day half-life of In-111 permits multiple-day sequential imaging. Several In-111 radiopharmaceuticals have proven clinically useful (e.g., In-111 oxine leukocytes for the evaluation of inflammatory or infectious disease). The somatostatin receptor binding peptide, pentetreotide (OctreoScan) labeled to In-111, binds to a variety of neuroendocrine tumors. In-111 capromab pendetide (ProstaScint) is a monoclonal antibody used for detection of recurrent prostate cancer.

Gallium-67 Citrate

Ga-67 citrate is transported and extracted like iron, localizing in tumors and inflammatory conditions. However, in many respects Ga-67 does not have favorable properties for scintigraphy. It has multiple photopeaks and the most abundant photon has the lowest energy (Table 1-2). In current practice, the lower three photopeaks (93 keV, 185 keV, 300 keV) are acquired. Nonetheless, "downscatter" from the higher energies degrades the image data in the lower windows.

Other disadvantages of Ga-67 include slow clearance from background tissues, necessitating delayed imaging at 48 hours (even ≥72 hours in some applications). Early excretion (<24 hours) through the kidneys and delayed excretion via the bowel make imaging in the abdomen problematic. Care must be taken to interpret the scintigraphic images with a full knowledge of how long after tracer administration the study was obtained. Laxatives may be required to clear confusing or obscuring activity from the colon.

Thallium-201

Thallium-201 became clinically available in the mid-1970s as a radiopharmaceutical for myocardial scintigraphy. Thallium behaves as a potassium analog, with high net clearance (~85%) in its passage through the myocardial capillary bed, which makes it an excellent marker of regional blood flow to viable myocardium.

The major disadvantage of thallium as a radioactive imaging agent is the absence of an ideal photopeak for imaging. The gamma rays at 135 keV and 167 keV occur in low abundance (Table 1-2). The emitted mercury characteristic x-rays in the range of 69–83 keV are acquired. The ability of the gamma scintillation camera to discriminate scattered events from primary photons is suboptimal at this energy. Because of the poor imaging characteristics of Tl-201, alternative Tc-99m labeled radiopharmaceuticals have been sought and are now available, although they also have their limitations, as discussed in the chapter on cardiac imaging.

Radioactive Inert Gases

Radioactive inert gases are used for pulmonary ventilation imaging. Xenon-133 (Xe-133) is a convenient agent to have on hand because of its 5.2-day half-life. Its major disadvantage is the relatively low energy of its principal photon (81 keV). This low energy dictates the performance of ventilation scintigraphy before Tc-99m perfusion scintigraphy. Nonetheless, Xe-133 is still a commonly used agent because of its superior distribution in the lung periphery of patients with chronic obstructive lung disease.

Xe-127 is theoretically superior to Xe-133 because of its higher photon energies (Table 1-2). Because its photon energies are higher than those of Tc-99m, the ventilation portion of a ventilation-perfusion study can be performed after the locations of any perfusion defects are known, which allows the examination to be tailored to the findings in individual patients. The high cost of producing Xe-127 has kept it from wide use.

Krypton-81m has potential advantages because of its high principal gamma emission of 190 keV and short half-life of 13 seconds allowing for postperfusion imaging and multiple view acquisition without concern for retained activity or radiation dose. However, the rubidium-81/krypton-81m generator system is relatively expensive and not commonly used because it must be replaced daily due to the generator's short half-life.

A host of other radionuclides have been used over the years. The radionuclides summarized in Fig. 1-1 are the most important in current practice.

RADIOPHARMACEUTICALS FOR POSITRON EMISSION TOMOGRAPHY

The physical characteristics of commonly used positron-emitting radionuclides are summarized in Table 1-3. Many radiopharmaceuticals have been described for use in positron emission tomography (PET) (Box 1-1). Carbon, nitrogen, and oxygen are found ubiquitously in biological molecules. It is thus theoretically possible to radiolabel just about any molecule of biological interest. Fluorine-18 (F-18) has the advantage of a longer half-life than C-11, N-13, or O-15 and has been used as a label for the glucose analog fluorodeoxyglucose (FDG). F-18 FDG has found widespread clinical application in whole body tumor imaging and, to a lesser extent, imaging of the brain and heart. Tumors derive their energy from glucose metabolism and the uptake of F-18 FDG is a marker of tumor metabolism and viability.

Rubidium-82 is available from a generator system with a relatively long-lived parent (strontium-82, $T_{1/2} =$

25 days) (*see* Table 1-4). Rubidium, like thallium, is a potassium analog and is used for myocardial perfusion imaging. Its availability from a generator system obviates the need for an on-site cyclotron for production. One limitation of Rb-82 is the high energy (3.15 MeV) of its positron emissions. This high energy results in a relatively long average path in soft tissue before annihilation, degrading the ultimate spatial resolution available with the agent. This feature is shared to a lesser extent by O-15.

The production of most positron-emitting radionuclides and their subsequent incorporation into PET radiopharmaceuticals is expensive, complex, and requires a cyclotron or other special accelerator and relatively elaborate radiochemical-handling equipment. In-house self-contained small cyclotrons with automated chemistry are available but are expensive for most clinical settings. However, the large clinical demand and the relatively long 2-hour half-life of F-18 FDG has resulted in its production and distribution by regional radiopharmacies.

Box 1-1   Positron Emission Tomography Selected Radiopharmaceuticals

PERFUSION AGENTS

Oxygen-15 carbon dioxide
Oxygen-15 water
Nitrogen-13 ammonia
Rubidium-82 chloride

BLOOD VOLUME

Oxygen-15 carbon monoxide
Carbon-11 carbon monoxide
Gallium-68 EDTA

METABOLIC AGENTS

Fluorine-18 sodium fluoride
Fluorine-18 fluorodeoxyglucose
Oxygen-15 oxygen
Carbon-11 acetate
Carbon-11 palmitate
Nitrogen-13 glutamate

TUMOR AGENTS

Fluorine-18 fluorodeoxyglucose
Carbon-11 methionine
Fluorine-18 fluorothymidine

RECEPTOR-BINDING AGENTS

Carbon-11 carfentanil
Carbon-11 raclopride
Fluorine-18 fluoro-L-dopa
Fluorine-18 spiperone

DISPENSING RADIOPHARMACEUTICALS

Normal Procedures

General radiation safety procedures should be followed in any laboratory (Box 1-2). The dispensing of radiopharmaceuticals is under a series of exacting rules and regulations promulgated by the FDA and NRC, as well as state pharmacy boards and hospital radiation safety committees. In brief, radiopharmaceuticals are prescription drugs that cannot be legally administered without being ordered by an authorized individual. The nuclear medicine physician and the radiopharmacy are responsible for confirming the appropriateness of the request, ensuring that the correct radiopharmaceutical in the requested or designated amount is administered to the patient, and keeping records of both the request and the documentation of the dosage administration.

Before any material is dispensed, all appropriate quality assurance measures should be carried out. These measures are described in detail earlier in the chapter for the Mo-99/Tc-99m generator system and Tc-99m-labeled radiopharmaceuticals. For other agents, the package

Box 1-2   Radiation Safety Procedures

Wear laboratory coats in areas where radioactive materials are present.
Wear disposable gloves when handling radioactive materials.
Monitor hands and body for radioactive contamination before leaving the area.
Use syringe and vial shields as necessary.
Do not eat, drink, smoke, apply cosmetics, or store food in any area where radioactive material is stored or used.
Wear personnel monitoring devices in areas with radioactive materials.
Never pipette by mouth.
Dispose of radioactive waste in designated, labeled, and properly shielded receptacles located in a secured area.
Label containers, vials, syringes containing radioactive materials. When not in use, place in shielded containers or behind lead shielding in a secured area.
Store all sealed sources (floods, dose calibrator sources) in shielded containers in a secured area.
Before administering doses to patients, determine and record activity.
Know what steps to take and who to contact (radiation safety officer) in the event of radiation accident, improper operation of radiation safety equipment, or theft/loss of licensed material.

insert or protocol for formulation and dispensing should be consulted to see what radiochromatography or other quality control steps must be performed before dosage administration. As a good standard of practice, quality control should always be performed, even when not legally required. Every dose should be physically inspected before administration for any particulate or foreign material, such as bits of rubber from the tops of multidose injection vials. Each dose administered to a patient must be assayed in a dose calibrator. The administered activity should be within ±20% of the prescription request.

Special Considerations

Pregnancy and Lactation

The possibility of pregnancy should be considered for every woman of childbearing age referred to the nuclear medicine service for a diagnostic or therapeutic procedure. Pregnancy alone is not an absolute contraindication to performing a nuclear medicine study. For example, pulmonary embolism is encountered in pregnant women and is associated with potential serious morbidity and mortality. Thus, the risk-to-benefit ratio of ventilation-perfusion scintigraphy is high and considered a safe procedure in this circumstance. The radiation dosage is kept at a minimum. Neither of the radiopharmaceuticals employed (Xe-133 or Tc-99m macroaggregated albumin) crosses the placenta in considerable amounts. On the other hand, radioiodine does cross the placenta. The fetal thyroid develops the capacity to concentrate radioiodine at approximately weeks 10–12 of gestation and cases of cretinism caused by in utero exposure to radioiodine-I-131 have been documented.

The management of women who are lactating and breastfeeding an infant is another special problem. The need to suspend breastfeeding is determined by the half-life of the radionuclide involved and the degree to which it is secreted in breast milk. Radioiodine is secreted by the breast and breastfeeding should be terminated altogether after the administration of I-131. For I-123, it has generally been recommended that breastfeeding could safely be resumed after 2-3 days. For Tc-99m agents, 12–24 hours is sufficient. Table 1-11 lists recommendations for the length of time breastfeeding should be discontinued after administration of various radiopharmaceuticals.

Dosage Selection for Pediatric Patients

A number of approaches have been proposed for scaling down the amount of radioactivity administered to children. There is no perfect way to do this because of the differential rate of maturation of body organs and the changing ratio of different body compartments to

Table 1-11 Recommendations for Radio-pharmaceuticals Excreted in Breast Milk

Radiopharma-ceutical	Administered activity MBq (mCi)	Counseling	Advised
Ga-67 citrate	185 (5.0)	Yes	Cessation
I-131 sodium iodide	0.74 (.02)	Yes	Cessation
I-123 sodium iodide	14.8 (.4)	Yes	2-3 d
I-123 MIBG	370 (10)	Yes	48 hr
Tl-201	111 (3)	Yes	96 hr
In-111 leukocytes	185 (5)	Yes	48 hr
Tc-99m MAA	148 (4)	Yes	12 hr
Tc-99m red blood cells in vivo	740 (20)	Yes	12 hr
Tc-99m pertechnetate	185 (5)	Yes	4 hr

Modified with permission from Stabin MG, Breitz HB: Breast milk excretion of radiopharmaceuticals: mechanisms, findings, and radiation dosimetry. *J Nucl Med* 41:863-873, 2000.

body weight. Empirically, body surface area correlates better than body weight for dosage selection. Various formulas and nomograms have been developed. Each laboratory should select a method and standardize its application.

An approximation based on body weight uses the formula:

$$\text{Pediatric dose} = \frac{\text{Patient weight (kg)}}{70 \text{ kg}} \times \text{Adult dose}$$

Another alternative is the use of Webster's rule:

$$\text{Pediatric dose} = \frac{\text{Age} + 1}{\text{Age} + 7} \times \text{Adult dose}$$

This formula is not useful for infants. Moreover, in some cases a calculated dose may not be adequate to obtain a diagnostically useful study and physician judgment must be used. For example, a newborn infant with suspected biliary atresia may require 24-hour delayed Tc-99m hepatobiliary iminodiacetic acid (HIDA) imaging, which is not feasible if the dose is too low. Therefore, a minimum dose for each radiopharmaceutical should be established.

Medical Event (Misadministration)

The definition and procedures for handling misadministrations of radiopharmaceuticals are set out in the Code of Federal Regulations (10 CFR-35). However, the terminology has changed. What was previously called a misadministration is now called a medical event. The code was revised in 2002. Many of the prior "misadministrations" no longer have to be reported to the NRC or state. A *medical event* is defined by the NRC rules and regulations as a radiopharmaceutical dose administration involving the wrong patient, wrong radiopharmaceutical, wrong route of administration, or an administered dose differing from the prescribed dose when: (1) the effective dose equivalent to the patient exceeds 5 rem to the whole body or 50 rem to any individual organ (Box 1-3) or (2) a diagnostic dose of I-131 sodium iodide exceeds 30 μCi.

The criteria just described show that medical events are extremely unlikely to occur as a result of any diagnostic nuclear medicine procedure. Most will be related to radioiodine I-131. However, after the occurrence of a medical event is recognized, regulations for reporting of the event and management of the patient should be followed. The details are determined in part by the kind of material involved and the amount of the adverse exposure of the patient. All medical events must be reported to the regulatory agency, the referring physician, and the affected patient. Complete records on each event must be retained and available for NRC review for 10 years.

Certain states, called Agreement States, have entered into regulatory agreements with the NRC that give them the authority to license and inspect by-product, source, or special nuclear material used or possessed within their borders. There are now 32 Agreement States and this number is growing. Although the NRC regulates byproduct (reactor-produced) material such as I-131 and Xenon-133, the states often regulate other radiation sources as well, such as cyclotron-produced radioactive material (F-18, Co-57, Ga-67, In-111, and Tl-201). The states, not the NRC, regulate the use of positron emission tomography.

Box 1-3   Annual Dose Limits for Radiation Exposure (NRC Regulations)

ADULT OCCUPATIONAL

5 rem (0.05 Sv) total effective dose equivalent
50 rem (0.5 Sv) to any organ or tissue or extremity
15 rems (0.15 Sv) to the lens of the eye

MINORS (<18 YEARS OF AGE) OCCUPATIONAL

10% of those for adult workers

EMBRYO/FETUS OCCUPATIONAL

0.5 rem (5mSv) during pregnancy

MEMBERS OF THE PUBLIC

0.1 rem (1 mSv)
2 mrem (0.02 mSv) in any hour (average)

Adverse Reactions to Diagnostic Radiopharmaceuticals

Adverse reactions to radiopharmaceuticals are much less common than adverse reactions to iodinated contrast media. Reactions are usually mild and, for the radiopharmaceuticals in use today, rarely fatal. The greatest concern of allergic reactions is for agents containing human serum albumin. Also, preparations of Tc-99m-sulfur colloid have a gelatin stabilizer derived from animal protein. These agents can be associated with allergic reactions. Of more recent concern is the possibility of reactions caused by the development of human antimouse antibodies (HAMA) after repeated exposure to radiolabeled antibody imaging agents. The concern over the development of HAMA and potential adverse consequences has been a factor in the FDA's slow approval for radiolabeled antibodies. However, several diagnostic and therapeutic radiolabeled antibodies have been approved, such as In-111 ProstaScint, Tc-99m NeutroSpec, In-111 and Y-90 Zevalin.

RADIATION ACCIDENTS (SPILLS)

In a busy nuclear medicine practice handling several dozen patient doses a day, as well as stock solutions of generator eluate, with most materials in liquid form, accidental spills of radioactive material occur from time to time. The spills are somewhat arbitrarily divided into minor and major categories, depending on the radionuclide and the amount spilled. For I-131, incidents involving activities up to 1 mCi are considered minor; spills above that level are considered major. For Tc-99m, Tl-201, and Ga-67, the threshold for considering a spill to be major is 100 mCi.

The basic principles of responding to both kinds of spills are the same (Box 1-4). For minor spills, people in the area are warned that the spill has occurred. Attempts are made to prevent the spread of the spilled material. Absorbent paper may be used to cover the spilled material if it is visibly identifiable. Minor spills can be cleaned up directly with appropriate technique, including use of soap and water, disposable gloves, and remote handling devices. All contaminated material, including gloves and other objects, should be disposed of in designated bags. The area should be continually surveyed until the reading from a Geiger-Müller survey meter is at background levels. All personnel involved should also be monitored, including their hands, shoes, and clothing. The spill should be reported to the institution's radiation safety officer.

For major spills, the area is cleared immediately. Attempts are made to prevent further spread with absorbent pads, and if possible the radioactivity is shielded. The room is sealed off and the radiation safety

1. Notify all persons in the area that a spill has occurred.
2. Prevent the spread of contamination by isolating the area and covering the spill (absorbent paper).
3. If clothing is contaminated, remove and place in plastic bag.
4. If an individual is contaminated, rinse contaminated region with lukewarm water and wash with soap.
5. Notify the radiation safety officer.
6. Wear gloves, disposable lab coat, and booties to clean up spill with absorbent paper.
7. Put all contaminated absorbent paper in labeled radioactive waste container.
8. Check the area or contaminated individual with appropriate radiation survey meter.

officer is notified immediately. The radiation safety officer typically directs the further response, including determination of when and how to proceed with cleanup and decontamination.

In dealing with both minor and major spills, an attempt is made to keep radiation exposure of patients, hospital staff, and the environment to a minimum. There are no absolute guidelines that provide a definitive approach to every spill. The radiation safety officer must restrict access to the area until it is safe for patients and personnel.

QUALITY CONTROL IN THE NUCLEAR PHARMACY

Selected quality control procedures for Tc-99m-labeled radiopharmaceuticals and for Mo-99/Tc-99m generator systems are described earlier in this chapter. Considerations of radiochemical and radionuclidic purity also apply to other single-photon agents and positron radiopharmaceuticals (Table 1-8). For example, radiochemical purity is a special concern with radioiodinated agents because of the potential for uptake of free radioiodine in the thyroid gland if the radiolabel disassociates from the carrier molecule. Additional quality control procedures in the nuclear pharmacy are aimed at ensuring the sterility and apyrogenicity of administered radiopharmaceuticals. Quality control monitoring of the performance of the dose calibrator is also important to ensure that administered doses are within prescribed amounts.

Sterility and Pyrogen Testing

Sterility implies the absence of living organisms (Table 1-8). *Apyrogenicity* implies the absence of metabolic products such as endotoxins. Because many radiopharmaceuticals are prepared just before use, definitive testing before they are administered to the patient is impractical, which doubles the need for careful aseptic technique in the nuclear pharmacy.

Autoclaving is a well-known means of sterilization. It is useful for sterilizing preparation vials and other utensils and materials but is not useful for any of the radiopharmaceuticals employed in clinical practice. When terminal sterilization is required, various membrane filtration methods are used. Special filters with pore diameters smaller than microorganisms have been developed for this purpose. A filter pore size of 0.22 μm is necessary to sterilize a solution. This size traps bacteria, including small organisms such as *Pseudomonas*.

Sterility testing standards have been defined by the USP. Standard media including thioglycollate and soybean casein digest media are used for different categories of microorganisms, including aerobic and anaerobic bacteria and fungi.

Pyrogens are protein or polysaccharide metabolites of microorganisms or other contaminating substances that cause febrile reactions (Table 1-8). They can be present even in sterile preparations. The typical clinical syndrome is fever, chills, joint pain, and headache developing minutes to a few hours after injection. The pyrogenic reaction lasts for several hours and alone is not fatal.

The USP has established criteria for pyrogen testing. The historical method involved injecting pharmaceutical samples into the ear veins of rabbits while measuring their temperature response. The current USP test uses limulus amebocyte lysate (LAL). The test is based on the observation that amebocyte lysate preparations from the blood of horseshoe crabs become opaque in the presence of pyrogens. The LAL test is more reliable, more sensitive, and easier to perform than the rabbit test.

Radiopharmaceutical Dose Calibrators

The dose calibrator is a key instrument in the radiopharmacy and is subject to quality control requirements. Four basic measurements are included: accuracy, linearity, precision or constancy, and geometry. All of these tests must be performed at installation and after repair.

Accuracy
Accuracy is measured by using reference standard sources obtained from the National Institute of Standards and Technology. The test is performed annually and two different radioactive sources are used. If the measured activity in the dose calibrator varies from the standard or theoretical activity by more than 10%, the device must be recalibrated.

Linearity

The linearity test is designed to determine the response of the calibrator over a range of measured activities. A common approach is to take a sample of Tc-99m pertechnetate and sequentially measure it during radioactive decay. Because the change in activity with time is a definable physical parameter, any deviation in the observed assay value indicates equipment malfunction and nonlinearity. An alternative approach is to use precalibrated lead attenuators with sequential measurements of the same specimen. This test is performed quarterly.

Precision or Constancy

The precision or constancy test is designed to measure the ability of the dose calibrator to repeatedly measure the same specimen over time. A long-lived standard such as barium-133 (356 keV, $T_{1/2}$ 10.7 years), cesium-137 (662 keV, $T_{1/2}$ 30 years), or cobalt-57 (122 kev, $T_{1/2}$ 271 days) can be used. The test is performed daily and observed values should be within 10% of the value for the reference standard.

Geometry

The geometric test is performed during acceptance testing of the dose calibrator. The issue is that the same amount of radioactivity contained in different volumes of sample can result in different measured or observed radioactivities. For a given dose calibrator, if readings vary by more than 10% from one volume to another, correction factors are calculated. For convenience, the correction factors are based on the most commonly measured volume of material, which is typically determined from day-to-day clinical use of the dose calibrator.

RADIATION DOSIMETRY

Exposure of the patient to radiation limits the amount of radioactivity that can be administered in the scintigraphic procedures performed in clinical nuclear medicine. In general, the exact radiation dose that an individual patient receives from a nuclear medicine procedure cannot be calculated. It is not practical to acquire the amount of data necessary to calculate the actual radiation absorbed dose for a particular patient. It includes the percent localization of the administered dose in each organ of the body, the time course of retention in each organ, and the size and relative distribution of the organs in the body. Such information is obtained from biodistribution studies and pharmacokinetic studies in experimental animals during the development and regulatory approval process for a new radiopharmaceutical. For each radiopharmaceutical, estimates of radiation absorbed doses are made as part of the approval process and may be taken as "average" or nominal levels of exposure (Table 1-12).

In brief, the radiation absorbed dose to any organ in the body depends on biological factors (percent uptake, biological half-life) and physical factors (amount and nature of emitted radiations from the radionuclide). Radiation doses are typically given in rads (radiation absorbed dose). One rad is equal to the absorption of 100 ergs per gram of tissue. The formula for calculating the radiation absorbed dose is:

$$D\,(r_k \leftarrow r_b) = \tilde{A}_b\,S\,(r_k \leftarrow r_b)$$

The formula states that the absorbed dose in a region k resulting from activity from a source region b is equal to

---

Table 1-12   Radiation Doses from Common Diagnostic Nuclear Medicine Procedures

Radionuclide (rem)	Agent	Activity, mCi	Highest dose (organ), rad	Effective dose equivalent
F-18	FDG	10	5.9 (bladder)	0.7
Ga-67	Citrate	5	11.8 (bone surface)	1.9
Tc-99m	HIDA	5	2.0 (gallbladder)	0.3
	HMPAO	20	2.5 (kidneys)	0.7
	MAA	4	1.0 (lungs)	0.2
	MDP	20	4.7 (bone surface)	0.4
	MAG3	20	8.1 (bladder wall)	0.5
	Sestamibi	20	2.7 (gallbladder)	0.7
	Tetrofosmin	20	2.7 (gallbladder)	0.6
	Sulfur colloid	8	2.2 (spleen)	0.3
In-111	Leukocytes	0.5	10.9 (spleen)	1.2
I-123	Sodium iodide (25% uptake)	0.2	2.6 (thyroid)	0.2
	MIBG	10.0	0.1 (liver)	0.07
Xe-133	Gas	15	0.06 (lungs)	0.04
Tl-201	Chloride	3	4.6 (thyroid)	1.2

SI conversion: 1 rem = 0.01 Sv; 1 mCi = 37 MBq.
From Siegel JA: *Guide for diagnostic nuclear medicine and radiopharmaceutical therapy.* Reston, VA, Society of Nuclear Medicine, 2004.

the cumulative radioactivity given in microcurie-hours in the source region ($\tilde{A}$) times the mean absorbed dose per unit of cumulative activity in rads per microcurie-hour (S). The cumulative activity is determined from experimental measurements of uptake and retention in the different source regions. The mean absorbed dose per unit of cumulative activity is based on physical measurements and is determined by the kind of radiations emanating from the radionuclide being used.

The total absorbed dose to a region or organ is the sum of the contributions from all source regions around it and from activity within the target organ itself. For example, a calculation of the absorbed dose to the myocardium in a Tl-201 scan must take into account contributions from radioactivity localizing in the myocardium and from radioactivity in the lung, blood, liver, intestines, kidneys, and general background soft tissues. The percentage uptake and the biological behavior of Tl-201 are different in each of those tissues. The amount of radiation reaching the myocardium is also different, depending on the geometry of the source organ and its distance from the heart. The formula is applied separately for each source region, and the individual contributions are summed.

Factors that affect the dosimetry between patients include the amount of activity administered originally, the biodistribution in one patient vs. another, the route of administration, the rate of elimination, the size of the patient, and the presence of pathological processes. For example, for radiopharmaceuticals cleared by the kidney, radiation exposure is greater in patients with renal failure. Another commonly encountered example is differing percentage uptakes of radioiodine in the thyroid depending on whether a patient is hyperthyroid, euthyroid, or hypothyroid.

Estimates of radiation-absorbed dose for each major radiopharmaceutical are provided in tabular form in the organ system chapters. The tables indicate the absorbed dose per unit of administered activity for selected organs.

SUGGESTED READING

Chilton HM, Witcofski RL: *Nuclear pharmacy: an introduction to the clinical application of radiopharmaceuticals,* Philadelphia, Lea & Febiger, 1986.

Kowalsky RJ, Perry JR: *Radiopharmaceuticals in nuclear medicine practice.* Norwalk, Conn, Appleton & Lange, 1987.

Ponto JA: The AAPM/RSNA physics tutorial for residents: radiopharmaceuticals. *Radiographics* 18:1395-1404, 1998.

Saha GB: *Fundamentals of nuclear pharmacy,* 4th ed. New York, Springer, 1998.

Siegel JA: *Guide for diagnostic nuclear medicine and radiopharmaceutical therapy.* Reston, VA, Society of Nuclear Medicine, 2004.

Simpkin DJ: The AAPM/RSNA physics tutorial for residents: radiation interactions and internal dosimetry. *Radiographics* 19:155-167, 1999.

Stabin MG, Breitz HB: Breast milk excretion of radiopharmaceuticals: mechanisms, findings, and radiation dosimetry. *J Nucl Med* 41:863-873, 2000.

Swanson DP, Chilton HM, Thrall JH: *Pharmaceuticals in medical imaging,* New York, Macmillan, 1990.

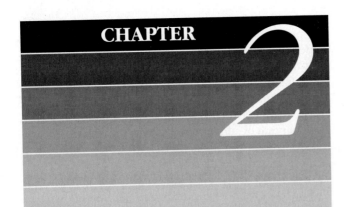

Physics of Nuclear Medicine

Medical imaging is based on the interaction of energy with biological tissues. The kind of diagnostic information available from each imaging modality is determined by the nature of these interactions. In conventional x-ray imaging, the differential absorption of x-rays in air, water, fat, and bone allows the distinction of these tissues in the image. In ultrasonography, the differing reflective properties of tissues are the basis for creating images. In magnetic resonance imaging, the differences in hydrogen content and in the chemical and physical environments of hydrogen nuclei provide the basis for distinguishing tissues.

In nuclear medicine, the body is imaged "from the inside out." Radiotracers, often in the form of complex radiopharmaceuticals, are administered internally. Diagnostic inference is gained by recording the distribution of the radioactive material in both time and space. Tracer pharmacokinetics and selective tissue uptake form the basis of diagnostic utility. To understand nuclear imaging procedures, one must understand a sequence of concepts, beginning with the physics of radioactivity, continuing through the process of detecting radiation and selecting appropriate radiopharmaceuticals, and ending with the uptake and distribution of those pharmaceuticals in health and disease.

ATOMS AND THE STRUCTURE OF MATTER

Atoms are the building blocks of molecules and are the smallest structures that represent the physical and chemical properties of the elements. Each atom consists of a nucleus surrounded by orbiting electrons (Fig. 2-1). The nuclei are composed of protons and neutrons, collectively referred to as *nucleons*. *Proton*s are positively charged particles weighing approximately 1.67×10^{-24} g. Their positive charge is equal in magnitude and opposite to the charge of an electron (Box 2-1). The element to which the atom belongs is determined by the number of protons in the nucleus. *Neutrons* are slightly heavier than protons and are electrically neutral, as the name implies.

A shorthand notation has been developed to describe or define specific atoms. The notation is as follows:

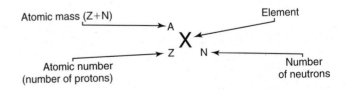

where X is the symbol for the element, Z is the number of protons, N is the number of neutrons, and A is the total number of neutrons and protons. Z is also referred to as the *atomic number* and A as the *mass number* or *atomic mass number*. A *nuclide* is an atom with a given number of neutrons and protons. A *radionuclide* is simply an unstable nuclide or nuclear species that undergoes radioactive decay.

Several terms help define special relationships between different nuclides. The term *isotope* is used to denote nuclides with the same number of protons (Z), that is, the same element but different numbers of neutrons (N). For example, the element iodine has more than 20 isotopes. All except one (I-127) are radioisotopes or radionuclides and several are of medical interest, including I-123, I-125, and I-131, which have the following notations:

$$^{123}_{35}\text{I}_{70} \qquad ^{125}_{35}\text{I}_{72} \qquad ^{131}_{35}\text{I}_{78}$$

Other special terms are: *isobar*, to indicate the same A but different N and Z; *isotone*, to indicate the same number of N but different Z and A; and *isomer*, to indicate different energy states in nuclides with identical A, Z, and N. The most important isomers in nuclear medicine are technetium-99 and technetium-99m, in which the *m* denotes a *metastable* or prolonged intermediate state in the decay of molybdenum-99 to technetium-99.

BOHR MODEL OF THE ATOM

In the classic Bohr model of the atom, electrons are arranged in well-defined orbits around the nucleus (Figs. 2-1 and 2-2). The number of orbital electrons in each atom equals the atomic number, Z (the number of protons in the nucleus). The closest orbit, referred to as the K shell, is followed by the L, M, and N shells and so forth. The maximum number of electrons in the K shell is 2, in the L shell is 8, in the M shell is 18, and in the N shell is 32, except that no more than 8 electrons can be in the outermost shell of an atom. Figure 2-2 is a simplified schematic of the Bohr model for potassium. The term *valence electron* is used to designate electrons in the outermost shell (Box 2-2). These electrons are important in defining the chemical properties of elements. For example, atoms with the outermost shell maximally filled are chemically unreactive (e.g., the inert gases helium, neon, argon, krypton, xenon, and radon).

Electrons have a negative charge equal to 1.6×10^{-19} coulomb; as previously noted, protons have a positive charge of equal magnitude. Electrons are bound in their

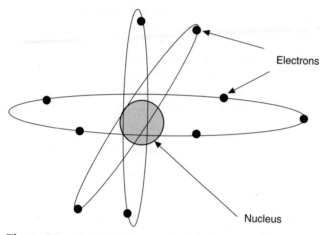

Figure 2-1 Bohr model of the atom. The nucleus contains protons and neutrons and has a radius of 10^{-14} m. The protons in the nucleus carry a positive charge. The orbital electrons carry a negative charge.

Box 2-1 **Summary of Physical Constants**	
Speed of light in a vacuum (c)	3.0×10^{8} m/sec
Elementary charge (e)	4.803×10^{-10} esu
1.602×10^{-19} coulomb	
Rest mass of electron	9.11×10^{-28} g
Rest mass of proton	1.67×10^{-24} g
Planck's constant (h)	6.63×10^{-27} erg sec
Avogadro's number	$6.02 \times 10^{23} \dfrac{\text{molecules}}{\text{gram mole}}$
1 electron volt (eV)	1.602×10^{-12} erg
1 calorie (cal)	4.18×10^{7} erg
1 Angstrom (Å)	10^{-10} m
Euler's number (e) (base of natural logarithms)	2.718
Atomic mass unit (U)	1.66×10^{-24} g (½ the mass of a carbon-12 atom)

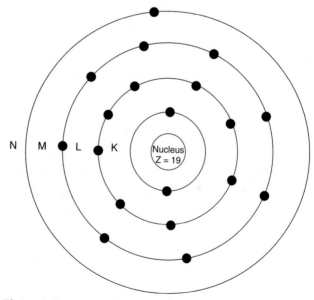

Figure 2-2 Potassium atom. Potassium has an atomic number of 19, with 19 protons in the nucleus and 19 orbital electrons.

orbits by the electrical force between their negative charge and the positive charge of the nucleus. The highest binding energy is in the electrons in the shell closest to the nucleus (K shell), with progressively lower binding energies in the more distant shells. Before an electron can be removed from its shell, the binding energy must be overcome. Interactions involving orbital electrons and ionizing electromagnetic radiation (x-rays and gamma rays) are central to the way medical images are made and to the quality of the images.

It has long been recognized that the Bohr model of the atom is too simplistic to portray many atomic phenomena accurately. Nuclear physicists have developed sophisticated wave mechanical or quantum mechanical models in which probability density functions are used to describe spatial and temporal properties of electrons. However, the Bohr model can still be used to describe the basic interactions of interest in nuclear medicine.

ELECTROMAGNETIC RADIATION

The term *electromagnetic radiation* or *electromagnetic waves* refers to energy in the form of oscillating electric and magnetic fields. Individual packets of electromagnetic radiation are referred to as *photons*. Photons with energy greater than 100 eV are classified as x-rays or gamma rays. Lower energy photons may be in the range of ultraviolet light, infrared, visible light, radar waves, or radio and television waves (Fig. 2-3). The unit of energy used to describe these electromagnetic waves or radiations is the *electron volt* (eV). One electron volt is defined as the kinetic energy of an electron accelerated through a potential difference of 1 volt (1 eV = 1.6×10^{-19} joules or 1.6×10^{-12} erg).

Mathematics of Electromagnetic Radiation

The relationship between the energy of x-rays and gamma rays (or other electromagnetic radiations) and their frequencies is given by E = $h v$, where v is the frequency and h is Planck's constant (*see* Box 2-1). Electromagnetic radiation travels with the speed of light (c). The relationship between frequency and wavelength is given by c = $v \lambda$, where λ is the wavelength. Rearranging this equation to solve for v and substituting it into the previous equation yields:

$$E = \frac{hc}{\lambda}$$

Box 2-2 Terms Used to Describe Electrons	
Term	**Comment**
Electron	Basic elementary particle
Orbital electron	Electron in one of the shells or orbits in an atom
Valence electron	Electron in the outermost shell of an atom; responsible for chemical characteristics and reactivity
Auger electron	Electron ejected from an atomic orbit by energy released during an electron transition
Photoelectron	Electron ejected from an atomic orbit as a consequence of an interaction with a photon (photoelectric interaction) and complete absorption of the photon's energy
Conversion electron	Electron ejected from an atomic orbit because of internal conversion phenomenon as energy is given off by an unstable nucleus

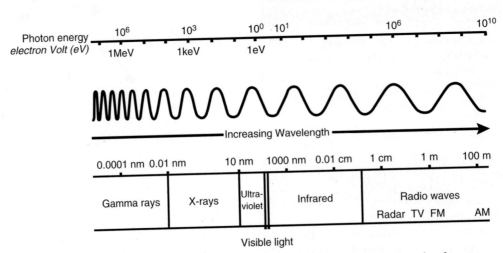

Figure 2-3   Electromagnetic energy spectrum. Photon energies (eV) and wavelengths of gamma and x-rays, ultraviolet, visible light, infrared, and radiowaves.

Taking wavelength in angstroms (Å) and energy in keV and substituting the numerical value for h and c, this becomes:

$$E(keV) = \frac{12.4}{\lambda(\text{Å})}$$

RELATIONSHIP OF MASS AND ENERGY

In 1905, Albert Einstein published his famous equation $E = mc^2$, where E is energy in ergs, m is mass in grams, and c is the velocity of light in a vacuum (3×10^8 m/sec). From this equation, it is possible to calculate the energy equivalent of the various subatomic particles. By definition the unified or universal *atomic mass unit* (U) is equal to one-twelfth the mass of a carbon-12 atom ($1 \text{ U} = 1.66 \times 10^{-24}$ g) (Box 2-1). Using this value for mass in Einstein's equation yields the following result:

$$E = (1.66 \times 10^{-24} \text{ g/U}) \times (3.0 \times 10^{10} \text{ cm/sec})^2$$
$$E = 1.5 \times 10^{-3} \text{ erg/U}$$
$$(1 \text{ erg} = 1 \text{ gcm}^2/\text{sec}^2)$$

Inserting the conversion factor between ergs and electron volts (Box 2-1) yields the relationship $1 \text{ U} = 931.5$ MeV. Table 2-1 provides the mass and energy relationships for the basic subatomic particles. The most important of these relationships in clinical nuclear medicine and positron emission tomography is the energy equivalence of the mass of an electron, which is 511 keV.

Mass Deficit and Nuclear Binding Energy

The relationships between mass and energy are of fundamental importance in nuclear physics. By carefully determining the weight of atomic nuclei, physicists have shown that the theoretical sum of the component nucleons is always greater than the actual observed mass of the respective atomic nuclei. The difference is known as the *mass deficit*. The *nuclear binding energy* is defined as the energy equivalent of the mass deficit.

Energy equal to the difference in nuclear binding energy of the pretransformation and posttransformation nuclei is released in atomic fusion and atomic fission. The energy of hydrogen and atomic bombs comes from energy released when trillions of new atomic nuclei are formed. That is, the aggregate mass deficit of the post-transformation nuclei after a fusion or fission reaction is greater than that of the original nuclei.

The concept of mass deficit is also fundamental to the use of radionuclides in medical imaging. As a more stable atomic configuration is formed in the radioactive decay process, the mass deficit always increases. In many radionuclide decay schemes, part of the mass deficit is given off in the form of energetic electromagnetic radiation (photons) that can be detected and used to form medical images.

RADIONUCLIDES AND THEIR RADIATIONS

Because of their physical properties, certain atoms are unstable and undergo radioactive decay. The daughter product in radioactive decay is always at a lower energy state than the parent. The energy difference or mass deficit between parent and daughter is equal to the total energy in the radiations emitted. For each radionuclide, the type of radiation given off, the energy of the radiation(s), and the half-life of the decay process are physical constants. These parameters are important in determining the suitability of a given radionuclide for medical use.

The types of radiation important in nuclear medicine are gamma rays, characteristic x-rays, negatrons (beta particles), positrons (beta particles), and alpha particles. By definition, the term *gamma ray* is used for photons originating in the nucleus and the term *x-ray* for photons originating outside the nucleus.

Among the lighter atomic elements, the number of protons and neutrons in the nucleus is roughly equal. As the atomic number Z increases, the ratio of neutrons to protons in stable nuclei increases. A plot of this ratio vs. atomic number defines an empirical "line of stability" (Fig. 2-4). That is, the neutron/proton (N/P) ratio is greater than 1 for stable nuclei in the middle and upper atomic numbers. This observation is important in predicting the mode of radioactive decay of unstable nuclides. In general, the decay process tends to return the daughter nucleus closer to the line of stability. That is, if an unstable nucleus contains more neutrons than do stable isotopes of the same element, the mode of decay will reduce the N/P ratio, and vice versa for nuclei with fewer neutrons than predicted by the line of stability.

A system of schematic diagrams has been developed to illustrate radioactive decay. Positive emissions (alpha particles and positrons) and electron capture cause the daughter nucleus to have a lower atomic number, which is indicated by an arrow pointing down and to the left (Fig. 2-5). Following negative emissions by beta minus particles (negatrons), the daughter nucleus has a higher atomic number, which is indicated by an arrow pointing down and to the right (Fig. 2-6).

Table 2-1	Mass-Energy Equivalence for Atomic Particles	
Particle	**Mass (U)**	**Energy (MeV)**
Electron	5.486×10^{-4}	0.511
Proton	1.0073	938.20
Neutron	1.0087	939.5

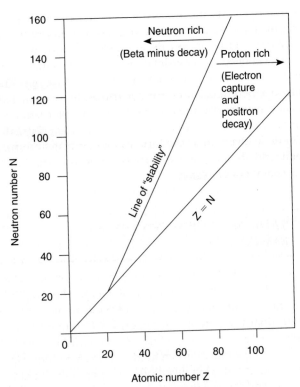

Figure 2-4 Ratio of neutrons to protons. For low atomic number elements, the two are roughly equal (Z = N). With increasing atomic number, the relative number of neutrons increases. Stable nuclear species tend to occur along the line of "stability."

Complete decay schemes can be complex, with multiple pathways from parent to daughter. For practical purposes, the decay schemes in this book are simplified to illustrate important general principles and specific aspects relevant to clinical nuclear medicine.

Alpha Decay

Alpha particles are essentially helium nuclei (i.e., two protons and two neutrons) with a +2 charge and an atomic mass number of 4. Alpha decay is common in the higher atomic number range of the periodic table of elements. For example, radium-226 (Ra-226) decays to radon-222 (Rn-222) by emitting an alpha particle (Fig. 2-5).

In the simplified scheme shown for Ra-226, three different alpha particles are shown (Fig. 2-5). One reaches the ground state of Rn-222 directly. The other two result in an excited state of Rn-222 with subsequent gamma ray emission to reach the ground state. In the complete decay scheme for Ra-226, additional alpha particles are present but they occur in low abundance.

In all radioactive decay processes, mass and energy are conserved. The *transition energy* is the total energy released during the decay process. For alpha decay, this energy is in the form of the kinetic energy of the alpha particle plus the energy released in the form of gamma radiation.

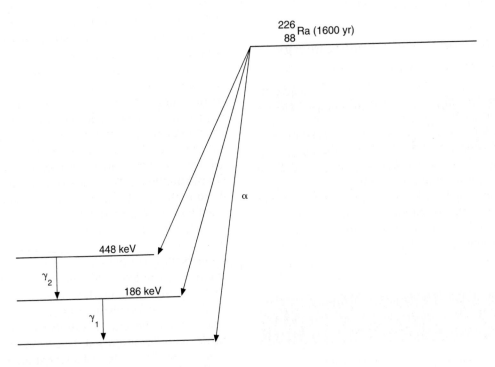

Figure 2-5 Decay scheme for radium-226. Decay is by alpha particle emission to the daughter product radon-222. The emission of an alpha particle results in a decrease in atomic number of 2 and a decrease in atomic mass of 4.

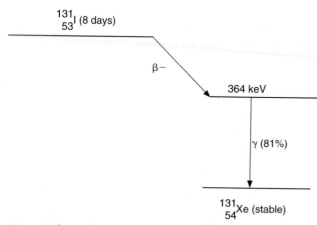

Figure 2-6   Decay scheme for iodine-131. Decay is by negatron emission. In negatron or beta minus decay the atomic mass does not change (isobaric transition). The atomic number increases by one. The daughter, xenon-131, has one more proton in the nucleus.

Alpha particles are undesirable in diagnostic applications because their range in soft tissue is a fraction of a millimeter. Therefore, they do not contribute to the image and result in high radiation to the patient without any contribution of diagnostic information. No currently used diagnostic radiopharmaceuticals include alpha-emitting radionuclides. On the other hand, a number of therapeutic agents have been designed to incorporate alpha particle emitters.

Beta Minus (β–) or Negatron Decay

The negatron decay process involves the conversion of a neutron into a proton, an electron, and a subatomic particle called an *antineutrino*. The electron is ejected from the atomic nucleus, thereby giving the decay process its name. The term *negatron* is used to distinguish negative electrons from positive electrons, or *positrons*. Negatrons and positrons are also referred to as "beta particles." Depending on their charge, they can also be referred to as beta minus (β–) or beta plus (β+) particles. Thus, negatron decay is also called *beta decay*. Negatrons or beta minus particles are identical to orbital electrons in both mass and charge, differing only in the fact that they originate from the nucleus of the atom.

The N/P ratio decreases as a result of negatron decay. This mode of decay could be predicted to occur in neutron-rich nuclei; that is, it occurs in nuclei with more neutrons than the stable species in the respective part of the atomic chart. For example, stable iodine has a mass number of 127 (53 protons, 74 neutrons). By comparison, I-131 has 78 neutrons. Because 78 neutrons is a higher number than stable iodine, I-131 undergoes beta minus decay (Fig. 2-6).

The transition energy in negatron decay is given off in the form of kinetic energy of the beta particle, the energy

in the antineutrino, and the energy in any associated gamma radiation. The maximum kinetic energy (E_{max}) that a beta particle can have is a physical constant of the decay process. Beta particles are emitted with a continuous spectrum of energies lower than the maximum. The mean kinetic energy of beta particles (E_β) is approximately one third of the maximum ($E_\beta = \frac{1}{3} E_{max}$). For beta particles with less than the maximum kinetic energy, the energy is shared between the beta particle and the antineutrino.

Again, a decay scheme can have more than one pathway from the parent to the daughter. For many radionuclides decaying by negatron decay, beta particles with different maximum kinetic energies are emitted. Because the total transition energy must be the same for each pathway, the energy of associated gamma radiation is also correspondingly different. For example, the decay scheme for I-131 presented in Fig. 2-6 illustrates only one pathway from parent to daughter, the one of most interest and importance in clinical practice. In reality, there are beta particles given off with six different energies and there are 19 different gamma rays. However, the most abundant gamma ray, with an energy of 364 keV, occurs in 81% of transitions (known as an abundance of 81%).

A number of beta-emitting radionuclides have been used in clinical nuclear medicine. I-131, the first radionuclide of importance in medicine, is still used. The disadvantage of beta emitters is the high radiation dose received by the patient from the beta particles. For radioiodine-131, this disadvantage becomes an advantage when the radionuclide is used as therapy for thyroid cancer and hyperthyroidism.

Positron Decay and Electron Capture

As the name implies, in *positron decay* a positive electron or positively charged beta particle is ejected from the nucleus, resulting in a decrease in the atomic number between the parent and the daughter nuclei and an increase in the N/P ratio. Positron decay occurs in nuclides that are neutron poor, with N/P ratios less than those occurring on the line of stability. Positron decay is illustrated in Fig. 2-7 for fluorine-18. The minimum transition energy required for positron decay is 1.02 MeV, which is the energy equivalent of the mass of two electrons. The transition energy in excess of the 1.02 MeV threshold is embodied in the kinetic energy of the positrons and any associated gamma rays. For positrons given off with less than maximum kinetic energy, the energy difference is in subatomic particles called *neutrinos*. In both positron and negatron decay, the neutrinos (or antineutrinos) carry away a substantial portion of the transition energy. The likelihood of neutrinos reacting in soft tissue is small and the energy in neutrinos is not important in calculating radiation dosimetry for clinical applications.

In unstable nuclei where the maximum available transition energy is less than 1.02 MeV, decay of neutron-poor radionuclides is by electron capture (Fig. 2-8). In *electron capture,* an electron from one of the orbital shells close to the nucleus is incorporated into the nucleus, converting a proton into a neutron. The captured electron is usually from the K shell. The resulting vacancy is filled by transition of an electron from a shell farther from the nucleus. The energy released from this electron transition appears either as characteristic x-radiation or as the kinetic energy of an Auger electron.

Some radionuclides decay by multiple modes, including electron capture, positron decay, and negatron decay (Fig. 2-9). The likelihood of electron capture increases as the available transition energy decreases. The probability of electron capture also increases with increasing atomic number.

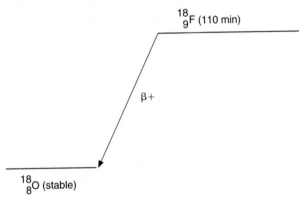

Figure 2-7   Decay scheme of fluorine-18 by positron emission. The daughter product, oxygen-18, has one fewer proton in the nucleus. Positron decay is another example of an isobaric transition without change in atomic mass between parent and daughter.

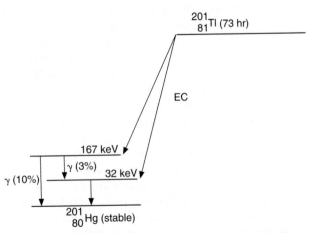

Figure 2-8   Thallium-201 decay by electron capture (EC). The daughter nucleus (mercury-201) has one fewer proton than the parent.

Isomeric Transition and Internal Conversion

No radionuclide undergoes true radioactive decay just by the emission of gamma radiation. However, in some decay schemes, there are intermediate species with measurable half-lives that exist in a *metastable* state. The concept of metastability is arbitrary. Most gamma rays are emitted almost immediately (10^{-12} seconds) after the primary decay process, whether it be alpha decay, negatron decay, positron decay, or electron capture. When the intermediate excited state lasts longer than 10^{-9} seconds, the term *metastable* is used and an *m* is placed after the mass number to indicate the phenomenon. The transition from the metastable state to the ground state is *isomeric* because the atomic number does not change and thus the transformation is from one isomer to another.

The most important example of a metastable state in nuclear medicine practice is technetium-99m (Tc-99m), which occurs in the decay of molybdenum-99 to technetium-99 (Figs. 2-10 and 2-11). The metastable state for Tc-99m has a half-life of 6 hours which allows ample time for the separation of the metastable species from the parent radionuclide and its subsequent use for clinical imaging procedures. Tc-99m is attractive from a radiation safety or health physics standpoint because it is essentially a pure gamma emitter not associated with primary

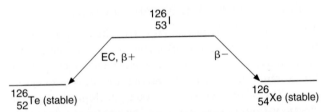

Figure 2-9   Iodine-126 decay through multiple processes. The diagram indicates decay by electron capture and by the emission of both positrons and negatrons.

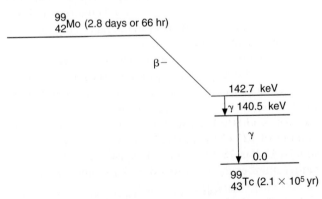

Figure 2-10   Decay scheme of molybdenum-99. Negatron emission to technetium-99.

particulate radiations. Its use as a radiolabel is associated with favorably low radiation dosimetry.

The energy released in isomeric transitions may be used to dislodge an orbital electron instead of being emitted as a gamma ray. This process is called *internal conversion* (Fig. 2-12). The kinetic energy of the electron (conversion electron) is equal to the difference between the gamma ray energy and the binding energy of the electron. The internal conversion process reduces the number of usable, detectable gamma photons for imag-

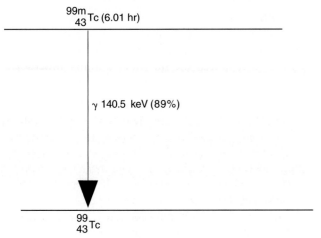

Figure 2-11 Isomeric transition of technetium-99m to technetium-99.

ing. It also results in a higher radiation dose to the patient because the conversion electron is absorbed in tissue close to its site of origin. In the "decay" of Tc-99m, a 140-keV gamma ray is given off 89% of the time and internal conversion accounts for most of the remaining transitions.

Gamma Ray Emission

Many radioactive decay processes result in the release of gamma rays or gamma photons, which are ionizing electromagnetic radiations that originate in the excited, unstable atomic nucleus. They have discrete energies defined by the decay scheme for the respective radionuclide and occur over a wide range of energies. Gamma rays most useful in conventional single-photon nuclear medicine applications have energies of approximately 80-400 keV. Nuclear medicine imaging equipment has been optimized for this energy range. Photons with energies less than 80 keV present difficulties because of their relatively high attenuation in tissue and their scattering properties. They are also less reliably localized by standard imaging devices because of the smaller amount of total energy available in the detection process. Gamma rays with energies significantly greater than 400 keV are progressively more difficult to image with conventional gamma cameras. The detection efficiency in gamma camera systems is less at higher energies. Spatial

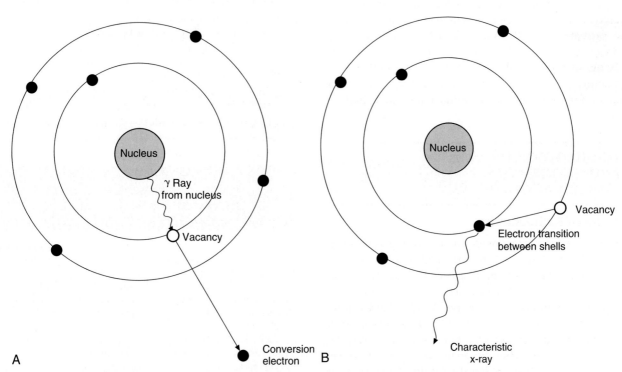

Figure 2-12 Internal conversion and characteristic x-ray emission. **A,** With internal conversion, an orbital electron is ejected from its shell, instead of the emission of a gamma ray. **B,** A characteristic x-ray is then given off as a consequence of the electron vacancy's being filled.

resolution is also lost through difficulty in collimating high-energy photons.

Characteristic Radiation and Auger Electrons

When an orbital electron is removed from its shell, it leaves a vacancy that is rapidly filled by a free electron or an electron from a shell farther from the nucleus. In this process, the "cascading" electron gives up energy as it fills in the vacancy and becomes more tightly bound. Most often, the energy that is given up by the electron is emitted in the form of electromagnetic radiation.

The electromagnetic radiations that arise in the process of filling a vacancy are called *characteristic radiations* or *characteristic x-rays* where applicable because their energy is uniquely defined by the difference in the binding energy of the donor shell and the shell where the vacancy is being filled (that is, the x-ray energy is "characteristic" of the respective transition) (*see* Fig. 2-12). In some applications of radionuclides, detection of characteristic x-rays is the primary means of forming the image or measuring the amount of radioactivity. An example of this is myocardial perfusion imaging with thallium-201 (Tl-201). The most abundant photons used for imaging are actually characteristic x-rays from mercury-201, the daughter product of Tl-201 decay.

An alternative process to the emission of characteristic radiation is the ejection of another electron by the energy released in filling a given vacancy. An electron ejected in this way is termed an *Auger electron* (Box 2-2). The probability of the emission of characteristic or fluorescent x-rays relative to Auger electrons is higher for more tightly bound electrons. Therefore, the emission of characteristic x-rays is more common for nuclei with a higher Z number and for electrons in the inner shells.

TERMINOLOGY, UNITS, AND MATHEMATICS OF RADIOACTIVE DECAY

Units of Radioactivity

Two systems for expressing decay or disintegration rates are in widespread use and are potentially confusing. The more widely-used system historically was based on the *curie*. This unit was based on the disintegration rate of 1 gram of radium and was defined as 3.7×10^{10} disintegrations per second (dps) (Box 2-3). It is now known that the disintegration rate of 1 gram of radium is slightly different than 1 curie, but the quantitative definition has been widely used throughout the world. Most medical diagnostic applications involve amounts of radioactivity in the microcurie (3.7×10^4 dps) or millicurie (3.7×10^7 dps) range.

An alternative to the curie in the international system (SI) of units is the becquerel (Bq), which is equal to 1 dps. The relationship between the curie and the becquerel is straightforward, but may be somewhat confusing to those used to the older term. One millicurie equals 37 million Bq, or 37 MBq. Both terminology systems are used widely in the literature (Table 2-2). However, the SI system is increasingly preferred.

Half-Life and Decay Constant

The mathematics of radioactive decay follow from direct physical measurements. The fundamental empirical observation determined early in the history of work with radionuclides is that the number of atoms undergoing decay during any finite period of time is proportional to

---

Box 2-3   Conversion of International System (SI) and Conventional Units of Radioactivity

CONVENTIONAL UNIT

1 curie (Ci) = 3.7×10^{10} disintegrations per second (dps)

SI UNIT

1 becquerel (Bq) = 1 dps

CURIES → BECQUERELS

1 Ci = 3.7×10^{10} dps = 37 GBq
1 mCi = 3.7×10^7 dps = 37 MBq
1 μCi = 3.7×10^4 dps = 37 KBq

BECQUERELS → CURIES

1 Bq = 1 dps = 2.7×10^{-11} Ci = 27 pCi
1 MBq = 10^6 dps = 2.7×10^{-5} Ci = 0.027 mCi
1 GBq = 10^9 dps = 27 mCi

Table 2-2   Conversion from Centimeter-gram-second (CGS) System to International System (SI) Units

	CGS unit	SI unit	Conversion factor
Work	erg	joule (J)	10^7
Radioactivity	curie (Ci)	becquerel (Bq)	3.7×10^{10}
Radiation absorbed dose	rad	gray (Gy)	100
Radiation exposure	roentgen (R)	coulomb/kg	2.58×10^{-4}
Roentgen equivalent man	rem	sievert (Sv)	100

the number of radioactive atoms in the sample. This proportion can be written:

$$\frac{-dN_t}{dt} \propto N_t$$

where N_t is the number of radioactive atoms in the sample at time t. The term dN_t/dt is mathematical notation expressing the change in the number of radioactive atoms over a short interval. The negative sign in the equation denotes that the number of radioactive atoms decreases over time.

For any given radioactive species, the equation may be rewritten as:

$$\frac{-dN_t}{dt} \lambda N_t$$

The term λ is the constant of proportionality and is a mathematical constant for each radionuclide. It is also called the *decay constant* and has units of 1/time.

The last equation can be rearranged and integrated and provides the classic equation:

$$N_t = N_0 e^{-\lambda t}$$

The term N_0 represents the number of radioactive atoms at time $t = 0$ and e is Euler's number, which equals ~2.718 (Box 2-1). In words, this equation says that the number of radioactive atoms at any later point in time (N_t) is equal to the product of the original number (N_0) times an exponential factor (e) that takes into account the rate of decay (λ) and the length of time after the initial measurement (t). Because the activity of the sample is proportional to the number of atoms in that sample (A = λN), the equation can be rewritten as:

$$A_t = A_0 e^{-\lambda t}$$

where A indicates activity in either curies or becquerels. The decay curve plotted on standard coordinates with time on the x-axis and activity on the y-axis for a radioactive sample shows an exponentially decreasing function that approaches but never reaches zero. On semilog graph paper, the function is a straight line with a slope equal to $-\lambda$ (Fig. 2-13).

From the preceding fundamental equations, it is possible to derive the concept of physical half-life, which turns out to be a more intuitive and useful way of describing radioactive decay than using the decay constant. The *half-life* is simply defined as the time required for the number of radioactive atoms in a sample to decrease by exactly one-half or 50%. Mathematically, the value of the half-life can be derived from the previous equations by substituting $N/2$ and $T_{1/2}$ on the two sides respectively as follows:

$$\frac{N_0}{2} = N_0 e^{-\lambda T_{1/2}}$$
$$\frac{1}{2} = e^{-\lambda T_{1/2}}$$

Because $e - 0.693 = 1/2$, this equation can be simplified to yield:

$$\lambda T_{1/2} = 0.693$$
$$T_{1/2} = \frac{0.693}{\lambda}$$

From the preceding equations, the decay constant has units of reciprocal time (e.g., $\sec^{-1}$ or hr^{-1}) and the physical half-life has units of time such as seconds, hours, days, or years. Radionuclides with long physical half-lives have smaller values for the decay constant. That is, the longer the physical half-life, the smaller the fraction of the radioactive atoms that undergoes disintegration in any given unit of time. From a practical standpoint, most radionuclides used in clinical nuclear medicine must have half-lives of hours or days, which permits shipping from the manufacturing site to the hospital, preparation of the radiopharmaceutical, and imaging. Use of shorter-lived agents is feasible in institutions with radionuclide production facilities such as cyclotrons or special accelerators.

In certain cases, radionuclides are obtained from "generator" systems, and the practical limitation is then the half-life of the parent compound. For example, the half-life of Tc-99m is 6 hours. The half-life of its parent,

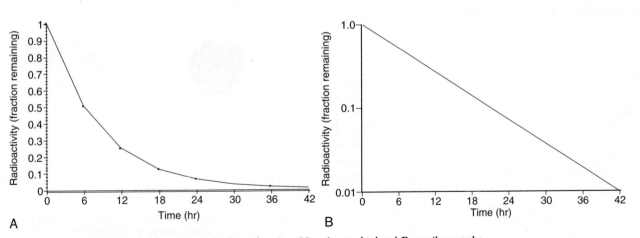

Figure 2-13   Decay plot for technetium-99m. **A,** standard and, **B,** semilog graphs.

molybdenum-99 (Mo-99), is 2.7 days (see Figs. 2-10 and 2-11). The Mo-99/Tc-99m generator system provides the dual advantage of a longer-lived parent, which permits commercial distribution and prolonged on-site availability, while the short half-life of the Tc-99m daughter reduces radiation exposure to the patient compared with longer-lived agents.

Mean Life

The concept of the mean life of a radionuclide is useful in thinking about radiation dosimetry. The mean life is given as:

$$\bar{t} = \frac{1}{\lambda}$$

or

$$\bar{t} = 1.44 \, T_{1/2}$$

The concept of mean life is more difficult to understand intuitively than the concept of physical half-life but may be thought of as the average length of time of the radioactive atoms in a sample before they undergo disintegration.

Biological Half-Life and Effective Half-Life

An important concept in determining radiation exposure to patients is the *biological half-life* and the corollary concept, *effective half-life*. The term *biological half-life* is used to describe the biological clearance of the radionuclide from a particular tissue or organ system. Thus the actual half-life or *effective half-life* of a radiopharmaceutical in a biological system is dependent on both the physical (p) half-life and the biological (b) clearance. Because physical decay and biological clearance occur simultaneously in parallel, the relationship between them and the effective half-life is given by:

$$\frac{1}{T_{1/2 \, \text{eff}}} = \frac{1}{T_{1/2 \, \text{p}}} + \frac{1}{T_{1/2 \, \text{b}}}$$

Rearranging terms, this becomes:

$$T_{1/2 \, \text{eff}} = \frac{T_{1/2 \, \text{b}} \times T_{1/2 \, \text{p}}}{T_{1/2 \, \text{b}} + T_{1/2 \, \text{p}}}$$

The concept of biological half-life is not as mathematically clear-cut as the physical half-life. It can vary among subjects and does not necessarily follow a regular exponential process. For example, the biological half-life of radioactivity in the bladder is determined by the time at which a patient chooses to void. The half-life of xenon-133 in the lung during pulmonary ventilation studies is determined by the rate and depth of respiration and by the presence of pulmonary disease. Nonetheless, the term biological half-life is useful in thinking about the amount of exposure the patient actually receives during a nuclear medicine procedure.

INTERACTIONS OF RADIATION WITH MATTER

Negatrons (Beta Particles)

Negatrons, or beta particles, cause ionization in tissues by electrostatic interactions with orbital electrons. They give up energy through a series of such interactions along a tortuous path. As a rule of thumb, the maximum penetration of beta particles in soft tissue in centimeters is equal to the maximum kinetic energy of the negatron in megaelectron volts divided by two. Thus, the radiation dose delivered by negatrons in soft tissue is relatively close to their source. For example, the maximum kinetic energy of the most abundant beta particle in the decay of I-131 is 0.606 MeV. The majority of the radiation dose delivered in I-131 therapy is within 0.3 cm of the location of the nucleus undergoing decay.

Positrons

Positrons also give up their kinetic energy through electrostatic ionizations. As the positron approaches thermal energy, it undergoes *annihilation* by combining with a negatively charged electron (Fig. 2-14). Two gamma photons are emitted 180 degrees apart. Each has an energy of 0.511 MeV, the energy equivalent of positron-electron mass. This unique phenomenon of annihilation radiation 180 degrees apart is the basis for positron emission tomography (PET).

Gamma Rays and X-Rays

Gamma rays and x-rays are attenuated in tissues through three processes. Photons can be completely absorbed by the *photoelectric effect* or in *pair production*. They can also undergo scattering or deflection from their original path by the *Compton effect or Compton-scattering* phenomenon, in which photons give up part of their original energy.

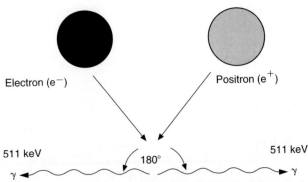

Figure 2-14 Positron annihilation. The mass of a positron and an electron is converted to energy in the form of two photons. The photons each have an energy of 0.511 MeV and are given off 180 degrees apart.

Pair Production

Pair production requires a photon with a minimum energy of 1.02 MeV. The photon energy is converted into one negative and one positive electron. Because the energy required is greater than the photon energies used in medical imaging, this form of attenuation is not important in nuclear medicine.

Photoelectric Absorption

Photoelectric absorption occurs when the total energy of an x-ray or gamma ray photon is transferred to an orbital electron (Fig. 2-15, A). The photon must possess energy greater than the binding energy of the electron. The elec-tron is displaced from its orbit or shell and is either lifted to a higher shell or ejected from the atom (Fig. 2-15, B). Ejected electrons are termed *photoelectrons*.

As a consequence of the photoelectric interaction, an electron cascade occurs to fill the vacancy, with the subse-quent emission of characteristic x-rays or Auger electrons (Fig. 2-15, C). Photoelectric absorption is most likely to occur when the photon energy is just above the electron binding energy. The kinetic energy of the photoelectron is equal to the difference between the energy of the inci-dent photon and the electron binding energy.

For a given absorbing material, as photon energy increases, the likelihood of a photoelectric event decreases.

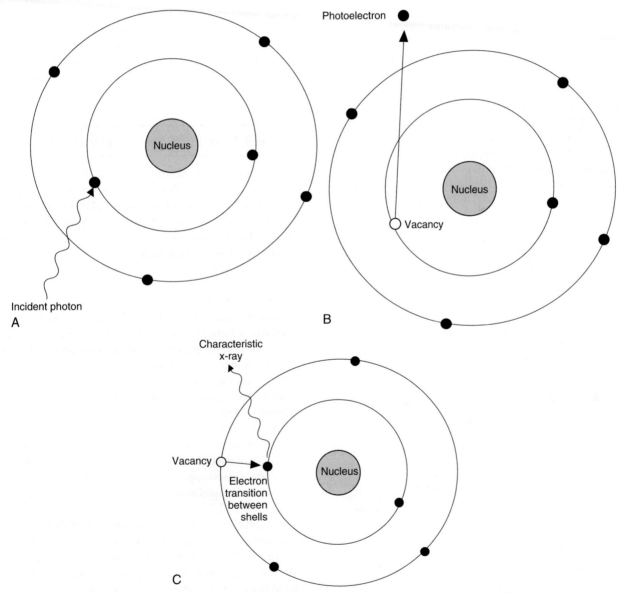

Figure 2-15   Photoelectric absorption. **A,** An incident photon interacts with an orbital electron. **B,** The electron is ejected from its shell, creating a vacancy. The electron is either ejected from the atom or moved to a shell farther from the nucleus. **C,** The orbital vacancy is filled by the transition of an electron from a more distant shell. A characteristic x-ray is given off as a consequence of this transition.

The photoelectric interaction is important in soft tissues up to an energy of approximately 50 keV. Radionuclides with associated photon energies lower than 50 keV are less desirable for clinical applications because of the high absorption of these photons in soft tissue owing to photoelectric interaction.

Although photoelectric absorption is undesirable in body tissues, it is fundamental to the detection of ionizing radiation. In both nuclear medicine and roentgenography, the creation of images depends on energy absorption in a detecting medium through the photoelectric interaction. For this reason, imaging systems typically are high-density, high-Z materials such as inorganic crystals, in which the likelihood of photoelectric absorption is high.

Compton Scattering and Compton Effect

In Compton scattering, a photon interacts with a weakly bound outer shell electron. Instead of being completely absorbed as in the photoelectric interaction, in the Compton process the photon is deflected from its original direction and continues to exist but at lower energy (Fig. 2-16). The energy difference is transferred to the recoil electron as kinetic energy. Compton scattering is the dominant mode of gamma ray and x-ray interaction in soft tissues between 30 keV and 30 MeV.

Because the Compton-scattered photon gives up energy in the interaction, its wavelength increases. The formula for this is:

$$\Lambda\lambda = 0.0243\,(1 - \cos\phi)$$

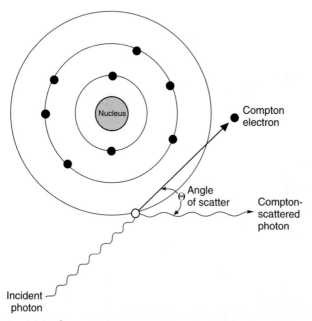

Figure 2-16   Compton scatter. An incident photon interacts with an outer or loosely bound electron. The photon gives up a portion of its energy to the electron and undergoes a change in direction at a lower energy.

where $\Lambda\lambda$ is the change in wavelength and the angle ϕ is the angle through which the photon is scattered. The angle of scatter can be minimal or up to 180 degrees (backscatter).

The significance of Compton scattering in nuclear imaging is that scattered photons reaching the imaging detector must be discriminated against and not allowed to form part of the image. Because Compton-scattered photons give up part of their energy, one way to discriminate against them is through setting an "energy window" for acceptance of events in the detector. However, photons scattered through a relatively narrow angle lose only small amounts of energy and may not be effectively excluded by pulse height analysis and the setting of an energy window. Thus, Compton-scattered photons contribute to the loss of spatial resolution in nuclear medicine images. The problem is progressively worse for lower energies because the lower the original photon energy, the less the change in energy for a given scattering angle.

STATISTICS OF RADIOACTIVE DECAY

The time of decay of any single unstable radioactive nucleus is unpredictable and is not influenced by the decay of other nuclei or the physical or chemical environment of the nucleus. Because radioactive decay is random, the actual observed number of nuclei undergoing decay in any given period is subject to statistical uncertainty; this uncertainty is a practical problem in clinical nuclear medicine. In any setting where a quantitative measurement is required, such as determining the amount of radioactivity in a radiopharmaceutical to be given to the patient or in a blood sample used in calculating a physiologic parameter or performing quality control of nuclear instrumentation, estimates of statistical certainty are necessary.

Radioactive decay follows *Poisson statistics* or the Poisson probability law. The Poisson probability density function is similar but not identical to the Gaussian or normal probability density function. Curves expressing the Poisson and Gaussian probability density functions are more closely matched as the number of observed events is increased and practically identical if the mean is greater than 20.

For data obeying the Poisson probability distribution, the standard deviation (SD) is given by $SD = \sqrt{r}$, where r is the true mean. Because the true mean is usually estimated from an average of a number of individual measurements, the estimated standard deviation is $SD(est) = \sqrt{r}$ (es).

Expressing standard deviation as a fraction or a percentage is often useful. The *fractional standard deviation* is simply $1\sqrt{r}$. The *percent fractional standard deviation* (% SD) is the fractional standard deviation × 100. For example, if 2500 counts are recorded in a picture element or "pixel" in an image, the fractional standard deviation of the measurement is $\frac{1}{\sqrt{2500}} = 0.2$. The percent fractional standard deviation is 2%. This equation can also be expressed as:

$$\%SD = \frac{100}{\sqrt{n}}$$

where *n* is the number of counts observed.

Calculation of standard deviation is useful in determining the number of counts to obtain in the measurement of a radioactive sample or in a scintigraphic image for statistical certainty. As the number of counts increases, the percent fractional or relative standard deviation decreases and the ability to distinguish a true difference in the amount of radioactivity in two different samples increases. Likewise, in imaging, as the number of counts per pixel increases, the likeliness of the observed differences in the image actually representing true differences in the amount of activity between two locations in the image increases.

SUGGESTED READING

Chandra R: *Nuclear medicine physics: the basics*, 6th ed. Baltimore, Williams & Wilkins, 2004.

Hendee WR: *Medical radiation physics*, 3rd ed. St. Louis, Mosby, 1992.

Johns HE, Cunningham JR: *The physics of radiology*, 4th ed. Chicago, Thomas Books, 1983.

Powsner RA, Powsner ER: *Essentials of nuclear medicine physics*, Malden, MA, Blackwell Science, 1998.

Cherry SR, Sorenson JA, Phelps ME: *Physics in nuclear medicine*, 3rd ed. Philadelphia, WB Saunders, 2003.

Weber DA, Eckerman KF, Dillman LT, Ryman JC: *MIRD: radionuclide data and decay schemes.* New York, Society of Nuclear Medicine, 1989.

Radiation Detection and Instrumentation

Detection of radioactivity is fundamental to the practice of nuclear medicine. The amount and type of radioactivity being administered to patients must be measured and documented, and the areas in which people work must be monitored to ensure safety to both health care personnel and patients. Radioactivity emanating from the patient must be detected to allow the temporal and spatial localization necessary to create scintigraphic images. The common denominator in all of the devices used in contemporary nuclear medicine practice for calibration of administered dosages, area monitoring, and imaging is the conversion of energy in the form of ionizing radiation into electrical energy. In modern imaging equipment, these electronic signals are often recorded and processed by dedicated nuclear medicine computer systems. Nuclear medicine imaging devices, including the gamma scintillation camera, can be thought of as specialized radiation detection devices, highly modified and adapted to record the temporal and spatial localization of radioactivity in the patient.

RADIATION DETECTION

Ionization Chambers, Proportional Counters, and Geiger-Müller Counters

One important approach to radiation detection is the use of an ionization chamber. The generic design concept is a gas-filled chamber with positive and negative electrodes, placed either at opposite sides of the chamber or in a concentric cylinder geometry. A potential difference is created between the two electrodes, but no current flows in the absence of exposure of the chamber to radiation. The interaction of ionizing radiation with the gas in the chamber creates positive and negative ions, which move to the electrodes and produce an electrical current.

The basic concept of the ionization chamber is extremely versatile, allowing specialized devices to be designed for specific applications. For example, the problem of detecting alpha and beta radiation is quite different from that of detecting gamma radiation because of differences in both their power to penetrate different materials and their likelihood of interaction with matter. In addition, the problem of surveying a wide area to determine the presence or absence of radiation is different from the problem of accurately calibrating the millicuries of activity to be administered to a patient. Three important subtypes of ionization chambers with nuclear medicine applications are the basic ionization chamber, the proportional counter, and the Geiger-Müller counter.

Basic Ionization Chambers

The voltage difference between the electrodes in the basic ionization chamber is calibrated to be just high enough to "harvest" all of the ions from the sensitive volume of the chamber, but not high enough that the ions in the chamber are accelerated to the point of creating additional secondary ionizations. As a result of this voltage calibration strategy, the current produced in any single event is very small and not measurable with any accuracy. Rather, the ionization chamber is used to measure the total current resulting from multiple events over a certain integration time in a given radiation detection setting.

A number of devices routinely used in nuclear medicine clinics operate on the principle of the ionization chamber. Radiation survey meters such as the cutie-pie, some pocket dosimeters, and radionuclide dose calibrators are all examples of specialized basic ionization chambers. The survey meters are typically calibrated to provide units of exposure such as milliroentgens per hour. Dose calibrators are set up to provide readings in the units of radioactivity used in clinical practice. Many laboratories now express these units in becquerels in response to a mandate from the U.S. Food and Drug Administration to use the International System as soon as possible; other laboratories have retained the Ci, mCi, and μCi convention. The amount of energy converted to electrical current per unit of radioactivity is unique for each radionuclide and radionuclide dose calibrators must be calibrated for the radionuclide to be measured.

Proportional Counters

The main difference between a proportional counter and the basic ionization chamber is greater applied voltage between the electrodes in the former. The higher voltage results in secondary ionizations in the sensitive volume of the chamber. The term *gas amplification* describes this phenomenon. Gas amplification can result in increased ionization by a factor of $10^3 - 10^6$. The resulting current pulse is large enough to be measured individually and is proportional to the energy originally deposited in the gas chamber. Typically, an inert gas such as helium or argon is used. The name of the device is based on the proportionality of total ionization to the total energy of the ionizing radiation. Proportional chambers do not have wide applicability in clinical nuclear medicine. They are used in research to detect alpha and beta particles.

Geiger-Müller Counter

In the Geiger-Müller counter, the voltage is increased even higher than in the proportional chamber application. Because of the high voltage, the initial ionization causes an "avalanche" of secondary ionizations, so that the gas is essentially completely ionized. This mode of operation of an ionization chamber allows detection of individual events but not their energy (i.e., pulse counting). Another important characteristic of the Geiger-Müller counter is detector dead time. Because the gas in the chamber is completely ionized, it takes a significant amount of time to become ready for the next event. Thus, Geiger-Müller counters are not useful in the presence of large amounts of radioactivity. They are good for detecting low levels of activity and are widely used as area survey meters and area monitors. They are valuable in detecting radiation contamination.

Scintillation Detectors: Thallium-Activated Sodium Iodide Crystals

The gas-filled ionization chambers described in the preceding section are not very sensitive to x-rays and gamma rays because of the low likelihood of ionizing interactions. The "stopping power" of gas is low. In current practice, thallium-activated sodium iodide crystals (NaI[Tl]) are used as the detector medium for single-photon imaging systems. These crystals are optically transparent and have sufficient stopping power for sensitive detection of gamma rays (Table 3-1).

As noted earlier, an important common denominator of many types of radiation detectors is the conversion of the ionizing radiation energy to electrical energy. Scintillation detector systems have an interesting conversion process. Gamma rays or x-rays enter the sodium iodide crystal and impart energy to valence electrons during photoelectric and Compton interactions. The imparted energy raises the electrons into the conduction band of the crystal lattice. The energy difference between the valence band and the conduction band is a few electron volts. As the electrons give up energy in the transition back from the conduction band to the valence band, photons of light are emitted. The light photons have a spectrum of energies; for sodium iodide crystals, the spectrum peaks at a wavelength of 4150 Å, or approximately 3 eV. The energy conversion efficiency in the NaI(Tl) crystal is approximately 13%. The remaining energy is dissipated in the crystal in the form of molecular motion or heat. The scintillation decay time or length of time for the scintillation event is approximately 1 μsec (10^{-6} seconds).

Thallium-activated sodium iodide crystals have become the preferred scintillation detector in many nuclear medicine applications for a number of reasons. The crystals are relatively inexpensive and allow great flexibility in

Table 3-1   Half-Value Layers of Selected Radionuclides

Radionuclide	Energy (keV)		Half-value layer (cm)		
			Lead	Water (soft tissue)	NaI
Tc-99m	140		0.028	4.50	0.265
Tl-201	69	Hg x-rays	0.0005	3.85	0.048
	81			0.048	0.069
I-131	364		0.220	6.35	1.500

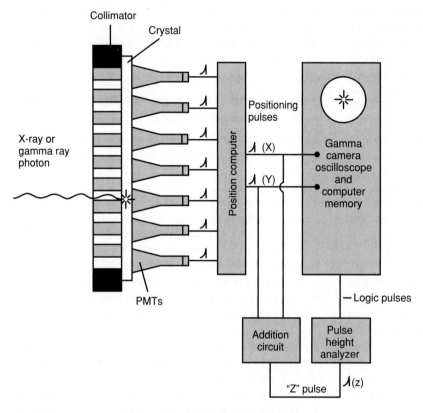

Figure 3-1   Schematic of gamma scintillation camera. The diagram shows a photon reaching the crystal through the collimator and undergoing photoelectric absorption. The photomultiplier tubes *(PMTs)* are optically coupled to the NaI(Tl) crystal. The electrical outputs from the respective photomultiplier tubes are further processed through positioning circuitry to calculate (*x, y*) coordinates and through addition circuitry to calculate the Z pulse. The Z pulse passes through the pulse height analyzer. If the event is accepted, it is recorded spatially in the location determined by the (*x, y*) positioning pulses.

size and shape. The stopping power of the sodium iodide crystals is good for the energy range used in clinical nuclear medicine for single-photon applications (i.e., 70–364 keV) (*see* Table 3-1). The thallium impurities in the sodium iodide crystal provide "activation centers" or luminescence centers that offer easier pathways for the return of the electrons from the conduction band of the crystal to the valence bands of atoms requiring electrons for electrical neutrality. Only a small amount of thallium impurity (0.1–0.4 mole %) is required in the sodium iodide crystal lattice to achieve the desired effect of making the scintillation process more efficient. The conversion efficiency of 13% is relatively high and the crystals are internally transparent to the light photons so that they reach the photocathodes. The disadvantages of

sodium iodide crystals are their fragility and their highly hydroscopic nature, necessitating hermetically sealed containers. In most applications, the crystal is sealed on all sides by a thin aluminum canister except on the photomultiplier tube side, which is covered by a quartz window to allow the scintillation photons to escape and reach the photomultiplier tubes.

The next step in the detection process is the interaction of the light photons arising in the crystal with the photocathode of a photomultiplier tube (Fig. 3-1). In the typical sodium iodide detector system, whether it is a simple probe or a gamma scintillation camera, the crystal is optically coupled to the photomultiplier tube by a light guide or light pipe to ensure the efficiency of light collection. The light photons dislodge electrons from the photocathode. These electrons are then accelerated by a series of electrodes (dynodes) in the photomultiplier tube. With each acceleration, the number of electrons is increased. The electrons are collected at the anode or collector of the photomultiplier tube. The multiplication factor is on the order of 3–6 per dynode stage and up to several million overall. The resulting voltage pulse from the photomultiplier tube is then available for further processing. This processing may take the form of amplification followed by pulse analysis to determine either the energy deposited in the crystal (pulse height analysis) or the spatial location of the event (position analysis) in the case of gamma scintillation cameras.

A key point to understand in the scintillation detection process is that proportionality is maintained at each step. That is, the number of light photons given off in the NaI(Tl) crystal is proportional to the energy deposited in the crystal from the x-ray or gamma ray, the number of electrons dislodged from the photocathode is proportional to the number of light photons, and the electrical output of the photomultiplier tube is proportional to the number of electrons dislodged from the photocathode. Thus, the height of the electrical pulse coming from the photomultiplier tube is proportional to the energy of the radiation absorbed in the crystal. This allows different radionuclides with different energies to be distinguished from one another by pulse height analysis. It also permits a distinction between primary photons and photons that have undergone Compton scatter events before detection. Compton-scattered photons are less energetic than the primary photons and have lower pulse heights. Recognizing Compton-scattered photons is critical in imaging applications of scintillation detection because only primary photons are desired to create the image.

Other Detection Devices

A host of other radiation detection devices are used in nuclear medicine and radiology including photographic film, which is used in personnel film badges, semiconductors, thermoluminescent and ultraviolet fluorescent detection devices, and chemical detectors that are useful for measuring cumulative radiation effects over a long period. They are not discussed here.

GAMMA RAY SPECTROMETRY AND PULSE HEIGHT ANALYSIS

The energies and relative abundance of the ionizing radiations given off by each radionuclide are physical constants. The proportionality between the energy of a gamma ray and the output of the electrical pulse from the photomultiplier tube provides a means for distinguishing between gamma rays (or x-rays) of different energies.

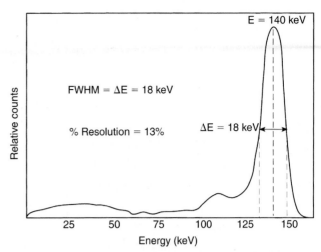

Figure 3-2   Spectrum for technetium-99m in air. The figure illustrates the concept of full width at half maximum (FWHM). For the particular detector system illustrated, the FWHM is 18 keV. The energy resolution of the detector system for Tc-99m is 13%.

However, the spectrum of recorded energies is more complex than would be predicted from the decay scheme because of Compton and photoelectric interactions both outside the NaI(Tl) scintillation detector and within the crystal. Recognizing the consequences of these interactions is important to the optimal use of counting and imaging instrumentation.

By convention, the energy spectra from x-ray and gamma ray detection are plotted with energy on the x-axis and the relative number of events is plotted on the y-axis (Fig. 3-2). The important relationships in gamma spectra are illustrated here for technetium-99m (Tc-99m) because it is the most commonly used radionuclide in clinical practice.

Photopeak

In a perfect detection system and with the complete absorption of the 140-keV gamma rays of Tc-99m in the detector, a single line would be recorded on the energy spectrum at exactly 140 keV. In practice, the 140-keV photopeak is recorded as a bell-shaped curve centered at 140 keV (*see* Fig. 3-2). The Gaussian distribution of recorded events stems from the statistical nature of the radiation detection process. Each step in the conversion of ionizing radiation to electrical current is subject to statistical fluctuation. Light photons are given off in the scintillation crystal with equal but random probability in all directions. Slightly different numbers of light photons impinge on the photocathodes between different absorption events. The number of electrons dislodged is also subject to statistical fluctuation, as is the electron amplification at each dynode stage in the photomultiplier tube.

The energy resolution of a detecting system can be expressed by the spread in the photopeak. A frequently

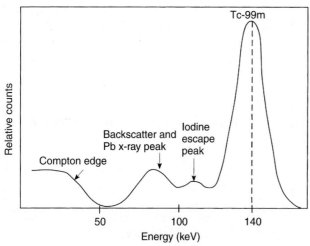

Figure 3-3   Energy spectrum for Tc-99m in air for a gamma scintillation camera with the collimator in place. Note the iodine escape peak at approximately 112 keV. The 180-degree backscatter peak at 90 keV merges with the characteristic x-ray peaks for lead (Pb). The Compton edge is at 50 keV.

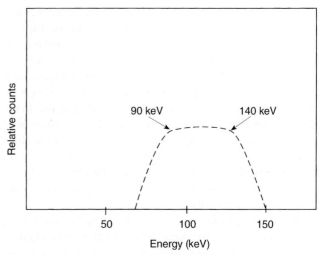

Figure 3-4   Compton scatter spectrum in soft tissue for single scattering events. Note that Compton-scattered photons have energy <140 keV but can be recorded above this level because of the imperfect energy resolution of the gamma camera.

used measure is full width at half maximum (FWHM), which is defined as the energy range encompassed by the bell-shaped curve halfway down from the apex of the photopeak (*see* Fig. 3-2). A typical gamma scintillation camera might have an FWHM equal to 14 keV for detecting Tc-99m. Energy resolution of a detecting system can also be expressed as a percentage of the photopeak energy, and the detector would be said to have an energy resolution of 10% (14/140). A narrower peak indicates better energy resolution and a greater ability to distinguish gamma rays with energies close to each other. The *photofraction* is the fraction of total counts in the entire spectrum within the photopeak.

Iodine Escape Peak

Photoelectric interactions occurring close to the edge of the sodium iodide crystal may result in the "escape" of iodine K-characteristic x-rays from the crystal. When this happens, the corresponding x-ray energy of approximately 28.5 keV is not deposited in the crystal and will result in a small peak on the energy spectrum at 112 keV (i.e., 140 − 28 keV) (Fig. 3-3). This peak, referred to as the *iodine escape peak,* can be observed with a Tc-99m source in air but is typically not observed in vivo because of the relatively much larger contribution from Compton-scattered photons from the patient in the recorded energy spectrum (Fig. 3-4).

Compton Valley, Edge, and Plateau

Not every photon entering a NaI(Tl) crystal undergoes photoelectric absorption. If a primary photon undergoes a Compton scatter interaction in the crystal with subsequent escape of the scattered photon, a smaller voltage pulse will be detected than those composing the photo-

peak. If the 140-keV gamma rays from technetium are used as the example, the maximum energy transferred to a recoil electron in the crystal occurs at the largest scattering angle (180 degrees) and is 50 keV. This energy is referred to as the *Compton edge.* The energy from 0–50 keV is called the *Compton plateau* or *continuum* and corresponds to the energy deposited by photons that scatter from 0–180 degrees before escaping the crystal (*see* Fig. 3-3). The portion of the energy spectrum between the Compton edge and the photopeak is the *Compton valley.* Some gamma rays undergo multiple Compton scatter events before escaping from the detector crystal. These events may be recorded in the region of the Compton valley. The energy relationships obviously differ for each radionuclide with differing photopeak energy.

Backscatter Peak

Another peak resulting from Compton scattering occurs when primary gamma photons undergo 180-degree scattering outside the detector and are then completely absorbed. The scattering can take place either in front of the detector or behind it if a gamma ray has initially passed completely through the crystal without being scattered or absorbed. From the previous section, it is apparent that for Tc-99m the backscatter peak occurs at 90 keV (140 − 50 keV) (*see* Fig. 3-3).

Lead Characteristic X-ray Peak

In most nuclear medicine applications, scintillation detectors are used in conjunction with lead collimators. The 140-keV primary photons of technetium are energetic enough to interact with the K shell electrons of lead. The resulting K-characteristic x-rays are in the range of 75–88 keV and are readily seen in the energy spectrum (Fig. 3-5).

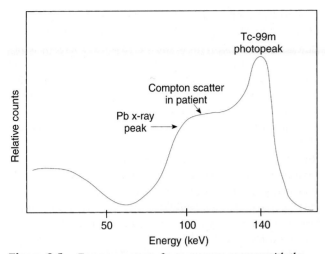

Figure 3-5 Energy spectrum from a gamma camera with the Tc-99m activity in the patient. Note the loss of definition of the lower limb of the Tc-99m photopeak. This spectrum can be thought of as a sum of the spectra in Figs. 3-3 and 3-4. This spectrum illustrates the difficulty of discriminating against Compton-scattered photons using pulse height analysis.

Coincidence or Sum Peaks

The likelihood of two separate events taking place simultaneously in the sodium iodide crystal increases with the amount of radiation present. If two events occur close enough in time, the detector system may record them as a single event. Two primary photons from Tc-99m that are detected in coincidence will appear at 280 keV on the energy spectrum. However, every combination of events is possible. That is, a primary photon can be detected in coincidence with a scattered photon of any energy or a lead characteristic x-ray, and so forth. For many detecting systems, the ability to discriminate or resolve different discrete energies decreases with increasing amounts of radiation exposure because the likelihood of coincidence events increases with increasing event rate.

Compton Scatter in the Patient

Degradation of clinical images is caused by Compton scatter in the patient and the inability of imaging systems to completely discriminate primary from Compton-scattered photons. For the gamma scintillation camera, up to 35% (or even more) of recorded events come from Compton-scattered photons. The energy spectrum for Tc-99m photons undergoing one scattering event in the patient ranges from 90 keV (i.e., 180 degree scattering angle) to just under the energy of the primary photon, 140 keV (*see* Fig. 3-4). In Tc-99m spectra obtained with radioactivity in the patient, the lower limb of the primary photopeak merges into the events owing to Compton scattering in the patient, which in turn merges with the lead K-characteristic x-ray peak (*see* Fig. 3-5).

IMAGING INSTRUMENTATION

The original instruments available for medical applications of radionuclides were handheld Geiger-Müller devices and simple scintillation probe systems. These systems did not allow spatial localization of radioactivity emanating from the body but did provide a means of crude overall counting. Early clinical applications in nuclear medicine were aimed at calculating the percentage uptake of radioiodine in the thyroid gland with these simple radiation detector systems.

Rectilinear Scanners

In the 1950s, probe systems were adapted into electro-mechanical devices called rectilinear scanners. The geometric field of view of the probe was focused or restricted through the application of collimating devices and the probes were mounted on mechanical transport systems to systematically traverse back and forth over an organ of interest. The original probe systems used calcium tungstenate crystals, which rapidly gave way to sodium iodide crystals for the radiation detection step. By the 1960s, rectilinear scanning systems were available with 3-, 5-, and 8-inch diameter detectors.

Gamma Scintillation Cameras

The rectilinear scanner has been replaced by the gamma scintillation camera invented by Hal Anger, also known as the Anger camera. The gamma camera offers far more flexibility than the rectilinear scanner and has been developed into a sophisticated series of imaging devices that permit dynamic and tomographic imaging, as well as conventional static planar imaging. The major components of the gamma scintillation camera are illustrated in Fig. 3-1. Perhaps the easiest way to understand the way gamma cameras work is to follow a photon through the radiation detection and spatial localization process, beginning with the origin of photons in the patient.

The Patient as a Source of Photons

Ideally, the flux of photons arriving at a radiation detector would be proportional to the number of photons emitted in the respective part of the body being imaged. This assumption would be valid only if the body part were a point source of radiation in air, which is clearly never the case in clinical practice. Additionally, a number of factors cause distortion of the photon flux reaching the gamma camera.

One may think of "good" photons as primary photons arising in the organ of interest and emitted parallel to the axis of the collimator field of view. These are the photons desired for creating the scintigraphic image. Good photons are reduced in number by absorption and scatter, which decreases the information available for creating the image (Fig. 3-6). In the clinical applications of nuclear medicine, many potentially useful photons are absorbed or scattered before they reach the detector.

Unwanted primary photons can arise from background radioactivity in tissues in front of or behind the structure of interest (*see* Fig. 3-6). These primary photons can travel directly to the detector and are then indistinguishable from photons arising in the body part of interest. They may be thought of as "bad" photons because they reduce image contrast and may distort quantitative data analysis. Background activity produced by primary photons is hard to correct. One major advantage of single-photon emission computed tomography (SPECT) is the increase in image contrast resulting from reduction in this kind of background activity superimposed on object activity.

Another source of bad photons is primary photons arising from the organ of interest, which travel "off axis" toward the detector. Radiation is given off isotropically (i.e., with equal probability in all directions) and only a small fraction of the total emitted photons are useful for forming the image. A principal function of collimators is to absorb off-axis photons (Fig. 3-7).

Compton scatter is a third source of bad photons (*see* Figs. 3-6 and 3-7). Photons originating in or adjacent to the organ of interest can scatter and subsequently travel toward the detector. Photons that undergo Compton scattering in the patient lose some of their energy and can be partially discriminated against by using pulse height analysis. However, this ability is far from perfect. For example, a 140-keV photon scattered through a 30-degree angle retains an energy of 135 keV. This energy would be accepted in a typical 20% energy window used for clinical imaging with Tc-99m.

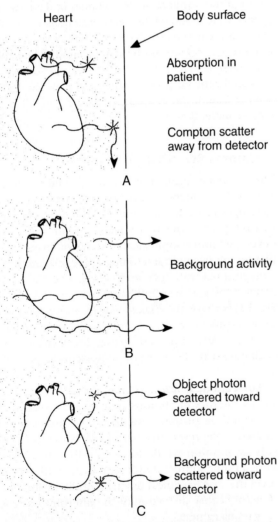

Figure 3-6   Patient as a source of photons. **A,** Absorption and scattering of primary photons in the body. These never reach the detector. **B,** Background activity arising from in front of, behind, and beside the organ of interest. **C,** Object and background photons scattered toward the detector.

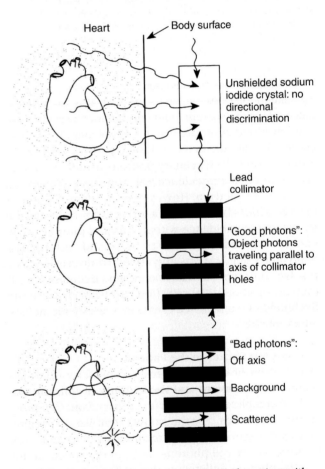

Figure 3-7   Interaction of photons arising in the patient with detector and parallel-hole collimator. The collimator provides directional discrimination for primary and scattered photons. It does not eliminate either background or scattered photons that travel toward the detector within the geometric acceptance field of view of the collimator. "Good" photons are primary (unscattered) photons that originate in the object and travel parallel to the axis of the collimator field of view. All other photons (i.e., background, scattered, off-axis) are undesirable in the image.

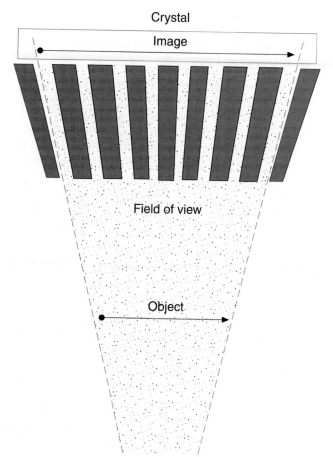

Figure 3-11   Converging-hole collimator. Objects are magnified.

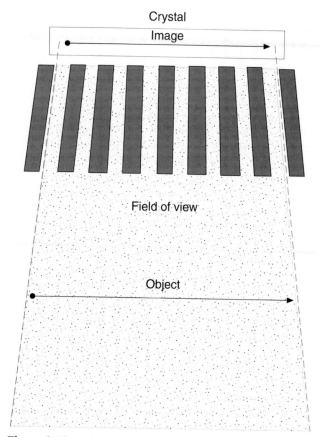

Figure 3-12   Diverging-hole collimator. Objects are minified.

minified to a different extent, depending on the distance between the respective location and the collimator.

In addition to the primary collimator designs, a number of specialty use collimators have been described. Parallel slant-hole collimators have found application in nuclear cardiology. Some nuclear medicine physicians favor a 30-degree caudal angulation for separating the left atrium from the left ventricle in radionuclide ventriculography. Rotating slant-hole collimators and multiple-pin-hole collimators have been used for limited angle emission computed tomography.

Gamma Ray Detection: The Sodium Iodide Crystal
Modern gamma scintillation cameras use thallium-activated sodium iodide crystals as the radiation detector (*see* Fig. 3-1). The desired event in the camera crystal is the complete photoelectric absorption of a primary photon that reached the crystal by traveling parallel to the geometric axis of the collimator field of view from its origin in the organ of interest in the patient. The likelihood of a photoelectric interaction and complete energy absorption in the sodium iodide crystal is greater at low energies and decreases at higher energies as Compton scatter becomes more likely (*see* Table 3-1).

As discussed in the section on radiation detection, the gamma ray energy is converted to light energy in the crystal. For every 140-keV technetium photon completely absorbed, approximately 4200 light photons are emitted with an average energy of 3 eV. One of the limitations of lower energy gamma rays, including those from Tc-99m, is the limited number of light photons available for subsequent event localization. Higher energy photons potentially provide more light photons and better statistical certainty for event localization. However, this is counterbalanced by the greater likelihood of an initial Compton scatter event in the crystal before a terminal photoelectric interaction. When multiple scattering events occur in the crystal before complete energy absorption, spatial resolution is reduced.

Signal Processing and Event Localization
The breakthrough concept in the design of the gamma scintillation camera is the use of an array of photomultiplier tubes behind the crystal for event localization. In the first commercial gamma camera, a 10-inch diameter sodium iodide crystal was optically coupled to a hexagonal array of 19 3-inch diameter photomultiplier tubes (Fig. 3-13).

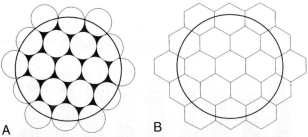

Figure 3-13 Circular (**A**) and hexagonal (**B**) photomultiplier tubes. The tubes are arrayed in a hexagonal configuration so that the distance from each tube to all of its nearest neighbors is identical. The switch from round to hexagonal tubes allows more complete coverage of the gamma camera crystal.

For each event, two kinds of signal processing are performed. First, the output from all of the photomultiplier tubes is summed for the purpose of pulse height analysis. This summed pulse is typically referred to as the *Z pulse*. It is used to determine whether the detected event is within the desired energy range and should be accepted into the formation of the image. If it is of lower or higher energy, it is discriminated against and rejected (*see* Fig. 3-1).

Simultaneously, the output of each photomultiplier tube is looked at in a different way. Each tube may be thought of as having *x* and *y* coordinates in a Cartesian plane, with the center of the central photomultiplier tube being the origin. Each photomultiplier tube then can be thought of as contributing either a positive or a negative value for *x* and *y* positioning. The photomultiplier tubes closest to the event collect the greatest number of light photons, with lesser contributions from more remote tubes. The logic circuitry of the camera is used to compute the most likely coordinates of the event location in the crystal by adding together all of the *x* and *y* pulses from the 19 photomultiplier tubes (*see* Fig. 3-1).

Image Recording

If the Z pulse indicates that a primary photon has been absorbed, an unblanking signal is sent to the image-recording device. On original cameras, the recording system was an oscilloscope with a Polaroid camera or 35-mm camera attachment. The *x* and *y* positioning signals provided the deflection coordinates for the cathode ray tube (CRT) and the event was recorded on film as a single flash of light from the screen. In modern cameras, the signals from the photomultiplier tubes are individually digitized by analog-to-digital converters (ADCs). The Z signal and the position signals are determined by a computer. If the Z signal is within the energy acceptance window (e.g., 133–147 keV for Tc-99m), the pixel in the computer matrix corresponding to the estimated position of the event is incremented. A typical image is created by recording 100,000–1,000,000 individual events.

Characteristics of Modern Gamma Scintillation Cameras

The original commercial gamma cameras had 10- to 12-inch-diameter crystals with a thickness of 0.5 inch. These cameras were designed in an era when I-131 (364 keV) was the most important radionuclide. In the ensuing 25 years, crystal sizes and shapes have changed. Large field-of-view cameras with 30–50 cm rectangular fields of view have become the standard.

A series of changes in the original gamma camera design has been aimed at improving spatial resolution. The crystal thickness can vary in modern cameras from 0.25–1 inch. The 0.25-inch crystal thickness is more suited to studies with lower energy radionuclides, such as Tc-99m and thallium-201. For Tc-99m with a 140-keV principal photon energy, the loss in sensitivity between 0.5- and 0.25-inch thickness is only 6% (*see* Table 3-1), whereas the spatial resolution is improved by 20%. For Tl-201, there is virtually no loss of sensitivity with the same 20% improvement in spatial resolution. However, for studies using gallium (93, 185, 300, 394 keV), indium-111 (172, 247 keV), or I-131 (364 keV), a ⅜-inch thick crystal is most commonly used.

SPECT imaging of fluoride-18 rekindled interest in thicker crystals. The detection efficiency for 511-keV photons increases from ~12% for ⅜-inch NaI(Tl) crystals to ~18% for 0.5-inch crystals. Crystal thicknesses of up to 1 inch are used in some cases.

The number of photomultiplier tubes used in gamma cameras has increased. The first step was to reduce tube diameter from 3 to 2 inches, which permitted use of 37 photomultiplier tubes for a standard field-of-view camera. Large field-of-view cameras are available with 55, 61, 75, and even 91 tubes. Another advance in photomultiplier tubes is the hexagonal photocathode, which allows the tubes to cover the crystal completely without leaving gaps between them (*see* Fig. 3-13). Light pipes have been replaced with direct coupling of the photomultiplier tubes to the crystal. The collection of more light photons reduces the statistical uncertainty in the (*x, y*) event localization logic circuitry.

An area that has received major attention over the years is field uniformity. The basic problem is that each photomultiplier tube behaves slightly differently and may drift in its performance over time. Field uniformity was not a major problem before SPECT but is now critical to prevent artifacts in SPECT images.

In addition to slight differences in photomultiplier tube response, subtle differences occur in the crystal itself and in the efficiency of the optical coupling of the photomultiplier tubes with the crystal. The collection efficiency is also very dependent on whether the initial

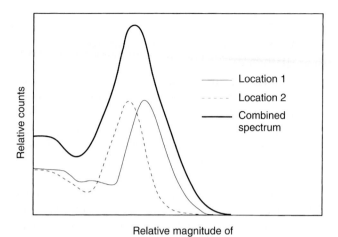

Figure 3-14 Slightly offset spectra from two different photomultiplier tubes in the gamma camera crystal and the combined spectrum. Especially in older gamma scintillation cameras, a wide energy acceptance window was necessary to encompass the variations in response across the crystal.

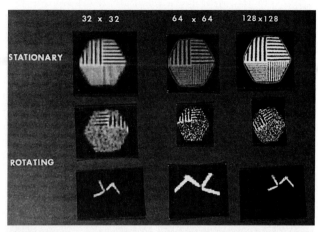

Figure 3-15 Four-quadrant bar phantom images obtained with the gamma camera stationary and during rotation. Note the degradation in bar phantom resolution in this early generation rotating SPECT system.

interaction occurred right above a photomultiplier tube or between tubes. For this reason, the energy spectrum that is collected from any one photomultiplier tube is different from all the other tubes (Fig. 3-14). The observed energy spectrum from the overall camera is made up of a sum of the slightly different spectra from each tube. This spectrum could be dramatically demonstrated in some cameras by setting an asymmetrical pulse height analyzer window over a photopeak to accentuate the differences in tube performance.

Although vendors have tried a number of approaches to match the performance characteristics of the photomultiplier tubes, problems persist. The current approach is to use computer correction of the response across the crystal. In effect, after the camera system is manufactured and tuned as well as possible, its actual performance relative to a known radioactive source energy and its imaging geometry are empirically mapped and correction factors are established for each small area of the detector.

The ZLC system introduced by Siemens a number of years ago is illustrative of attempts to correct for spatial variation in energy response and for small nonlinearities. The Z signals are corrected by empirically measuring a 128×128 energy response matrix. Each Z signal is then corrected by a factor, ΔZ, obtained for its respective pixel location in the matrix before the pulse reaches the pulse height analyzer. The corrected pulse $(Z + \Delta Z)$ is then analyzed. Each event is energy corrected on the fly during image acquisition.

For linearity correction, a rectilinear grid is imaged, and a $4k \times 4k$ lookup table of correction factors for spatial localization is created. Each event is positioned in the image based on ΔX and ΔY correction factors corresponding to the observed location of the event.

More recently, several strategies for automatic and active photomultiplier tube adjustment have been introduced. In one system, light-emitting diodes of known output are used to measure and fine-tune photomultiplier tube response as often as 10 times per second. This approach is advantageous for applications in which the camera head is rotating, because photomultiplier tube performance can be affected by changes in alignment to the earth's magnetic field (Fig. 3-15). Each gamma camera vendor has taken a different approach to the energy response and spatial localization problems. The unifying theme is increasing sophistication in making corrections event by event.

In the best contemporary cameras, the recording of each event is corrected separately for location and energy. This kind of event-by-event correction permits the use of asymmetrical windows. The advantage of an asymmetrical window offset to the high side of the photopeak is reduction in scattered photons accepted in the image. However, unless energy correction is performed properly, the response across the image will vary depending on photomultiplier tube response. Events in areas of lower output tubes will be underrepresented in the image, whereas events in areas with higher output tubes will be overrepresented (Fig. 3-16). Further advances from commercial vendors have led to automatic tuning systems and online adjustment systems for photomultiplier and overall system response.

The past 15 years has seen an explosion in the number and kinds of gamma cameras on the commercial market. Mobile cameras, whole body imaging systems, and cameras adapted to special nuclear cardiology applications are available, as are camera systems with multiple detector heads for SPECT and whole body imaging.

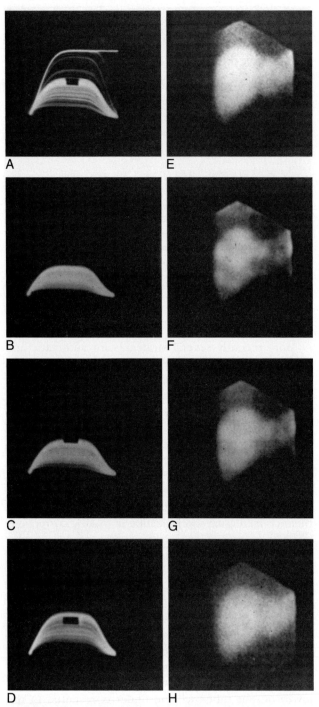

Figure 3-16 Effect of different photopeak window settings. All images are from the same patient. **A–D,** The energy spectrum from the patient. The location of the energy window is indicated by the black rectangle superimposed over the spectral lines. **E–H,** The resulting liver image. **E,** A symmetrical window centered at the proper photopeak. **F–G,** The energy window is offset to the high side. **H,** The window is offset to the low side. Note the loss of homogeneity in the liver in **F** and **G** with a geometric pattern of hot and cold areas owing to the location pattern of the photomultiplier tubes. Scatter is decreased, as indicated by the lower counts coming from the heart region, but the images are grossly misleading. In **H,** the image is degraded by excessive scatter and loss of spatial resolution. Note the blurring of the liver margin.

Gamma Camera Quality Control

Gamma scintillation cameras are complex devices with physical, mechanical, and electronic components. Malfunction or breakage of any of these components can be catastrophic to system performance and may not be recognized from a review of clinical images. For these reasons, a number of comprehensive and sophisticated procedures have been developed over the years to ensure adequate camera performance. The ones used most often in routine clinical practice are summarized in Box 3-1. In addition to these, the National Electrical Manufacturers Association (NEMA) has developed a comprehensive set of tests to measure camera performance.

Field Uniformity

One fundamental parameter that requires daily assessment is the uniformity of response of the gamma camera across its entire field of view (Fig. 3-17). A source of radioactivity of appropriate energy is used to test the camera response. Measurements made with the collimator in place are referred to as *extrinsic,* and those made without the collimator are referred to as *intrinsic.*

The specific method for assessing field uniformity varies. For example, a uniform disk or flood source in a phantom can be used to measure extrinsic field uniformity. With this approach, the radioactive source is placed at or on the surface of the gamma camera collimator. To measure intrinsic field uniformity, a point source of radioactivity is positioned at the center of the crystal at a distance from the uncollimated crystal face. The rule of thumb is that the source should be at a distance at least equal to five times the size of the field of view to acquire a uniform image. For example, if the camera has a 40-cm field of view, the point source should be placed at least 200 cm away. In the case of fixed dual-detector SPECT systems, it is impossible to get the source the necessary distance from the camera, and thus the acquired image has higher counts in the center than on the edges. In this case, a correction can be applied to correct for this geometric nonuniformity so that instrumentational nonuniformities can still be evaluated. Typically, 1000k–5000k counts are obtained to evaluate field uniformity for planar imaging.

For extrinsic field uniformity testing, most laboratories use either a phantom filled with a uniform solution of Tc-99m or a permanent disk source of uniformly distributed cobalt-57 (Co-57; $T_{1/2}$ 270 days, 122 keV). The standard practice is to obtain a flood image with each camera every day before it is used for clinical studies. In laboratories where obtaining the daily flood image with the collimator in place is more practical, obtaining an intrinsic flood image weekly is still useful, and vice versa for laboratories that routinely acquire flood images without the collimator in place.

Box 3-1 Gamma Camera Quality Control Summary

Parameter	Comment
DAILY	
Uniformity	Flood field; intrinsic (without collimator) or extrinsic (with collimator)
Window setting	Confirm energy window setting relative to photopeak for each radionuclide used with each patient
WEEKLY	
Spatial resolution	Requires a "resolution" phantom (parallel line equal spacing, four-quadrant bar, orthogonal hole) and standardized protocol
Linearity check	Qualitative assessment of bar pattern linearity
PERIODIC (BIANNUALLY OR WHEN A PROBLEM IS SUSPECTED)	
Collimator performance	High count flood with each collimator
Energy registration	For cameras with capability of imaging multiple energy windows simultaneously
Count rate performance and count rate linearity	More important in cameras with "count skimming" or "count addition" correction circuitry
Energy resolution	Easiest in cameras with built in multiple-channel analyzers
Sensitivity	Count rate performance per unit of activity

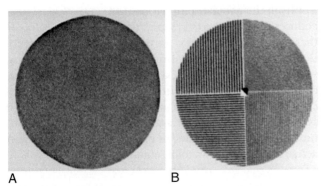

A   B

Figure 3-17   Flood source and four-quadrant bar phantom. Images of the flood source **(A)** and bar phantom **(B)** from a well-tuned gamma scintillation camera with the collimator off. The flood image shows slight mottling but no focal or localized areas of increased or decreased activity within the center of the field of view. The slightly increased activity along the rim is a common characteristic of gamma cameras seen on intrinsic flood images. The smallest bars are partially discernible on the bar phantom image. They have a spacing of 3 mm. The bar images show good linearity.

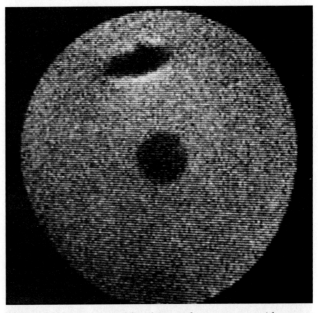

Figure 3-18   Abnormal flood. Image from a camera with a nonfunctioning central photomultiplier tube and a crystal defect.

The image obtained in the field uniformity examination should be carefully inspected. A well-tuned camera with proper photomultiplier tube and correction circuitry performance should provide a flood image with a highly uniform appearance. Some minor mottling with slightly increased intensity in regions corresponding to photomultiplier tubes is acceptable (Fig. 3-17). Photomultiplier tube drift or even the failure of a photomultiplier tube can be recognized as an area of decreased activity (Fig. 3-18). Cracked crystals are readily identified and even damage to a collimator can be detected. The soft lead in collimators is often protected by a covering but can still be subject to denting, causing bending and distortion of the septa.

Spatial Resolution and Linearity

Bar phantoms are routinely used to evaluate image resolution and linearity in the clinic setting. With modern gamma cameras, a weekly assessment is sufficient. The phantoms are constructed of parallel lead strips encased in a plastic holder. Resolution is defined by the ability to discriminate between two distinct points. For routine clinical gamma camera quality control, visual assessment is adequate. The subjective spatial resolution is expressed in terms of the smallest bar pattern visible on the image. In a properly functioning camera, all groups of bars in the bar phantom pattern should appear straight and parallel (*see* Fig. 3-17). Some distortion is typically seen at the edge of the field of view.

A four-quadrant bar phantom is most commonly used. In this phantom, the lead strips are thinner and spaced closer in sequential quadrants (*see* Fig. 3-17). The phantom is chosen so that the quadrant with the narrowest lead strips appears slightly blurred. The phantom is positioned on the collimator face with the center of the four-quadrant pattern corresponding to the center of the camera. A uniform Tc-99m flood source is then placed on the bar phantom. Four images are obtained at sequential 90-degree rotations between positions. Care must be taken not to position the bars on the collimator in such a way that an interference or *moiré pattern* occurs (Fig. 3-19).

An alternative is the parallel-line equal-spacing bar phantom. When this device is used, two images are necessary. Because signals from the photomultiplier tubes are processed through two essentially independent positioning circuits (*x* and *y*), degradations can occur in a selective direction. Another alternative is the orthogonal-hole test pattern (*see* Fig. 3-19). It is designed so that only a single image is required. Regardless of the phantom chosen, when trouble is suspected, the procedure should be repeated with and without the collimator.

The spatial resolution of gamma cameras is expressed quantitatively as the full width at half maximum (FWHM) of a line spread function. A line spread function is obtained by first imaging a narrow line source of radioactivity on the collimator (extrinsic) or crystal face (intrinsic), followed by determining a count profile or histogram perpendicularly across it. This histogram is called the *line spread function.* In an imaging system with perfect spatial resolution, the line spread function would have a single spike corresponding to the radioactive line source. In practice, a bell-shaped curve is seen.

FWHM is simply the distance encompassed by the curve halfway down from its peak. This measurement is the same as previously discussed for describing energy resolution. By analogy, a narrower peak indicates better spatial resolution and therewith the ability to resolve objects close to each other. In modern gamma cameras, intrinsic resolution (collimator off) approaches 3-mm FWHM or less. An estimate of FWHM can be made using the four-quadrant bar phantom by determining the smallest discernible bars and then multiplying the size of the bars by a factor of 1.7.

Clinical Use of the Gamma Scintillation Camera

Applying the gamma scintillation camera to clinical procedures requires the development of *imaging protocols* that define the diagnostic purpose, the radiopharmaceutical to be used, patient preparation, and the imaging sequence. These issues are discussed in the organ system chapters for the major scintigraphic studies. The protocols include selection of collimator, timing of image acquisition after radiopharmaceutical administration, time per image or number of counts to be recorded, and actual images or views to be obtained.

Window Setting

A quality control issue sometimes overlooked in the clinical application of gamma cameras is the setting of the energy window. The most common approach is to use a symmetrical window centered at the energy peak of the radionuclide label being used in the imaging procedure. For Tc-99m, the most common recommendation is to use a 20% window centered at 140 keV. The acceptance range for this window is 126–154 keV. In gamma cameras with energy correction circuitry, setting an asymmetrical window to reduce Compton scatter may be possible. Using a narrower window of 10–15% for higher resolution imaging may also be desirable. These approaches should be undertaken with caution for older gamma cameras because of the problem of nonuniform response across the crystal, which is discussed in some detail in a previous section.

The most conservative approach is to confirm the window setting for each radionuclide used during the course of a day and then to reconfirm the window

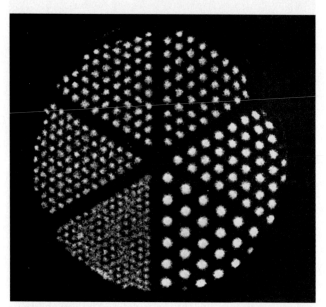

Figure 3-19 Moiré patterns. Note the abnormal pattern in the three triangles on the left in an image of a "hot spot" phantom. The distortion is especially marked in the lower left triangle.

setting before imaging each patient. Setting the energy window ("peaking in the camera," "setting the peak") should be done with a radioactive source in air and *not* by using radioactivity in the patient. The spectrum from the patient includes scatter that can shift the perceived location of the photopeak.

False positive and false negative interpretations may occur because of artifacts and loss of resolution, respectively, with incorrect window settings. Occasionally, the window is inadvertently left at the setting for a Co-57 flood source (122 keV). Figure 3-20 illustrates the degradation of image quality in a Tc-99m diphosphonate bone study resulting from this error.

Another practical problem of window setting occurs in cameras that image multiple photopeaks simultaneously. Care must be taken to ensure that the image data from the different photopeaks are correctly registered together on the clinical image. Figure 3-21 illustrates incorrect and correct multipeak registration for a Ga-67 flood image.

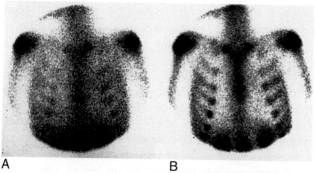

A   B

Figure 3-20 Incorrect photopeak setting. **A,** Image obtained with a 20% window set at 122 keV, the energy of the cobalt-57 flood source. The image quality is dramatically improved in **B,** which was obtained at the correct window setting for technetium-99m.

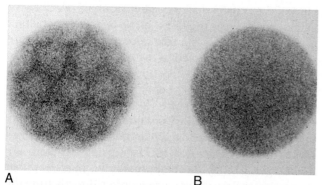

A   B

Figure 3-21 Spatial misregistration. Gallium-67 flood images obtained using multiple photopeaks. **A,** Artifacts in the flood image caused by spatial misregistration. **B,** The properly registered image shows good uniformity.

COMPUTERS IN NUCLEAR MEDICINE

Computers in nuclear medicine were first used clinically with the development of gated blood pool imaging in the mid-1970s. Subsequently, the computer has become a primary image acquisition and processing device and it is used for image management and formatting, in addition to its integral role for dynamic studies and SPECT. Currently, all state-of-the-art gamma cameras have computers as fundamental components of the system.

Creation of the Digital Image

The x and y pulses generated in the gamma scintillation camera logic circuitry define event location. In older cameras, these pulses are in analog form and must be converted to digital form for computer processing. To accomplish this, an analog-to-digital converter is interposed between the gamma camera and the computer. Some modern cameras convert the (x, y) signals to digital form within the camera's own electronic circuitry. The Z pulse is used in computer data acquisition to indicate that a particular event should be accepted for storage.

Two fundamentally different modes have been used to acquire and store digitized data: list (serial) mode and frame (histogram) mode. In the list mode approach, each pair of digitized (x, y) position signals is stored separately and sequentially in computer memory. The "list" is simply a line of data flowing into computer memory. If time information is desired, additional time markers are inserted into the list. Physiological signals such as the R wave on the electrocardiogram can also be recorded (Fig. 3-22).

The *list mode* approach offers great flexibility. For example, data from each cardiac cycle can be analyzed separately. If a particular beat was caused by an arrhythmia, the data from that beat can be excluded from the desired data from normal sinus beats. Alternatively, data from beats caused by particular types of arrhythmias can be analyzed separately. The major disadvantage of list mode is that it requires a large amount of computer memory to store the study data. It also requires additional time to process data into an image format after acquisition is complete.

In the alternative *histogram* or *frame mode* of data acquisition the digitized (x, y) pairs are used to locate the picture element to which they belong. The image may be thought of as a grid or matrix superimposed on the analog data (Fig. 3-23). The x and y numbers determine which matrix element encloses the location of the original event. At the end of data collection, rather than having discrete information on each event, each matrix location has a number corresponding to the total events accumulated throughout the imaging period.

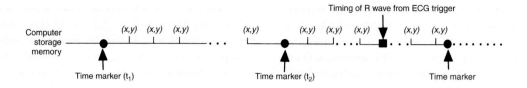

(x,y) = coordinates of each individual scintillation

Figure 3-22   List mode data acquisition.

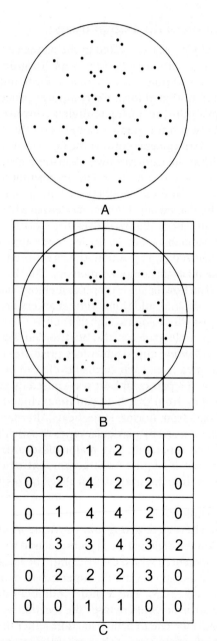

A

B

C

Figure 3-23   Digital image. Analog image (**A**) has 6 × 6 matrix superimposed (**B**). The number of events (dots) in each pixel is recorded to create the digital matrix (**C**).

Frame mode is much more sparing of computer memory. It has the further advantage that the data are immediately ready for display or analysis, without postprocessing or formatting. Physiological signals can still be used to control data collection as in multigated cardiac studies. However, once recorded, data from arrhythmic beats cannot be excluded. Dynamic studies can be acquired by using multiple frames as a function of time.

A larger matrix results in better potential spatial resolution but also requires longer time to achieve adequate counting statistics in each pixel. Most studies in current practice are obtained in a 128 × 128 matrix, although 64 × 64 and 218 × 218 matrixes are also used.

Data Analysis

Computer recording of image data greatly facilitates quantitative analysis. Specific types of analyses are discussed in the respective organ system chapters. A recurring requirement in data analysis is the definition of a "region of interest." These regions can be defined by the computer operator or through the use of automated region of interest definition programs. The latter are often used to define the area of the left ventricle of the heart in calculating ejection fractions.

The computer can make various calculations on the pixels in regions of interest. In most applications, the total count within the region is of greatest value. This kind of data analysis allows calculation of quantitative parameters such as the left ventricular ejection fraction or the percentage of the total glomerular filtration rate attributable to the left versus the right kidney.

Data Display and Formatting

Clinics with contemporary computer systems frequently use them to archive image data and to control image-formatting devices such as laser printers. There are advantages of using the computer for this purpose rather than using analog imaging or recording directly from the gamma camera cathode ray tube. Images may be windowed and centered to provide the optimum gray scale after the fact. Also, the same image data may be viewed with and without secondary image processing, including background subtraction or contrast enhancement. It is also possible to view correlative images for other modalities on the system. For example, a SPECT brain scan can be compared to an MR image acquired on the same patient. The computer is invaluable for looking at dynamic data. This capability is most important for viewing the beating heart in nuclear cardiology. It also has value in performing time lapse photography for other applications, such as localizing the site of bleeding in gastrointestinal bleeding detection studies or assessing biliary dynamics during hepatobiliary imaging studies.

SUGGESTED READING

Chandra R: *Nuclear medicine physics: the basics,* 6th ed. Baltimore, Williams & Wilkins, 2004.

Hendee WR: *Medical radiation physics,* 3rd ed. St. Louis, Mosby, 1992.

Hutton BF, Barnden LR, Fulton RR: Nuclear medicine computers: applications. In *Nuclear medicine in clinical diagnosis and treatment,* 3rd ed. Ell PJ, Gambhir SS, Eds. New York, Churchill Livingstone. 2004, pp 1793-1814.

Johns HE, Cunningham JR: *The physics of radiology,* 4th ed. Chicago, Thomas Books, 1983.

Powsner RA, Powsner ER: *Essentials of nuclear medicine physics,* Malden, MA, Blackwell Science, 1998.

Cherry SR, Sorenson JA, Phelps ME: *Physics in nuclear medicine,* 3rd ed. Philadelphia, WB Saunders, 2003.

Weber DA, Eckerman KF, Dillman LT, Ryman JC: *MIRD: radionuclide data and decay schemes.* New York, Society of Nuclear Medicine, 1989.

Single-Photon Emission Computed Tomography (SPECT) and Positron Emission Tomography (PET)

RADIONUCLIDE TOMOGRAPHY

Conventional or planar radionuclide imaging suffers a major limitation in loss of object contrast as a result of background radioactivity. In the conventional planar image, radioactivity underlying and overlying an object is superimposed on radioactivity coming from the object. The fundamental goal of tomographic imaging systems is a more accurate portrayal of the distribution of radioactivity in the patient, with improved definition of image detail. The Greek *tomo* means "to cut"; tomography may be thought of as a means of "cutting" the body into discrete image planes. Tomographic techniques have been developed for both single-photon and positron tomography.

Rectilinear scanners with focused collimators represent a crude type of tomography; the count rate sensitivity is greatest in the collimator focal plane, and therefore more weight is given to radioactivity arising in that plane than in planes superficial or deep to it. However, this is not "true" tomography because the blurred out-of-plane activity contributes to the image.

Restricted angle or longitudinal (frontal) tomography shares the phenomenon of the rectilinear scanner: inplane data are kept in focus, with blurring of out-of-plane data. Restricted angle or longitudinal tomography is analogous to conventional x-ray tomography, in which the relative positions of the film and x-ray source remain constant for the desired image plane but move relative to each other in the overlying and underlying planes, blurring the out-of-plane structures. A number of restricted angle systems were in vogue in the late 1970s and early 1980s, including seven-pinhole collimator systems, pseudorandom coded aperture collimator systems, and various rotating slant-hole collimator systems.

Rotating gamma camera tomographic systems offer the ability to perform true transaxial tomography. The most important characteristic is that only data arising in the image plane are used in the reconstruction or creation of the tomographic image. Rotational single-photon emission computed tomography (SPECT) shares this feature with x-ray computed tomography (CT) and positron emission tomography (PET). This is an important characteristic because it offers a higher image contrast than with tomographic systems, which merely blur the out-of-plane data.

SPECT

With use of conventional radiopharmaceuticals, SPECT allows true three-dimensional (3D) image acquisition and display. Reconstruction of cross-sectional slices has traditionally used filtered backprojection, the same methodology used for CT. However, newer systems offer iterative approaches to image reconstruction.

Instrumentation

The most common approach to rotational SPECT is to mount one or more gamma camera heads on a special rotating gantry. Original systems used a single head, but systems with two, three, and even four heads have been developed. Today, two-headed systems are the most common commercially available SPECT systems. In particular, two-headed systems that allow flexibility in orientation between the heads have become popular. For body imaging, the heads are typically arrayed parallel to each other; for cardiac applications, they are often placed at right angles (Fig. 4-1)

Multiple heads are desirable because they allow more data to be collected in a given period. Rotational SPECT is "photon poor" compared with x-ray CT. Therefore, it is desirable to collect as many counts as possible and complete imaging within a reasonable time because of radiopharmaceutical pharmacokinetics and limits of the patient's ability to remain still. Thus, a study of Tl-201 distribution in the heart should be accomplished before significant redistribution occurs.

In addition to the special gantry that permits camera head rotation, modifications have been necessary for rotational SPECT. Photomultiplier tube performance can be affected by gravitational and magnetic fields. These change depending on rotational angle, and subtle alterations in photomultiplier tube energy response can degrade images. Magnetic shielding of photomultiplier tubes reduces this problem.

Rotational SPECT has highlighted the need to improve every aspect of gamma camera system performance. Flood field nonuniformities are translated as major artifacts in tomographic images because they distort the data obtained from each view or projection. Desirable characteristics for SPECT are an intrinsic spatial resolution (full width at half maximum [FWHM]) of 3 mm, linearity distortion of 1 mm or less, uncorrected field uniformity within 3%, and corrected field uniformity within 1%.

All contemporary rotational SPECT systems have online uniformity and energy correction. Nonlinearities in photomultiplier tube energy response degrade both gamma camera energy resolution and spatial resolution. Degraded energy resolution is devastating because 35% or more of recorded events can represent Compton-scattered photons. Poor energy resolution degrades the ability to reject scattered photons on the basis of pulse height analysis. It also degrades spatial resolution through decreased accuracy of determining x and y event localization coordinates.

Image Acquisition

Box 4-1 summarizes factors that must be considered in performing rotational SPECT. In addition to standard gamma camera quality control, confirmation is needed that the axis of rotation corresponds to the center of the matrix in the computer. Incorrect alignment results in a blurring of the image or poorer resolution.

Collimator Selection

Collimator selection is generally limited to those supplied by the system vendor. As discussed previously, for

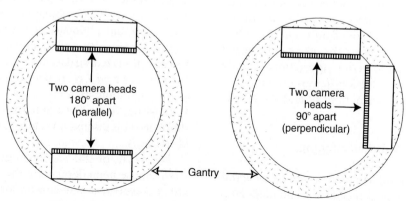

Figure 4-1   Two configurations for dual-headed SPECT systems.

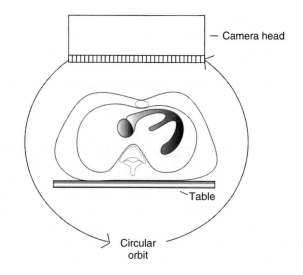

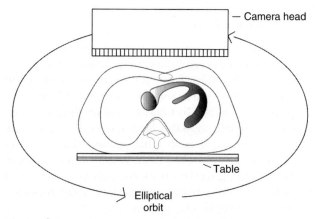

Figure 4-2   Circular orbit *(top)* and elliptical orbit *(bottom)*.

a given septal thickness and hole diameter, collimators with longer channels have higher resolution and lower sensitivity. Even though SPECT is relatively photon poor, collimator selection should favor higher resolution whenever possible. This means selecting the high-resolution collimator over a high-sensitivity or general purpose collimator for studies using Tc-99m. The multiheaded systems permit the operator to trade the improved count rate sensitivity for improved resolution by using ultra-high-resolution collimators.

Special collimator options are available for imaging the brain. Fan-beam and cone-beam collimators permit more of the camera crystal to be used for radiation detection. The fan- and cone-beam collimators are similar in geometry to converging collimators. They cause magnification of the object being imaged when it is placed proximal to the focal point of the respective collimators. The resulting geometric distortion of the image data must be taken into account during image reconstruction.

Orbit

The orbit selected depends on the organ of interest and whether the system being used offers a noncircular orbit capability. The ideal orbit keeps the gamma head as close to the organ of interest as possible because, for parallel-hole collimators, the resolution is best at the face of the collimator. Most imaging is still done using circular orbits but contemporary systems permit the use of customized noncircular orbits, which better approximate body contours (Fig. 4-2). Orbit selection attempts to minimize the distance between the camera head and the object being imaged.

Arc of Acquisition, Angular Sampling, and Matrix Size

The choice of angular sampling interval and arc of acquisition depend on the clinical application and collimator selection. For body imaging applications, the arc of acquisition is typically a full 360 degrees. For studies with Tc-99m-labeled agents it is often feasible to use a high-resolution collimator and to acquire data in a 128 × 128 matrix with an angular increment of 3 degrees or a total of 120 angular projections. If these studies are performed with a general purpose or lower resolution collimator, a 64 × 64 matrix is typically selected with an angular sampling increment of 6 degrees for a total of 60 angular projections or 4 degrees for a total of 90 angular projections. These combinations of sampling increment, matrix size, and collimator selection "balance" the resolution of the respective parameters. For imaging of tumors and infections with gallium-67 (Ga-67) or indium-111 (In-111) tracers, a 64 × 64 matrix is selected with a 6-degree angular sampling increment. (Note that in some SPECT systems, 64, 96, or 128 angular projections are used. For simplicity, this discussion refers to 60, 90, and 120 projections only.)

The merits of 180- vs. 360-degree rotation for cardiac studies have been debated in the literature. A minimum arc of 180 degrees is necessary for true transaxial tomography. Proponents of the 180-degree approach argue that

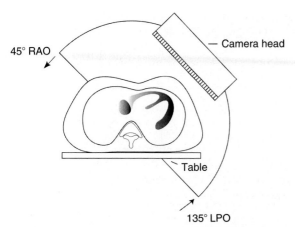

Figure 4-3   The 180-degree arc frequently used for cardiac imaging.

because the heart is close to the anterior chest wall, the best data are available by imaging in a 180-degree arc typically spanning 135-degree left posterior oblique to 45-degree right anterior oblique (Fig. 4-3). The use of 180-degree arcs for cardiac SPECT is widely accepted in clinical practice, particularly for cardiac imaging when attenuation correction is not used.

Another question is whether to use continuous data acquisition or "step-and-shoot" acquisition. Continuous acquisition has the advantage of not wasting time during movement of the camera head from one angular sampling position to the next. However, the data are blurred by the motion artifact of the moving camera head. The resulting tradeoff between sensitivity and resolution favor step-and-shoot acquisition for most clinical applications. Exceptions are applications with rapidly changing tracer distribution and when determination of overall tracer concentration is more important than spatial resolution.

Imaging Time

Most clinical protocols require a total imaging time of 20–40 minutes. Correspondingly, the time per projection is usually 15–30 seconds, but as much as 40–60 seconds may be needed for relatively photon-poor studies with Ga-67 and In-111.

Patient Factors

A major limitation in data acquisition time is the ability of the patient to remain still throughout the imaging procedure. Within accepted limits for dosimetry and radiation exposure, a larger administered dosage allows for more available counts. Although clinically accepted limits for administered radioactivity should never be exceeded, the radiation risk vs. benefit must take into account the likelihood of obtaining a diagnostic quality image. The goal of obtaining higher counting statistics is meaningless if the patient moves, causing data between the different angular sampling views to be misregistered. Currently available

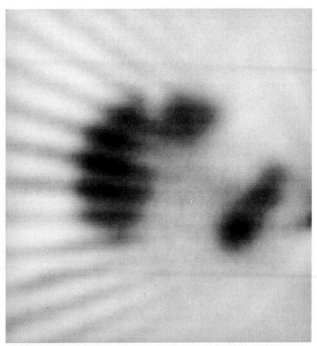

Figure 4-4   SPECT artifact caused by injection site activity. Degraded SPECT image of the liver and spleen caused by including activity at the injection site in the imaging field of view. The starburst artifact is due to backprojection of the hot spot activity across the image. In this case, the degree of activity in the injection site could not be accommodated in the reconstruction algorithm.

motion correction programs correct the data in one dimension (vertical motion) but not three dimensions.

Patient compliance is improved by taking time during setup to position the patient comfortably. For scans of the head, the patient's arms can be in a natural position at the sides. For rotational SPECT studies of the heart, thorax, abdomen, or pelvis, the arms are typically raised out of the field of view so that they do not interfere with the path of photons toward the detector. In all applications, it is important to keep the injection site out of the field of view to prevent artifacts resulting from residual or infiltrated activity (Fig. 4-4).

Image Reconstruction

Each commercially available SPECT system takes a somewhat different and proprietary approach to the image reconstruction process. Filtered backprojection has been the standard method for SPECT reconstruction. However, newer systems now offer iterative approaches for reconstruction. Reconstruction is accomplished either in the spatial domain or in the frequency domain after Fourier transformation of the raw data. All approaches to reconstruction use mathematical filters that alter the raw data to facilitate tomographic image creation. Although reconstruction of SPECT images is highly analytical, it is also an art. Different observers prefer differ-

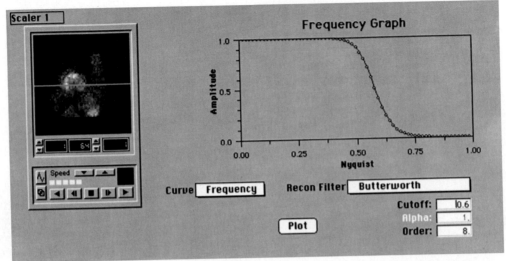

Figure 4-5   Frequency graph of image profile data. The graph corresponds to the cursor in the image on the left after Fourier transformation. The frequencies are scaled as a fraction of Nyquist. Their frequencies could also be scaled in terms of cycles per pixel or cycles per centimeter. Nyquist 1.00 corresponds to 0.5 cycle/pixel.

ent characteristics in the final images that are determined by operator-adjustable parameters, including filtering.

Before a discussion of the image reconstruction process, the following terms should be defined.

Spatial Domain

The *spatial domain* is the one in which we live. Its terminology is that of counts per pixel, and measurements of pixel size are in millimeters or centimeters.

Fourier Transformation and Frequency Domain

The French mathematician Fourier demonstrated that any continuous function, such as projection profiles, in the spatial domain can be approximated within an arbitrarily determined value by the sum of a series of trigonometric functions of varying frequencies and amplitudes. This process is known as *Fourier transformation*. After Fourier transformation, the data are said to reside in the *frequency domain*, reflecting the periodicity of trigonometric functions. Figure 4-5 is a frequency graph of image data after Fourier transformation. One *cycle* of a periodic function is the interval from peak to peak. High-frequency phenomena have short cycles and vary rapidly, and low-frequency phenomena have longer cycles. The distance between maximum and minimum values in a periodic function is termed the *amplitude* (Fig. 4-6).

One way to consider the Fourier transform is that it is a plot of the amplitude as a function of frequency of the trigonomic functions (sines and cosines). When added, these functions yield the spatial domain representation of interest. In the frequency domain, low frequencies yield the overall shape of the object and high frequencies yield the sharp corners and fine detail associated with the object.

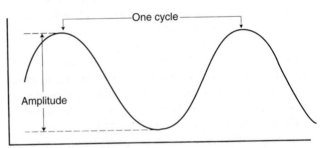

Figure 4-6   A periodic function. One cycle is the distance from peak to peak. Amplitude is the distance from peak to trough.

The advantage of working with image data in the frequency domain is the relative simplicity of the mathematical manipulations once the data have been transformed. Less computing power and computational time are required than to perform reconstructions on the raw data in the spatial domain. As computing power is becoming less expensive, this relative advantage is fading.

Angular Projection (View)

The term *angular projection* (or *view*) refers to the standard planar images obtained at each angle of SPECT acquisition. The SPECT raw data set typically has 60–120 angular projections, corresponding to angular increments between 6 degrees and 3 degrees, respectively. Figure 4-7 illustrates the detector in two sampling positions.

Projection Profile (Slice Profile)

The angular projections exist in the computer as either 64×64 or 128×128 matrices. A *projection profile*, also referred to as a *slice profile*, represents the data in one row of the matrix. The raw data for a given tomographic slice come from all the projection profiles corresponding

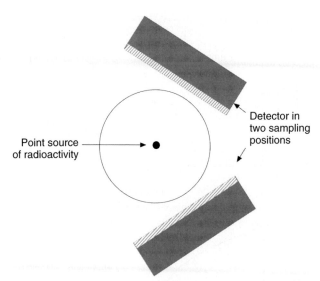

Figure 4-7   Acquisition positions. Point source of radioactivity with the detector illustrated in two sampling positions. Typically 60–120 sampling positions are used for SPECT.

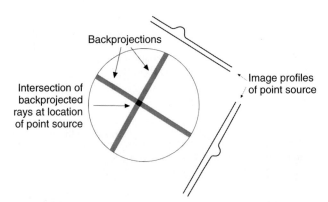

Figure 4-8   Backprojection for two rays obtained at different sampling angles. The respective counts for the rays are projected for each pixel along their paths. Note the summation at the point of intersection.

to that slice in the angular projection views. Thus, a study with 60 angular projections yields 60 projection profiles as the input data for reconstruction of each tomographic image (Fig. 4-8).

Ray Sum
The value of each pixel in a projection profile is called the *ray sum*. It is equal to the total activity recorded from the corresponding ray perpendicular to the camera face in the plane of interest.

Nyquist Frequency
The *Nyquist frequency* is the highest frequency that can be resolved in the image, based on the resolution characteristics of the imaging system and the parameters selected for data acquisition. For SPECT, the Nyquist frequency is equal to 0.5 cycle/pixel (1 Nyquist = 0.5 cycle/pixel). The Nyquist frequency can also be expressed in cycles per centimeter. Thus, for an acquisition matrix with 6 mm pixels, the Nyquist frequency would equal approximately 0.8 cycle/cm (0.5 cycle/pixel = 0.5 cycle/0.6 cm = 0.8 cycle/cm). The Nyquist frequency is an important consideration in the design and selection of filters used in the tomographic reconstruction process.

Backprojection
The concept of backprojection is fundamental to the reconstruction of tomographic images from the raw data. *Backprojection* takes the line data from the projection profiles and projects it back into a two-dimensional (tomographic) image. In simple backprojection in the spatial domain, the count values or ray sums in each pixel of the projection profiles corresponding to a given tomographic slice are first redistributed equally along the corresponding rays (*see* Fig. 4-8). The distribution is equalized along the ray because there is no way of telling from what depth the counts originated. These recorded values for each ray from all sampling angles are added together at their intersections in the tomographic image plane. That is, at each pixel in the tomographic image plane, rays from all of the angular projections intersect, and the count value given to the pixel is the sum of the values assigned to all the rays intersecting at that point (*see* Fig. 4-8). *Hot spots* are associated with high count values in the backprojected rays intersecting at their corresponding location. *Cold spots* do not contribute to counts in the individual ray projections and the cumulative value of the corresponding summation is less.

If one performs only simple backprojection, satisfactory tomographic images are not obtained. Reconstructing a point source results in a "star" artifact with exaggerated borders of the point source itself and starburst ray artifacts emanating from it (Fig. 4-9). In the frequency domain, in which reconstruction is performed, a mathematical (ramp) function is applied to the projection data that allows for tomographic reconstruction.

Filters
To solve the problem of the star artifact that arises from simple backprojection and to address issues of background and noise, image data are "filtered." The filters are mathematical functions designed for enhancement of desired characteristics in the image. These include elimination of the star artifact, background subtraction, edge enhancement, and suppression of statistical noise by selectively emphasizing certain frequency components of the image. A good analogy is the audio graphic equalizer that allows one to selectively enhance or minimize certain frequency components in order to improve the quality of the audio signal. Spatial filters can work in much

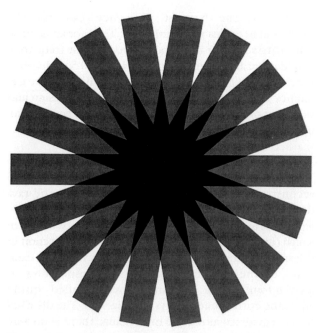

Figure 4-9   Star artifact resulting from simple backprojection. The star results from the multiple summations in the areas of intersection of the backprojected rays.

the same way, allowing the user to improve the image quality by enhancing and minimizing certain frequencies.

Low-pass filters selectively let through low frequencies and filter out high frequencies in the data; the opposite applies for *high-pass filters*. Background activity, including the star artifact, resides in the low-frequency portion of the spectrum. Statistical noise exists at all frequencies but becomes dominant at higher frequencies. Thus, using a high-pass filter will improve the fine detail of the image but may also lead to more image noise.

In diagrams of filter functions in the frequency domain, the amplitude is plotted on the *y*-axis and the frequency is plotted on the *x*-axis (Fig. 4-10). The frequencies and amplitudes under the filter function are "passed" by the filter. Since Fourier series are by definition infinite, a *cutoff frequency* is also defined for practical purposes and is typically equal to the Nyquist frequency. This makes sense because frequencies higher than the Nyquist frequency cannot contribute additional information to the image. Restricting the filter function to a cutoff frequency simplifies the calculations.

As the name implies, the *ramp filter* has the shape of a straight line extending up from the origin when graphed in frequency space (*see* Fig. 4-10). By inspecting the area under the curve, one can see that ramp filters are high-pass filters. Ramp filters are applied in filtered backprojection reconstruction algorithms to suppress the star artifact and low-frequency noise. They also eliminate low frequencies from the signal.

The ramp filter takes care of the star artifact and low-frequency background, but other filters are used to sup-

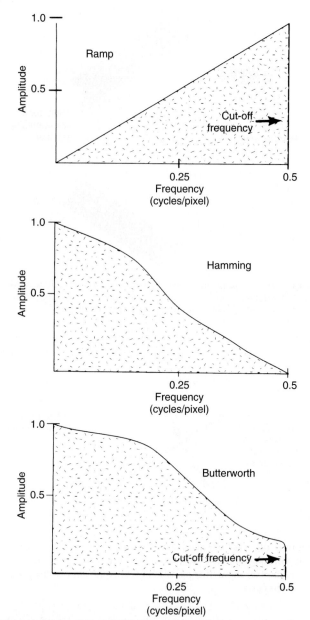

Figure 4-10   Ramp, Hamming, and Butterworth filters. The ramp filter is a "high-pass" filter designed to reduce background activity and the star artifact. Hamming and Butterworth filters are "low-pass" filters designed to reduce high-frequency noise.

press high-frequency noise. Many of these filters have been named after their inventors, and such names as Butterworth, Hamming, Hanning, and Hann are frequently seen in the literature (*see* Fig. 4-10). These low-pass filters eliminate higher frequency noise components. Too little filtering of high-frequency noise results in images with excessively grainy texture. Too much filtration of high-frequency data results in oversmoothing of images with loss of edge definition (Fig. 4-11). Areas where radioactivity concentrations change rapidly, such as the borders of organs, are represented in the high-frequency data, and oversmoothing blurs borders.

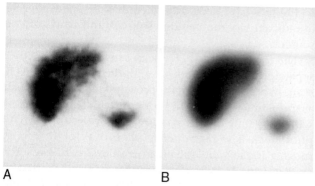

Figure 4-11   Effects of different filters on the appearance of SPECT liver and spleen images. **A,** The filter has resulted in excessive noise texture in the image. **B,** The filter has oversmoothed the image, with loss of detail.

The *Butterworth filter* is commonly used because it both smoothes noise and preserves edges. It is particularly flexible because it allows the operator to select two defining parameters, the cut-off frequency and the order. The *cutoff frequency* is sometimes called the power of the filter and, as described previously, is the maximum frequency that a filter will pass. For the Butterworth filter, the *order* is a parameter that controls the shape or slope of the filter.

Reconstruction in the Frequency Domain

With the foregoing concepts in hand, it is possible to describe the entire reconstruction process as it applies to filtered backprojection in frequency space or the frequency domain (Fig. 4-12). First, the individual projection profiles undergo Fourier transformation into frequency

space. A ramp filter is applied to the transformed profiles. Then smoothing and edge enhancement/preservation filters are applied. The filtered profiles are then summed from all projection angles akin to backprojection. Finally, an inverse Fourier transform is applied to the data to create the reconstructed image in the spatial domain. Alternatively, the inverse Fourier transformation can be performed after filtration and the back-projection accomplished in the spatial domain.

Other Reconstruction Techniques

With the availability of increasing computer power, iterative methods are increasingly used for the reconstruction of SPECT and other tomographic images. In the iterative approach, an initial set of tomograms is reconstructed. This 3D data set is then used to create a new set of reprojection images. If the reconstruction process were perfect, the reprojection images would be identical to the initial projection images. Because this is not the case, the difference between the original projection and the reprojection images based on tomographic reconstruction is used as input for another iteration of reconstruction. This process can go on as long as is practical or until there is no further convergence between the reprojection views based on the tomographic data and the initial projection images.

Each iteration takes about as long as one implementation of filtered backprojection. Because early algorithms required tens if not hundreds of iterations to achieve an acceptable image, these were considered too slow for routine clinical use. However, with newer, more efficient

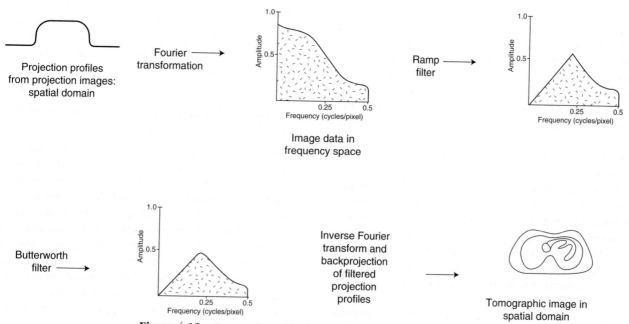

Figure 4-12   Steps in filtered backprojection reconstruction for SPECT.

algorithms and more powerful, faster computers, iterative reconstruction can now be performed in a reasonable amount of time for routine clinical use.

Ordered subset expectation maximization (OSEM) is a commonly used form of iterative reconstruction that speeds the process using limited subsets of data. Iterative reconstruction techniques offer the flexibility to include corrections for system performance (e.g., scatter correction and resolution degradations) and are finding use in various approaches to attenuation correction.

Attenuation Correction

A special problem of SPECT imaging is the attenuation of radioactivity in tissue. Photons emitted from deeper within the subject are more likely to be absorbed in the tissue than those emitted from the periphery. Therefore, the signals from these tissues are "attenuated." To obtain an image where the signal is not depth dependent, one must therefore perform an attenuation correction. Evidence is increasing that certain studies, such as myocardial perfusion imaging, benefit from attenuation correction. There are two fundamentally different approaches to the problem. Both are designed to create an image attenuation correction matrix, where the value of each pixel represents the correction factor that should be applied to the corresponding data in the reconstructed image.

For solid organs such as the liver, in which an assumption of near uniform attenuation can be made, an analytical or mathematical approach such as the Chang algorithm can be used. After the object is initially reconstructed, an outline of the body part is made on the computer for each tomographic slice. From this outline, the depth and therefore the appropriate correction factor for each pixel location can be computed.

The theoretical attenuation coefficient for Tc-99m in soft tissue is 0.15 per centimeter. (This applies only to "good" geometry, that is, a point source with no scatter into the ray. The observed value for Tc-99m in the abdomen is 0.12 per centimeter and in the brain is 0.13 per centimeter.) Thus, at a depth of 7 cm in a liver SPECT study, almost 60% of the corresponding activity is attenuated. The observed count value would have to be multiplied by a factor of 2.5 ($0.4 \times 2.5 = 1$) to correct for attenuation.

The major limitation of the analytical approach occurs when multiple types of tissue, each with a different attenuation coefficient, are in the field of view. Cardiac imaging is the most important example. The soft tissues of the heart and thorax are surrounded by the air-containing lungs and the bony structures of the thorax. To correct for nonuniform attenuation, a transmission scanning approach is used for attenuation correction. In essence, a CT scan of the thorax is obtained using a radionuclide source rather than an x-ray tube. Innumerable specific techniques have been described that use sheet sources of radioactivity, moving line sources, and arrays of line sources.

The transmission SPECT scan can be obtained either separately or simultaneously with the diagnostic SPECT scan. In the simultaneous approach, a radionuclide such as gadolinium-153 (Gd-153) or cobalt-57 (Co-57) is used with a separate energy window set for the appropriate photopeak. The high-energy photopeak of Gd-153 is roughly 100 keV and the energy of Co-57 is 122 keV. For studies using Tc-99m, correction for crosstalk caused by downscatter from the 140-keV photons is done first, and then the radionuclide transmission CT image is reconstructed using the kinds of SPECT reconstruction techniques described previously. This image is then normalized and scaled for the difference between the energy of the transmission source and the 140-keV photon energy of Tc-99m. The resulting image is an attenuation map of the thorax that can be applied pixel by pixel to correct for the effects of attenuation.

It is hoped that this approach will address two lingering problems with cardiac SPECT. For men, scans often show decreased activity in the inferior wall, possibly resulting from attenuation by overlapping organs beneath the diaphragm. For women, overlying breast tissue can significantly distort SPECT data by differential attenuation. Both of these can lead to loss of signal from certain portions of the myocardium. Appropriately applied attenuation correction can correct for this and lead to a more accurate diagnosis.

Another approach to nonuniform attenuation correction is the use of hybrid SPECT-CT imaging systems. In these systems, the SPECT camera is interfaced with a CT scanner. The image from the CT scans can thereby be used as the transmission image used for attenuation correction. The CT scan can also be used for anatomical correlation of the functional SPECT data. Several of the SPECT camera manufacturers have recently introduced such hybrid devices.

Image Reformatting: Transaxial, Sagittal, Coronal, and Oblique Views

A particular advantage of gamma camera rotational SPECT is that a volume of image data is collected at one time. This permits the acquisition of multiple tomographic slices simultaneously and the registration of the data between planes. Interslice filtering is also used to reduce artifacts in reformatted data. In addition to the standard transaxial images, other image planes that have special relevance to the organ of interest can be reconstructed. For example, sagittal and coronal images can be directly generated from the transaxial images.

The resorting or reformatting approach is particularly valuable in cardiac imaging (Fig. 4-13). The orientation

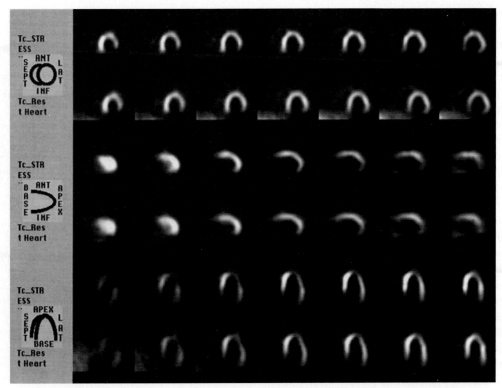

Figure 4-13 Cardiac SPECT images reformat data into multiple planes. The top two rows are short-axis views obtained perpendicular to the long axis of the left ventricle. The middle two rows are horizontal long-axis images, and the bottom two rows are vertical long-axis images. The patient has a large fixed perfusion defect involving the inferior wall of the left ventricle. The ability to reformat the data allows more precise and accurate localization of abnormalities.

of the heart varies among patients. The heart usually has a horizontal orientation in shorter subjects and a more vertical orientation in taller ones. Image planes both perpendicular and parallel to the long axis of the heart would be more useful. This is readily accomplished with a volume data set. The computer operator defines the geometry of the long axis of the heart. The computer is programmed to resort the data to create cardiac long-axis and short-axis planes oblique to the transaxial slices. The optimum angulation is highly variable among patients, reflecting the differing orientation of the heart.

A useful strategy is to reproject the tomographic data as a sequence of planar images having the same fields of view as the original angled sampling images. Viewing the reconstructed projection images in cinematic mode gives an excellent 3D display of the data. An additional advantage of using the reconstructed data is that overlying structures can be removed before the data are reprojected and selected features in the data can be emphasized. For example, in Tc-99m pyrophosphate imaging of the heart, the ribs can be subtracted from the 3D data set before the data are reprojected. The ribs no longer obscure the cardiac activity. Another advantage of using reprojection rather than tomographic images is that this technique provides a better overall orientation of the heart in the chest.

A *maximum intensity projection scan* (MIPS) can be created by reprojecting the hottest point along each particular ray for any given projection. These MIPS images emphasize areas of abnormally increased accumulation while providing a better overall orientation of the abnormality to the skeleton than individual tomographic slices. In some cases, the MIPS images are distance weighted to make activity that is further from the viewer appear less intense, thereby enhancing the 3D effect. Looking at individual transaxial tomograms can be confusing without knowing a lesion's location relative to surrounding structures.

Quality Assurance

The projection data from all SPECT scans should be inspected before image reconstruction. Excessive patient motion degrades the quality of SPECT scans because of misregistration of data in the different angular projections. Patient motion can be assessed in a number of ways. When the angular unprocessed projections are viewed in a cinematic closed loop display, excessive patient motion is readily detected as a flicker or discontinuity in the display. Some laboratories use radioactive marker sources placed on the patient to assess motion.

Another approach is to view a sinogram of a slice. Sinograms are constructed by placing the projection profiles for a given tomographic slice in a stack. The borders of the sinogram should be smooth and interslice changes in intensity should be small; any discontinuity indicates motion of the patient (Figs. 4-14 and 4-15). Only up-and-down motion can be corrected.

Rotational SPECT requires maximum performance from the gamma camera. All standard quality control procedures are observed, as well as several additional points (Box 4-2). The alignment of the detector, gantry, and imaging table is critical. In transaxial rotation, the basic assumption is that the face of the collimator is truly parallel to the axis of rotation. If it is off-axis, the tilted field of view of the collimator will result in misregistered data. Similarly for multihead cameras, the detector heads must be aligned with each other for correct registration of data. Another fundamental assumption is that the center of rotation corresponds to the center of the image matrix in the computer. If the center of rotation is offset, it manifests as degradation in resolution.

The gamma camera–computer interface is particularly important in rotational SPECT. The pixel size must be carefully calibrated. Attenuation correction depends on depth estimates, and a change in pixel size will change distance and therefore attenuation correction factors. Pixel size is adjusted by the setting of the analog-to-digital converters and should be checked in both

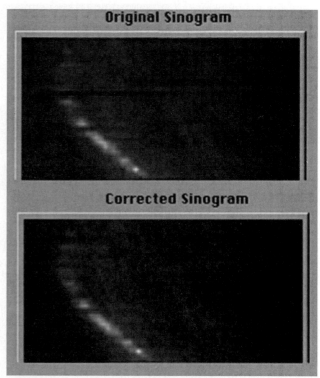

Figure 4-15 Sinogram illustrating multiple gaps in the sequential profile data. Compare these discontinuities with the regular progression of data in Figure 4-14. The discontinuities indicate unwanted motion of the object from one sampling position to the next.

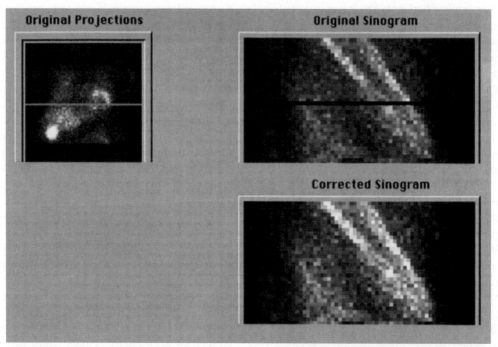

Figure 4-14 Sinogram from a myocardial perfusion study. The sinogram corresponds to the level of the cursor in the image on the left. Note the regular progression in the data across the projection profiles, indicating stability and lack of unwanted movement of the heart from one projection view to the next.

the x and y dimensions. Pixel width should be identical in the x and y directions. The y-axis determines slice thickness, and a difference in x and y pixel dimensions will create problems in reformatting image data into oblique planes. A shift in the performance of the analog-to-digital converters can result in movement of the center of rotation.

Field uniformity corrections are critical in SPECT imaging. Detector nonuniformity results in *bull's-eye* or *ring artifacts*. The usual count flood image of 1 million to 5 million obtained for planar imaging is inadequate for uniformity correction in SPECT imaging. For large field-of-view cameras and a 64×64 matrix, 30 million counts are acquired (roughly 10,000 counts per pixel) in the image to achieve the desired relative standard deviation of 1%. For a 128×128 matrix, four times this amount or 120 million counts must be acquired to achieve the same level of statistical precision.

Acquiring this number of counts requires a significant amount of time. The temptation to use very large amounts of radioactivity should be avoided because high count rates can also result in degraded performance of gamma camera electronics and in the recording of spurious coincidence events. Conservatively, the correction floods should be obtained at 20,000 counts per second, or less. The radioactivity in the flood itself must have a uniformity within 1%. Water-filled sources are subject to problems of incomplete mixing and introduction of air bubbles, as well as bulging of the container. For these reasons, Co-57 sheet sources are more convenient and more reliable than water-filled sources.

PET

PET is a form of tomography made possible by the unique fate of positrons. When positrons undergo annihilation by combining with negatively charged electrons, two 511-keV gamma rays are given off in opposite directions 180 degrees apart. In contrast to SPECT imaging, which detects single events, in PET imaging two detector elements on opposite sides of the subject are used to detect paired annihilation photons. If the photons are detected at the same time (or "in coincidence"), the event is assumed to have occurred along the line connecting the two detectors involved. Thus, the direction of the photons can be determined without the use of absorptive collimation.

Coincidence detection leads to at least a 100-fold increase in the sensitivity of PET relative to conventional nuclear medicine imaging and explains the higher quality of images as compared to SPECT. The counts occurring between a single pair of detectors can be considered a ray sum just as in SPECT, and thereby projections can be generated that can be reconstructed just as in SPECT. Both filtered backprojection and iterative approaches such as OSEM can be used to reconstruct the data (Fig. 4-16).

Instrumentation

Instrumentation for PET has undergone several generations of development. Early systems had a single ring

Box 4-2	Quality Assurance in Single-Photon Emission Computed Tomography

Parameter	Comment
Center of rotation	Should match center of image matrix in the computer; look for horizontal shift on x-axis
Pixel size	X and y dimensions should be equal; any change in pixel size requires recalibration of attenuation correction factors
Uniformity	Counts of 3 million for routine intrinsic and extrinsic uniformity checks; 30 million for input for uniformity correction
Spatial resolution and linearity	Weekly per usual gamma camera quality control
Detector head alignment	Camera face parallel to axis of rotation
Head matching	Alignment of multiple heads for correct event localization

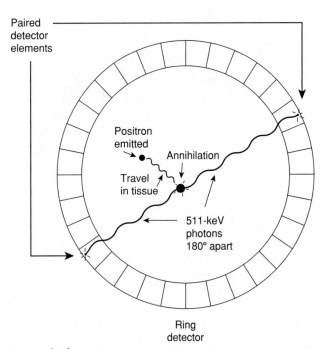

Figure 4-16 PET ring detector. After emission, positrons travel a short distance in tissue before the annihilation event. The 511-keV protons are given off 180 degrees apart.

with multiple detectors and generated a single tomographic section at a time. Now, PET typically consists of many rings of multiple detectors. Each detector in the ring is typically paired with multiple other detectors on the opposite side of the detector ring. These detectors, or the arc of detectors, are selected to encompass the field of view of the object or organ being imaged (Fig. 4-17).

Multiple-ring systems were rapidly developed, allowing a volume to be imaged simultaneously. Early systems with three to eight rings of detectors typically had septa inserted between the tomographic planes to shield the detectors from crosstalk from activity arising outside of the plane of interest. These multiple-ring systems with septa inserted between the tomographic planes are often referred to as *two-dimensional systems*.

The technical development of PET instrumentation has now reached the point where systems have as many as 32 rings of detectors with the capability of creating a simultaneous tomographic section for each ring and an additional section between each pair of rings, for a total of 63 simultaneously acquired tomographic images.

Contemporary systems have retractable septa between the planes and are referred to as *3D systems*. This design greatly increases system sensitivity. However, with larger patients, scatter and the presence of random coincidences can limit the quality of the 3D PET images. The concept of pairing each detector with multiple detectors on the opposite side of the ring has been retained with these systems and extended to pairings between different rings.

Gantry Size

Similar to the history of x-ray, CT, and magnetic resonance imaging, the first PET scanners were designed for head imaging. The early PET systems had a typical diameter of 60 cm. Current systems are suitable for head and body imaging, with a typical diameter of 100 cm.

Detector Materials

The density and effective atomic number (Z) for NaI(Tl) crystals are not ideal for "stopping" or detecting the 511-keV gamma rays used in PET imaging. Bismuth germinate oxide (BGO) is approximately twice as dense with an effective Z of 74, compared with an effective Z of 50 for NaI(Tl). BGO detectors have been used extensively in PET imaging applications for this reason. Other detector materials that have found application include cesium fluoride and barium fluoride. These have much faster resolution than BGO but are not as dense (Table 4-1).

New detector materials, such as lutetium oxyorthosilicate (LSO) and gadolinium oxyorthosilicate (GSO), are currently in use in several state-of-the-art PET scanners. They combine the high density of BGO with far better time resolution and superior light yield. This material shows promise as the detector material of choice for the future.

Coincidence Detection

Special circuitry in the PET tomograph allows detection of two gamma ray photons given off by a single positron annihilation event. The two events are considered to be from the same event if they are counted within the coincidence timing window. The coincidence window is on the order of 10 nsec. Thus, when events are registered in paired detectors within 10 nsec of each other, they are accepted as true coincidence events. If a recorded event is not matched by a paired event within the coincidence time window, the data are discarded. This approach effectively provides "electronic collimation" to define the

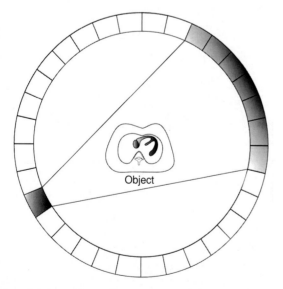

Figure 4-17 Pairing of detectors. In the PET tomograph, each detector is paired with multiple detectors on the opposite side of the ring to create an arc encompassing the object. This multiple-pairing strategy increases the sensitivity of the device.

Table 4-1	Characteristics of Positron Emission Tomography Detector Materials		
Material	**Density**	**Effective Z**	**Delay time (nsec)**
Bismuth germinate oxide (BGO)	7.13	74	300
Gadolinium oxyorthosilicate (GSO)	6.71	59	60
Lutetium oxyorthosilicate (LSO)	7.40	66	40
Sodium iodide (NaI[T1])	3.67	50	230

tomographic image planes. By not having to physically collimate the detector elements, PET tomographs offer much higher sensitivity than would otherwise be the case.

One of the problems in the coincidence approach is the presence of paired random events that appear to the detection circuitry as paired annihilation photons (Fig. 4-18). Paired random events are two photons arising from two different positron annihilation events and are therefore not useful in reconstructing the true location of tracer distribution. As the amount of radioactivity in

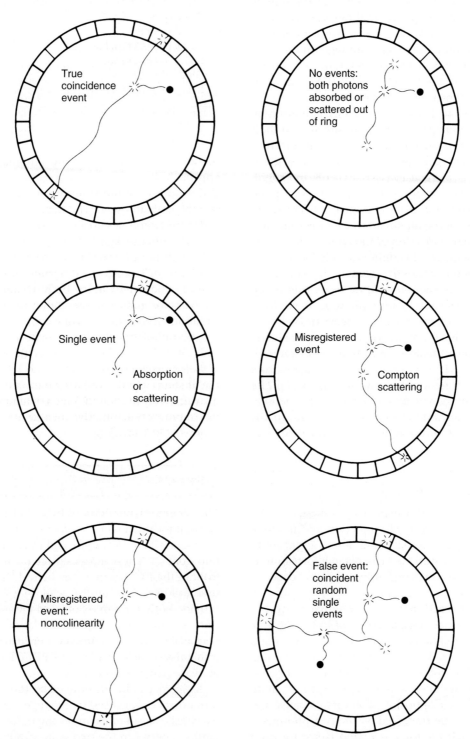

Figure 4-18   Different possibilities in positron decay and event detection with PET. The wanted event is a true coincidence event. Single events are easily rejected but contribute to processor dead time. Misregistered events caused by noncolinearity are difficult to discriminate. "False events" may be incorrectly accepted if the two photons are intercepted in paired detectors.

the field of view increases and the count rate increases, the number of falsely recorded paired random events also increases.

Spatial Resolution

The spatial resolution of modern PET tomographs is excellent. Specialized experimental devices approach 1.5-mm resolution (FWHM) as measured by a line source in air. Resolution under clinical scanning conditions is superior in PET compared with SPECT. Resolution for clinical studies is in the 6- to 8-mm FWHM range with high-end contemporary PET scanners.

The ultimate spatial resolution of PET is limited by two physical phenomena related to positrons and their annihilation. First, positrons are given off at different kinetic energies. Energetic positrons such as those given off in the decay of oxygen-15 (O-15), Ga-68, and rubidium-82 (Rb-82) may travel several millimeters in tissue before undergoing annihilation (Fig. 4-16). Thus, the detected location of the annihilation event is some distance from the actual location of the radionuclide. This travel in tissue degrades the ability to truly localize the biodistribution of the radioactive agent in the patient.

The second phenomenon limiting resolution is the noncolinearity of the annihilation photons. In addition to the energy equivalent of the rest mass of two electrons, the annihilation event incorporates residual kinetic energies of the positron and the negative electron with which it combines. This results in a small deviation from true colinearity along a single ray (see Fig. 4-18). The angle by which the gamma rays depart from the theoretical 180-degree colinearity results in a 1- to 2-mm spatial uncertainty in event localization for clinical whole body PET scanners.

Image Reconstruction

Image reconstruction in PET uses many of the same principles as SPECT. Filtered backprojection and iterative reconstruction algorithms have both found application. In three-dimensional systems, crossplane information is incorporated into the "in-plane" or "direct plane" data.

Attenuation Correction and Quantitative Analysis

A unique and important characteristic of PET is the ability to correct for attenuation of the 511-keV gamma rays in tissue. The basis of this ability is the fact that attenuation and therefore coincidence detection of positron annihilation are independent of the location along a given ray between opposite detectors. Because the total amount of tissue traversed by the two photons is a constant for each ray, the correction factor for each coincidence line can be determined empirically by performing a transmission scan. The observed count rate obtained along each ray during the actual scan is cor-

---

Box 4-3 Quantitative Measurements by Positron Emission Tomography

Regional (absolute) radionuclide localization
pH
Blood flow
Blood volume
Oxygen extraction fraction
Oxygen metabolism
Glucose metabolism
Receptor binding and occupancy

---

rected by dividing it by the attenuation factor. This approach to attenuation correction assumes that the patient does not move between the transmission scan and the emission scan. The transmission scan must have sufficient counting statistics to avoid introducing statistical error into the data.

The ability to correct for attenuation improves the quality of PET images and permits absolute quantification of radioactivity in the body. Quantitative analysis is the basis for numerous metabolic, perfusion, and biodistribution measurements. For example, a therapeutic drug can be radiolabeled with a positron-emitting radionuclide. With knowledge of the specific activity of the radiolabeled drug and the ability to correct for attenuation, the absolute uptake and distribution of the drug can be quantitatively measured. Box 4-3 summarizes several of the important quantitative measurements used in applications of PET imaging.

PET-CT

The recent introduction of hybrid PET-CT scanners has allowed for the direct correlation of the functional information available from PET and the anatomical information from CT. These devices place the CT scan directly in front of the PET scanner. The helical CT scan is acquired first, followed by the PET scan. The CT scan can then provide both a transmission scan for attenuation correction as well as anatomical correlation. Because the CT scan can be acquired much faster than a traditional PET transmission scan, the use of PET-CT can substantially increase patient throughput.

Artifacts can be introduced by the CT-based attenuation correction caused by misregistration between the two image sets. For example, the difference in breathing patterns between the two scans can make it difficult to register the two studies in the area of the diaphragm. However, PET-CT has been extremely useful in anatomically defining both pathology and normal anatomy on the PET scan. Areas of increased FDG uptake can be more easily correlated with a metastatic lymph node or shown to be associated with a region of brown fat or intestine. For these reasons, the use of PET-CT has increased dramatically in the few years and will most likely continue to grow into the future.

COMPARISON OF PET AND SPECT

The advantages of PET are superior sensitivity and resolution and a far greater flexibility of incorporating positron labels into biomolecules. PET scanners are considerably more expensive than SPECT systems and also require the presence of an onsite cyclotron for a full range of applications.

SPECT has significant cost advantages. SPECT systems are smaller and easier to place within hospitals. SPECT has a singular advantage in being applicable to the most commonly performed procedures in nuclear medicine, including myocardial perfusion imaging with either thallium-201 (Tl-201) or Tc-99m and oncological imaging with Ga-67 citrate.

SPECT CAMERA IMAGING OF 511 keV POSITRONS (SPECT-PET)

The feasibility of imaging positron-emitting radionuclides with SPECT systems has been widely explored. The use of this approach has been established with greatest applicability to studies of the heart and certain tumors using fluorine-18 fluorodeoxyglucose (F-18 FDG).

Although initially imaged with very high-energy collimators, noncollimator systems incorporating coincidence detection circuitry have been developed for and used with dual-headed SPECT devices. Spatial resolution is considerably better when coincidence detection is used. These systems became commercially available.

SPECT-PET was initially conceived as a way to bring PET to those who did not have a dedicated PET system. Gamma cameras were available in all nuclear medicine clinics and this minimized the high initial cost of PET systems. However, with the rapid growth and acceptance of dedicated PET systems, current SPECT-PET systems will probably be replaced by dedicated PET systems and it likely will be looked back upon as a temporary historical bridge between SPECT and PET. On the other hand, it is conceivable that systems may be developed in the future that can perform both functions optimally.

SUGGESTED READING

Celler A, Sitek A, Stoub E, et al: Multiple line source array for SPECT transmission scans: simulation, phantom and patient studies, *J Nucl Med* 39: 2183–2189, 1998.

Chandra R: *Nuclear medicine physics: the basics,* 6th ed. Baltimore, Williams & Wilkins, 2004.

Freeman LM, Blauflox MD: The coming age of PET (part 1). *Semin Nucl Med* 28, 1998.

Freeman LM, Blaufox MD: The coming age of PET (part 2). *Semin Nucl Med* 28, 1998.

Hichwa RD: Production of PET radioisotopes and principles of PET imaging. In Henkin RE, editor: *Nuclear medicine,* St Louis, 1996, Mosby, pp 279-291.

Patton JA, Rollo FD: Basic physics of radionuclide imaging. In *Freeman and Johnson's clinical radionuclide imaging,* 3rd ed. Freeman LM, Ed. New York, Grune & Stratton, 1984.

Patton JA, Turkington TG: Coincidence imaging with a dual-head scintillation camera, *J Nucl Med* 40: 4432-4441, 1999.

Phelps ME, Mazziotta JC, Schelbert HR: *Positron emission tomography and autoradiography: principles and application for the brain and heart.* New York, Raven Press, 1986.

Powsner RA, Powsner ER: *Essentials of nuclear medicine physics.* Malden, MA, Blackwell Science, 1998.

Reivich M, Alavi A: *Positron emission tomography.* New York, Alan R Liss, 1985.

Rollo FD: *Nuclear medicine physics, instrumentation and agents.* St. Louis, Mosby, 1977.

Simmons GH: *The scintillation camera.* New York, Society of Nuclear Medicine, 1988.

Cherry SR, Sorenson JA, Phelps ME: *Physics in nuclear medicine,* 3rd ed. Philadelphia, WB Saunders, 2003.

Votaw JR: The AAPM/RSNA physics tutorial for residents: physics of PET, *Radiographics* 15: 1179-1190, 1995.

Yester MV: Theory of tomographic reconstruction. In *Nuclear medicine.* Henkin RE, Ed. St Louis, Mosby, 1996, pp 222-231.

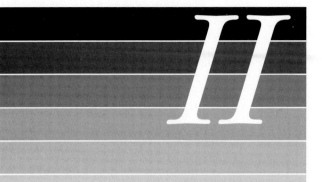

CLINICAL NUCLEAR MEDICINE

CHAPTER 5

Endocrine System

THYROID SCINTIGRAPHY AND FUNCTION STUDIES

Thyroid studies were among the first nuclear medicine procedures. When iodine-131 became available to the medical community in the United States after World War II, thyroidologists quickly recognized that the percentage uptake of radioiodine at a fixed point in time after administration was a measure of thyroid function. This measurement was further enhanced by suppression and stimulation interventions aimed at determining thyroid autonomy and thyroid functional reserve. By the early 1950s, gamma scintillation detectors had been coupled to mechanical devices to produce scans of the thyroid gland. These scans and uptake studies stimulated the early development of the nuclear medicine field. Therapy with radioiodine has been a primary objective since the beginning of nuclear medicine. Thyroid diagnostic studies and therapy principles serve as the physiologic basis for much that we do today and hope to do in the future.

Thyroid Anatomy and Physiology

The thyroid follicular cell synthesizes, stores, and secretes thyroid hormones. An understanding of iodine metabolism, thyroid physiology, and the diseases that result in disordered pathophysiology of the thyroid is needed for the optimal performance and proper interpretation of thyroid uptake studies and thyroid scintigraphy.

Anatomy

The thyroid gland is located at the anterior superior aspect of the trachea just below the thyroid cartilage and extends laterally, superiorly and inferiorly (Fig. 5-1). The name of the gland is derived from the Greek word for

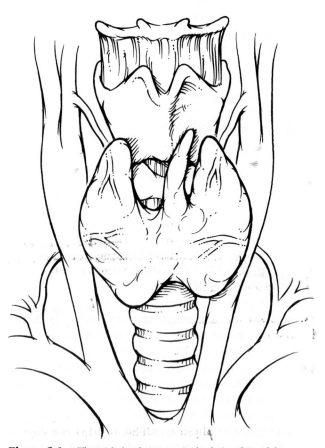

Figure 5-1   Thyroid gland. Anatomical relationship of the thyroid gland to the thyroid and cricoid cartilages and other adjacent anatomical structures.

shield. Because of its embryological development from pharyngeal pouches and descent, ectopic tissue can be found anywhere from the foramen caecum at the base of the tongue to the myocardium. The pyramidal lobe extends towards the hyoid bone and is a remnant of the thyroglossal duct.

The normal adult thyroid gland weighs approximately 15–20 g. The gland consists of many follicles of varying size lined by epithelium made up of cuboidal and columnar follicular cells, which secrete toward the large lumen of the follicle containing colloid (Fig. 5-2). The thyroid gland is 50–75% colloid by weight.

Physiology

Iodine is essential for synthesis of thyroid hormones. After oral ingestion, iodine is rapidly reduced to iodide in the upper small intestine. More than 90% of the iodide is systemically absorbed within 60 minutes of oral ingestion. It distributes in the blood as an extracellular ion similar to chloride. Most leaves the extracellular space through thyroid extraction (20%) or urinary excretion (80%). Some is taken up by the salivary glands and gastric mucosa, which secrete into the gastrointestinal tract.

Iodide Trapping and Organification

The thyroid follicular cell traps iodide by means of a high-energy sodium iodide "thyroid pump" that concentrates iodine intracellularly at 25–500 times the plasma concentration. Trapping can be blocked competitively by monovalent anions (e.g., perchlorate). In the normal thyroid, organification promptly follows trapping (*see* Fig. 5-2). The iodide is oxidized by thyroid peroxidase at the follicular cell colloid interface to neutral iodine, which binds to tyrosine residues on thyroglobulin. These mono- and di-iodinated tyrosines (MIT, DIT) couple to form T_3 and T_4, which are stored in the colloid filled follicular lumen. Organification can be blocked by drugs such as propylthiouracil and methimazole.

Thyroid Hormone Storage and Release

Thyroid stimulating hormone (TSH) initiates iodide uptake and organification, as well as release of thyroid hormone through hydrolysis of thyroglobulin. Thyroglobulin does not normally enter the bloodstream except during disease states (e.g., thyroiditis or thyroid cancer). The normal thyroid gland contains a 1-month supply of hormone, thus drugs blocking hormone synthesis (e.g., propylthiouracil) do not become fully effective in controlling hyperthyroidism until intrathyroidal stores are depleted.

Thyroid-Pituitary Feedback

The thyroid-pituitary feedback mechanism is very sensitive to circulating serum thyroid hormone levels and is the dominant method of adjusting TSH secretion (Fig. 5-3). When serum thyroid hormone levels are increased, the serum TSH is suppressed; when serum thyroid hormone levels are low, serum TSH increases. The major hormone released by the thyroid is T_4, which is

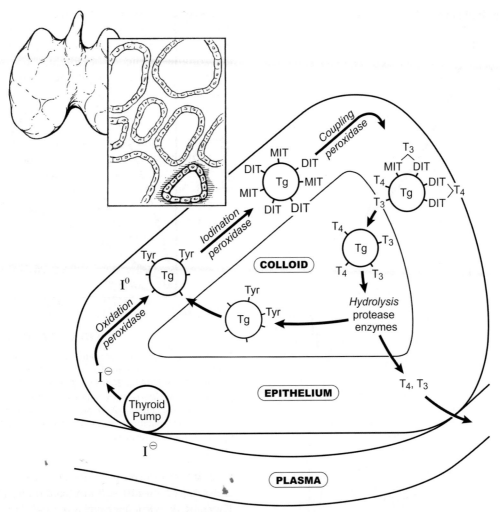

Figure 5-2   Iodine metabolism. The thyroid follicular cell epithelium extracts (traps) iodide from the plasma via the thyroid pump and organifies it. The iodide (I^-) is converted to neutral iodine (I^0) which is then incorporated into thyroglobulin-bound tyrosine molecules as mono or diiodotyrosine (MIT, DIT). Coupling of the iodotyrosines results in T4 and T3 bound to the thyroglobulin which is transported to and stored in the colloid until T4 and T3 are released into the plasma by proteolytic enzymes.

transported to peripheral tissues by thyroid-binding proteins and converted to the more metabolically active T_3 at peripheral tissue site of action.

Radiopharmaceuticals

Radioiodine

Because radioiodine is selectively trapped and organified by the thyroid and incorporated into thyroid hormone, radioactive iodine is an ideal physiological radiotracer, providing clinically important physiological information regarding thyroid function. I-123 and I-131 are the two radiopharmaceuticals used clinically.

Because of the rapid absorption, prompt uptake, and organification of iodine, radioactivity is detectable in the thyroid gland within minutes and normally reaches the thyroid follicular lumen by 20–30 minutes. A progressive increase in thyroid uptake normally occurs over 24 hours (Fig. 5-4). The time delay between radioiodine ingestion and imaging (e.g., 2–6 hours for routine I-123 thyroid imaging and 1–3 days for I-131) is dictated more by the desire for background clearance and a high target-to-background ratio than by slow gland uptake.

Radioiodine is also taken up in the salivary glands, stomach, and to a lesser extent, choroid plexus. It is not concentrated in these organs. The kidneys and gastrointestinal tract serve as the excretory route (Fig. 5-5).

Iodine I-131

Physics   The physical half-life of I-131 is 8 days. It undergoes beta minus decay and emits a principle primary gamma photon of 364 keV (Table 5-1). The 364-keV gamma photons are not optimal for modern-day gamma

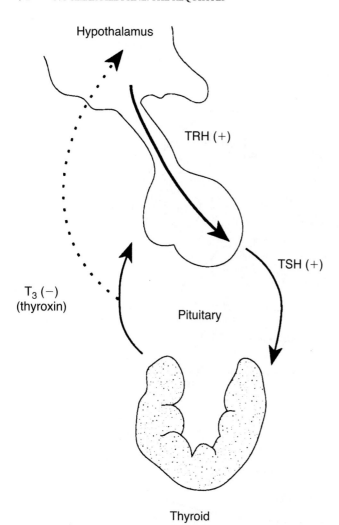

Figure 5-3   Thyroid-pituitary feedback loop. The normal thyroid is under the control of thyroid-stimulating hormone (TSH). The hypothalamic production of thyroid-releasing hormone (TRH) and the pituitary release of TSH are decreased or suppressed as circulating levels of thyroid hormone increase.

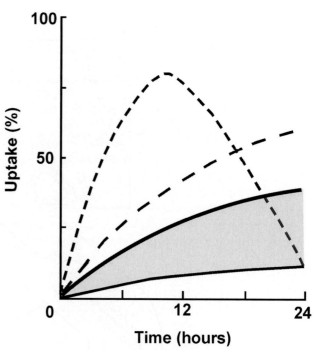

Figure 5-4   Thyroid radioiodine uptake. Radioiodine uptake normally increases progressively over 24 hours (gray area) and is between 10 and 30% at 24 hours. A typical Graves' hyperthyroid patient is noted by the broken line above the normal range with 24-hour uptakes ranging from 50–80%. Some patients with Graves' disease have rapid iodine turnover which is depicted by the top curve, with early elevated uptake but mildly elevated or normal uptake at 24 hours.

cameras. Camera count detection sensitivity for I-131 is poor; approximately half of the photons penetrate the typical three-eighths-inch crystal and thus are not detected. Septal penetration of the collimator by the high-energy emissions results in image degradation. High-energy beta particles are also emitted, the principle one being 0.606 MeV.

Dosimetry   The high-energy beta emissions and long physical half-life of I-131 result in relatively high radiation to the patient, particularly to the thyroid (approximately 1 rad/μCi) (Table 5-2). This high radiation-absorbed dose severely limits the dose that can be administered, further impacting on image quality.

Iodine I-123

Physics   I-123 decays by electron capture with a half-life of 13.2 hours. The principal gamma emission is a 159 keV photon which is well-suited for gamma cameras. There are a small percentage of higher energy

emissions (2.4% 440–625 keV) and 0.15% (625–784 keV). There are no particulate emissions (*see* Table 5-1).

Dosimetry   Methods used for I-123 production in the United States today result in long-lived radionuclide impurities. In the past, I-123 was contaminated with I-124 and I-125. However, commercially available I-123 produced by MDS Nordian in Canada is 99.9% I-123. The maximal levels of identified impurities are Te-121 (0.05%) and I-125 (0.06%). The thyroid receives 1.5–2.6 rads (15–25% RAIU) from a 200 μCi dose of I-123 (Table 5-2). The considerably lower radiation dosimetry of I-123 compared to I-131 allows administration of 200–400 μCi of I-123 for routine thyroid scanning compared to 50 μCi of I-131. This higher administered dose results in considerably better image quality.

Tc-99m Pertechnetate

Because of Tc-99m pertechnetate's low cost and ready availability from molybdenum-99/Tc-99m generator systems, it has long served as an alternative to radioiodine for thyroid scintigraphy.

Physics

The 140-keV photopeak of Tc-99m is ideal for use with the gamma camera. It has a short 6-hour half-life and no particulate emissions (*see* Table 5-1).

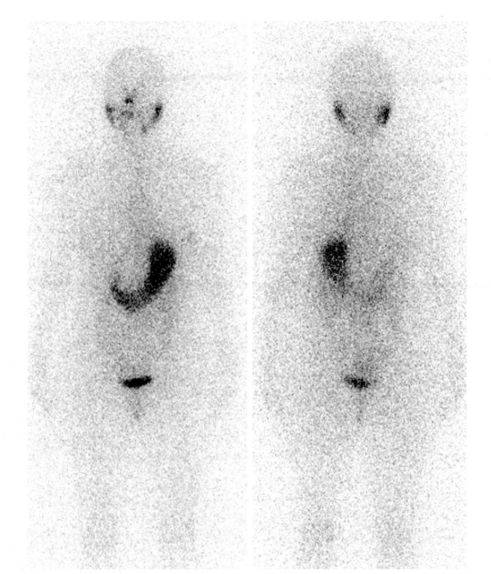

Figure 5-5   Radioiodine distribution within the body. I-123 thyroid whole body scan of patient post total thyroidectomy for thyroid cancer who has received radioactive iodine therapy in the past, thus no thyroid is seen. Otherwise, the distribution at 24 hours is normal with salivary gland and gastric uptake and urinary excretion.

Pharmacokinetics

In contrast to the oral administration of radioiodine, Tc-99m pertechnetate is administered intravenously. Tc-99m is trapped by the thyroid in an identical manner as iodide, but it is not organified nor incorporated into thyroid hormone. Because it is not organified, it is not retained in the thyroid. Thus, thyroid imaging is performed at peak uptake 20–30 minutes after injection.

Dosimetry

The lack of particulate emissions and the short half-life of 6 hours results in relatively low radiation dosimetry to the thyroid (*see* Table 5-2). Thus, the allowable administered activity of Tc-99m pertechnetate (3–5 mCi) is considerably higher that I-123 for routine thyroid scans. The large photon flux provides high quality images.

Which Radiopharmaceutical to Use

I-131 is not used for routine thyroid scans because of its poor image quality and high radiation dosimetry. On the other hand, its long half-life permits delayed imaging that improves the target-to-background ratio, increasing detectability of substernal goiter and thyroid cancer.

Table 5-1 Physical Characteristics of Thyroid Radiopharmaceuticals

	Tc-99m pertechnetate	I-123	I-131
MODE OF DECAY	Isometric transition	Electron capture	Beta minus
PHYSICAL HALF-LIFE (T½)	6 hr	13.2 hr	8.1 days
PHOTON ENERGY	140 keV	159 keV	364 keV
ABUNDANCE	89%	83.4%	81%
BETA EMISSIONS			606 keV

Table 5-2 Dosimetry of Thyroid Radiopharmaceuticals

	Tc-99m pertechnetate (rads/5 mCi, cGY/185 MBq)	I-123 (rads/200 μCi, cGY/7.5 MBq)	I-131 (rads/50 μCi, cGy/3.7 MBq)
THYROID	0.600	1.5 to 2.6*	39.000 to 65.000*
BLADDER WALL	0.430	0.070	0.150
STOMACH	0.250	0.050	0.085
SMALL INTESTINE	0.550	0.030	0.003
RED MARROW	0.100	0.060	0.007
TESTIS	0.050	0.027	0.006
OVARIES	0.150	0.072	0.009
TOTAL BODY	0.070	0.009	0.035

*Lower estimate assumes a 15% RAIU and higher estimate assumes a 25% RAIU, both at time of calibration.

However, for reasons discussed later, I-123 is replacing I-131 even for these indications. The high-energy beta emissions of I-131 make it very useful for radiotherapy of Graves' disease, toxic nodules, and thyroid cancer. Tc-99m pertechnetate is sometimes preferred for thyroid scanning in children because of its low radiation dosimetry and high count rate.

Special Considerations and Precautions

Food and Medications Containing Iodine
Stable iodine contained in foods and medications can interfere with radionuclide thyroid studies (Box 5-1). Expansion of the iodine pool due to ingestion or parenteral administration of iodine containing agents results in a reduced percent radioiodine uptake (%RAIU) by the

thyroid. Increasing amounts of iodine in the normal diet over the years has resulted in a lower normal value for the %RAIU. Numerous noniodine-containing drugs also affect thyroidal uptake (*see* Box 5-1).

Suppression of uptake by exogenous iodine may preclude successful imaging or accurate uptake measurements. As little as 1 mg of stable iodine can cause marked reduction of uptake and 10 mg can effectively block the gland (98% reduction). Radiographic contrast media are a common source of iodine that interferes with radioiodine thyroid studies. A food and drug history should be obtained from all patients prior to undergoing thyroid imaging and uptake studies.

Chronic renal failure impairs iodide clearance, expands the iodide pool, and thus lowers the %RAIU. Hypothyroidism slows clearance of radioactive iodine from the body; hyperthyroidism increases the clearance rate.

Pregnancy
The fetal thyroid concentrates radioiodine after 10–12 weeks of gestation. Radioiodine crosses the placenta and significant exposure of the fetal thyroid can occur after therapeutic doses to the mother, resulting in fetal hypothyroidism and even cretinism.

Nursing Mother
Radioiodine is excreted in human breast milk. Because of its long half-life, nursing should be discontinued after diagnostic or therapeutic studies with I-131. With I-123, it has generally been recommended that breastfeeding may resume after 2–3 days. With Tc-99m pertechnetate, nursing can be resumed after 24 hours.

Patient Information
Thyroid studies must always be interpreted in light of the patient's clinical history, thyroid physical examination, and, importantly, with knowledge of the patient's serum thyroid function studies.

Methodology for Thyroid Uptake Studies and Thyroid Scans

Thyroid uptake studies and thyroid scans are often performed at the same clinic visit. However, they are usually acquired with different instrumentation, providing different but complementary information. Thyroid scans are acquired with a gamma camera. Thyroid uptake studies are most commonly acquired with a nonimaging gamma scintillation probe detector. Camera-based methods are sometimes used and will be discussed. A thyroid uptake provides quantitative information regarding the percent of the administered activity taken up by the thyroid.

Thyroid Uptake

Radioiodine Percent Uptake
Both I-131 and I-123 can be used for calculation of the %RAIU or the percent of the administered radioactive

Box 5-1   Drugs, Foods, Radiographic Contrast Agents, and Therapies that Decrease or Increase the %RAIU

DECREASED UPTAKE	DURATION OF EFFECT
Thyroid Hormones	
Thyroxine (T$_4$)	4-6 weeks
Triiodothyronine (T$_3$)	2 weeks
Excess Iodine (Expanded Iodine Pool)	
Saturated solution of potassium iodide	2-4 weeks
Some mineral supplements, cough medicines, and vitamin preparations	2-4 weeks
Iodine food supplements	
Iodinated drugs (e.g., amiodarone)	Weeks to months
Iodinated skin ointments	2-4 weeks
Congestive heart failure	
Renal failure	
Radiographic Contrast Media	
Water-soluble intravascular media	2-4 weeks
Oral cholecystographic agents	4 weeks to indefinite
Fat-soluble media (lymphography)	Months to years
Noniodine-Containing Drugs	Variable
Adrenocorticotropic hormone, adrenal steroids	
Monovalent anions (perchlorate)	
Penicillin	
Antithyroid drugs	
Propylthiouracil (PTU)	3-5 days
Methimazole (Tapazole)	5-7 days
Bromides	
Goitrogenic foods (e.g., cabbage, turnips)	
Prior radiation to neck	
INCREASED UPTAKE	
Iodine Deficiency	
Pregnancy	
Rebound after therapy withdrawal (thyroid hormones, antithyroid drugs)	
Lithium	

iodine taken up by the thyroid. Clinical indications for uptake determinations are few, but important (Box 5-2).

Indications   The most common clinical indication for a %RAIU study is to aid in the differential diagnosis of newly diagnosed thyrotoxicosis. In most cases, the referring physician seeks to differentiate Graves' disease, the most common cause for thyrotoxicosis (Box 5-3), from other causes (e.g., thyroiditis, the second most common cause). Therapy of Graves' disease is quite different than that for other causes. The %RAIU is elevated in Graves' disease, but suppressed or decreased in most other causes of thyrotoxicosis with diffuse goiter, such as thyroiditis (Box 5-4).

The %RAIU is also often used for the calculation of an I-131 therapy dose for Graves' disease (Box 5-5).

Methodology   Medications that might interfere with thyroid uptake should be discontinued for an appropriate length of time (*see* Box 5-1). Patients should have nothing by mouth for 4 hours prior to the study to assure good radioiodine absorption. I-123 and I-131 are usually administered in capsule form rather than liquid. The unit-dosed capsule formulation minimizes airborne exposure of radioiodine to technologists and is convenient for handling.

When a scan is not needed, 5-10 µCi I-131 or 50-100 µCi I-123 is adequate for an uptake because of the probe's high detection sensitivity compared to a gamma camera. When a scan is indicated, both can be performed using the scan dose of I-123 (200-300 µCi). The standard %RAIU uptake is acquired at 24 hours. In some

Box 5-2 Clinical Indications for Thyroid Scintigraphy and Uptakes

THYROID SCANS

Determination of functional status (cold, hot) of thyroid nodule

Detection of ectopic thyroid tissue (lingual thyroid)

Differential diagnosis of mediastinal masses (substernal goiter)

Thyroid cancer whole body scan

THYROID UPTAKES

Differential diagnosis of thyrotoxicosis

Estimate I-131 therapy dose for Graves' disease

Together with whole body thyroid cancer scans

Estimate residual thyroid postsurgery

Estimate I-131 therapeutic effectiveness

Follow-up for recurrence

Box 5-3 Clinical Frequency of Various Causes for Thyrotoxicosis

Graves' disease	70%
Thyroiditis	20%
Toxic multinodular goiter	5%
Toxic adenoma	5%
Others	<1%

Box 5-4 Differential Diagnosis of Thyrotoxicosis-based Increased or Decreased %RAIU

INCREASED UPTAKE

Graves' disease
Multinodular toxic goiter
Hashitoxicosis
Central hypothyroidism
Hydatiform mole, trophoblastic tumors, choriocarcinoma
Metastatic thyroid cancer

DECREASED UPTAKE

Subacute thyroiditis
   Granulomatous thyroiditis (de Quervain's)
   Silent thyroiditis
   Postpartum thyroiditis
Iodine-induced thyrotoxicosis (Jod-Basedow)
Amiodarone-induced thyrotoxicosis
Thyrotoxicosis factitia
Struma ovarii

Box 5-5 Calculation of Thyroid Percent Uptake of Radioiodine I-123 and I-131

1. **PRELIMINARY MEASUREMENTS**

   Place dose capsule in neck phantom and count for 1 minute

   Count patient's neck and thigh (background) for 1 minute

2. **ADMINISTER ORAL DOSE CAPSULE**

3. **UPTAKE MEASUREMENT AT (OPTIONAL: 2–6 HOURS AND) 24 HOURS**

   Count patient's neck for 1 min

   Count patient's thigh for 1 min

4. **CALCULATION AT SELECTED UPTAKE INTERVALS AT (OPTIONAL: 2–6 HOURS AND) 24 HOURS**

$$\%RAIU = \frac{\text{Neck (background corrected) counts/min}}{\text{Dose capsule (decay corrected and background corrected) counts/min}} \times 100$$

Correction is also routinely made for room background. In the past, a standard dose capsule was also counted initially and at uptake intervals and used for decay correction. However, in most modern systems, decay is automatically calculated by the probe computer system.

clinics, a 2–6 hour uptake is also routinely performed. In some clinics, only a 2–6 hour uptake is done.

A nonimaging gamma scintillation probe detector is used for radioiodine thyroid uptake studies. It has a 2-cm thick × 2-cm diameter sodium iodine crystal with an open cone-shaped single-hole lead collimator coupled to a photomultiplier tube and electronics.

Room background activity is determined. The radioiodine capsule is placed in a Lucite neck phantom and activity counted with the probe detector placed at a standardized distance of 30 cm (Fig. 5-6). The capsule is administered to the patient. The probe is placed 30 cm from the anterior surface of the patient's neck, such that the entire gland can be detected by the probe but most extrathyroidal activity is not. The patient's neck (background) is counted (Fig. 5-7).

At the uptake times (2–6 hours and/or 24 hours), counts are obtained for the neck and the patient's thigh (background). The percent radioiodine uptake is calculated according to this formula:

$$\%RAIU = \frac{\text{Neck counts/min (background corrected)}}{\text{Administered dose capsule counts/min (background and decay corrected)}} \times 100$$

In the past, a standard reference capsule similar in activity to the administered capsule was counted initially and

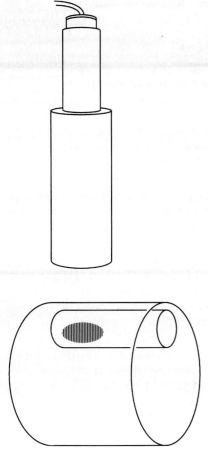

Figure 5-6   Uptake probe: neck lucite phantom. The gamma detector is placed at a standard distance of 30 cm from the neck phantom which contains the capsule dose of radioiodine to be administered to the patient.

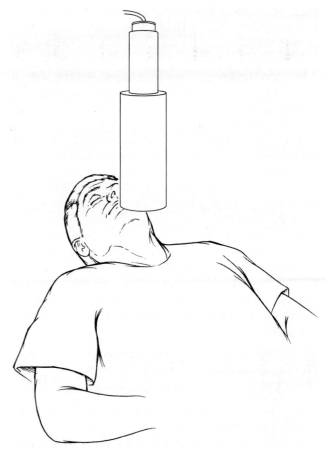

Figure 5-7   Uptake probe: patient. The detector is positioned 30 cm from the patient's thyroid.

at the uptake intervals. The purpose of the standard was to correct for decay. A dose-to-standard ratio was determined to correct for the difference in standard and administered dose. In present-day uptake probe-computer systems, decay is automatically corrected.

Normal Values   The %RAIU increases progressively over 24 hours (*see* Fig 5-4). In the United States, the normal range is approximately 10–30% (8-35% in some laboratories) at 24 hours. Before widespread iodine supplementation in bread and table salt, the normal range was substantially higher. The normal range for the 2-6 hour %RAIU is 4-15%.

The early 2–6 hour %RAIU can serve two purposes. An occasional patient with Graves' disease has rapid iodine turnover within the thyroid, resulting in a normal or only mildly elevated 24 hour %RAIU but a very high 2–6 hour value (*see* Fig 5-4). Thus an early uptake confirms that the %RAIU is indeed elevated, and furthermore may suggest that a higher therapy dose is needed

because of the rapid turnover and shorter residence time in the thyroid.

In some clinics, the 2–6 hour %RAIU is used to predict the 24-hour uptake so that a therapy dose can be estimated, ordered, and available for administration at 24 hours. The dose can be adjusted based on the 24 hour uptake. Other clinics treat immediately after the 2–6 hour %RAIU.

Another use of the %RAIU is in conjunction with whole body thyroid cancer scans (i.e., to quantify residual thyroid tissue uptake after thyroidectomy or I-131 therapy, therapeutic effectiveness, or recurrence). For whole body thyroid cancer scans, a camera-based method is used to calculate the %RAIU. A standard with calibrator-measured activity is also imaged. Regions of interest are drawn for the thyroid, background, and standard. The uptake is calculated at the time of whole body imaging (24–48 hours).

Tc-99m Pertechnetate Uptake

The advantages of using Tc-99m pertechnetate as an alternative to radioiodine to calculate an uptake include its favorable radiation dosimetry, a particular consideration for children (*see* Table 5-2), and that the study can be completed within 30 minutes with uptake results available soon thereafter. The disadvantages of the Tc-99m pertechnetate uptake include a less well-defined normal range, the standard practice of calculating the therapy dose based on the radioiodine uptake, and the lack of software for this calculation on some newer camera computer systems.

Methodology A scintillation probe is not used for a Tc-99m uptake because of the high neck and body background. This is a gamma camera technique for calculating the percent uptake, similar to that used for thyroid cancer scans. Before and after injection of the Tc-99m pertechnetate, the syringe is imaged with the gamma camera (preinjection counts minus postinjection residual counts = administered counts). Twenty minutes after injection, the thyroid scan is acquired on computer. Regions of interest are drawn on computer for the thyroid, thyroid background, and the syringes. Areas of interest are normalized for pixel size and thyroid and syringe counts are normalized for time of acquisition. The percent uptake is calculated:

$$\text{Tc-99m pertechnetate percent uptake} = \frac{\text{Thyroid counts} - \text{Background counts}}{\text{Injected counts} - \text{R counts}} \times 100$$

Normal Tc-99m uptake ranges from 0.3–4.5%. Accuracy is less than with the %RAIU.

A simple qualitative approach has been used to estimate uptake by obtaining images with the salivary glands in the same field-of-view as the thyroid. In the euthyroid patient, relative uptake in the salivary and thyroid glands is similar. With hyperthyroidism, thyroid uptake is considerably greater than salivary gland uptake.

Thyroid Scintigraphy

The thyroid scan depicts the entire gland in a single image and permits direct correlation of physical findings with abnormalities in the image. The combination of gamma camera and pinhole collimator offers the flexibility of obtaining multiple-view high-resolution images of the thyroid. Pinhole collimator magnification provides image resolution superior to parallel-hole collimators in the range of 5 mm, compared to 1–2 cm with a parallel-hole collimator.

Thyroid Examination

The thyroid gland should be routinely examined by palpation at the time of imaging in order to estimate the size of the gland and to confirm the presence and location of nodules. A radioactive marker source (122-keV Cobalt-57 or Tc-99m) can then be placed over the palpated nodule for anatomical and functional correlation.

Methodology

Thyroid I-123 and Tc-99 Pertechnetate Scans Clinical indications for thyroid scintigraphy are listed in Box 5-2 and discussed later in the section entitled *Clinical Indications for Thyroid Scintigraphy*.

Procedure Radioiodine is administered orally. The usual I-123 thyroid scintigraphy dose is 200–300 μCi. The scan is usually acquired at 2–6 hours after administration but may be acquired at the time of the 24-hour %RAIU. The higher count rate obtainable at 2–6 hours allows for shorter imaging time and better image quality. The low count rate at 24 hours requires longer acquisition time which increases the likelihood of patient movement. With Tc-99m pertechnetate, 3–5 mCi is administered intravenously and imaging begins 20–30 minutes after injection.

For both radiopharmaceuticals, a standard or large field-of-view gamma camera is used, equipped with a pinhole collimator (Fig. 5-8) that has an interchangeable lead pinhole insert of 3- to 6-mm in internal diameter placed in its distal aspect. Smaller diameter inserts provide higher resolution but lower sensitivity.

A 15–20% photopeak window is set at 159 keV for I-123 and at 140 keV for Tc-99m. Imaging protocols for thyroid imaging for the two radiopharmaceuticals are similar and described in more detail in Boxes 5-6 and 5-7.

The patient is positioned supine with the neck hyperextended so that the plane of the thyroid gland is parallel to the crystal face of the camera. The thyroid gland should fill approximately two-thirds of the field of view. This is achieved with a 6–8 cm distance from the collimator

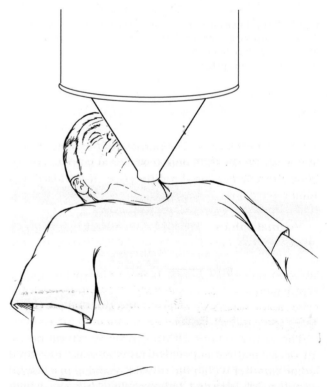

Figure 5-8   Pinhole collimator. The gamma camera with a pinhole collimator is placed close to the thyroid to permit maximal magnification. The thyroid gland should fill approximately two thirds of the field of view.

Box 5-6 Tc-99m Pertechnetate Thyroid Imaging: Protocol Summary

PATIENT PREPARATION

Discontinue any medications that interfere with thyroid uptake of Tc-99m pertechnetate.
Nothing by mouth for 4 hours prior to study.

RADIOPHARMACEUTICAL

Tc-99m pertechnetate, 3–5 mCi (111–185 MBq) intravenously

TIME OF IMAGING

20 min after radiopharmaceutical administration

IMAGING PROCEDURE

Gamma camera with a 3- to 6-mm aperture pinhole collimator and a 20% energy window centered at 140 keV.
Position the patient supine with the chin up and neck extended.
Position the collimator so that the thyroid fills about two thirds of the diameter of the field of view.
Obtain anterior, 45-degree LAO and RAO views (move the collimator rather than the patient).
Obtain 250k counts per view.
Mark the chin and suprasternal notch.
Note the position and mark palpable nodules and surgical scars.
Place marker sources lateral to the thyroid to calibrate size.

Box 5-7 Iodine-123 Thyroid Imaging: Protocol Summary

PATIENT PREPARATION

Discontinue any medications that interfere with thyroid uptake of radioiodine.
Nothing by mouth for 4 hours prior to study.

RADIOPHARMACEUTICAL

I-123, 100–400 µCi (3.7–15 MBq), orally in capsule form

TIME OF IMAGING

At 4–6 or 24 hours

IMAGING PROCEDURE

Use a gamma camera with a 3- to 6-mm aperture pinhole collimator and a 20% energy window centered at 159 keV.
Position the patient supine with the chin up and the neck extended.
Position the collimator so that the thyroid fills about two-thirds of the diameter of the field of view.
Obtain anterior, 45-degree LAO and RAO views (move the collimator, if possible, rather than the patient).
Obtain 100k–250k counts per view.
Mark the chin and suprasternal notch.
Note the position and mark palpable nodules and surgical scars.
Place marker sources lateral to the thyroid to calibrate size.

to the surface of the neck. Magnification increases as the pinhole collimator approaches the neck.

On one image, a radioactive marker (Tc-99m or Cobalt-57) or computer cursor is placed at the sternal notch and on the right side (Figs. 5-9 and 5-10). A 4- to 5-cm line source marker or two point sources 4–5 cm apart may be placed on the neck just lateral to the thyroid lobes and parallel to their long axis (Fig. 5-11) to estimate the size of the thyroid and nodules. Because of the three-dimensional nature of the gland and pinhole collimator distortion, this is an approximate measurement and does not obviate physical exam size estimation.

Images are routinely obtained in the anterior, right anterior oblique (RAO), and left anterior oblique (LAO) views (see Fig. 5-9). Each image is obtained for 100,000 counts. It is preferable for the patient to remain in one position while the camera and collimator are moved to the different projections, thus making images more reproducible between patients and resulting in less image distortion and patient motion.

Additional images with a radioactive marker may be indicated to determine whether a palpable nodule takes up the radiopharmaceutical (i.e., a hot or cold nodule). Special care should be taken to avoid the parallax effect of a pinhole collimator. The *parallax effect* results in a change in the relationship between a near and distant object when viewed from different angles. With a pinhole collimator, this can result in misregistration of the relationship between the nodule and the marker or, in the case of a suspected substernal goiter, the suprasternal notch marker and the thyroid. The effect can be minimized in several ways. One method is to obtain an image with the collimator at an increased distance from the thyroid (see Fig. 5-9), decreasing the effect of magnification and distortion. A second method is to place the marker region of interest in the center of the field-of-view. Finally, a parallel-hole collimator might be used for the marker image.

Iodide I-131 Scan Because of the high radiation dose the thyroid with I-131, clinical indications for I-131 thyroid scans are limited to confirming the thyroid origin of a mediastinal mass (substernal goiter) and for thyroid cancer scintigraphy. The advantage of I-131 is that delayed imaging allows for improved target-to-background ratio, thus improving detectability.

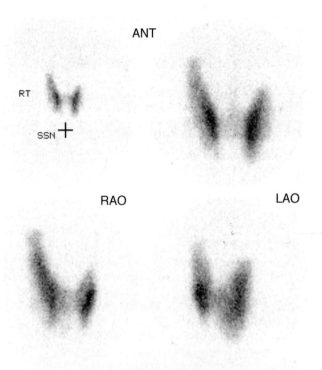

ANT

RT

SSN +

RAO   LAO

Figure 5-9   Normal I-123 thyroid scan. On the initial image, the collimator is placed at a greater distance from the neck than the other images. A computer cursor marks the suprasternal notch (SSN) and the right side (RT). The collimator is moved closer to the neck to acquire the anterior, right anterior oblique and left anterior oblique views, which have greater magnification and resolution.

For the substernal goiter, 50 μCi I-131 is administered orally. A large-field-of-view gamma camera equipped with a high-energy parallel-hole collimator is used. A 20–30% window is centered at 364 keV. A radioactive marker should be placed at the suprasternal notch as discussed previously (*see* Fig. 5-11)

Thyroid Cancer Scan   Thyroid cancer cells are hypofunctional compared to normal thyroid tissue and thus take up radioiodine to a lesser degree. This is the reason that cancer nodules appear cold on routine thyroid scans.

To maximize thyroid cancer cell uptake, TSH stimulation is necessary. For decades, this has been done through endogenous stimulation of TSH by making the patient hypothyroid by total thyroidectomy and radioactive iodine therapy. Endogenous stimulation of TSH requires discontinuation of thyroid hormone (i.e., 4–6 weeks off Synthroid and 2 weeks without Cytomel). The serum TSH should be greater than 30 IU before radioiodine can be administered. Alternatively, recombinant TSH (Thyrogen) can stimulate uptake without thyroid hormone withdrawal. A low-iodine diet is an ancillary method used to increase uptake by decreasing the iodine pool.

Iodine-131   For many years, 5–10 mCi of I-131 was the usual administered dose for whole-body thyroid cancer scans. However, because of reports of thyroid "stunning" after the diagnostic dose, the recommended dose

was reduced to 2 mCi. With diagnostic doses greater than 5 mCi, this stunning of thyroid cells decreases subsequent therapeutic dose uptake.

When Thyrogen (recombinant TSH) is used as an alternative to endogenous TSH stimulation, the dose is raised to 4 mCi because uptake is 50% of that seen with thyroid hormone withdrawal. The explanation is that thyroid hormone withdrawal and the resulting hypothyroidism causes renal insufficiency with reduced radioiodine clearance and increased iodine uptake. Thyrogen doses do not have that advantage.

Thyrogen is given on two consecutive days as an intramuscular injection of 0.9 mg. On the third day, radioiodine is administered. Imaging is performed on day 5 for I-131 and day 4 for I-123. Serum thyroglobulin, a tumor marker for thyroid cancer, is drawn on day 5.

A large field-of-view gamma camera equipped with a high-energy parallel-hole collimator is used with a 20–30% window centered at 364 keV. Imaging is usually performed 48 hours after oral administration. For detection of thyroid carcinoma, the most important view is the anterior image of the head, neck, and chest. However, whole body views are desirable because thyroid metastases may occur outside this field of view (e.g., in the bones of the skull, humeri, and femurs, liver, and brain). Spot imaging requires 10–20 minutes per view. The pinhole collimator allows for high-resolution views of the neck, which is most helpful when there is intensive uptake in the thyroid bed and associated "star" artifact (Fig. 5-12) due to septal penetration of the parallel-hole collimator. Since pinhole collimators do not have septa, neck uptake can be resolved without this artifact.

Iodine-123   I-123 is increasingly replacing I-131 for whole body thyroid cancer scans. Stunning is not an issue with I-123, image quality is better, and the study is completed at 24 hours. One might expect I-123 to detect fewer tumors than I-131 because of the earlier imaging period (24 rather than 48 hours). However, investigations have shown similar ability to detect metastases, possibly because of the higher photon flux with I-123. The orally administered dose of I-123 is typically 1.5–2 mCi.

Clinical Indications for Thyroid Uptake Studies

Thyrotoxicosis

Thyrotoxicosis is characterized by hypermetabolism due to increased circulating thyroid hormone. *Hyperthyroidism* is thyrotoxicosis caused by a hyperfunctioning thyroid gland (e.g., Graves' disease or toxic nodular goiter) (Box 5-8). Examples of thyrotoxicosis not caused by a hyperfunctioning thyroid gland are subacute thyroiditis, thyroiditis factitia, and struma ovarii.

Clinical Diagnosis

The symptoms of thyrotoxicosis are those of increased metabolism such as weight loss, tachycardia, palpitations,

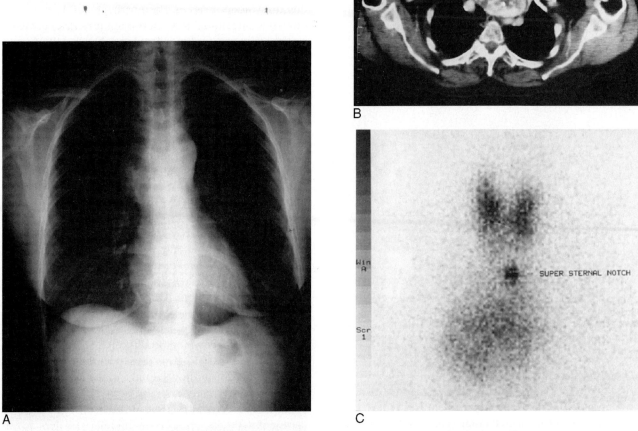

Figure 5-10   Substernal goiter. **A,** Chest radiograph reveals a superior mediastinal mass. **B,** Computed tomography confirms the presence of the mass, which demonstrates inhomogeneous density. **C,** Subsequent I-131 scintigraphy reveals a large substernal goiter. A radioactive marker is placed at the suprasternal notch.

heat intolerance, hyperhidrosis, and anxiety. However, these symptoms are nonspecific and require confirmation with serum thyroid function studies. A suppressed serum thyroid stimulating hormone (TSH) less than 0.1 mU/L is the most sensitive test for diagnosis of thyrotoxicosis. The suppressed TSH is caused by negative feedback on the pituitary from the elevated serum thyroid hormone. The only exception to a suppressed TSH with thyrotoxicosis is a rare hypothalamic or pituitary etiology.

Differential Diagnosis

The clinical history and physical exam may suggest the etiology of thyrotoxicosis. For example, recent upper respiratory infection and a tender thyroid would suggest subacute thyroiditis, whereas exophthalmus and pretibial edema is consistent with Graves' disease. However, in many cases, the diagnosis is uncertain. The %RAIU can help with this differential diagnosis.

%RAIU Interpretation

The %RAIU does not define thyroid function per se. An increased %RAIU is not diagnostic of hyperthyroidism. Patients with iodine deficiency, dyshormonogenesis (organification defects), or chronic autoimmune thyroiditis may have elevated %RAIU despite clinical euthyroidism or even hypothyroidism (Box 5-9). The %RAIU must be interpreted in light of the patient's serum thyroid function studies.

Normally, iodine uptake is dependent on pituitary-produced TSH stimulation. For many causes of thyrotoxicosis, radioiodine uptake will be suppressed (less than 1–2%) (e.g., in subacute thyroiditis, iodine-induced thyroiditis, and thyrotoxicosis factitia [*see* Box 5-8]). However, iodine uptake will be increased despite the suppressed TSH if the thyroid has autonomous function independent of pituitary feedback, the most common cause being Graves' disease. Thus, the clinical utility of the %RAIU for thyrotoxicosis lies in the confirmation or exclusion of Graves' disease as the cause of a toxic diffuse goiter.

The %RAIU has been used in conjunction with various pharmacologic interventions described in the later section *Other Thyroid Function Studies*. These include the T3 suppression test, TSH stimulation test, and perchlorate washout test. Although these interventions nicely delineate underlying pathophysiological processes, they are rarely requested in current practice due to various advancements in diagnosis and therapy.

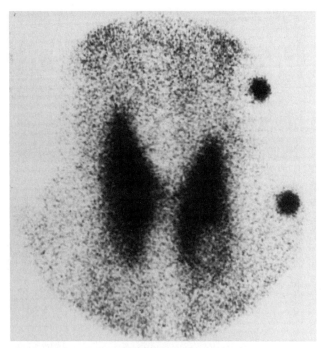

Figure 5-11 Solitary cold nodule. A palpable nodule corresponds to the cold defect in left lower lobe on the thyroid scan. Radioactive markers are placed 4 cm apart on the left side as an aid to approximate the size of gland.

Diseases with Increased %RAIU

The list of diseases producing thyrotoxicosis with an "elevated" uptake (*see* Box 5-4) includes entities where the uptake may be in the normal range (e.g., toxic nodules). This can be viewed as elevated in the sense that the normal response to thyrotoxicosis is suppression of TSH by T-4 feedback to the pituitary with subsequent suppression of iodine uptake and thus %RAIU.

Graves' Disease Between 70% and 80% of patients presenting with thyrotoxicosis have Graves' disease as the etiology. This autoimmune disease is most commonly seen in middle-aged females but also occurs in children and the elderly. Thyroid-stimulating immunoglobulins similar to TSH bind to the follicular cells causing hyperplasia and autonomous thyroid hyperfunction.

The diagnosis of Graves' disease is often straightforward, such as thyrotoxicosis, diffuse goiter without nodules, characteristic exophthalmopathy, and pretibial dermopathy. However, in many patients the diagnosis is suspected but uncertain. An elevated %RAIU, usually in the range of 50-80%, confirms the diagnosis of Graves' disease and excludes most other causes. A Tc-99m pertechnetate uptake in Graves' disease is typically greater than 4.0%. A thyroid scan is often not necessary to confirm Graves' disease if physical examination or sonography is consistent with diffuse goiter without nodules.

Multinodular Toxic Goiter Sometimes referred to as *Plummer's disease*, multinodular goiter often presents in older patients with tachyarrhythmias, weight loss,

depression, anxiety, and insomnia. The hypermetabolism may exacerbate other medical problems. The natural history of individual autonomously functioning thyroid follicular adenomas is hemorrhage and necrosis, ultimately becoming nonfunctioning nodules. However, the time course is prolonged and variable, and the disease requires prompt therapy. Physical examination of the thyroid or ultrasonography can confirm nodularity but not function. Serum thyroid function tests make the diagnosis of thyrotoxicosis not infrequently T-3 toxicosis.

The %RAIU is often only moderately elevated; it can even be in the high normal range. The thyroid scan has the classical picture of high uptake within hyperfunctioning nodules but suppression of the extranodular tissue due to pituitary feedback and TSH suppression. Therapy with radioactive iodine I-131 is the usual treatment.

Single Autonomously Functioning Thyroid Nodule Toxic nodules occur in only 5% of patients with a solitary palpable nodule. Most are nonfunctioning. This entity occurs more frequently in the elderly and those living in iodine deficient regions. Once an autonomous nodule grows to a size of 2.5-3.0 cm, it produces enough thyroid hormone to cause clinical thyrotoxicosis. Therapy is often with radioactive iodine, although surgery is a treatment choice. The %RAIU is usually in the normal range and the thyroid scan shows uptake in the nodule but suppression of the remainder of the gland.

Chronic Thyroiditis (Hashitoxicosis) Hashimoto's disease commonly presents in middle-aged females as goiter or hypothyroidism. Much less frequently, patients manifest initially or later in the course of the disease with thyrotoxicosis (3–5% of cases), so-called Hashitoxicosis. Histopathologically, lymphocytic infiltration is predominant. Some consider Hashitoxicosis to be an overlap syndrome with Graves' disease.

The gland is diffusely and symmetrically enlarged. It is nontender, firm, and usually without nodules. Serum antithyroglobulin and antimicrosomal antibodies are elevated. During the thyrotoxic phase, the %RAIU is increased, similar in degree to Graves' disease. The thyroid scan typically shows diffuse increased uptake. Radioactive iodine I-131 is the usual therapy.

Rare Causes A *pituitary adenoma* secreting TSH is a rare cause of hyperthyroidism. An even rarer condition is resistance of the pituitary to thyroid hormone feedback. In both cases, the TSH is elevated. *Hydatiform mole, trophoblastic tumors,* and *choriocarcinoma* may manifest symptoms of hyperthyroidism. Human chorionic gonadotropin (HCG) is a weak TSH-like agonist. The serum level of HCG correlates with the severity of hyperthyroidism. Serum TSH is suppressed and the %RAIU is elevated. Hyperthyroidism secondary to *metastatic thyroid cancer* is quite rare, usually occurring with follicular carcinoma.

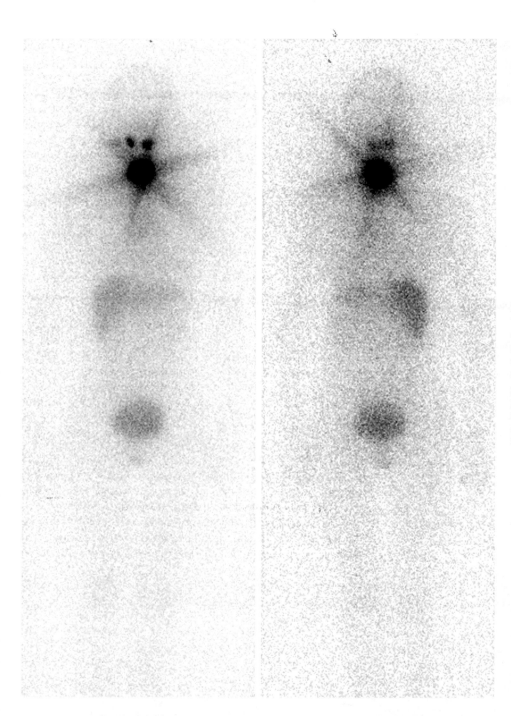

Figure 5-12   Star artifact. Whole body thyroid cancer scan obtained seven days after high-dose I-131 therapy. The intense uptake in the thyroid bed results in a star artifact caused by septal penetration of the high energy photons through the septa of the collimator. Note liver uptake caused by metabolized thyroid hormone.

Diseases with Suppressed %RAIU

Subacute Thyroiditis   The most common reason for thyrotoxicosis associated with a decreased %RAIU is subacute thyroiditis. There are several causes for the disease. *Granulomatous thyroiditis* (de Quervain's) is characteristically preceded by several days of upper respiratory illness and presents with a tender thyroid. Histopathologically, granulomas are seen on biopsy. *Silent thyroiditis,* commonly seen in elderly patients, is not a granulomatous process nor is it associated with respiratory symptoms or thyroid tenderness. Often, elderly patients present with arrhythmia and normal size

thyroid. *Postpartum thyroiditis* occurs within weeks or months of delivery. A mild goiter is often palpated in patients with subacute thyroiditis.

The decreased %RAIU associated with subacute thyroiditis is the result of an intact pituitary feedback mechanism, not because of damage and dysfunction of the gland (Fig. 5-13). Uptake is suppressed in the entire gland, but the disease is often patchy or regional.

During the initial stage of subacute thyroiditis, stored intracellular thyroid hormone is released into the blood. This is caused by increased cell permeability as a result of the inflammatory process. As the inflammation resolves,

Box 5-8 Classification of Thyrotoxicosis Based on Thyroid Hyperfunction or No Thyroid Hyperfunction

Thyroid hyperfunction

A. Abnormal thyroid stimulator
  1. Graves' disease
  2. Trophoblastic tumor
    a. Hydatiform mole, choriocarcinoma uterus or testes
B. Intrinsic thyroid autonomy
  1. Hyperfunctioning adenoma
  2. Toxic multinodular goiter
C. Excess production of TSH (rare)

No thyroid hyperfunction

A. Disorders of hormone storage
  1. Subacute thyroiditis
  2. Chronic thyroiditis with transient thyrotoxicosis
B. Extrathyroid source of hormone
  1. Thyrotoxicosis factitia
  2. "Hamburger toxicosis" (epidemic caused by thyroid gland contaminated hamburger meat)
  3. Ectopic thyroid tissue
    a. Struma ovarii
    b. Functioning follicular carcinoma

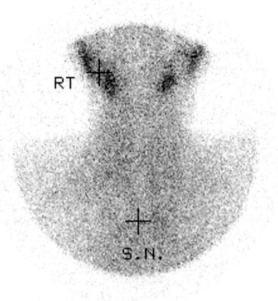

Figure 5-13 Subacute thyroiditis. Suppressed Tc-99m thyroid uptake in patient presenting with new onset thyrotoxicosis.

serum thyroid hormone levels decrease and often fall into the subnormal range with a resulting rise in TSH. It is not uncommon for patients to become hypothyroid, during the recovery phase, manifested by a high TSH. The level of the %RAIU depends on the damaged thyroid's ability to respond to TSH stimulation. The hypothyroidism usually resolves over weeks and months and the TSH and %RAIU return to normal. The rapidity of this process depends on the degree of damage. The %RAIU depends on the stage of the disease (Fig. 5-14).

Iodine-Induced Thyrotoxicosis (Jod-Basedow) In the past, this condition occurred with the introduction

Box 5-9 Relationship of Thyroid Uptake to Thyroid Function

	Thyroid Uptake		
THYROID FUNCTION	**INCREASED**	**NORMAL**	**DECREASED**

Thyrotoxicosis	Graves' disease
	Hashitoxicosis
		Antithyroid drugs
		  Propylthiouracil
		  Methimazole
			Expanded iodide pool
			Subacute thyroiditis, thyrotoxic phase
			Thyrotoxicosis factitia
			Antithyroid drugs
			Struma ovarii

Euthyroid	Rebound after antithyroid drug withdrawal Recovery from subacute thyroiditis Compensated dyshormonogenesis		Decompensated dyshormonogenesis
Hypothyroid	Decompensated dyshormonogenesis Hashimoto's disease	Hashimoto's disease after I-131 therapy Subacute thyroiditis, recovery phase decompensated dyshormonogenesis	Hypothyroidism: primary or secondary

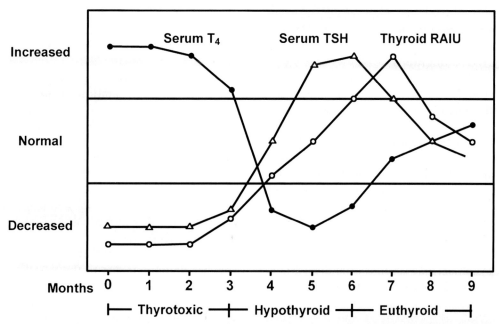

Figure 5-14   Clinical course of subacute thyroiditis. Typical evolving pattern of the serum T_4, TSH and %RAIU over 9 months, from initial presentation to resolution. When the patient initially presents, the T_4 is elevated and TSH and RAIU are suppressed. Once there is no more thyroid hormone to release, thyroid function may be poor due to inflammatory damage to the gland and the TSH and RAIU will rise. With time, most patients become euthyroid and the values normalize.

of iodized salt into the diet in iodine deficient areas (goiter belts). Today it most commonly occurs in patients who have received iodinated contrast media during a computed tomography (CT) exam. The iodine induces a thyroiditis. The %RAIU is usually near zero. Occasionally, the iodine load causes activation of subclinical Graves' disease or toxic multinodular goiter and the uptake is elevated rather than suppressed.

Amiodarone-Induced Thyrotoxicosis Amiodarone is an antiarrhythmic drug containing 75 mg iodine per tablet. It has a physiological half-life of more than 3 months and its effects may last even longer. Hyperthyroidism or hypothyroidism occurs in up to 10% of patients on the drug. Two types of thyrotoxicosis are seen: type I, which is iodine-induced (Jod-Basedow) in patients with preexisting nodular goiter or subclinical Graves' disease, and type II, which is more common and results in a destructive thyroiditis. In the latter, the %RAIU is near zero. In the former, the uptake may be elevated.

Thyrotoxicosis Factitia This is not a rare cause of clinical hyperthyroidism. The thyroid hormone may have been prescribed by a physician or surreptitiously taken by the patient for weight loss. Oftentimes the patients are healthcare workers.

Struma Ovarii Approximately 1–2% of benign ovarian teratomas have functioning thyroid tissue as a major component. In rare instances, this tumor produces sufficient thyroid hormone to cause thyrotoxicosis. The

diagnosis is suspected in a patient with a concomitant pelvic mass. The normal cervical thyroid is suppressed. The ectopic thyroid tissue can be visualized with radioiodine or Tc-99m pertechnetate.

I-131 Therapy Dose Calculation for Graves' Disease This important clinical indication for a %RAIU is discussed in the *Radioiodine Therapy* section later.

Radioiodine Uptake on Thyroid Cancer Scans The %RAIU is frequently calculated at the time of whole body thyroid cancer imaging. It can provide an estimate of postthyroidectomy residual thyroid prior to I-131 ablation therapy and on follow-up scans to quantify the effectiveness of I-131 therapy. The amount of uptake seen visually on the whole body thyroid scan can be misleading because of the variability of background clearance and the windowing used for "optimal" viewing.

Clinical Indications for Thyroid Scintigraphy

Thyroid scans have been used diagnostically for decades for the evaluation of various types of thyroid disease. They are requested less today than in the past because of the availability of other thyroid imaging modalities and the aggressive use of diagnostic percutaneous aspiration biopsy of thyroid nodules. Because of the thyroid scan's functional nature, scintigraphy still provides valuable clinical information for many patients.

Normal Thyroid Scintigraphy

Thyroid scans should always be correlated with physical examination of the thyroid gland and interpreted with knowledge of the patient's thyroid function studies and other imaging studies.

The normal thyroid has a butterfly shape with lateral lobes extending along each side of the thyroid cartilage (*see* Fig. 5-9). The lateral lobes are connected by an isthmus that crosses the trachea anteriorly below the level of the cricoid cartilage. However, the appearance of the gland is quite variable from patient to patient. The right lobe is often larger than the left. The lateral lobes measure 4–5 cm from superior to inferior poles and are 1.5–2 cm wide. The pyramidal lobe ascends from the isthmus or adjacent part of either lobe (more often the left lobe) to the hyoid bone.

The normal gland has homogeneous and uniform distribution of radiotracer throughout. Some increased intensity may be seen in the middle or medial aspects of the lateral lobes, owing to the thickness of the gland in this location. The amount of activity in the isthmus varies greatly, with little or no activity in some patients and prominent activity in others. In normal adults, the thin pyramidal lobe is usually not seen.

The salivary glands are routinely seen on Tc-99m pertechnetate imaging at 20 minutes postinjection. However, they are not usually seen on I-123 scans imaged at 4 hours because the radiopharmaceutical has cleared. Higher generalized background is seen on Tc-99m pertechnetate compared to I-123 imaging.

Esophageal activity can be problematic with either agent. It is frequently not in the midline, being displaced by the trachea and cervical spine when the neck is hyperextended in the imaging position. It is more often seen just to the left of midline and can usually be confirmed by having the patient swallow water to clear the esophagus, followed by repeat imaging (Fig. 5-15).

Abnormal Thyroid Scintigraphy

A systematic interpretation of the thyroid scintigram requires assessment of thyroid size and configuration and the identification of focal abnormalities. These include hot and cold nodules and extrathyroidal activity in the neck or mediastinum. The thyroid scan allows for correlation of palpable abnormalities with scintigraphic findings. This is frequently critical in assigning significance to a palpable abnormality. Radionuclide markers can aid in confirming that the palpated nodule correlates with the scintigraphic finding.

Gland size can be estimated using the thyroid scan but this has limitations due to the scan's two-dimensional nature and the magnification and distortion caused by pinhole collimation. However, image appearance and surface radiomarkers provide some indication of size. Enlargement seen on the scan is often accompanied by a change from a relatively concave to a convex appearance of the lobes.

The major clinical applications for thyroid scintigraphy are listed in Box 5-2. The specific scan findings seen in various disease processes are discussed in this section.

Thyroid Nodule

Thyroid nodules are quite common. They occur more often in women than men. The incidence of both benign and malignant nodules increases with age. Determining whether a nodule is benign or malignant is a common clinical problem. A nodule presenting in a young person, a male, or with recent nodule growth increases concern for malignancy. The presence of multiple nodules decreases the likelihood of malignancy. A nodule in a patient with Graves' disease requires evaluation (Fig. 5-16).

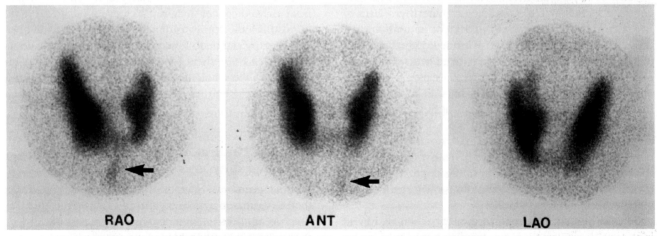

RAO ANT LAO

Figure 5-15 Esophageal activity. Anterior *(ANT)* and right and left anterior oblique *(RAO, LAO)* views obtained with Tc-99m pertechnetate. Note the esophageal activity below the thyroid to the left of midline *(arrows)*.

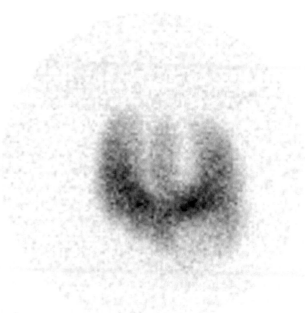

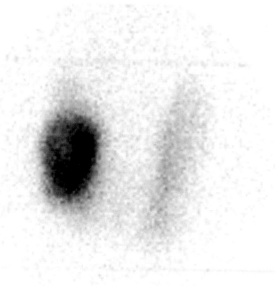

Figure 5-16   Cold thyroid nodule and Graves' disease. Patient presented with a palpable nodule in the inferior aspect of the left lobe. TSH was suppressed and T4 elevated. I-123 thyroid scan shows a non-functional nodule. The gland is full and the pyramidal lobe prominent. The nodule must be evaluated prior to radioiodine therapy.

Figure 5-17   Toxic (hot) thyroid nodule. Patient presented with suppressed TSH, elevated T4 and a palpable nodule in the right lobe of the thyroid. Uptake in the nodule is intense and the remainder of the gland is suppressed.

Radiation to the head and neck or mediastinum is associated with an increased incidence of thyroid cancer, particularly in children. Several decades ago, external radiation therapy was used to shrink asymptomatic enlarged thymus glands and to treat enlarged tonsils, adenoids, and acne. This radiation therapy, usually in the range of 10–50 rads, was associated with an increased incidence of thyroid cancer. The radiation released at Hiroshima, Nagasaki, and Chernobyl also resulted in an increased incidence of thyroid cancer.

Radiation exposure up to 1500 rads increases the incidence of thyroid nodules and cancer. The mean latency period is approximately 5 years. For radiation greater than 1500 rads, the risk decreases, presumably due to tissue destruction. High doses of radiation used in the therapy of malignant tumors are more likely to cause hypothyroidism.

Ultrasonography

Nodules can be confirmed on sonography when suspected on physical exam. Sonography can also detect additional nodules to the palpated one and determine whether a nodule is solid or cystic. Purely cystic lesions are benign; however, cancer cannot be excluded if the cyst has a soft tissue component or cystic degeneration.

Fine Needle Aspiration (FNA)

Aspiration biopsy is often performed today without prior scintigraphy because it is a more direct means of establishing the histology of solitary nodules. This procedure is often performed in the endocrinologist's office.

Sonographic-guided biopsy is used for nonpalpable nodules. Although aspiration biopsy is subject to sampling error, the overall accuracy is high. Benign follicular neoplasms cannot always be distinguished histopathologically from follicular cancer.

Thyroid Scintigraphy

The thyroid scan is more sensitive than physical examination for detecting nodules. Although ultrasonography is more sensitive than scintigraphy for detection of small nodules, the natural history and clinical significance of small nodules seen only on sonography is uncertain. The data used to assign risk to hot or cold nodules is based on scintigraphy correlation with pathology.

The thyroid scan does not diagnose nodules per se. A hot or cold region on the scan may be due to various other pathologies discussed later (e.g., thyroiditis and scarring). A nodule is diagnosed by physical examination of the thyroid or detected by an anatomical imaging modality (e.g., ultrasonography, CT, or MRI).

Thyroid scintigraphy can determine the functional status of a nodule detected by physical examination or anatomical imaging. Thyroid nodules are classified scintigraphically as *cold* (hypofunctioning compared to adjacent normal tissue) (Figs. 5-11 and 5-16), *hot* (hyperfunctioning with suppression of the extranodular gland) (Fig. 5-17), *warm* (increased uptake compared to adjacent tissue but without suppression of the extranodular tissue (Fig. 5-18), or *indeterminate* (palpable but not visualized on scintigraphy). The scan can also show the presence of multiple nodules (multinodular goiter) (Fig. 5-19). This interpretation

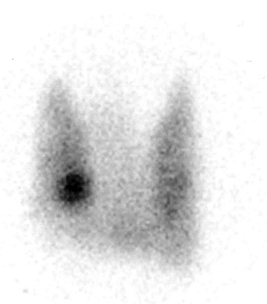

Figure 5-18   Warm thyroid nodule in euthyroid patient. Patient presented with a palpable 1.5 cm nodule. Increased uptake is seen in the inferior aspect of the right lobe of the thyroid. The extranodular gland is not suppressed. The patient had normal thyroid function tests. Thus, the nodule may be autonomous but it is not a toxic nodule.

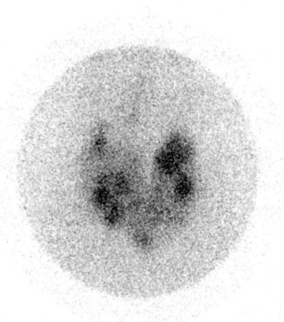

Figure 5-19   Multinodular goiter. The patient has multiple thyroid nodules and thyromegaly by examination. There are increased and decreased regions of uptake in full (convex borders) gland. The patient is euthyroid. The extrathyroidal tissue is not definitely suppressed.

system can provide a relative risk assessment for malignancy (Box 5-10).

Cold Nodule

Greater than 85–90% of thyroid nodules are cold (hypofunctional) on thyroid scintigraphy, that is, they have decreased uptake compared to adjacent thyroid tissue. Many have benign etiologies, such as simple cysts, colloid nodules, thyroiditis, hemorrhage, necrosis, and infiltrative disorders such as amyloid or hemochromotosis (Box 5-11). However, a significant subgroup of patients with cold nodules has malignancy as the etiology.

Box 5-10   Likelihood of Thyroid Cancer in Nodule Based on Thyroid Scintigraphy

NODULE	LIKELIHOOD OF THYROID CANCER
Cold	15–20%
Indeterminate	15–20%
Multinodular	5%
Hot	<1%

Box 5-11   Differential Diagnosis for Thyroid Nodules

Cold nodules (non-functioning)
  Benign
    Colloid nodule
    Simple cyst
    Hemorrhagic cyst
    Adenoma
    Thyroiditis
    Abscess
    Parathyroid cyst or adenoma
  Malignant
    Papillary
    Follicular
    Anaplastic
    Medullary
    Hürthle cell
    Lymphoma
    Metastatic carcinoma
      Lung
      Breast
      Melanoma
      Gastrointestinal
      Renal
Functioning nodules (warm or hot)
  Adenomas
  Hyperfunctioning adenomas

The incidence of thyroid carcinoma in a single cold nodule is reported to be as high as 40% in surgical series but as low as 5% in general medical series. Overall, the incidence of cancer in a cold thyroid nodule is generally considered to be approximately 15–20%. With multinodular goiters, the incidence of malignancy in cold nodules is lower, less than 5%. Enlarging nodules or "dominant" nodules (i.e., those that are distinctly larger than the other nodules in a multinodular goiter) require further evaluation because of relatively increased risk.

Hot and Warm Nodules

Radioiodine uptake within a nodule denotes function. A functioning nodule is very unlikely to be malignant. Less than 1% of hot nodules harbor malignancy. The term *hot nodule* should be reserved for those that not only have high uptake in the nodule scintigraphically, but also have suppression of extranodular tissue (*see* Fig. 5-17). If extranodular tissue is not suppressed, it should be referred to as a warm nodule.

Hot nodules are caused by toxic adenomatous nodules. Warm nodules may be caused by autonomous hyperfunctioning adenomas. However, they are not toxic, that is, they are not producing enough thyroid hormone to cause thyrotoxicosis and thus TSH is not suppressed. A warm nodule may also be due to nonautonomous hyperplastic tissue or even normal functioning tissue surrounded by poorly functioning thyroid. Differentiation can be made by administration of thyroid hormone (thyroid suppression test). Autonomous nodules cannot be suppressed (see *T-3 Suppression Test*). However, the suppression test is rarely needed in current practice.

Large hot nodules greater than 2.5–3.0 cm usually produce overt hyperthyroidism. Some patients with smaller nodules have subclinical hyperthyroidism, which can be confirmed by a suppressed serum TSH but normal T_4. In the past, a small autonomous nodule might be followed clinically because some stabilize, whereas others regress or undergo involution (Fig. 5-20). Increasingly, nodules are treated at an early stage because of the low incidence of regression and increased awareness of adverse consequences associated with subclinical hyperthyroidism (e.g., bone mineral loss).

Radioiodine I-131 is the usual therapeutic method of choice for toxic nodules. Radiation is delivered selectively to the hyperfunctioning tissue while sparing suppressed extranodular tissues. The suppression of normal tissue results in a low incidence of posttherapy hypothyroidism. After successful treatment of the nodule, the suppressed tissue regains function. Surgery, usually lobectomy, may be indicated if there are local symptoms or cosmetic concerns.

Indeterminate Nodule

When a palpable or sonographically detected nodule greater than a centimeter in size cannot be differentiated

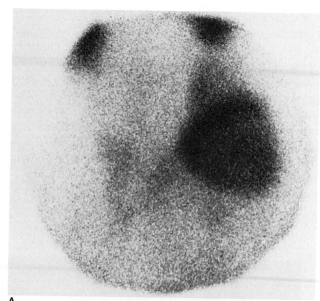

A

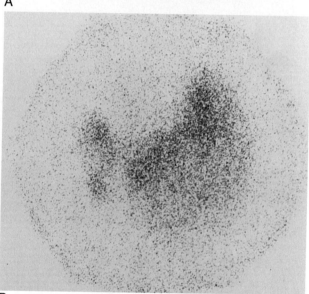

B

Figure 5-20   Spontaneous resolution of a hot nodule. **A,** Thyroid scan reveals a large, hot nodule in the left lobe of the thyroid. The center of the nodule appears to have less intense tracer activity than the periphery, suggesting central degeneration. **B,** Follow-up scan 1 year later reveals complete involution of the hot nodule, with residual distortion of the gland.

by thyroid scan as hot or cold compared to surrounding normal thyroid, it is referred to as an indeterminate nodule. A cold nodule arising from the posterior aspect of the gland may have normal glandular activity superimposed over the nodule, making it appear to have normal uptake. For management purposes, an indeterminate nodule has the same significance as a cold nodule. The possibility of an indeterminate nodule highlights the need for close correlation between physical and scintigraphic findings.

Discordant Nodule

Discordance in appearance between radioiodine and Tc-99m pertechnetate scans is seen in a small minority of patients. A nodule may appear hot on pertechnetate imaging but cold on radioiodine imaging because Tc-99m pertechnetate is trapped but not organified (Fig. 5-21). This discordance occurs in approximately 5% of hot nodules seen on Tc-99m pertechnetate scans. Because some thyroid cancers maintain trapping but not the organification function, a single hot nodule identified on Tc-99m pertechnetate imaging should not be considered a functioning nodule until confirmed by radioiodine studies.

Still, a minority of discordant nodules are malignant (20%). The discordant nodule is a drawback to the use of Tc-99m pertechnetate for routine thyroid scintigraphy.

Goiter

The term *goiter* refers to thyroid gland enlargement, but it is often qualified to indicate the cause of the enlargement (e.g., toxic nodular goiter, colloid goiter, or diffuse toxic goiter [Graves' disease]) (Box 5-12).

Graves' Disease vs. Multinodular Toxic Goiter

In a patient with newly diagnosed thyrotoxicosis, the physical exam can usually differentiate the diffuse goiter

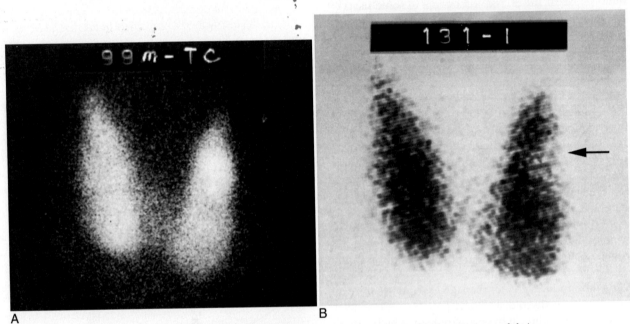

A   B

Figure 5-21 Discordant nodule. **A,** Tc-99m pertechnetate scan reveals a functioning nodule in the left upper pole. **B,** In the corresponding iodine-131 scintigram the nodule is cold. Thus the nodule can trap but not organify iodine. This requires further work-up.

Box 5-12 Conditions Associated with Goiter

Graves' disease: Autoimmune disease associated with hyperthyroidism and exophthalmos. Patients have diffuse hyperplasia of the thyroid gland and thyroid-stimulating immunoglobulins (TSIs).

Plummer's disease: Hyperthyroidism associated with toxic nodular goiter (one or more nodules).

Hashimoto's disease (Hashimoto's thyroiditis): Form of thyroiditis and autoimmune disorder often leading to hypothyroidism. Patients may rarely experience transient hyperthyroidism ("Hashitoxicosis").

de Quervain's disease: Subacute thyroiditis, with granulomatous infiltration and destruction of thyroid cells. Transient hyperthyroidism early in course.

Riedel's struma (Riedel's thyroiditis): Chronic fibrous replacement of the thyroid gland.

Jod-Basedow phenomenon: Induction of thyrotoxicosis in a euthyroid individual after exposure to large amounts of iodine. Occurs in areas of endemic iodine-deficient goiter or after use of iodine contrast agents.

Wolff-Chaikoff effect: Paradoxical blocking of iodine incorporation into thyroid hormone resulting from large amounts of iodine.

Marine-Lenhart syndrome: Graves' disease with incidentally functioning nodules that are responsive to thyroid-stimulating hormone but are not responsive to TSIs.

of Graves' disease (Fig. 5-22) from a multinodular toxic gland (*see* Fig. 5-19). The thyroid scintigram can help make the distinction. Toxic nodular goiter has the characteristic scintigraphic pattern of increased uptake that corresponds to palpable nodules and suppression of extranodular thyroid tissue. This contrasts with the diffuse homogenous increased uptake of Graves' disease. The pyramidal lobe, a paramedian structure arising superiorly from the isthmus (right or left lobe), is also usually well visualized (*see* Fig. 5-22) with Graves' disease.

Colloid Nodular Goiter

Before the addition of iodine supplements to salt and food, goiter was endemic in the northern United States around the Great Lakes, and still occurs in some parts of the world. These endemic goiters were typically composed of colloid nodules (colloid nodular goiters) and most were benign.

The pathogenesis of nodule formation in these patients is iodine deficiency-induced hyperplasia followed by the formation of functioning nodules that undergo hemorrhage and necrosis replaced by lakes of colloid. Repetition of this process over time leads to glandular enlargement, with nonfunctioning colloid nodules as the dominant histopathological feature. The typical scintigraphic appearance of benign multinodular colloid goiters is inhomogeneous uptake of tracer with cold areas of various sizes (Fig. 5-23).

Substernal Goiter

Most substernal goiters are extensions of the thyroid into the mediastinum. As they enlarge, they may cause symptoms of dyspnea, dysphagia, or stridor. Many are asymptomatic and incidentally detected as an anterior upper mediastinal mass on CT. A radioiodine scan can confirm the thyroid origin of this mass (*see* Fig. 5-10).

Scintigraphy   Tc-99m pertechnetate is not suited for this purpose because of its high mediastinal blood pool activity. The ability to perform delayed imaging after tissue and blood pool clearance of background activity is the advantage of I-131 for evaluation of a substernal goiter. Iodine uptake in substernal goiters is often poor and the highest target-to-background ratio possible is desirable. Imaging at 24–48 hours is sometimes necessary.

The rationale for the use of I-131 rather than I-123 for evaluating a substernal goiter has been that I-123 would be attenuated by the sternum. However, attenuation with I-123 is only in the range of 10–20%. In most cases, I-123 can provide similar information with better image quality and lower radiation to the patient.

The usual cervical location of the thyroid gland should always be imaged when searching for a substernal goiter because most demonstrate continuity with the cervical portion of the gland, although some patients have only a fibrous band connecting the substernal and cervical thyroid tissues.

Ectopic Thyroid Tissue

The thyroglossal duct runs from the foramen caecum at the base of the tongue to the thyroid. If it fails to migrate

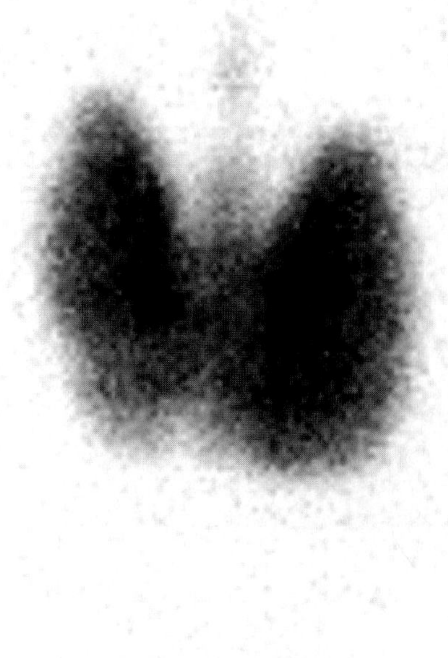

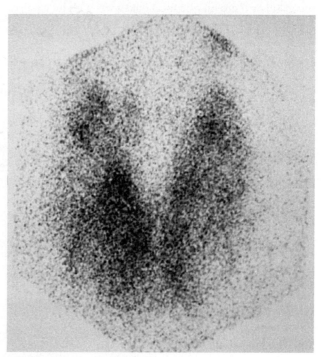

Figure 5-22   Graves' disease. Large goiter with high uptake. The %RAIU was 65%. Note the pyramidal lobe.

Figure 5-23   Colloid nodular goiter. Goiter with inhomogeneous tracer distribution and focal cold areas corresponding to nodules.

from its anlage, lingual or upper cervical thyroid tissue can present in the neonate or child as a midline mass with or without obstructive symptoms and often accompanied by hypothyroidism. Ectopic thyroid tissue may also be mediastinal (substernal goiter) or even pelvic/ovarian (struma ovarii).

Scintigraphy

The typical appearance of a *lingual thyroid* is a focal or nodular accumulation at the base of the tongue and absence of tracer uptake in the expected cervical location (Fig. 5-24). However, lingual thyroids usually function poorly. Lateral thyroid rests are also often hypofunctional. However, rests can function, hyperfunction, or be involved with adenocarcinoma of the thyroid. Functioning ectopic thyroid tissue should be considered metastatic until proven otherwise.

Subacute Thyroiditis

This entity is discussed in the section *Thyrotoxicosis*. With hyperthyroidism, the scan shows only suppression (*see* Fig. 5-13). During recovery phases, the appearance of the thyroid is variable and depends upon the severity and distribution of the disease (Fig. 5-25). The scintigram may show inhomogeneity of uptake, regional areas of hypofunction, or even focal hypofunction.

Chronic Thyroiditis (Hashimoto's Thyroiditis)

Scintigraphic findings are highly variable. Diffuse enlargement is usual, although the scan may be normal early in the process. Uptake may be inhomogeneous throughout the gland or there may be focal cold areas without a palpable nodule. The pyramidal lobe is often seen in Hashimoto's disease.

Acute Thyroiditis

Suppurative bacterial infection is the usual cause for this rare condition. The thyroid is typically enlarged and tender. Focal abscesses will appear as cold regions scintigraphically. *Reidel's struma* is an uncommon form of thyroiditis where all or part of the gland is replaced by fibrous tissue. No uptake is seen in the region of fibrous tissue.

Thyroid Cancer

Whole body thyroid cancer scintigraphy has long been used for well-differentiated papillary and follicular thyroid cancer. It is often performed post-thyroidectomy prior to radioiodine I-131 therapy and for evaluating response therapy (Fig. 5-26). The most common sites of metastasis are locally in the lymph nodes of the neck, lung, mediastinum, and bones (Fig. 5-27). Medullary carcinomas and anaplastic carcinomas do not concentrate radioiodine and are not detected with conventional thyroid scintigraphy.

Whole body thyroid cancer scanning requires patient preparation. The traditional approach is to withdraw hormone replacement therapy for 4-6 weeks so that patients may achieve a maximal endogenous thyroid-stimulating hormone (TSH) response (>30 U/ml). To minimize symptoms of hypothyroidism, patients are sometimes switched to short-acting triiodothyronine (T_3), which is discontinued 2 weeks prior to the scan.

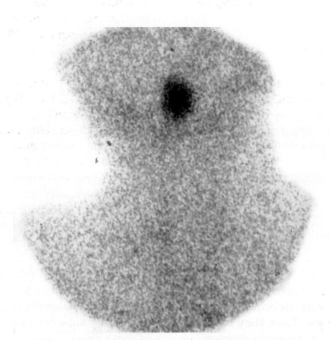

Figure 5-24   Lingual thyroid. Hypothyroid infant with neck mass. Scan (anterior view) shows prominent uptake within the neck mass and no thyroid in region of thyroid bed.

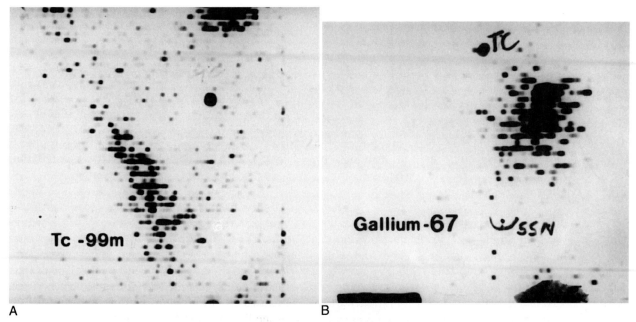

Figure 5-25   Resolving subacute thyroiditis. **A,** Tc-99m pertechnetate scan in a patient with resolving subacute thyroiditis affecting the left lobe. The patient is now moderately hypothyroid. There is lack of tracer uptake in the left lobe and decreased accumulation in the right lobe. **B,** Corresponding gallium-67 scintigram reveals marked focal accumulation in the area of the left lobe, indicating inflammatory nature of the process.

Imaging with I-131 is typically performed 48 hours after I-131 diagnostic dose administration (Box 5-13). More lesions are demonstrated in this time than at 24 hours due to background clearance and the higher target-to-background ratio. Serum thyroglobulin levels are also measured during maximum TSH stimulation (a sensitive tumor marker). For I-123, whole body imaging is acquired at 24 hours (Box 5-14).

Postthyroidectomy, it is not uncommon to have high intensity uptake in the thyroid bed (*star artifact*), which may preclude good visualization of the neck or mediastinum. The artifact is caused by septal penetration of high-energy photons through the collimator (*see* Fig. 5-12). A pinhole collimator that has no septa can better resolve the high intensity uptake in the neck. In the postoperative state, uptake in the neck may be due to residual normal thyroid or to thyroid cancer. The scan cannot make the distinction. Activity outside the thyroid bed is very likely metastatic.

Other Thyroid Imaging Radiopharmaceuticals

Tl-201 and Tc-99m Sestamibi
Both radiotracers are nonspecific tumor imaging agents. Uptake of these radiopharmaceuticals occurs in benign as well as malignant conditions. Thus, they have not found widespread application in the initial diagnosis of thyroid cancer. Some advocate their use for thyroid can-

cer follow-up imaging, where differentiating uptake in normal tissue and benign lesions from tumor is not an issue. One advantage is that patients need not discontinue thyroid hormone replacement therapy before imaging. This approach has mainly found acceptance for locating metastases in patients with increased serum thyroglobulin levels and negative radioiodine whole body scintigrams. F-18 fluorodeoxyglucose (FDG) positron emission tomography (PET) imaging is rapidly taking over that indication.

F-18 Fluorodeoxyglucose (FDG)
The sensitivity of F-18 FDG PET for detection of well-differentiated thyroid cancer metastases is not high (~70%) and thus not generally used for routine thyroid cancer imaging. Its major indication has been in patients who have had negative I-131 whole body scans but elevated serum thyroglobulin levels. In these patients, the tumor has dedifferentiated into a higher grade tumor. Many of these patients have focal uptake of F-18 FDG at the site of metastasis (Fig. 5-28). A higher-grade tumor increases the likelihood of FDG uptake. Localization of the tumor allows for surgical resection or evaluation of response to therapy.

On whole body FDG PET performed for staging or surveillance of other oncologic tumors, focal F-18 FDG uptake is occasionally seen in the thyroid. This finding usually indicates thyroid pathology. Up to one-half of these patients have incidental primary thyroid cancers diagnosed. Other causes of focal uptake include

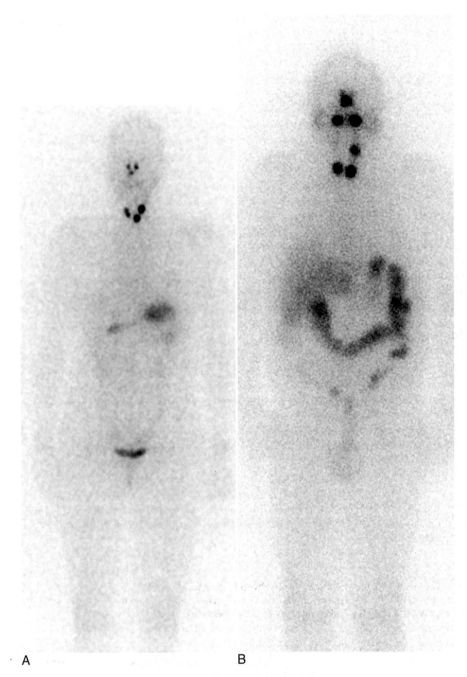

Figure 5-26   Whole body I-123 thyroid cancer scans pre- and post-I-131 ablation therapy. **A,** The postthyroidectomy, pre-I-131 ablation therapy scan shows uptake limited to three focal areas in the thyroid bed. There are no local or distant metastases. Normal stomach and urinary clearance. **B,** Seven days post-I-131 therapy, there has been no significant change from the pretherapy scan, except for liver uptake due to metabolism of I-131 labeled thyroid hormone.

A   B

metastatic cancer, benign follicular adenoma, and thyroiditis. Diffuse gland uptake can be seen with thyroiditis and Graves' disease.

I-131/I-123 Metaiodobenzylguanidine (MIBG)

Some medullary carcinomas of the thyroid demonstrate I-123 or I-131 MIBG uptake. However, the sensitivity is low (~30%). MIBG localizes in neurosecretory storage vesicles of chromaffin cells. Soft tissue metastases are better visualized than skeletal metastases. The low sensitivity precludes a routine role for MIBG in the workup of medullary thyroid cancer.

Indium-111 Somatostatin Receptor Scintigraphy

Medullary carcinoma of the thyroid is a neuroectodermal tumor. However, unlike many neuroendocrine tumors, sensitivity for detection of medullary carcinoma of the thyroid with In-111 somatostatin receptor scintigraphy (OctreoScan) is low (<50%).

Other Thyroid Function Studies

Most of these classical pharmacologic interventions are not commonly used today and are of historical interest, but are pertinent to an understanding of

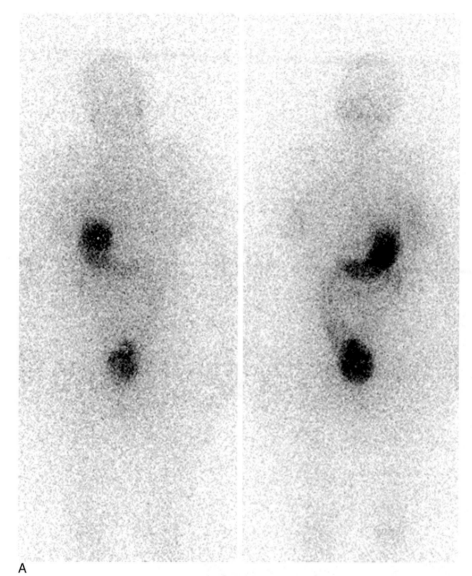

A

Figure 5-27   Lung metastases seen post-I-131 therapy. Follicular thyroid carcinoma treated with total thyroidectomy and I-131 ablation three years prior. Serum thyroglobulin level is now elevated. **A,** I-123 whole body pre-therapy scan shows no uptake in the neck or elsewhere to suggest metastases.

Continued

thyroid physiology and interpretation of present-day studies.

T₃ Suppression Test

The test's clinical utility was for diagnosing patients with borderline Graves' disease and autonomous functioning glands. In the T_3 suppression test, a baseline 24-hour uptake is obtained. The patient then receives 25 mcg of T_3 four times a day for 8 days. The 24-hour uptake is repeated beginning on day 7. A normal response to thy-

roid suppression is a fall in the percentage of uptake to less than 50% of the baseline value and less than 10% overall. An autonomously functioning gland will not suppress. Very sensitive tests for TSH levels are now used and can accurately detect early hyperthyroidism.

TSH Stimulation Test

The test has been used to distinguish primary from secondary (pituitary) hypothyroidism. Failure to respond to exogenous TSH is indicative of primary hypothyroidism.

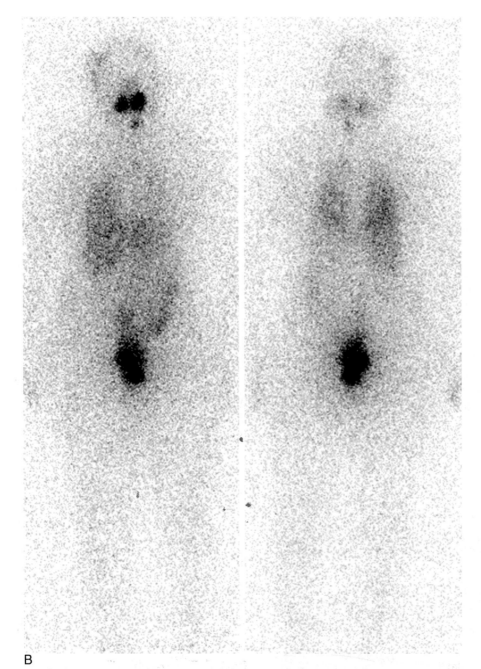

B

Figure 5-27, cont'd   B, After 150 mCi of I-131, the scan shows uptake diffusely throughout both lung fields consistent with miliary lung metastases.

Patients with secondary hypothyroidism have increased radioiodine uptake after TSH stimulation. The stimulation test is performed by first determining a baseline 24-hour radioiodine percent uptake. The patient then receives TSH intramuscularly. The %RAIU is repeated beginning the next day. In healthy subjects and patients with hypopituitarism the uptake should double, whereas those with primary hypothyroidism show no response.

Perchlorate Discharge Test
The perchlorate discharge test demonstrates dissociation of the trapping and organification functions in the

Box 5-13 Iodine-131 Whole Body Imaging for Thyroid Cancer: Protocol Summary

PATIENT PREPARATION

Discontinue thyroid hormone for a sufficient period (T_4 for 6 weeks, T_3 for 2 weeks) to ensure maximum endogenous thyroid-stimulating hormone response (>30 µU/mL).

RADIOPHARMACEUTICAL

Withdrawal: 2 mCi (74 MBq), orally
Thyrogen: 4 mCi (148 MBq)

IMAGING TIME

At 48 hours.

PROCEDURE

Use a wide field-of-view gamma camera with computer acquisition.
Use a high-energy parallel-hole collimator and a 20% window centered at 364 keV.
Whole body scan and a 20-min spot view to include head, neck, and mediastinum.
Calculate a percent radioactive iodine uptake.

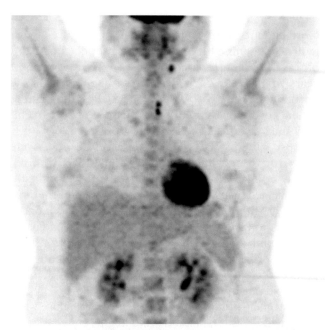

Figure 5-28 F-18 FDG PET scan for thyroid cancer. Patient had negative I-123 whole body scan but elevated serum thyroglobulin. The FDG PET scan shows focal uptake in the left neck as well as abnormal uptake in the paratracheal region, consistent with dedifferentiated tumor metastases.

thyroid. This occurs with congenital enzyme deficiencies, in chronic thyroiditis, and during therapy with propylthiouracil. The patient receives a tracer dose of radioiodine. The percent uptake is measured at 1–2 hours. One gram of potassium perchlorate is then given orally and the percent uptake is measured hourly. A washout greater than 10% suggests an organification defect.

Box 5-14 Iodine-123 Whole Body Imaging for Thyroid Cancer: Protocol Summary

PATIENT PREPARATION

Discontinue thyroid hormone for a sufficient period (T_4 for 6 weeks, T_3 for 2 weeks) to ensure maximum endogenous thyroid-stimulating hormone response (>30 µU/mL).

RADIOPHARMACEUTICAL

Withdrawal: 1.5 mCi (56 MBq), orally
Thyrogen: 2 mCi (74 MBq)

IMAGING TIME

At 24 hours.

PROCEDURE

Use a wide field-of-view gamma camera with computer acquisition.
Use a high-energy parallel-hole collimator and a 20% window centered at 364 keV.
Whole body scan and a 20-min spot view to include head, neck, and mediastinum.
Calculate a percent radioactive iodine uptake.

Radioiodine Therapy

Graves' Disease

Pharmacologic and Surgical Therapy

Patients with newly diagnosed Graves' disease are often treated with beta-blockers, which provide prompt symptomatic relief. More specific therapy with thiourea antithyroid drugs that block organification, such as propylthiouracil (PTU) and methimazole (Tapazole), reduce thyroid hormone production. These drugs are used to "cool" the patient down, render them euthyroid, and provide time to consider further therapeutic options. Patients may take these drugs for 6–12 months. These drugs have a rather high incidence of adverse effects (50%), the most serious being liver dysfunction and agranulocytosis. The latter side effects are not common but quite serious, thus the drugs are rarely administered for longer than a year. Thyroidectomy is a rather uncommon form of therapy for Graves' disease.

Radioactive Iodine

Most patients with Graves' disease are treated with radioactive iodine I-131, some early after diagnosis and others 6–12 months later (Box 5-15). There is over 50 years of experience with use of therapeutic I-131. Endocrinologists have become comfortable with treating patients, even children, with I-131 because of its high efficacy and low incidence of adverse affects.

Most patients with Graves' disease are effectively treated with one therapeutic dose of I-131. Approximately 10% require a second treatment. Symptomatic improvement is usually noted by 3 weeks after therapy. However, the full therapeutic effect takes 3–6 months because stored hormone must first be released and used. The exophthalmos of Graves' disease is not controlled by thiourea drugs or radioactive iodine. Some evidence suggests exacerbation of exophthalmos with I-131 therapy, so steroids are often administered.

In women, pregnancy must be ruled out before I-131 therapy. Because the fetal thyroid begins concentrating iodine at 10–12 weeks of gestation, cretinism may occur after therapeutic doses of I-131 given during pregnancy. Women should be counseled to avoid pregnancy for 3–6 months after therapy in case retreatment is indicated.

Most patients eventually become hypothyroid and need replacement hormone therapy. Hypothyroidism can occur within several months or decades after therapy. A greater administered dose causes earlier onset of hypothyroidism, and vice versa.

Various approaches have been used for selecting an I-131 dose for therapy of Graves' disease. One approach is to prescribe a standard I-131 dose in the range of 8–15 mCi. Overall, this usually works well. However, factors such as the size of the gland and the %RAIU may result in very different radiation doses to the thyroid in different patients. Generally, large glands require a relatively higher therapeutic dose and patients with a high %RAIU require a lower dose.

A commonly used formula takes both of these factors, gland size and %RAIU, into consideration (Box 5-16):

$$\text{I-131 administered dose} = \frac{\text{gram size of thyroid gland} \times 100\text{–}180 \ \mu\text{Ci/gm}}{24\text{-hour \%RAIU}}$$

This approach calculates an individual therapy dose for each patient with Graves' disease. An estimation of the gram weight of the gland is required. A normal gland weighs 15–20 gm. Patients with Graves' disease often have glands in the range of 40–80 gm and larger. There is considerable interphysician variability in gland size estimation.

The other variable in this calculation is the μCi/gm dose. Often in the past, referring physicians requested low I-131 doses to minimize the radiation to the patient (e.g., 60–80 μCi/gm tissue). Referring physicians are increasingly comfortable with the safety of higher doses (120–180 μCi/gm tissue) and prefer the increased likelihood of success with a single therapeutic dose. Early onset hypothyroidism is also often preferred by some because it is inevitable in any event and prompt replacement therapy can be instituted.

In patients demonstrating rapid radioiodine turnover in the gland (i.e., high 4-hour but normal or near-normal 24-hour %RAIU), a higher I-131 dose than would be

---

Box 5-15 Indications for Iodine-131 Therapy

INDICATED

Graves' disease (diffuse toxic goiter)
Plummer's disease (toxic nodular goiter)
Functioning thyroid cancer (metastatic)

NOT INDICATED

Thyrotoxicosis factitia
Subacute thyroiditis
"Silent" thyroiditis (atypical, subacute, lymphocytic, transient, postpartum)
Struma ovarii
Thyroid hormone resistance (biochemical/clinical manifestations)
Secondary hyperthyroidism (pituitary tumor, ectopic thyroid-stimulating hormone, trophoblastic tumors [human chorionic gonadotropin])
Thyrotoxicosis associated with Hashimoto's disease ("Hashitoxicosis")
Jod-Basedow phenomenon (iodine-induced hyperthyroidism)

Box 5-16 Calculation of Iodine-131 Therapeutic Dose for Graves' Hyperthyroidism

INPUT DATA

Gland weight: 60 g
24-hour uptake: 80%
Desired dose to be retained in thyroid (selected to deliver 8000 to 10,000 rads to thyroid): 100 μCi/g

CALCULATIONS

$$\text{Required dose (}\mu\text{Ci)} = \frac{60 \text{ g} \times 100 \ \mu\text{Ci/g}}{0.80} = 7500$$

$$\text{Dose (mCi)} = \frac{7500}{1000} = 7.5 \text{ mCi}$$

calculated using the 24-hour %RAIU should be considered. This indicates a shorter residence time within the thyroid.

Some patients report local neck pain, tenderness, and swelling after I-131 therapy due to radiation thyroiditis. Thyroiditis results in release of thyroid hormone and poses the risk of thyroid storm, although this is rare. Patients with florid disease and those treated with higher amounts of radioactivity are at greater risk. In older patients who have preexisting heart disease and in patients otherwise at risk, medical therapy with thiourea drugs can be carried out for several months to deplete thyroid hormone before radioiodine therapy. Beta blockers are often used both before and after therapy to minimize this risk.

Other secondary effects of radiation exposure (e.g., secondary cancers, infertility, abnormal offspring) have been a concern. Evidence collected over a half-century of I-131 therapy has shown no statistically significant difference in the frequency of these events between patients receiving I-131 therapy and patients treated by surgery for Graves' disease. I-131 therapy does not reduce fertility and congenital defects are not increased in the children of treated individuals. Patients treated with I-131 have a somewhat higher incidence of leukemia than the general population.

Toxic Nodular Goiter

Patients with hyperthyroidism caused by a toxic multinodular goiter are generally more resistant to therapy with radioiodine than patients with diffuse toxic goiter (Graves' disease). The reason is uncertain. Radioiodine turnover may be higher in these nodules, leading to a lower retained dose. Thus the dose of radioiodine should be increased by at least 50% over what would be given for Graves' disease. An empirical dose, often in the range of 20–25 mCi, is often given. Because extranodular tissue in the thyroid is suppressed, it is spared from radiation and usually resumes normal function after successful therapy. Patients with a single toxic nodule are often treated similarly. A more sophisticated approach would be to use the formula described for Graves' disease (see Box 5-16). In place of the estimated gland size for Graves' disease, replace it with a calculation of the volume of the nodule (V = 4/3 Πr^3).

Thyroid Cancer

Radioactive iodine I-131 has also been used extensively in the treatment of differentiated thyroid cancer. It is not useful for treating anaplastic and medullary cancers. Postsurgical ablation of normal thyroid remnants reduces local recurrences and allows the patient to be followed with serum thyroglobulins and radioiodine whole body thyroid cancer scans. Patients with residual or recurrent differentiated thyroid cancer have improved survival with I-131 treatment.

Patients are prepared for therapy by discontinuing thyroid hormone therapy. A diagnostic scan is usually done to establish the presence of residual thyroid tissue or metastatic disease. Serum thyroglobulin levels are also measured. In the past, patients had to remain hospitalized and isolated until retained whole body activity was less than 30 mCi. The Nuclear Regulatory Commission has published new rules (10CFR 20 and 35) for release of patients based on the likely exposure to others. The release criterion state that no person should receive more than 5 millisieverts (0.5 rem) from exposure to a released I-131 treated patient. In general, this allows for considerably higher release activity. At some centers, the majority of patients are now treated on an outpatient basis.

Radiation safety instructions are discussed with the patient and family. Patient specific information regarding limiting close contact and preventing exposure to others is provided.

A whole body scan 7 days after the therapeutic dose is generally routine. Metastatic disease not seen on the pretherapy diagnostic scan may be detected due to the high therapy administered dose. After therapy, the patient is placed back on thyroid hormone replacement and suppressive therapy. Retreatment is usually not considered for at least 6 and usually 12 months to avoid bone marrow damage.

Metastatic disease most commonly occurs locally in the neck. Distant metastases have a predilection for the lung and skeleton. Brain and liver metastases are less common. Therapeutic doses vary somewhat by institution; however, regional neck metastases typically receive 75–100 mCi and lung and bone metastases receive 150–200 mCi. Follow-up imaging is usually carried out at yearly intervals until all detected metastases are eliminated with repeat therapy. Concern about bone marrow suppression and leukemia increases as the total dose approaches 500 mCi. Doses greater than 1000 mCi are rarely administered.

PARATHYROID SCINTIGRAPHY

Parathyroid scintigraphy has changed over the years from a procedure with a variable reported accuracy that was considered unnecessary by many surgeons to a much improved imaging methodology with good accuracy, which has become accepted by endocrinologists and neck surgeons as part of the routine preoperative workup of hyperparathyroidism. The importance of preoperative parathyroid imaging has paralleled the growth of minimally invasive surgery and the use of intraoperative gamma probe methodology.

Anatomy and Embryology

There are usually four parathyroid glands, two upper and two lower, measuring approximately 6 mm × 3 mm and weighing 35–40 gm. A fifth supernumerary gland occurs in 10% of individuals. Rarely, there may be only two glands or as many as eight.

The *inferior parathyroid glands* arise from the third branchial pouch and migrate caudally with the thymus. Their location is somewhat variable with 60% located just posterior to the lower thyroid poles, 25% in the cervical portion of the thymus gland, and a minority within the thyroid gland or at various positions from the angle of the jaw to the arch of the aorta (Fig. 5-29). The *superior glands* arise from the fourth branchial pouch and migrate with the thyroid. They are usually just posterior to the upper thyroid lobes. Only 1% are ectopic, located between the thyroid and esophagus, within the carotid sheath, behind the innominate vein, or in the posterior mediastinum.

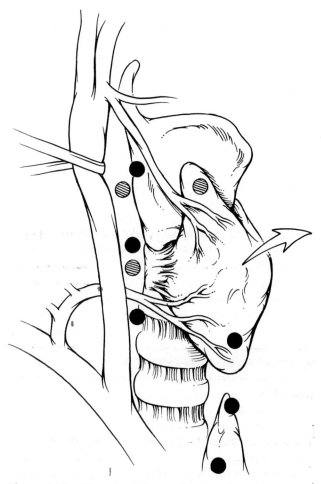

Figure 5-29   Normal and aberrant location of parathyroid glands. The superior pair of glands (*striped circles*) often lie within the fascial covering of the posterior aspect of the thyroid gland outside the capsule, although rarely intrathyroidal. Most are adjacent to the thyroid or cricothyroid cartilage, rarely retropharyngeal or retroesophageal. Inferior glands (*black circles*) are more variable. Many are located inferior, lateral or posterior to the lower pole of the thyroid gland. They are commonly found in the thyrothymic ligament or even in the cervical thymus. A small percent migrate to the superior mediastinum. Rare ectopic glands are found superiorly. Arrow indicates retraction of the thyroid.

There are two types of cells in the parathyroid. The predominant functioning cell is the chief cell which produces parathormone (PTH). It has little cytoplasm or mitochondria. The oxyphil cells have a higher proportion of mitochondria and are increased in number in diseased glands.

Pathophysiology

Hyperparathyroidism

Increased synthesis and release of parathyroid hormone (PTH) from the chief cells of a single gland or multiple glands characterizes this disease. PTH is an 84-amino acid polypeptide synthesized, stored, and secreted by the parathyroid glands. The hormone is responsible for calcium and phosphorus homeostasis by its action on bone, small intestine, and the kidneys. Sporadic parathyroid adenomas are caused by somatic mutations with subsequent clonal expansion of the mutated cells. Primary hyperplasia is a polyclonal proliferation. In patients with familial multiendocrine neoplasia (MEN syndrome), hyperparathyroidism is secondary to a multiglandular hyperplasia.

Primary hyperparathyroidism is caused by abnormal parathyroid gland or glands that secrete excessive PTH. Greater than 85% of patients with primary hyperthyroidism have adenomas as the cause (Box 5-17). Most of the others have multigland hyperplasia. Less than 1% of patients with hyperparathyroidism have carcinoma of the parathyroid gland. They tend to have marked elevations in serum calcium associated with palpable neck mass, bone pain, fractures, and renal colic.

Secondary hyperparathyroidism occurs in patients with renal insufficiency. It is an appropriate compensatory mechanism to increase the serum calcium level, which is low in patients with renal failure. Despite the elevated serum PTH, the serum calcium level remains below normal levels.

Tertiary hyperparathyroidism occurs in patients with renal failure when one or more of the glands become autonomous and produces hypercalcemia.

Clinical Presentation

In the past, patients often presented with nephrolithiasis and osteitis fibrosa cystica associated with osteoporosis, pathologic fractures, and brown tumors. Many had gastrointestinal and neuropsychiatric symptoms. Today,

Box 5-17 Etiology of Hyperparathyroidism	
Adenoma	85%
Hyperplasia	10%
Ectopic	<5%
Carcinoma	<1%

most patients are asymptomatic and diagnosed during routine blood test screening. The diagnosis is suspected clinically because of an elevated serum calcium level and a reduced serum inorganic phosphate. There are numerous other causes of hypercalcemia. The most common is malignancy. Others include vitamin D intoxication, sarcoidosis, and thiazide diuretics.

Diagnosis

The diagnosis of primary hyperparathyroidism is made clinically. An elevated parathormone level in a patient with hypercalcemia is diagnostic of primary hyperparathyroidism. Most other causes of hypercalcemia, except parathyroid carcinoma, have reduced parathormone levels. Imaging is performed for localization, not diagnosis.

Treatment

Bone mineral density loss caused by hyperparathyroidism is of increasing concern and early surgical resection is an increasingly common practice. The standard operation has been bilateral neck exploration with removal of the adenoma. Hyperplasia usually requires removal of 3.5 glands. Increasingly, minimally invasive surgery is being performed, which permits a shortened operation time and fewer complications. The latter approach requires preoperative imaging for localization. Some surgeons now use a gamma probe in the operating suite to help localize the hyperfunctioning gland(s).

Post-operative recurrence rates are in the range of 5–10%. Common reasons for surgical failure include: (1) an abnormal location of the tumor within the neck or mediastinum, (2) failure to recognize hyperplasia, or (3) an undiscovered fifth gland. Re-exploration has an increased morbidity and poorer success rate than the primary procedure. Thus preoperative imaging is particularly valuable in this group of patients.

Preoperative Noninvasive Imaging

Various imaging techniques have been used to preoperatively localize hyperfunctioning parathyroid glands. The accuracy of ultrasonography, computed tomography, and magnetic resonance imaging are inferior to present-day methods of performing scintigraphy. The other imaging modalities are particularly insensitive for detecting ectopic and mediastinal glands. Numerous different scintigraphic protocols have been used over the years. Tl-201/Tc 99m pertechnetate imaging has long been abandoned in favor of Tc-99m sestamibi protocols.

Radiopharmaceuticals

Selenium-75 selenomethionine was the first radiopharmaceutical used for parathyroid scintigraphy in 1965. This amino acid analog of methionine is incorporated into areas of protein synthesis. Image quality was poor and accuracy was suboptimal.

The thallium-201/Tc-99m pertechnetate subtraction technique was used in the 1980s. Tl-201 is a nonspecific tumor imaging agent taken up by both benign and malignant tumors, including hyperfunctioning parathyroid glands. Being a blood flow agent, it is also avidly taken up by normal thyroid. Tc-99m pertechnetate is only extracted by thyroid tissue.

With commonly used methodology, Tl-201 was administered first and a neck image acquired on computer. Then Tc-99m pertechnetate was administered and another image acquired. The Tc-99m activity was then computer subtracted from the Tl-201 (Fig. 5-30). This method has been abandoned because of the poor imaging characteristics of thallium-201, difficulties associated with patient motion and computer image registration, variable reported accuracy, and the advent of Tc-99m sestamibi.

Technetium-99m Sestamibi and Tc-99m Tetrofosmin

Mechanism of Uptake

Tc-99m sestamibi (Cardiolite), like Tl-201, is a cardiac imaging agent. Sestamibi is a lipophilic cation and member of the isonitrile family (hexakis 2-methoxyisobutyl isonitrile). The mechanism of uptake is probably related to high cellularity and tumor vascularity. It localizes within the cytoplasm and mitochondria of the cell because of electrical potentials. The large number of mitochondria oxyphil cells of parathyroid adenomas may be responsible for its avid uptake and slow release compared to surrounding tissue. Tc-99m tetrofosmin is similar to Tc-99m sestamibi in its mechanism of uptake; however, data are more limited.

Pharmacokinetics

Tc-99m sestamibi has higher uptake than Tl-201, superior image quality, and lower radiation dosimetry. Peak accumulation occurs at 3–5 minutes with a half-time clearance of approximately 60 minutes. In addition, sestamibi has interesting washout characteristics. Tc-99m sestamibi usually clears slower from hyperfunctioning parathyroid tissue than adjacent thyroid tissue. This is the rationale for early (10 min) and late (2 hour) imaging. By delayed imaging, the thyroid has usually cleared, leaving uptake in the hyperfunctioning parathyroid tissue (Fig. 5-31).

Methodology

Tc-99m sestamibi, 20–25 mCi, is injected intravenously. The study is commonly performed in two phases, early planar imaging at 10 minutes and late planar imaging at 2 hours after injection (Box 5-18). This permits diagnosis by observing the differential washout from the thyroid and hyperfunctioning parathyroid. Some centers use pinhole imaging of the neck and parallel hole imaging of the chest in order not to miss a mediastinal adenoma; others use only one large field of view using a high-resolution parallel hole collimator. Dual-isotope techniques using I-123 thyroid subtraction are used at some centers. Single-photon emission computed tomography (SPECT) is increasingly being performed. Because the length of

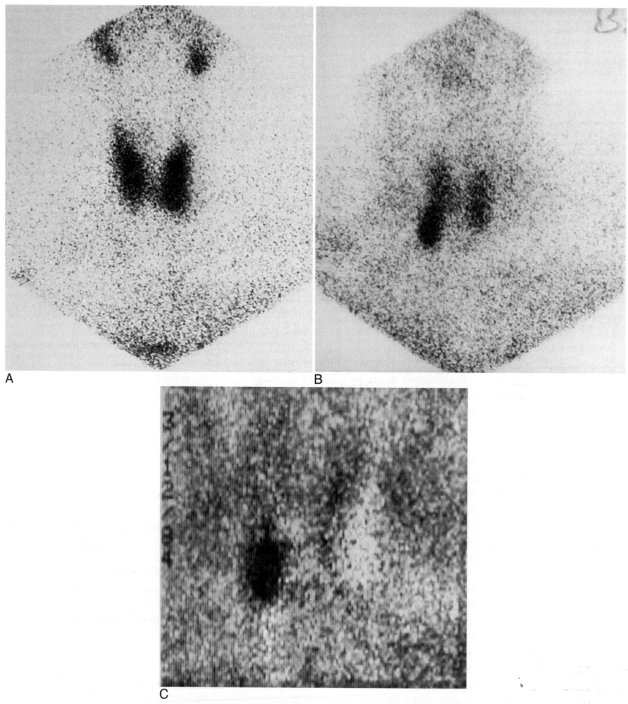

Figure 5-30 Thallium-21/Tc-99m pertechnetate parathyroid subtraction scan. Patient has hypercalcemia and increased serum parathormone level. **A,** Tc-99m pertechnetate scintigraphy in a patient is essentially normal. **B,** Corresponding Tl-201 scintigraphy reveals an apparent area of increased uptake adjacent to the lower pole of the right lobe. **C,** Subtraction of the Tc-99m pertechnetate study from the Tl-201 study confirms the presence of the parathyroid adenoma.

time for acquisition is long, only one imaging period is commonly used (Fig. 5-32).

Image Interpretation
Initial images at 10–15 minutes after injection show prominent thyroid uptake. Many times, focal uptake is seen in a parathyroid adenoma at this time point. On delayed imaging, much of the thyroid uptake has washed out and the typical finding of a hyperfunctioning parathyroid gland is a focus of residual activity in the neck with a high target-to-background ratio. On occasion, multiple adenomas or hyperplastic glands may be seen (Fig. 5-33).

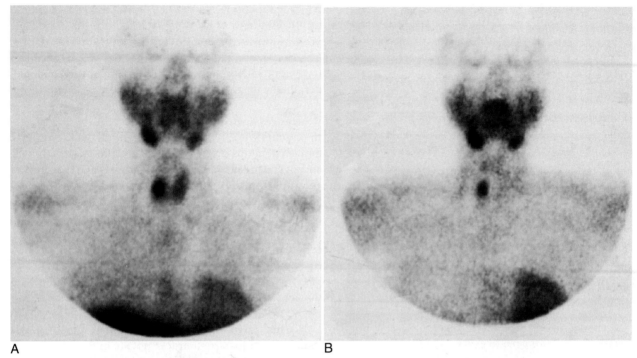

Figure 5-31   Tc-99m sestamibi parathyroid scan. Patient has hypercalcemia and increased PTH. **A,** Early imaging at 15 minutes with Tc-99m sestamibi reveals somewhat asymmetrical activity in the region of the thyroid gland. **B,** Delayed imaging at 2 hours demonstrates washout of thyroid activity and a parathyroid adenoma.

In a minority of patients, the washout rate of the thyroid and hyperfunctioning parathyroid will be similar. However, often in these cases, the parathyroid adenoma can be seen as a distinct focus with a background of thyroid activity. Although adenomas are most commonly detected contiguous to the thyroid or occasionally intrathyroidal, they may be ectopic, anywhere from high in the neck down to the mediastinum. The advantage of SPECT is increased sensitivity (although direct comparison data is limited) and better anatomical localization (e.g., defining a retrotracheal gland) (*see* Fig. 5-32).

Accuracy

The sensitivity for detection of parathyroid adenomas larger than 300 mg in size is greater than 85–90% but is less for smaller adenomas. The most common cause for a false negative study is the small size of the adenoma. The sensitivity for detection of hyperplasia is considerably lower than adenoma (~50–60%). The most common cause for a false positive study is a thyroid adenoma.

ADRENAL SCINTIGRAPHY

Different radiopharmaceuticals are available for scintigraphic imaging of the adrenal cortex and the adrenal medulla. Adrenocortical scintigraphy was used before the development of CT and MRI. Nuclear imaging studies of the adrenal cortex are not frequently performed in current practice but retain a limited role for assessing the functional status of adrenocortical tissue when other imaging studies are indeterminate. However, scintigraphic studies of the adrenal medulla and related tissues have found an increasing role in contemporary practice.

Adrenocortical Scintigraphy

The most common indication for adrenocortical scintigraphy is hypercortisolism (Cushing's syndrome or Cushing's disease). Less common indications include hyperaldosteronism (Conn's syndrome) and adrenal-virilizing tumors. These hormones are derived from different layers of the adrenal cortex: the zona fasciculata, zona glomerulosa, and zona reticularis, respectively.

Radiopharmaceuticals

I-131-6β-iodomethyl-19-norcholesterol (NP-59) localizes in the adrenal cortex as a result of the transport and receptor systems for serum cholesterol bound to low-density lipoprotein (LDL). Factors affecting cholesterol uptake into the adrenal also affect uptake of the radiopharmaceutical. Thus, elevated serum cholesterol reduces the percent uptake. Increases in plasma adrenocorticotropic hormone (ACTH) result in increased radiocholesterol uptake. The radiopharmaceutical is stored in adrenocortical cells and is esterified but not incorporated into adrenal hormones.

Box 5-18 Tc-99m Sestamibi Parathyroid Imaging: Protocol Summary

PATIENT PREPARATION
None

RADIOPHARMACEUTICAL
20 mCi (740 MBq), intravenously

TIME OF IMAGING
Early scans at 15 minutes
Delayed scans at 2 hours

IMAGING PROCEDURE
Planar
Use a high-resolution collimator and a 20% window
    centered at 140 keV.
Position the patient supine with the chin up and neck
    extended.
Place markers on the chin and sternal notch.
Obtain anterior and 45-degree left and right anterior
    oblique views, 300k counts per view.

SPECT IMAGING
Position patient as above.
Use a high-resolution collimator and a 20% window
    centered at 140 keV.
Use dual-headed SPECT camera: 360-degree contoured
    acquisition arc, 3-degree angular
Sampling increment, 15–30 sec per view, 128 × 128
    matrix with 1.5 zoom, Hanning or Butterworth filter.
Reconstruct transaxial, coronal, and sagittal planes.
Reproject images at each sampling angle.

The uptake of I-131-6β-iodomethyl-19-norcholesterol is progressive over several days after tracer administration. Background clearance is also relatively slow, and for routine or baseline studies, imaging is typically performed several days after tracer injection. Background tissues demonstrating significant localization include the liver, colon, and gallbladder.

Patients should be pretreated for at least 1 day with iodine (e.g., SSKI, 1 drop three times a day or equivalent) to block uptake of free radioiodine in the thyroid. This is continued for 7 days (Box 5-19).

I-131-6β-iodomethyl-19-norcholesterol is usually given in a dose of 1 mCi/1.7 m^2 of body surface area. The dose is administered intravenously over 1–2 minutes. For hypercortisolism, imaging is acquired at 48 hours after radiopharmaceutical injection. For other indications, imaging is initiated at 4–5 days because the lower level of uptake requires more time for background clearance and because of the suppression protocol described later.

A large field-of-view gamma scintillation camera with a high-energy parallel-hole collimator is used and a 20% window is centered at 364 keV. A standard imaging time of 20 minutes per view is used. The most important view is posterior and includes both adrenal glands. Anterior views may be helpful to assess adrenal asymmetry. Lateral views can help differentiate normal gallbladder uptake from activity in the right adrenal gland.

Suppression Studies

In patients with hyperfunctioning of the zona glomerulosa (hyperaldosteronism) or the zona reticularis (hyperandrogenism), it is desirable to suppress ACTH secretion and thus uptake of radiocholesterol in the zona fasciculata site of cortisol production. Without suppression, normal high uptake in the zona fasciculata would make interpretation of uptake by the zona glomerulosa or reticularis quite difficult. Suppression is accomplished by administering dexamethasone, 4 mg per day (2 mg bid) for 7 days before radiopharmaceutical administration and continuing until imaging is completed.

Normal Adrenocortical Scintigram

In normal subjects, radiotracer uptake in the adrenal cortex increases over the first 2 days after injection. Background activity is still relatively high at this time, especially in the liver, and imaging may be delayed until day 4 or 5.

The two adrenal glands are not anatomically symmetrical and often have different scintigraphic appearances. The right adrenal typically sits at the superior pole of the right kidney and is slightly cephalad to the left adrenal gland. The right adrenal gland appears round and in most subjects is slightly more intense than the left because of its more posterior location in the body and less soft tissue attenuation. Liver activity is also superimposed. The left adrenal gland typically lies at the anteromedial border of the left kidney and may extend inferiorly to the renal hilum. It appears more caudad and has an oval rather than a round configuration. The left adrenal gland frequently appears less intense because of its more anterior location and the lack of additive background liver activity.

Cushing's Syndrome

The scintigraphic pattern of uptake depends on the etiology of hypercortisolism (Fig. 5-34). In Cushing's disease, caused by a pituitary adenoma with increased production of ACTH, there is bilateral early visualization of the adrenal glands (Fig. 5-35). Ectopic ACTH production would produce a similar scintigraphic pattern, although it is not a common indication for scintigraphy. Unilateral visualization is classically seen in patients with glucocorticoid-producing adrenal adenomas (Fig. 5-36). The autonomous production of cortisol in the adenoma feeds back to shut off pituitary ACTH secretion and thereby shuts off uptake in the contralateral adrenal gland

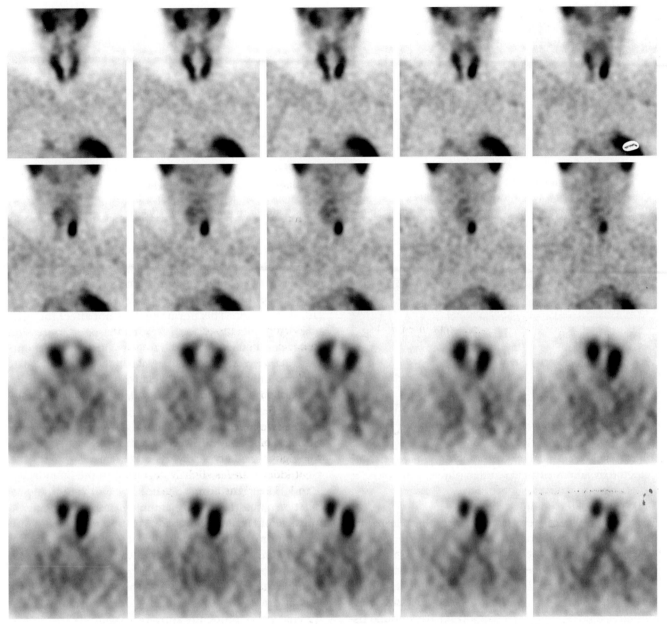

Figure 5-32   SPECT sestamibi parathyroid scan. Preoperative hyperparathyroidism. Sequential coronal *(above)* and transverse *(below)*. Posterior inferior parathyroid adenoma.

(Fig. 5-37). Adrenal macronodular hyperplasia is an uncommon form of hypercorticalism in which there is autonomous function of both adrenal glands and bilateral uptake scintigraphically, although often somewhat asymmetrically.

Nonvisualization of both adrenal glands in patients with Cushing's syndrome indicates adrenal carcinoma. The tumors can be quite large and are often first manifested clinically with signs and symptoms of hormone excess. However, the function per gram of tumor tissue is typically low and tracer uptake is insufficient to visualize the tumor.

The contralateral adrenal gland is not visualized because the excessive cortisol production shuts down pituitary ACTH secretion. Biochemical proof of hypercortisolism and CT demonstration of a large lesion in the adrenal are considered sufficient evidence and scintigraphy is not needed. However, if CT findings are negative or equivocal, adrenocortical scintigraphy can be helpful.

One use of adrenocortical scintigraphy in patients with Cushing's syndrome, even in the era of MRI and CT, is in the detection of postsurgical *adrenal remnants*. These remnants may cause recurrent disease and be difficult

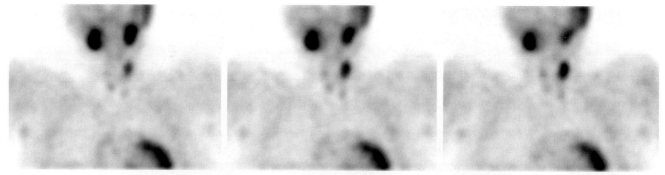

Figure 5-33 Tertiary hyperparathyroidism with four glands detected.Tc-99m sestamibi scan in patient with renal failure and elevated calcium. SPECT coronals with four abnormal foci, the left superior parathyroid gland being the largest, but also the left inferior, right superior and right inferior glands detected. Confirmation of scintigraphic findings at surgery.

Box 5-19	Iodine Available for Thyroid Radiation Protection
Lugol's solution	6.3 mg/drop
Supersaturated potassium iodide (SSKI)	38 mg/drop
Quadrinol	145 mg/tab
Potassium iodide capsules	130 mg/capsule

to localize in a surgically altered anatomy. They can be detected by adrenocortical scintigraphy.

Hyperaldosteronism

The principal clinical question in aldosteronism is the distinction of adenoma from hyperplasia. Aldosteronomas are typically small and CT or MRI often is not diagnostic. Aldosterone is produced in the zona glomerulosa of the adrenal cortex. This hormone does not affect the pituitary–ACTH feedback loop. Dexamethasone suppression scan is necessary for scintigraphic evaluation of patients with aldosteronism. Normal uptake in the zona fasciculata can obscure asymmetry caused by small nodules and adenomas in the zona glomerulosa. Scintigraphy is performed over several days. Early (<5 days) unilateral "breakthrough" indicates aldosteronoma. Bilateral, delayed breakthrough typically indicates hyperplasia.

Androgen Excess

The adrenal glands may be the source of excessive production of androgen. Scintigraphic patterns are similar to those found in aldosteronism. That is, patients with bilateral hyperplasia demonstrate bilateral breakthrough on

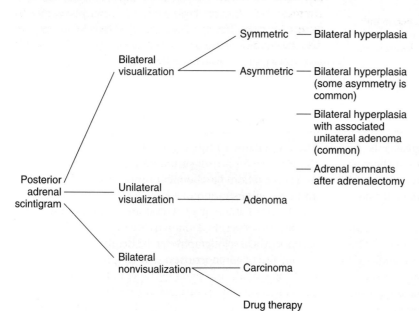

Figure 5-34 Cushing's syndrome: NP-59 diagnostic patterns. I-131 norcholesterol (NP-59) can aid in the differential diagnosis. Diagnostic patterns in patients with biochemically proven Cushing's syndrome include unilateral uptake for adenomas, bilateral uptake for pituitary etiology, and no uptake for adrenocortical carcinoma.

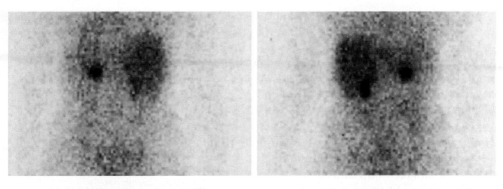

Posterior   Anterior

Figure 5-35   Adrenal adenoma. Adrenocortical scintigraphy in the posterior view reveals unilateral uptake in the left adrenal gland in a patient with adrenal adenoma. The anterior view shows uptake in the adenoma as well as in the gallbladder that was confirmed by a lateral view.

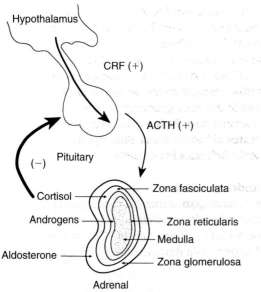

Figure 5-36   Pituitary–adrenal feedback loop. Function in the zona fasciculata is stimulated by adrenocorticotropic hormone (ACTH). Pituitary secretion of ACTH decreases as circulating levels of cortisol increase. CRF, corticotropin-releasing factor.

dexamethasone suppression scans and adenomas are characterized by marked scintigraphic asymmetry.

Incidentalomas

I-131 MIBG has been used as an aid in determining the etiology of a nodule found incidentally (e.g., on CT). Uptake in the nodule signifies a functioning nodule and not metastatic disease.

Adrenomedullary Scintigraphy

Adrenomedullary scintigraphy has proven useful in the management of patients with functional adrenergic tumors, including paragangliomas, neuroblastomas, and pheochromocytomas. Pheochromocytomas are paragangliomas that arise in the adrenal medulla. Paragangliomas are associated with a number of important familial syndromes, including multiple endocrine neoplasia (MEN) type IIA (medullary carcinoma of the thyroid, pheochromocytoma, and hyperparathyroidism) and MEN type IIB (medullary carcinoma of the thyroid, pheochromocytoma,

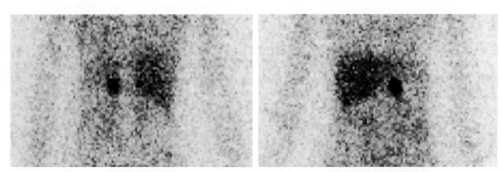

Figure 5-37   I-131 MIBG localizes pheochromocytoma. Adrenomedullary scintigraphy reveals unilaterally increased uptake in the region of the left adrenal due to pheochromocytoma. The patient had elevated nor- and metanephrines.

and ganglioneuromas), von Hippel-Lindau disease, and neurofibromatosis.

Radiopharmaceuticals

Scintigraphic studies of the adrenergic nervous system became possible with meta-iodo-benzyl-guanidine (MIBG), a norepinephrine analogue. Localization is via the type I, energy-dependent, active amine transport mechanism. The tracer is taken up and localized in cytoplasmic storage vesicles in presynaptic adrenergic nerves. In addition to the uptake in the adrenal medulla and other adrenergic and neuroblastic tumor tissues, the tracer localizes avidly in other organs with rich adrenergic innervation, including the heart, salivary glands, and spleen. Both I-131 and I-123 have been used as radiolabels. I-123 has the advantage of a lower radiation dose to the patient, whereas I-131 allows for delayed imaging.

Technique

MIBG is taken up rapidly by adrenergic tissues. To achieve a sufficient target-to-background ratio, imaging is typically delayed for 24–48 hours, usually longer.

For studies with I-131 or I-123 MIBG, patients are given a blocking dose of saturated solution of potassium iodide (SSKI). The usual adult dose of I-131 MIBG is 0.5 mCi/1.7 m². The tracer is administered intravenously over 15–30 seconds. When MIBG is radiolabeled with I-123, up to 10 mCi/m² can be administered with the same radiation dose to the patient as from 0.5 mCi/m² of I-131 MIBG.

Initial images with I-131 MIBG may be obtained at 24 hours. The optimal imaging time is 48 hours after injection, and 72-hour imaging is possible. A wide field-of-view gamma scintillation camera equipped with a high-energy parallel-hole collimator is used. Imaging is typically for 20 minutes. The views obtained are determined by the clinical condition under evaluation. For pheochromocytoma, the posterior view of the mid-abdomen with the region of the adrenal glands is most important. Additional images from the pelvis to the base of the skull are indicated to detect extra-adrenal pheochromocytoma (paraganglioma) and neuroblastomas.

With I-123 MIBG, initial images may be obtained at 4 hours, although images at 24 hours are superior. SPECT is feasible with I-123 MIBG. The significantly lower radiation dose and superior image quality is a major advantage for children with neuroblastoma.

Precautions

A number of drugs interfere with MIBG uptake and a drug history should be obtained before imaging. Interfering drugs include tricyclic antidepressants, reserpine, guanethidine, certain antipsychotics, cocaine, and the alpha- and beta-blocker labetalol (Table 5-3).

Table 5-3 Drugs Known or Expected to Reduce MIBG Uptake

KNOWN (PATIENT MUST BE OFF PRIOR TO SCANNING)

Antihypertensive/Cardiovascular

Labetalol, reserpine
Calcium-channel blockers (diltiazem, nifedipine, verapamil)

Tricyclic Antidepressants

Amitriptyline and derivatives
Imipramine and derivatives
Doxepin, amoxapine, loxapine (antipsychotic agent)

Sympathomimetics

Phenylephrine, phenylpropanolamine, pseudoephedrine, ephedrine

Cocaine

EXPECTED (MAY INTERFERE BUT NEED NOT BE CEASED PRIOR TO SCANNING)

Antihypertensive/Cardiovascular

Adrenergic neurone blockers (bethanidine, debrisoquine, bretylium, guanethidine)

"Atypical" Antidepressants

Maprotiline, Trazodone

POSSIBLE

Antipsychotics (major tranquilizers)

Phenothiazines (chlorpromazine, triflupromazine, promethazine, etc.)
Thioxanthenes (chlorprothixene, thiothixene)
Butyrophenones (droperidol, haloperidol, pimozide)

Sympathomimetics

Amphetamine and related compounds
Beta-sympathomimetics: albuterol, isoetharine, isoproterenol, metaproterenol, terbutaline
Dobutamine, dopamine, metaraminol, tetrabenazine

NO EFFECT

Antihypertensive/Cardiovascular

Alpha-blockers (clonidine, phenoxybenzamine, phentolamine, prazosin)
Alpha-methyldopa
Angiotensin converting enzyme inhibitors (captopril, enalapril)
Beta-blockers (does not include labetalol)
Digitalis glycosides, diuretics

Analgesics

Major (morphine and other opioids), minor (aspirin, acetaminophen)

Hypnotics, minor tranquilizers

Normal MIBG Scintigraphy

With the usual doses used for I-131 MIBG imaging, only faint visualization of the normal adrenal medulla is achieved in 10% of patients. The normal adrenal medulla is visualized more frequently with I-123 MIBG. Early images reveal activity in the spleen, heart, salivary glands, and liver. These areas clear with time. Some bladder activity may be visualized because of free radioiodine. The colon is also seen transiently in 20% of cases.

Clinical Applications

The greatest clinical experience with MIBG is in the evaluation of patients with suspected pheochromocytoma. However, it has an important role in the evaluation and follow-up of patients with neuroblastoma.

Pheochromocytoma

The characteristic appearance is unilateral focal uptake in the tumor (Fig. 5-38). Sensitivity for detection of pheochromocytoma is approximately 90%, with specificity being greater than 95%. In approximately 10% of patients, pheochromocytoma is bilateral. In 10–20% of patients, the tumors are extra-adrenal and are referred to as *paragangliomas*. Pheochromocytomas are increasingly seen with other neuroectodermal disorders, including neurofibromatosis, tuberous sclerosis, Carney's syndrome, and von Hippel-Lindau disease. Paragangliomas may be found from the bladder up to the base of the skull.

Scintigraphy with MIBG is not a screening procedure for pheochromocytoma and should be applied only after biochemical tests suggest the diagnosis. Many centers first use CT to evaluate the adrenal glands. If an adrenal mass is demonstrated, the diagnosis is inferred and further workup before surgery is often unnecessary. MIBG is particularly helpful in surveying the entire body for extraadrenal tumors and metastatic disease.

Adrenomedullary hyperplasia develops in patients with MEN type IIA. This condition is difficult to diagnose with CT or MRI. MIBG scintigraphy is uniquely suited to detect medullary hyperplasia and has been used to assist decision making for timing of surgery.

Neuroblastoma

This malignant tumor of neural crest origin occurs in young children, usually less than 4 years of age. Seventy percent of tumors originate in the retroperitoneal region, either from the adrenal or the abdominal sympathetic chain. However, 20% occur in the chest, deriving from the thoracic sympathetic chain. More than 90% of neuroblastomas produce catecholamines.

Bone scans have traditionally been used to detect metastases. However, a common location for metastases is in the metaphyseal region, which can be hard to detect because of the high uptake in growth plates. MIBG has superior sensitivity for detection of metastases compared to the bone scan because these tumors initially involve

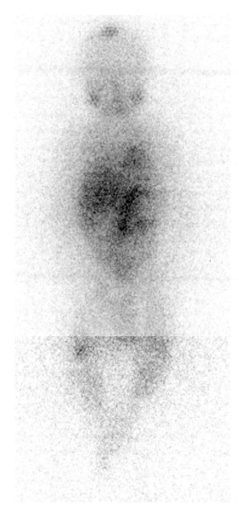

Figure 5-38   I-131 MIBG: neuroblastoma follow-up. Two-year-old with stage 4 neuroblastoma status post left retroperitoneal mass resection, bone marrow transplant, and monoclonal antibody therapy. The 48-hour I-131 scan shows a large left upper intra-abdominal mass seen with greatest uptake at the periphery. Bone metastases in the skull and right femur.

the bone marrow. The combination of the two results in the highest sensitivity for detection.

The sensitivity for MIBG for neuroblastoma is greater than 90%, with a high degree of specificity. MIBG is used for staging (Fig. 5-39), detecting metastatic disease, and following the patient's response to therapy. Whole body scanning is routine for imaging patients with this disease. The higher count rate, better image quality, and lower dosimetry of I-123 MIBG makes it preferable over I-131 MIBG in children.

Other tumors demonstrating uptake of MIBG include carcinoid tumors and medullary carcinoma of the thyroid. However, the sensitivity for tumor detection is lower than for neuroblastoma or pheochromocytoma.

The high uptake of MIBG in these tumors has led investigators to attempt therapy with I-131 MIBG. Therapeutic

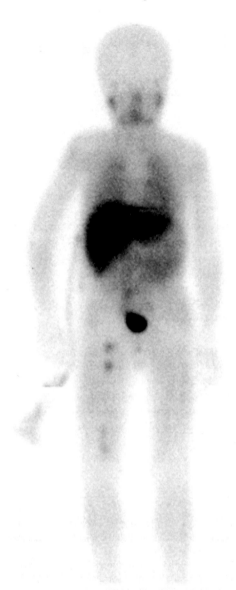

Figure 5-39 I-123 MIBG: neuroblastoma follow-up. A 4-year-old with metastatic neuroblastoma since age 2. Postresection of right adrenal mass and adenopathy, chemotherapy, radiation, stem cell transplant. Large intra-abdominal tumor mass. I-123 4-hour scan only because family refused 24-hour imaging. Considerable background uptake in lungs, abdomen, and soft tissue. Focal uptake in the proximal and distal femur. An intra-abdominal tumor mass was seen on SPECT (not shown). Nephrostomy tube in place for urinary obstruction.

applications are still investigational and restricted largely to patients in whom prior conventional therapies have failed.

SUGGESTED READING

Thyroid Imaging and Function Studies

Chapman EM: History of the discovery and early use of radioactive iodine. *JAMA* 250: 2042-2044, 1983.

Filesi M, Signore A, Ventroni G, et al: Role of initial iodine-131 whole-body scan and serum thyroglobulin in differentiated thyroid carcinoma metastases. *J Nucl Med* 39: 1542-1546, 1998.

Freitas JE: Changing concepts in the management of thyroid cancer. In *Nuclear medicine annual*. Leonard M. Freeman, Ed. Philadelphia, Lippincott Williams & Wilkins, 2003, pp. 101-130.

Grunwald F, Schomburg A, Bender H, et al: Fluorine-18–fluorodeoxyglucose positron emission tomography in the follow-up of differentiated thyroid cancer. *Eur J Nucl Med* 23: 312-319, 1996.

Gulec MG, Rubello D, Boni G, et al: Preoperative localization and radioguided parathyroid surgery. *J Nucl Med* 44: 1443-1458, 2003.

Intenzo CM, dePapp AE, Jabbour S, et al: Scintigraphic manifestations of thyrotoxicosis. *Radiographics* 23: 857-869, 2003.

Intenzo CM, Capuzzi DM, Jabbour S, et al: Scintigraphic features of autoimmune thyroiditis. *Radiographics* 21: 957-964, 2001.

Park HM, Perkins OW, Edmondson JW, et al: Influence of diagnostic radioiodines on the uptake of ablative dose of iodine-131. *Thyroid* 4: 49-54, 1994.

Shankar LK, Yamamoto AJ, Alavi A, Mandel SJ: Comparison of I-123 scintigraphy at 5 and 24 hours in patients with differentiated thyroid cancer. *J Nucl Med* 43: 72-76, 2002.

Smith JR and Oates E: Radionuclide imaging of the thyroid gland: patterns, pearls, and pitfalls. *Clin Nucl Med* 29: 181-193, 2004.

Uematsu H, Sadato N, Ohtsubo T, et al: Fluorine-18-fluorodeoxyglucose PET versus thallium-201 scintigraphy evaluation of thyroid tumors. *J Nucl Med* 39: 453-459, 1998.

Adrenal Scintigraphy

Gelfand MJ: Meta-iodobenzylguanidine in children. *Semin Nucl Med* 23: 231-242, 1993.

Gross MD, Shapiro B, Frances IR, et al: Scintigraphic evaluation of clinically silent adrenal masses using adrenocortical scintigraphy. *J Nucl Med* 35: 1145-1152, 1994.

Hay RV, Shapiro B, Gross MD: Scintigraphic imaging of the adrenals and neuroectodermal tumors. In *Nuclear medicine*. Henkin RE, Boles MA, Dillehay GL, et al, Eds. St Louis, Mosby, 1996.

Sisson JC: Scintigraphic localization of pheochromocytomas. *N Engl J Med* 305: 12-17, 1981.

Parathyroid Scintigraphy

Civelek AC, Ozalp E, Donovan P, Udelsman R: Prospective evaluation of delayed technetium-99m sestamibi SPECT scintigraphy for preoperative localization of primary hyperparathyroidism. *Surgery* 131: 149-157, 2002.

Perez-Monte JE, Brown ML, Shah AN, et al: Parathyroid adenomas: accurate detection and localization with Tc-99m sestamibi SPECT. *Radiology* 201: 85-91, 1996.

Taillefer R, Boucher Y, Potvin C, Lambert R: Detection and localization of parathyroid adenomas in patients with hyperparathyroidism using a single radionuclide imaging procedure with technetium-99m sestamibi (double-phase study). *J Nucl Med* 33: 1801-1807, 1992.

CHAPTER 6

Skeletal Scintigraphy

BONE SCAN INTRODUCTION

The skeleton is an active, constantly changing organ. It is made up of inorganic calcium hydroxyapatite crystal, $Ca_{10}(PO_4)_6(OH)_2$, and an organic matrix of collagen and blood vessels. Bone responds to injury and disease with increased turnover and attempts at self-repair. This physiologic process can be imaged with a radiotracer that localizes to areas of bone formation.

Bone scans have used the technetium-99m labeled diphosphonates such as Tc-99m methylene diphosphonate (Tc-99m MDP) for decades to perform skeletal imaging. The bone scan is a versatile tool that can image malignant and benign processes. The bone scan is highly sensitive for disease, is readily available, and can image the entire skeleton at reasonable cost. Therefore, skeletal scintigraphy (Fig. 6-1) remains popular despite technological advances in magnetic resonance imaging (MRI), computed tomography (CT), and positron emission tomography (PET).

The major drawback of this exam is its low specificity. Numerous benign processes (e.g., arthritis) cause increased radiotracer uptake by increasing blood flow and osteogenic activity. Often the location and patterns of

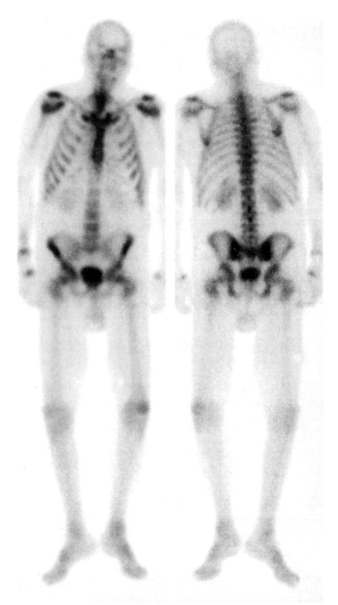

Figure 6-1 Normal Tc-99m methylene diphosphonate (MDP) whole body bone scan. A high level of anatomic detail can be visualized. Some areas of increased uptake are normally seen in the adult including activity in the joints.

abnormalities can guide interpretation. However, it is essential to know the patient's history, understand when radiographic correlation is necessary, and know how to use it.

Radiopharmaceuticals

History

It has long been known that certain radioisotopes localize to bone. In the 1920s, devastating cancers were reported in women who painted luminescent watch dials with radium.

These women ingested the bone seeker, Radium-226, when licking their brushes to tip them. Since then, numerous bone-seeking agents have been studied and abandoned. This includes Phosphorus-32, radioisotopes of calcium, several rare earth elements, and isotopes of gallium, barium, samarium, and strontium. Gallium-67 is still used in tumor and infection imaging. Fluorine-18 (F-18) is an analog of the hydroxyl ion found in calcium hydroxyapatite and avidly localizes to bone. It was the agent of choice for skeletal scintigraphy until the advent of the Tc-99m phosphonates in the 1970s.

An ideal radiopharmaceutical for skeletal scintigraphy must be inexpensive, remain stable, rapidly localize to bone, quickly clear from the background soft tissues, and have favorable imaging and dosimetry characteristics. These parameters were essentially met in the 1970s when technetium-99m, already desirable for gamma camera imaging studies, was combined with members of the phosphate family.

These radiopharmaceuticals are classified by the type of phosphate bond. The first of these agents, pyrophosphates and then the longer-chain polyphosphates, were soon replaced by the diphosphonates (Fig. 6-2). The diphosphonates are more stable in the body and have better background clearance than pyrophosphates or polyphosphates. The diphosphonate agents include Tc-99m hydroxyethylidene diphosphonate (Tc-99m HEDP), Tc-99m hydroxymethylene diphosphonate (Tc-99m HMDP or HDP), and Tc-99m methylene diphosphonate (Tc-99m MDP). The ability of each diphosphonate to detect lesions has been studied. Although some differences are present, Tc-99m MDP and Tc-99m HDP are both excellent agents.

Preparation

Tc-99m MDP can be prepared from a simple kit. Technetium-99m, in the form of sodium pertechnetate (NaTcO$_4$), is obtained from a molybdenum-99 generator and injected into a vial containing methylene diphosphonate, stabilizers, and stannous ion. Stannous tin acts as a reducing agent which allows the technetium-99m to form a chelate bond with the methylene diphosphonate carrier molecule.

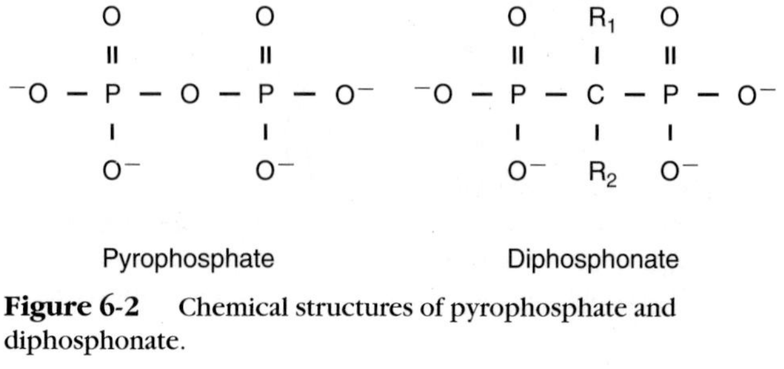

Pyrophosphate   Diphosphonate

Figure 6-2 Chemical structures of pyrophosphate and diphosphonate.

Incomplete labeling may occur if air is introduced into the vial causing hydrolysis of the stannous ion (from Sn II into Sn IV). If not enough stannous ion is available to reduce the technetium ion, free technetium pertechnetate ("free tech") will result, causing image degradation as a result of increased soft tissue uptake distribution and uptake in thyroid, stomach, and salivary glands (Fig. 6-3). Occasionally, the excess Sn II may form a partly colloidal radiopharmaceutical, which can accumulate in the reticuloendothelial system of organs such as the liver. Tc-99m MDP should be used within 2–3 hours of preparation or radiopharmaceutical breakdown may also yield technetium pertechnetate.

Uptake and Pharmacokinetics

After intravenous injection, Tc-99m MDP rapidly distributes into the extracellular fluid and is quickly taken up into the bone. Tc-99m MDP accumulates primarily in relation to osteogenic activity levels, although the amount of blood flow plays a part. Activity is much higher in areas of active bone formation compared with mature bone. Tc-99m MDP binding occurs by chemoadsorption in the hydroxyapatite mineral component of the osseous matrix. Uptake in areas of amorphous cal-

cium phosphate may account for Tc-99m MDP uptake in sites outside the bone, such as dystrophic soft tissue ossification.

Approximately 50% of the dose is localized to the bone with the remainder excreted by the kidneys. Although peak bone uptake occurs approximately 1 hour after injection, highest target-to-background ratios are seen after 6–12 hours. This must be balanced with the relatively short 6-hour half-life of Tc-99m and patient convenience. Therefore, images are typically taken 2–4 hours after injection. Serum radiotracer levels at this time are down to 3–5% of the injected dose in patients with normal renal function. It should be noted that the half-life of Tc-99m effectively limits imaging to within approximately 24 hours of injection.

Decreased localization is seen in areas of reduced or absent blood flow or infarction. Diminished uptake is also seen in areas of severe destruction that can occur in some very aggressive metastasis (Fig. 6-4). Photon deficient areas are sometimes referred to as "cold."

Dosimetry

Estimates of absorbed radiation doses are listed in Table 6-1. The radiation dose to the bladder wall, ovaries, and testes depends on the frequency of voiding. The dosimetry provided assumes a 2-hour voiding cycle. Significantly higher doses result if voiding is infrequent. Radiopharmaceuticals are administered to pregnant women only if clearly needed on a risk-versus-benefit basis. Tc-99m is excreted in breast milk so breastfeeding should be stopped for 24 hours.

Imaging Protocol

An example protocol is listed in Box 6-1. There are several modifications possible in skeletal scintigraphy protocols. It must first be determined if a three-phase bone scan is needed to assess blood flow and soft tissue activity for

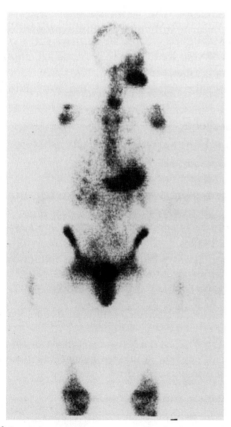

Figure 6-3   Free pertechnetate in the radiopharmaceutical preparation. This has resulted in uptake in stomach, thyroid gland, and salivary glands. Salivary activity has entered the oropharynx on this 3-hour delayed image.

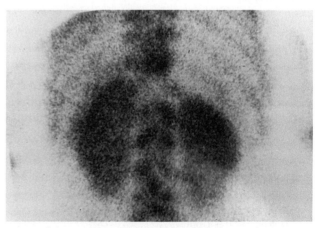

Figure 6-4   Complete destruction of the L1 vertebral body with corresponding photon-deficient (or cold) lesion.

Table 6-1 Radiation Absorbed Dosimetry from Technetium-99m medronate (Tc-99m MDP)

Organ	Radiation Dose (rads/mCi) (cGy/37 MBq)
Skeleton	0.035
Marrow	0.0280
Kidneys	0.04
Bladder	0.13
Testes	0.008
Ovaries	0.008
Whole body	0.0065

Box 6-1 Skeletal Scintigraphy: Protocol Summary for Whole Body Survey and SPECT

PATIENT PREPARATION AND FOLLOW-UP

Patient should be well hydrated

Patient should void immediately before study and should void frequently after procedure (reduces radiation dose to bladder wall)

Patient should remove metal objects (jewelry, coins, keys) before imaging

DOSAGE AND ROUTE OF ADMINISTRATION

20 mCi (740 MBq) technetium-99m diphosphonate adult dose (standard)

Intravenous injection (site selected to avoid known or suspected pathological condition)

Adjust dosage for pediatric patients (Webster's rule or weight adjusted; Minimum 74 MBq [2 mCi])

TIME OF IMAGING

Begin imaging 2–4 hr after tracer administration

PROCEDURE

Anterior and posterior views of the entire skeleton

Obtain a minimum of 1000k counts per view for "whole body" imaging systems

Obtain 300k–500k counts per image if multiple spot views are used

Use the highest resolution collimator that permits imaging in a reasonable length of time

Obtain high-count (1000k) spot views or SPECT for more detail

SPECT*

Acquisition: contoured orbit, 128 × 128 matrix, 6-degree intervals, 15–30 sec/stop

Reconstruction: filtered backprojection, Butterworth filter; cut-off 0.4, power 7

*Selection of SPECT acquisition and reconstruction parameters depends greatly on available equipment and software.

---

cases of infection and trauma. The injection site should be chosen to avoid any suspected pathology. Also, if comparison with the opposite hand may be needed at any time, injection in a site such as the foot should be considered.

Although many diagnostic questions can be answered with routine delayed imaging, the three-phase bone scan is helpful in addressing several problems. The most frequent indication for three-phase imaging is to assess for possible osteomyelitis. However, it is also beneficial in the evaluation of a painful hip prosthesis, trauma, bone graft status, and reflex sympathetic dystrophy. The technique for dynamic scanning is summarized in Box 6-2.

If dynamic three-phase scanning is to be performed, the area in question is positioned under the camera for the injection. A 20 mCi (740 MBq) bolus of Tc-99m MDP is injected intravenously. The first phase consists of serial 2–5 second dynamic images acquired for 60 seconds. Then blood pool or soft tissue second-phase images are obtained of this region. Additional blood pool images can be taken in any area of secondary interest, such as in patients with arthritis or multiple stress injuries. Delayed images constitute the third phase of a three-phase bone scan. The delayed images can be done without flow images for routine studies, such as the assessment of metastatic disease.

After injection, the patient should be instructed to drink several cups of fluid to improve soft tissue clearance and to void frequently to decrease radiation dose to the critical organ, the bladder. The patient returns 2–4 hours later for delayed images and voids immediately

---

Box 6-2 Three-Phase Skeletal Scintigraphy: Protocol Summary

RADIOPHARMACEUTICAL DOSAGE AND ROUTE OF ADMINISTRATION

Standard tracer and dosage are used and given as a bolus injection

PROCEDURE

The gamma camera is positioned before radiopharmaceutical administration immediately over the site of the suspected pathological condition

FLOW PHASE

Dynamic 2- to 5-sec images are obtained for 60 sec after bolus injection

BLOOD POOL AND TISSUE PHASE

Immediate static images for time (5 min) or counts (300k)

SKELETAL PHASE

Delayed 300k–1000k images at 2–4 hr

before scanning. Care must be used as urinary contamination frequently causes confusion or masks potential lesion sites. All metal (such as coins or belts) should be removed and sites of trauma or surgery noted.

Imaging is done with a low-energy, high-resolution collimator. Delayed planar images can be obtained either by a whole body scan or by spot views. The whole body scan offers the advantage of a more rapid seamless coverage of the entire body as the camera moves over the patient at a predetermined rate. Spot views, on the other hand, can provide greater detail due to higher resolution and can better define pathology by using different fixed camera positions (Fig. 6-5). In most centers, a whole body scan is performed with high count spot views reserved for symptomatic areas or suspicious appearing regions.

Other modifications to consider are special views obtained using magnified pinhole collimation and single photon emission computed tomography (SPECT). Magnified images with a pinhole collimator or converging collimator are commonly used in cases of osteonecrosis of the hips and trauma to the carpal

bones. Pinhole images may also be needed in children to better visualize the joints. Three-dimensional assessment of the bones with SPECT allows for high-contrast images that can be formatted in transaxial, sagittal, and coronal planes. SPECT is most useful in spinal and facial bones, where it allows better localization of uptake. This includes determining if there is involvement of the facets or vertebral pedicle. SPECT increases contrast of cold and hot lesions, which improves sensitivity. Sometimes in spondylosis, all images including MRI and planar bone scans are normal, but SPECT is positive (Fig. 6-6).

Normal and Altered Distribution

The normal bone scan varies dramatically with the age of the patient. Most notably, the growing skeleton will concentrate radiotracer at all active growth plates (Fig. 6-7). These areas are often the critical sites in child abuse, primary bone tumors, and osteomyelitis. Therefore, it is essential that children are immobilized and positioned

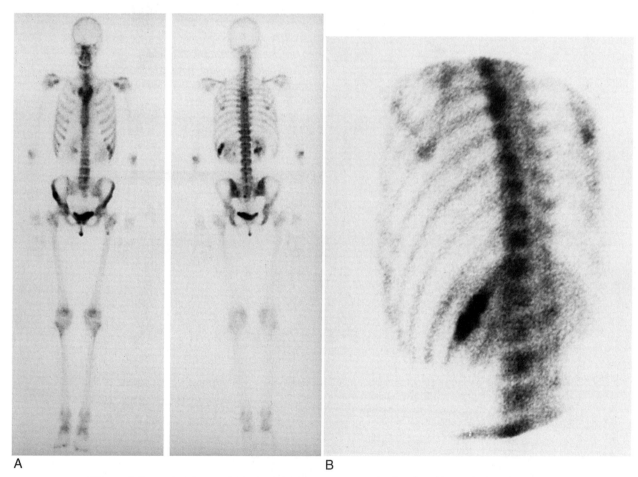

A   B

Figure 6-5   **A,** Anterior and posterior whole body images of a patient with carcinoma of the breast. Whole body images have the advantage of depicting the entire skeleton in a single view. Note the abnormal uptake in one of the left lower posterior ribs. **B,** High count density spot view of left posterior ribs from the patient in **A.** The location and appearance of the lesion are better delineated in the spot view. Tracking along the rib is classic for a metastatic lesion.

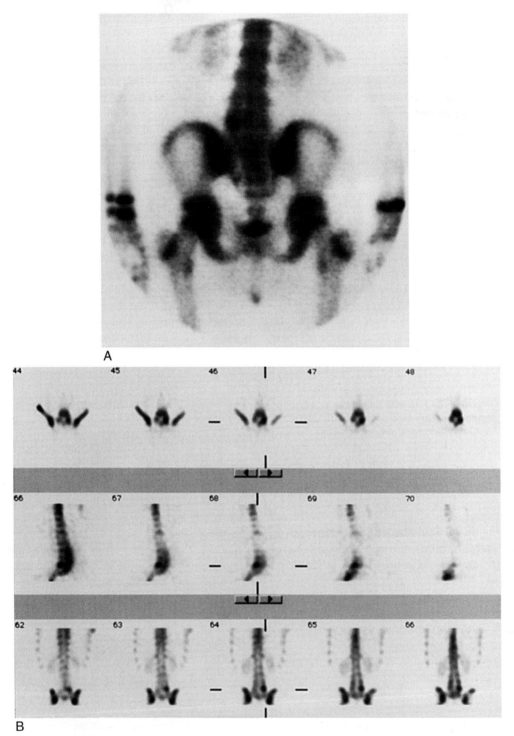

Figure 6-6   Added value of SPECT imaging. **A,** A 24-year-old athlete with chronic low back pain and negative radiographs and MRI had a near normal planar bone scan. **B,** SPECT images (transaxial, sagittal, and coronal) reveal asymmetry with focal increased uptake in the right L4-5 facet typical for spondylolysis. SPECT may be the only test that reveals the etiology of the patient's pain.

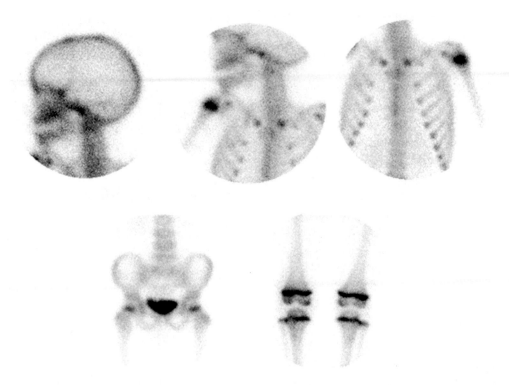

Figure 6-7   Normal radiotracer distribution in the immature skeleton. An anterior whole body image shows increased uptake in the growth centers. Uptake is seen in the anterior rib ends, sternal ossification centers, and major joints.

symmetrically. By adulthood, growth plate activity diminishes and disappears.

There are numerous areas that are normal or expected variants depending on age and history. Some bones such as those of the sacroiliac joints normally appear to have intense uptake. Other areas are more intense because of configuration and proximity to the camera, such as the iliac wings. The sternum often has residual ossification centers and the normal sternomanubrial joint may have increased uptake. The costochondral junction is a common site of benign uptake.

The skull is highly variable in appearance and may show increased uptake in the frontal bone from benign hyperostosis frontalis interna. The lateral orbits often show normal increased and sometimes asymmetric activity where the sphenoid ridge meets the calvarium.

The normal lordotic curvature of the spine causes portions of the vertebra closest to the camera to appear "hotter" than other areas. The joints may be mildly asymmetric due to use and arthritis. For example, the sternoclavicular joints typically accumulate activity, and it has been noted that handedness affects intensity of shoulder uptake.

The soft tissues are a critical component of scintigram analysis. The patient's body habitus must be considered as soft tissue attenuation from breast or abdomen changes intensity of the underlying bones. It is essential to examine the soft tissues for areas of abnormal uptake and evidence of surgery such as mastectomy. It is normal to see activity in the kidneys and bladder; absence of activity must be explained. If the renal cortical activity is equal to or greater than the lumbar spine, a renal abnormality or concomitant drug therapy should be suspected (Box 6-3).

CLINICAL USES OF SKELETAL SCINTIGRAPHY

Metastatic Disease

A significant fraction of patients with known malignancy develop osseous metastasis (Box 6-4). Patients may present with bone pain (50-80%) and elevated alkaline phosphatase (77%) but these findings are nonspecific. The evaluation of osseous metastatic disease is the most common use of skeletal scintigraphy. Bone scan may be used for staging, restaging, and monitoring therapy effectiveness. The decision on which patients will need a bone scan depends on factors such as the type and stage of tumor, history of pain, and radiographic abnormalities.

Box 6-3 Reported Causes of Bilaterally Increased and Decreased Renal Visualization on Skeletal Scintigrams

INCREASED UPTAKE

Nephrotoxic antibiotics
Urinary tract obstruction
Chemotherapy (doxorubicin, vincristine, cyclophosphamide)
Nephrocalcinosis
Hypercalcemia
Radiation nephritis
Acute tubular necrosis
Thalassemia

DECREASED UPTAKE

Renal failure
Superscan
    Metastatic disease
    Metabolic bone disease
        Paget's disease
        Osteomalacia
        Hyperparathyroidism
        Myelofibrosis
Nephrectomy

Box 6-4 Incidence of Osseous Metastasis by Tumor Type

Breast	50-85%
Neuroblastoma	80%
Prostate	50-70%
Hodgkin's lymphoma	50-70%
Ewing's sarcoma	60%
Lung	30-50%
Renal cell	30-50%
Thyroid	40%
Melanoma	30-40%
Bladder	15-25%
Osteosarcoma	25%
Wilm's	≤10%

Over 90% of osseous metastasis distribute to the red marrow. In adults, red marrow is found in the axial skeleton and the proximal portions of the humeri and femurs. As the tumor enlarges, the cortex becomes involved. The body responds by attempts at repair. The Tc-99m MDP binds to these regions in areas of bone deposition. Therefore, scans image the bone response to the tumor and not the tumor itself (Fig. 6-8). Even a 5% bone turnover can be detected by bone scan. Radiographs, on the other hand, require a minimum mineral loss of a 50% before a lesion is visualized. MRI is more sensitive than bone scan because signal changes in the marrow from the tumor can be visualized directly. However, whole body MRI is not widely available and generally not practical at this time.

Bone scan is said to be 95% sensitive, but this sensitivity depends on several factors related to tumor type. Areas which are predominantly osteoblastic are easily seen as areas of increased activity. Lesions which are mostly osteoclastic or lytic are more difficult to detect as they will appear cold or isointense. Sensitivity is highest for prostate cancer, which is mainly osteoblastic. The detection of breast and lung cancer is also very high, although these tumors are more mixed in their lesion pattern. When bone scan fails to detect the more aggressive or lytic lesions in lung or breast cancer, F-18 FDG PET can often detect bone marrow abnormalities. The sensitivity of bone scan is low for tumors that are predominantly lytic, such as multiple myeloma and renal cell carcinoma, as well as those which are contained in the marrow, such as lymphoma.

Metastatic Disease in Specific Tumors

Prostate Carcinoma

Skeletal scintigraphy is very sensitive in the detection of metastatic disease from prostate cancer. Until the introduction of the prostate specific antigen (PSA) blood test, bone scan was considered the most sensitive technique for detecting osseous metastasis. Serum alkaline phosphatase measurement detects only half the cases detected by scintigraphy. Radiographs may be normal 30% of the time.

The likelihood of an abnormal scintigram correlates with the clinical stage, Gleason score, and PSA level. In early stage I disease, scintigrams demonstrate metastasis less than 5% of the time. The incidence increases to 10% in stage II and 20% in stage III disease. In patients with PSA levels less than 10 ng/ml, bone metastases are rarely found (<1% of the time). Skeletal scintigrams are still indicated for symptomatic patients and for evaluation of suspicious areas seen radiographically. With increasing PSA levels, the chance of detecting metastatic disease increases.

Breast Carcinoma

Despite increased screening with mammography, a large number of patients with breast cancer present with advanced disease. Mean survival is only 24 months among those with confirmed bone disease. Autopsy studies have shown osseous metastases in 50-80% of patients with breast carcinoma. Like prostate cancer, stage of disease correlates with the incidence of osseous metastases on bone scan: 0.5% in stage I, 2-3% in stage II, 8% in stage III, and 13% in stage IV. Bone scans are not generally performed in patients with stage I or II disease.

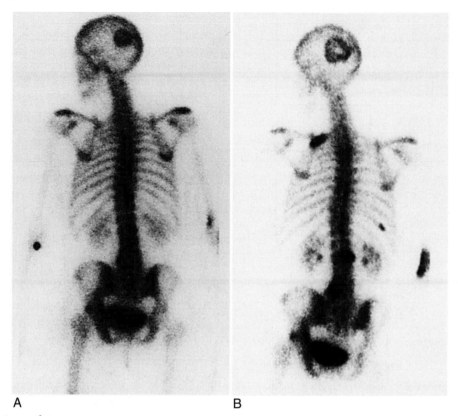

A   B

Figure 6-8   Progression of skeletal metastases. **A,** Initial skeletal scintigram in a patient with multiple skeletal metastases, including the skull. Note the intense uptake in the calvarial lesion with a small area of decreased uptake centrally. **B,** Several months later, the metastatic disease has progressed in the axial skeleton, the calvarium, and ribs. The overall diameter of the skull lesion has increased and the central photon-deficient area is much larger. The increased uptake is in bone at the margin of the metastatic lesion.

Although skeletal scintigraphy has a high sensitivity for breast carcinoma, it may not detect all lesions, such as those contained in the marrow or more lytic lesions.

Lung Carcinoma

Although up to 50% of patients dying from a primary lung cancer have osseous metastasis at autopsy, there is no complete agreement on when to use skeletal scintigraphy. Staging is generally done with CT, surgery (including mediastinoscopy and video-assisted thoracoscopic surgery [VATS]), and increasingly with F-18 FDG PET. Skeletal scintigraphy is useful in a patient who develops pain during or after treatment. However, it appears less useful in cases of local and mediastinal invasion or with advanced disease where therapy will be palliative, although it may also be helpful in planning radiation therapy.

Scintigraphic Patterns in Metastatic Disease

The scintigraphic patterns encountered in skeletal metastatic disease are summarized in Box 6-5. A deci-

> **Box 6-5   Scintigraphic Patterns in Metastatic Disease**
>
> Solitary focal lesions
> Multiple focal lesions
> Diffuse involvement ("superscan")
> Photon-deficient lesions (cold lesions)
> Normal (false negative)
> Flare phenomenon (follow-up studies)
> Soft tissue lesions (tracer uptake in tumor)

sion tree algorithm for the workup of patients with proven non osseous tumors is described in Fig. 6-9. The classic pattern of metastatic disease is that of multiple, focal lesions distributed randomly in the skeleton (Fig. 6-10). Although this typical pattern provides a high degree of clinical certainty as to the diagnosis, several other etiologies can also have multiple areas of uptake (Box 6-6). These must be differentiated from osseous

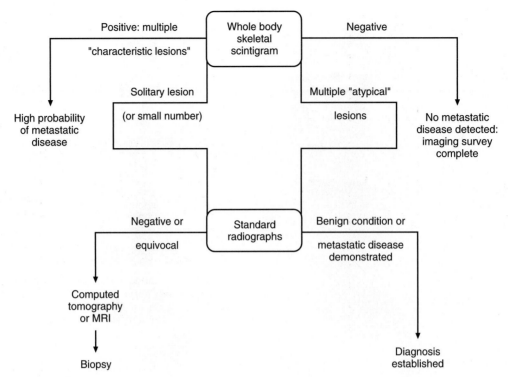

Figure 6-9 Simplified algorithm for the workup of patients with suspected skeletal metastasis.

metastasis. The key is to recognize the different features and patterns of these other etiologies. Final diagnosis may depend on correlation with anatomical imaging.

Osteoarthritic changes are routinely seen and often can be identified by classic locations. These include the medial compartment of the knee, hand, and wrist (especially at the base of the first metacarpal), shoulder, and bones of the feet (Fig. 6-11). The patella frequently shows increased uptake due to chondromalacia and degenerative change. Arthritic changes are frequently bilateral and on both sides of the joint. Degenerative changes in the spine are more problematic because both metastasis and arthritic changes occur in the same location.

Caution must be exercised when assessing uptake in the spine. The spatial resolution of planar images is not sufficient to determine the region of the vertebral body involved. SPECT may localize a lesion to the pedicle that is the typical location of metastasis. A bone scan lesion in the central vertebral body, even when near the end plate and disc space, could be degenerative or malignant and may require short term follow-up. Radiographic and CT correlation often identify the etiology of the uptake as degenerative changes: facet hypertrophy, disc space narrowing, and osteophyte formation. Sometimes MRI can add useful information in this difficult situation.

The findings of trauma can mimic the appearance of metastasis. Patients should be closely questioned for any history of trauma. In the ribs, a vertical alignment of focal abnormal uptake in several or successive ribs is classic for trauma. The nonrandom pattern is not expected in metastatic disease (Figs. 6-12 and 6-13). A metastatic lesion tracks along the bone as seen in Fig. 6-5 rather than remaining focal. Radiographic correlation may show the cortical disruption or callous formation. Because bone scan frequently detects fractures not seen on radiographs, correlation with CT or short-term follow-up bone scan may be needed if no fracture is seen on the radiograph. Persistently positive skeletal activity from old trauma poses another interpretive problem.

A number of other etiologies can cause multifocal abnormalities. Infarctions in sickle cell anemia can cause multiple areas of increased and decreased uptake. Cushing's disease and osteomalacia, for example, frequently cause disproportionate rib lesions as compared with other areas. Osteoporosis may result in dorsal kyphosis and classic fractures such as the vertebral insufficiency fractures and the H-type fracture of the sacrum. Paget's disease, which is addressed later in the chapter, may be differentiated from metastasis by an expansion of the bone and classic locations.

Solitary Lesions

Metastatic disease may present as a solitary bone lesion (Fig. 6-14). The chance that a solitary lesion is due to malignancy varies by location (Box 6-7). Uptake in a rib in a patient with known malignancy has a 10–20% chance

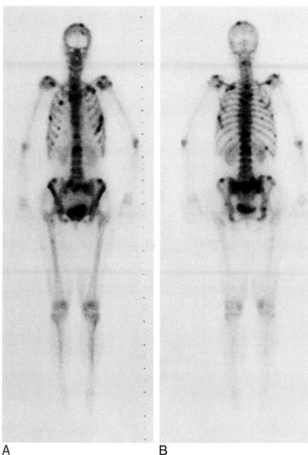

A   B

Figure 6-10   Widespread metastases. Anterior **(A)** and posterior **(B)** whole body scintigrams in a patient with widely distributed metastatic disease. Lesions are present in the skull, spine, ribs, pelvis, and extremities.

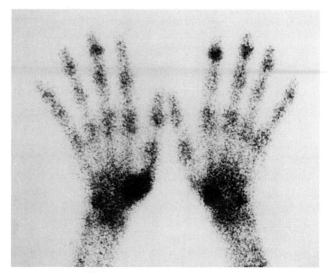

Figure 6-11   Characteristic appearance of osteoarthritis in the hands and wrists. Uptake is increased in multiple distal interphalangeal joints and is particularly intense at the base of the first left metacarpal, a characteristic place for osteoarthritis.

Box 6-6 Differential Diagnosis of Multiple Focal Lesions (Listed in Order of Decreasing Likelihood)

Metastatic disease
Arthritis
Trauma, osteoporotic insufficiency fractures
Paget's disease
Other metabolic bone disease
Osteomyelitis
Numerous other conditions (fibrous dysplasia, multiple enchondromas, infarction)

---

of being malignant, whereas uptake in the central skeleton has a much higher likelihood of being malignant. Focal rib uptake is likely due to fracture, whereas uptake extending along the rib is likely tumor. Common benign causes for a solitary focus of uptake are arthritis and trauma. Some benign bone lesions such as enchondroma, osteoma, fibrous dysplasia, osteomyelitis, and monostotic Paget's disease can also cause solitary abnormalities.

Superscan

A problematic scintigraphic pattern is the "superscan" or "beautiful bone scan." In some patients with prostate cancer and breast cancer, the entire axial skeleton is involved. Uptake may be uniform enough to appear deceptively normal (Fig. 6-15). The differential diagnosis of the superscan pattern is provided in Box 6-8. This is a less common interpretive problem than in the past due to improved technology and image quality, and it should be possible to discriminate diffuse metastasis. Classically, absent or faint visualization of the kidneys is seen with a superscan. However, the soft tissues (including the kidneys) may clear normally if the patient is imaged later than the usual imaging time. Reviewing the available radiographs on each patient will help prevent any mistake.

Flare Phenomenon

Another potentially perplexing pattern is seen in some bone scans done on patients undergoing cyclical chemotherapy. When a patient has a good response to chemotherapy, the bone scan may paradoxically worsen, with a "flare" of increased activity (Fig. 6-16). To add to the confusion, these patients may experience increased pain. If these lesions are followed radiographically, increased sclerosis is seen over 2–6 months because this is an osteoblastic response as the bone begins to heal. This is the same time frame that the bone scan typically shows increased uptake. The flare phenomenon reinforces the fact that tracer uptake is not in the tumor but rather in the surrounding bone.

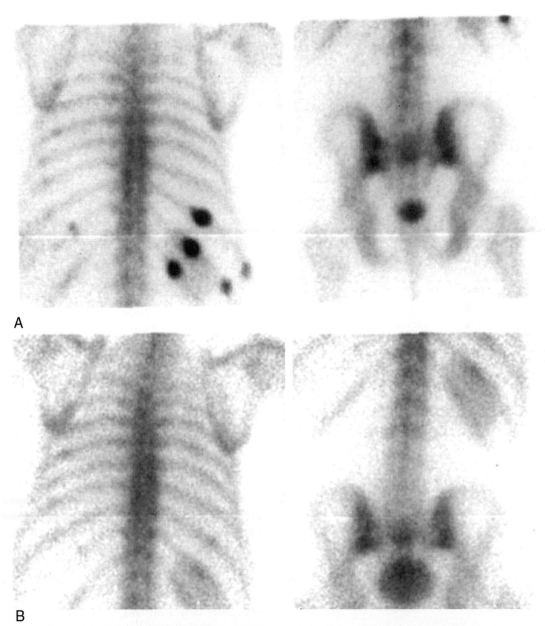

Figure 6-12   Typical appearance of rib fractures. **A,** Posterior views of the chest reveal focal uptake in a vertical alignment in the right lower ribs and a recent left nephrectomy with resection of some lower left ribs. **B,** A follow-up study 18 months later shows resolution of the right rib uptake as the fractures healed.

Cold Lesions

Lesions that are aggressive or purely lytic, as well as areas completely replaced by tumor, may show decreased uptake (*see* Fig. 6-4). A list of possible etiologies of cold defect is provided in Box 6-9. These "cold" or photon deficient areas may be difficult to spot because of overlying or adjacent uptake. Often, these cold areas are bordered by a rim of increased uptake. Another cause for an area of decreased uptake is radiation therapy changes. These are commonly geometric in shape, conforming to the radiation port.

Extraskeletal Uptake in Soft Tissues

A number of common soft tissue neoplasms exhibit varying degrees of skeleton-seeking tracer uptake in both the primary tumor and soft tissue metastases. The mechanism of localization is thought to be a combination of ossification in the tumor and binding to macromolecules. The degree of uptake is not sufficient to use the Tc-99m-labeled bone agents as primary tumor imaging agents. Tumors most commonly seen are carcinoma of the breast, lung, melanoma, neuroblastoma, metastatic colon carcinoma to liver, and some malignant pleural effusions.

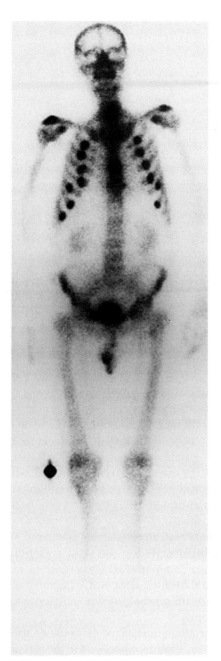

Figure 6-13   Multiple rib fractures bilaterally. The pattern of linearly aligned lesions is highly characteristic for trauma and would be unusual as a pattern for metastatic disease.

Soft tissue uptake must be differentiated from bone pathology (Fig. 6-17 and Fig. 6-18).

Imaging Findings in Specific Tumors

Breast Carcinoma

Skeletal scintigraphy is highly sensitive in breast cancer. Patients may show local invasion of the ribs or disseminated disease. Another important pattern to recognize is involvement of the sternum via the internal mammary

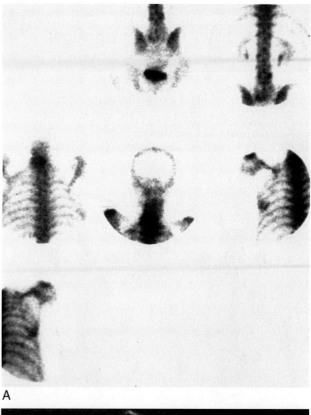

A

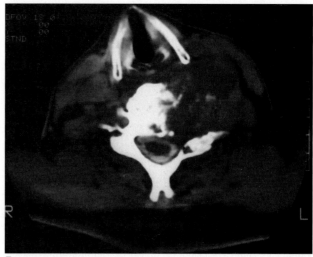

B

Figure 6-14   Suspected metastatic disease on bone scan. **A,** Posterior spot views show that a solitary area of abnormally increased uptake can be seen in the lower cervical spine. **B,** Computed tomographic scan obtained at the level of scintigraphic abnormality reveals extensive destruction of the corresponding vertebral body and demonstrates the clinically palpable soft tissue mass in the neck.

nodes. Although activity in the sternum is most often benign, there is a high incidence of metastatic disease in breast cancer patients (>80%). Metastatic disease to the soft tissues may be seen (*see* Fig. 6-18) and increased uptake may be present in malignant pleural effusions.

Box 6-7	Metastatic Disease Presenting as a Solitary Focus in Patients with Known Cancer
Spine and pelvis	60–70%
Skull	40–50%
Rib	10–20%
Sternum (in breast carcinoma)	75%

Box 6-8	Differential Diagnosis for Superscan Pattern

COMMON

Metastases (prostate, breast)
Renal osteodystrophy
Delayed Images

LESS COMMON

Severe hyperparathyroidism (rare primary)
Osteomalacia
Paget's disease

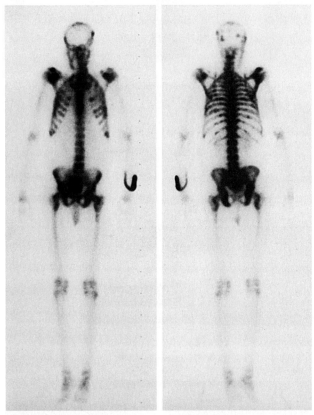

Figure 6-15 "Superscan" of a patient with prostatic carcinoma. In this case, the uptake is nonuniform enough that the abnormality is easily seen. The images show an increased skeletal uptake, largely in the axial skeleton. Soft tissue activity is decreased. The kidneys are faint. The bladder is well-visualized, indicating that failure to see the kidneys is not due to absence of tracer excretion through them. Rather, the uptake in the skeleton is so intense that the kidney activity is below the windowing threshold.

Lung Carcinoma

Interesting patterns of disease may occur on scintigrams in lung cancer. Because these tumors can easily invade the vasculature, arterial metastases are more common. These tumor emboli can reach the distal extremities. Thus, appendicular involvement is more common with aggressive lung cancer than cancer of the breast or prostate. Also, a characteristic periosteal change is seen

in lung cancer due to hypertrophic osteoarthropathy (Figs. 6-19 and 6-20). This is most often seen as linear, parallel "track" uptake in the medial and lateral margins of the long bones, but may be patchy or show skip areas. The patella, scapula, skull, clavicles, and hands and feet may be involved.

Neuroblastoma

Neuroblastoma has a neural crest origin and is the most common solid tumor to metastasize to bone in children (Fig. 6-21). Tc-99m MDP scintigraphy is twice as sensitive as radiographs on a lesion-by-lesion basis. MRI better determines the extent of a lesion than bone scan. I-131 or I-123 MIBG scanning is more sensitive than bone scan for metastases, although the combination of both gives the highest sensitivity.

Lesions are typically multifocal and in the metaphyses. However, involvement in the skull, vertebrae, ribs, and pelvis is also common. Early involvement may be symmetric and therefore difficult to diagnose on the bone scan due to the normal intense activity in the ends of growing bones.

A unique characteristic of neuroblastoma is the avidity of Tc-99m diphosphonates for the primary tumor. Approximately 30–50% of primary tumors are demonstrated scintigraphically. Occasionally, neuroblastomas are discovered in children undergoing radionuclide imaging to evaluate another condition. Particular attention should be paid to the abdomen.

Other Tumors of Epithelial Origin

Numerous other tumors metastasize to bone. The sensitivity for renal cell carcinoma is low and best assessed on skeletal survey or by MRI. Likewise, thyroid cancer is rarely detected on skeletal scintigraphy and is better evaluated with iodine-131 or, if noniodine avid, by F-18 FDG PET.

Gastrointestinal tract and gynecological cancers do not commonly metastasize to bone early in their courses. Late disease involves bone by direct exten-

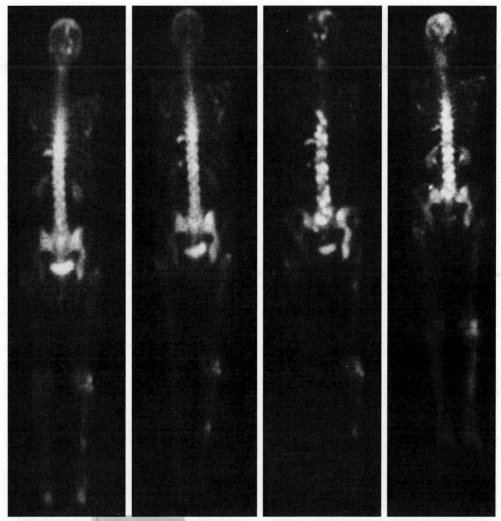

Figure 6-16   Flare phenomenon. Ten-month sequence of posterior whole body scintigrams of a patient undergoing chemotherapy for carcinoma of the breast. Note the increased intensity of uptake in the skull, spine, and pelvis, especially between the second and third images in the sequence. Although the scintigram appears worse, the patient was improving clinically with reduced bone pain and radiographic evidence of healing.

sion. The success of therapy, including chemotherapy, in controlling gastrointestinal tumors has led to an increase in cases with skeletal involvement. Due to longer survival and control of local and regional metastases that usually cause death, bone metastases can manifest.

Primary Tumors

Malignant Tumors

Primary bone tumors have avid uptake of the bone-seeking radiopharmaceuticals (Fig. 6-22). These tumors include the primary neoplasms, osteosarcoma, Ewing's sarcoma, and chondrosarcoma. However, skeletal scintigraphy is seldom used in the workup of primary bone neoplasms because it does not address the questions the orthopedic

surgeon needs answered: assessment of soft tissue extension or definition of tumor margins. MRI is the primary modality for osteosarcoma evaluation (Fig. 6-23). Although most primary bone tumors are monostotic, the occasional polyostotic involvement would be missed without a whole body survey of some kind (Fig. 6-24). Both thallium-201 and technetium-99m sestamibi have been used for sarcoma imaging. They may help to determine if the primary tumor is high- or low-grade and serve as a baseline so that it can be used to evaluate response to therapy. The increased uptake in FDG PET of high-grade tumors has been investigated but has not found a significant clinical role.

Multiple Myeloma

The most common primary bone tumor in adults is multiple myeloma. It is a tumor of the marrow and typically involves the vertebrae, pelvis, ribs, and skull. Radiographs

Box 6-9 Differential Diagnosis of a Cold Defect

Metal artifact (pacemaker, prosthesis)
Radiation changes
Barium in bowel
Vascular
   Early avascular necrosis
   Early infarct
Multiple myeloma
Osseous metastasis
   Renal cell carcinoma
   Thyroid carcinoma
   Anaplastic tumors
   Neuroblastoma
   Breast and lung carcinoma
Tumor marrow involvement
   Lymphoma
   Leukemia
Benign tumors, cysts

may only show osteopenia or a permeative pattern that can be confused with metastatic disease. Although bone scan will show some of the lesions as areas of decreased and sometimes increased uptake, radiographs are more sensitive overall for detecting disease. The lower sensitivity of bone scan relates to the lack of reactive bone formation in response to the lesions.

Leukemia

Bone scan plays a very limited role in the evaluation of leukemia. Patients with leukemia imaged with Tc-99m MDP may show focal increased uptake in areas of marrow infiltration. In blast crisis, diffusely increased uptake that is greater at the ends of the long bones may be present.

Lymphoma

Hodgkin's disease will involve the skeleton approximately one third of the time and the bone scan may show focal or diffuse uptake of Tc-99m MDP. Skeletal scintigraphy is less useful in non-Hodgkin's lymphoma. In general, lymphoma is best evaluated with gallium-67, F-18 FDG PET, and CT.

Histiocytosis

The sensitivity of bone scan varies with the spectrum of disease in histiocytosis. Although uptake is reliably seen in eosinophilic granuloma, detection of histiocytosis is limited, with lesions seen from one-third to two thirds of the time. Frequently, decreased uptake is shown.

Benign Bone Tumors

Usually, benign bone tumors are characterized by their radiographic appearance. The role of skeletal scintigraphy is very limited in general, although understanding is critical as benign tumors may be encountered during imaging for other reasons. Some benign tumors have intense uptake similar to malignant tumors. These include osteoid osteomas, giant cell tumors, and fibrous dysplasia. Most benign bone tumors are variable in appearance. Table 6-2 lists some of the benign bone tumors and their appearance on bone scan.

Osteoid Osteoma

Scintigraphy is very useful in identification of an osteoid osteoma. Classically, these lesions present in adolescents and young adults with severe pain at night. They commonly occur in the proximal femur and spine and may be difficult to detect with conventional radiography,

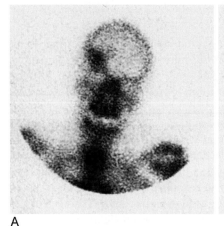
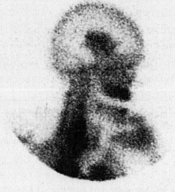
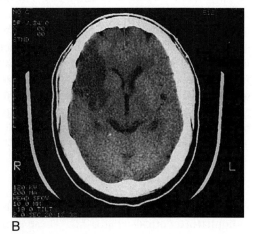

A   B

Figure 6-17   **A,** Tc-99m MDP uptake in a right parietal stroke. **B,** CT confirms the etiology of the uptake is intracranial and not in the skull.

especially in the spine. The diagnosis on radiographs can be made if a central lucent nidus is seen surrounded by sclerosis (Fig. 6-25). Skeletal scintigraphy is very sensitive as the lesion will show increased uptake (Fig. 6-26). SPECT adds to this sensitivity and is particularly useful in the spine. Surgeons can use an intraoperative probe to localize the lesion with its increased activity. However, CT has largely eliminated the need for the bone scan in the work up of osteoid osteoma.

Other Indications

Bone scan may be useful in assessing an atypical bone island on radiographs. If the sclerotic lesion on radiograph does not show increased scintigraphic activity, it is unlikely to be malignant.

Osteochondromas are common cartilage-containing benign tumors. They may show variable uptake that diminishes as the skeleton matures. Rarely, osteochondromas will show malignant transformation, usually into a chondrosarcoma. This degeneration occurs less than 1% of the time in a solitary lesion and less than 5% of the time in hereditary multiple osteochondromatosis (hereditary multiple exostoses). Although bone scan can exclude malignancy if no increased uptake is seen, the presence of increased activity does not differentiate benign from malignant lesions. Any new uptake in a lesion that previously had none is suspicious. Osteochondromas are usually best evaluated with CT and MRI.

Enchondromas usually present as a cystic lesion in the hands or a sclerotic area reminiscent of a bone infarct elsewhere. They are benign but can degenerate into a malignant tumor. This degeneration is more common in multiple enchondromatosis (Ollier's disease). Bone scan may help identify multiple lesions, but the role is otherwise very limited.

Bone Dysplasias

Numerous bone dysplasias demonstrate increased skeletal tracer uptake (Figs. 6-27 and 6-28). Fibrous dysplasia is the most commonly encountered of these and may be monostotic or polyostotic (*see* Fig. 6-28). The degree of increased tracer uptake is typically high, rivaling that seen in Paget's disease. Distinguishing features are the younger age of the patient and the different pattern of involvement. When Paget's disease involves a long bone, it invariably extends to at least one end of the bone. Fibrous dysplasia frequently does not involve the end of the bone. Other dysplasias associated with increased tracer uptake are listed in Box 6-10.

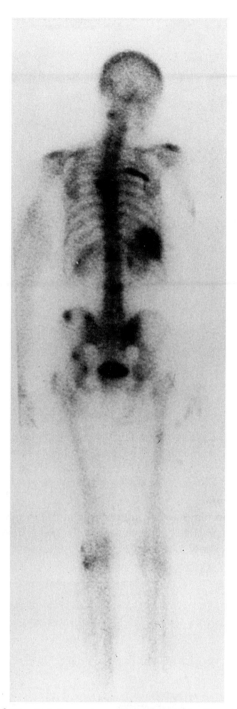

Figure 6-18   Soft tissue metastasis in breast cancer. Posterior scintigram of a patient with breast carcinoma. The patient has multiple skeletal metastases. Uptake is intense in the soft tissue liver metastasis. The uptake projects just superolateral to the right kidney.

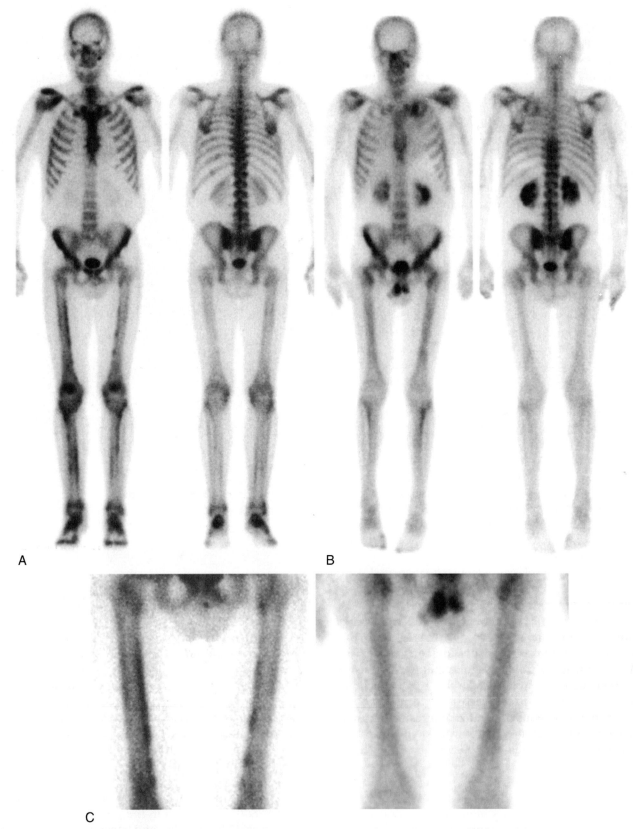

Figure 6-19   Hypertrophic osteoarthropathy in a patient with bronchogenic lung carcinoma.
A, Planar whole body scintigrams reveal the classic pattern of uptake in the periosteal region of the long bones. **B,** Follow-up scan 9 months later shows increased activity in a treated left apical lung mass. Radiation therapy changes of decreased uptake in the upper thoracic spine are seen. With successful treatment, the findings of hypertrophic osteoarthropathy have resolved. **C,** Spot views of the femurs more clearly show the abnormal uptake (*left*) that later resolves more clearly (*right*).

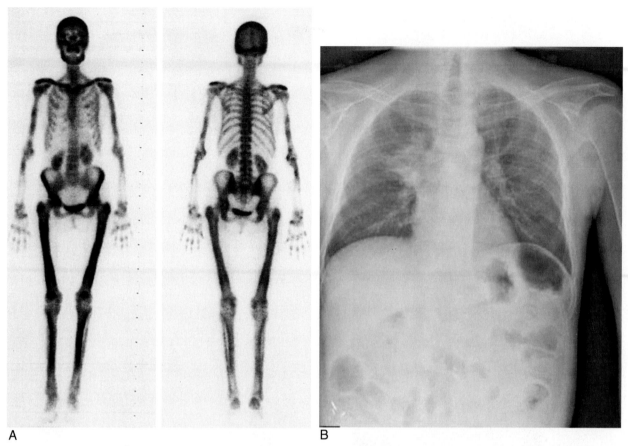

Figure 6-20   **A,** Florid hypertrophic osteoarthropathy. The bones of the upper and lower extremities are diffusely involved, as are the clavicles, mandible, and skull. Although the pattern may be confusing, the patient did not have skeletal metastatic disease. Involvement of the extremities is one clue. **B,** Chest x-ray reveals a bronchogenic carcinoma in the right upper lobe just above the right hilum.

Continued

Metabolic Bone Disease

A number of metabolic conditions can result in marked bone scan abnormalities (Box 6-11). The patterns of metabolic bone disease must be recognized to avoid confusion with pathology such as metastatic disease. However, there is no role for bone scan in the diagnosis and management of these diseases.

Inadequate osseous mineralization results in osteomalacia. This gives the bones a washed-out, chalky appearance with decreased trabeculae on radiographs. Osteomalacia, hyperparathyroidism, renal osteodystrophy and hypervitaminosis D can all cause patterns of increased scintigraphic uptake.

Problems with vitamin D metabolism can cause rickets. Although this affects adults, the changes are most striking in a growing skeleton. Radiographs may show changes at the growth plates (frayed, widened, cupping) of the proximal humerus, distal femur, distal tibia, and distal forearm. Significant changes are seen in the costochondral junctions. Striking "beading" of the costochondral junction may be seen (Fig. 6-29).

Hyperparathyroidism

Hyperparathyroidism, renal osteodystrophy, osteomalacia, and hypervitaminosis D can all result in various patterns of increased uptake in the skeleton, and Generalized increased tracer uptake may be seen throughout the skeleton (Fig. 6-30; Box 6-12). An increased skeleton-to-soft tissue ratio and poor renal visualization may create an appearance similar to a superscan seen in metastatic disease.

The bone scan in long standing renal osteodystrophy often has the most extreme appearance. Increased activity is typically seen in the periarticular regions, skull, mandible, maxilla, and sternum. These same findings may be seen to a varying degree in secondary hyperparathyroidism and osteomalacia. For example, pseudofractures are often present in osteomalacia and demonstrate avid radiopharmaceutical uptake

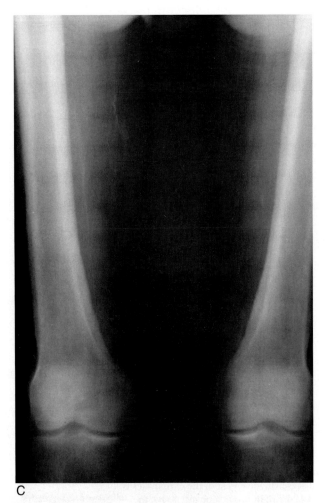

C

Figure 6-20, cont'd   C, Radiograph of the femurs shows characteristic periosteal new bone bilaterally on both the medial and lateral aspects of the femoral shaft.

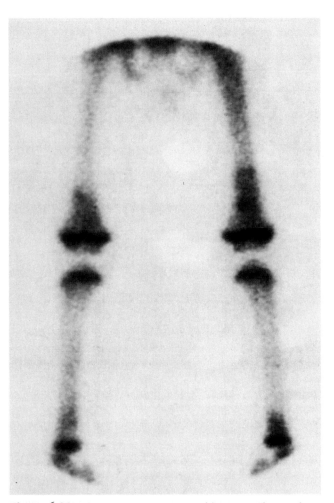

Figure 6-21   Bone metastases in neuroblastoma. Abnormal tracer localization is present in both femurs and distal tibial metaphyses, more extensive on the left than the right.

(Fig. 6-31). Extraskeletal uptake may be seen. Soft tissue uptake in the lungs may be caused by an increased serum calcium-phosphate ratio. In hyperparathyroidism associated with renal failure, a classic pattern of uptake is seen in the lungs, stomach, and kidneys. These organs are all involved in acid-base metabolism (Fig. 6-32).

Osteoporosis

Although inadequate osseous mineralization results in osteomalacia, osteoporosis is a decrease in bone mass. This results in an increase in fragility due to decreased bone mineral content and architectural deterioration. On radiographs, the bones have a washed-out appearance with decreased trabeculae.

Skeletal scintigraphy does not have a role in the diagnosis of osteoporosis but is useful in surveying the entire skeleton for osteoporotic insufficiency fractures. Because these may be asymptomatic, the ability to survey the entire skeleton is advantageous. Compression fractures of the spine are common and may show abnor-

mal uptake before radiographic changes (Fig. 6-33). These insufficiency osteoporotic fractures may show persistent uptake for months or years, so it can be difficult to determine if the fracture is acute.

Sacral insufficiency fractures are also common and are often difficult to diagnose radiographically or by CT. The most common pattern is the H or butterfly pattern, with a horizontal band of increased uptake across the body of the sacrum and two vertical limbs of activity in the sacral alae (Fig. 6-34). Several pattern variations may be seen, including asymmetry of the alar activity. Less severe fractures may show only horizontal linear uptake.

Paget's Disease

Paget's disease may be included in the metabolic bone disease category, although the exact etiology is not entirely understood. A chronic bone disease of the elderly, it causes enlarged, coarsened bones. The diagnosis can usually be made by radiographs, although CT and MRI can be used to assess complications of Paget's.

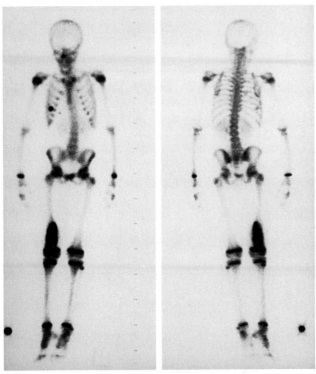

Figure 6-22   Osteosarcoma of the right distal femur. The degree of tracer accumulation in the lesion is striking. The increased blood flow induced by the osteosarcoma results in increased tracer delivery to the entire limb. This "extended" or augmented pattern of uptake adds to the difficulty in using the skeletal scintigram to determine the margins of primary bone tumors. (The focal activity over the right ribs is a marker.)

A bone scan is useful for the evaluation of the extent of disease. When it is found incidentally, the patterns of Paget's disease must be recognized.

The scintigraphic appearance is striking, with intensely increased tracer localization (Figs. 6-35 and 6-36). The expansion of bone demonstrated radiographically is not well-assessed by scintigraphy, owing to the lower resolution of the technique and the "blooming" appearance of very intense areas of uptake, but it is certainly suggested on the images. The pelvis is the most commonly involved site, followed by the spine, skull, femur, scapula, tibia, and humerus. The increased uptake is seen in all phases of the disease: the early resorptive, mixed, and sclerotic phases. In osteoporosis circumscripta, a characteristic rim of increased uptake borders the lesion.

Skeletal Trauma

Skeletal scintigraphy is able to demonstrate abnormalities early after direct trauma (Figs. 6-12 and 6-37). The bone scan findings from trauma may persist for quite some time. This may create problems when using skeletal scintigraphy for another purpose, such as the detection of metastatic disease.

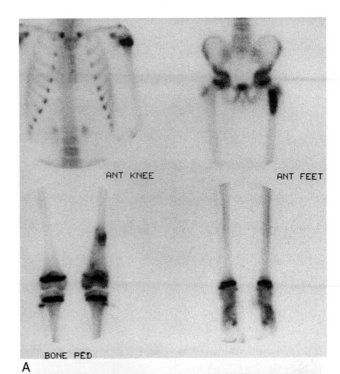

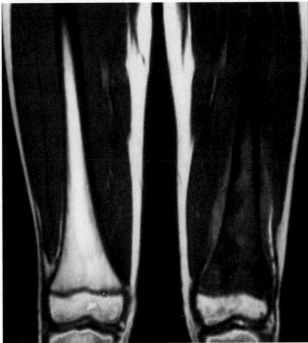

Figure 6-23   **A,** Osteosarcoma of the left distal femur and a metastatic lesion in the left proximal femur. **B,** Coronal T1-weighted MRI. Superior anatomical information about the osseous and soft tissue extent of the tumor. However, it missed the second lesion in the proximal femur which was out of the field of view.

Detection of Fractures

Approximately 80% of fractures can be visualized by 24 hours after trauma. The earliest scintigraphic appearance is diffusely increased uptake, most likely the result of hyperemia at the fracture site. After 3 days, 95% of

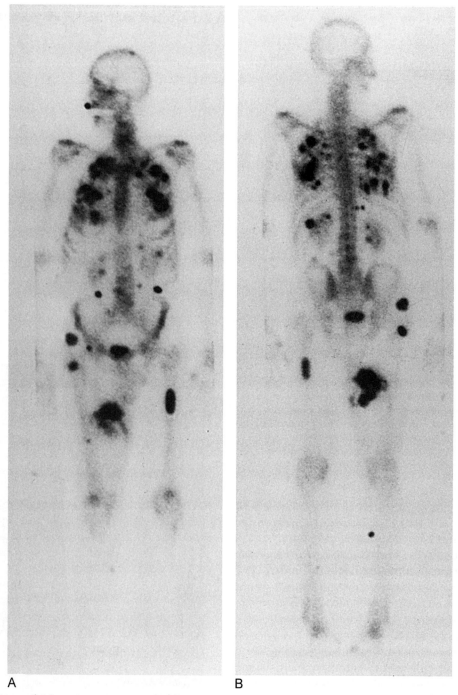

A   B

Figure 6-24   **A–B,** Extraosseous osteosarcoma arising in the right medial thigh area. The tumor is widely disseminated with skeletal metastases, soft tissue metastases, and pulmonary metastases. This study is a dramatic example of the ability of skeletal scintigraphy to survey the entire body.

fractures are positive on scintigraphy; in patients under the age of 65, essentially all fractures are positive by this time. Advanced age and debilitation are factors contributing to a lack of visualization or delayed visualization of fractures. The maximum degree of fracture uptake occurs 7 or more days after trauma and delayed imaging in this time frame is recommended in difficult or equivocal cases. In the past, skeletal scintigraphy was frequently performed to evaluate radiographically occult hip fractures. This role has largely moved to MRI, which is highly sensitive and often provides additional information.

The time a fracture takes to return to normal on the bone scan depends on its location, its stability, and the

Table 6-2 Benign Bone Lesions on Skeletal Scintigraphy

Degree of Uptake	Malignancy Potential	Comments
INTENSE UPTAKE		
Aneurysmal bone cyst	No	Donut sign pattern
Chondroblastoma	Almost always benign	Bone scan positive does not diagnose malignancy
Giant cell tumor	10%	
Fibrous dysplasia	<1%	
Osteoma	No	Gardner's syndrome
Osteoid osteoma	No	Osteoblastoma >2 cm
ISOINTENSE/MILD UPTAKE		
Bone island	No	
Enchondroma	Solitary: <20% long bones	
	Multiple enchondromatosis: <50%	
Nonossifying fibroma	No	
VARIABLE UPTAKE		
Osteochondroma	<1%	
HEREDITARY MULTIPLE EXOSTOSES		
Hemangioma	No	Prominent trabeculae diagnostic
Eosinophilic granuloma	No; least aggressive histiocytosis group	Monostotic /Polyostotic
LOW UPTAKE		
Unicameral bone cyst	No	

degree of damage to the skeleton. Some 60–80% of nondisplaced uncomplicated fractures revert to normal in 1 year and over 95% revert in 3 years (Table 6-3). However, there are many instances in which displaced fractures remained positive indefinitely (e.g., involvement of a joint by posttraumatic arthritis causes prolonged abnormal uptake). Patients undergoing metastatic skeletal survey should be routinely asked about prior trauma. In a prospective study by Kim, nearly half of patients being evaluated for skeletal metastatic disease reported previous fractures. In all, 26% of the fracture sites were positive at the time of scintigraphic examination, including 16 (16%) of 98 sites where the trauma had occurred more than 5 years before. Structural deformity and posttraumatic arthritis were the most common reasons for prolonged positive studies.

Iatrogenic Trauma

Iatrogenic trauma to either the skeleton or soft tissues may result in abnormal uptake on the bone scan. The key to correct interpretation is an accurate history. Craniotomy typically leaves a rim pattern at the surgical margin that may persist for months postoperatively. Rib retraction during thoracotomy can elicit periosteal reaction and increased uptake without actual resection of bone being involved. Bone resections are recognized as photon-defi-

cient areas, although small laminectomies are usually not appreciated scintigraphically.

Areas of the skeleton receiving therapeutic levels of external beam ionizing radiation (typically ≥4000 rads) characteristically demonstrate decreased uptake within 6 months to 1 year after therapy. The threshold for the effect is on the order of 2000 rads. The mechanism is probably decreased osteogenesis and decreased blood flow to postirradiated bone. The scintigraphic hallmark is a geometrical pattern of regionally decreased tracer uptake (*see* Fig. 6-19*B*). An increase in uptake immediately after therapy may be seen due to hyperemia.

Child Abuse

The generally high sensitivity of skeletal scintigraphy would seem to make it an ideal survey test in cases of suspected child abuse. In practice, however, the sensitivity is somewhat disappointing. This probably relates to the timing of injury in relation to scintigraphy. Older fractures may have healed and may not be seen scintigraphically, and skeletal scintigraphy has been reported to miss calvarial fractures in young children. In child abuse, radiographic skeletal survey is more sensitive than bone scintigraphy because of its ability to demonstrate old fractures. Scintigraphy should be reserved for cases of suspected child abuse in which radiographs are unrevealing.

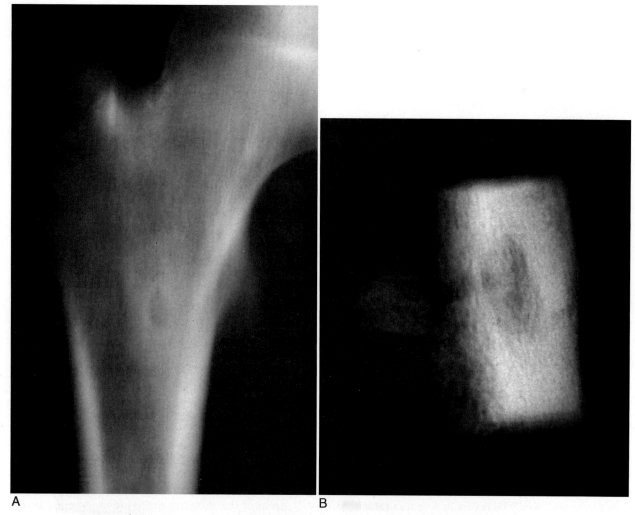

A   B

Figure 6-25   Osteoid osteoma: radiograph. **A,** Conventional tomogram of the right proximal femur reveals a characteristic radiolucent nidus surrounded by sclerotic bone. **B,** Specimen radiograph confirms the complete excision of the nidus.

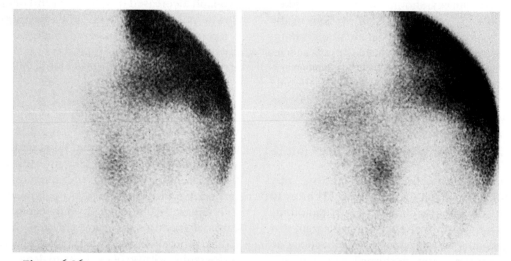

Figure 6-26   Osteoid osteoma: pinhole images. Internal and external rotation pinhole spot views of the proximal femur in a patient with suspected osteoid osteoma. An area of abnormally increased uptake demonstrated just lateral to the lesser trochanter confirms the clinical suspicion.

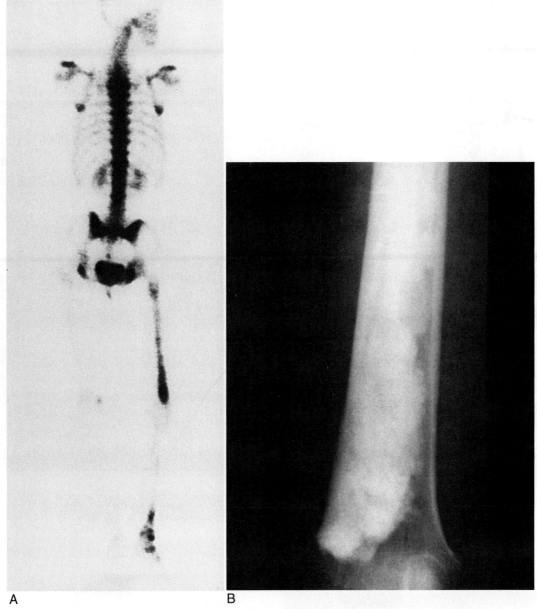

A   B

Figure 6-27   Melorheostosis. **A,** Posterior whole body image showing intensely increased uptake in a somewhat patchy distribution involving the right femur. **B,** Radiograph of the distal femur reveals the characteristic intensely sclerotic lesion of melorheostosis, often characterized as having the appearance of dripping candle wax.

In these cases, symmetric positioning of the patient is critical.

Complex Regional Pain Syndrome
Complex regional pain syndrome, previously known as reflex sympathetic dystrophy, is a complex disorder with a variable presentation. It is an exaggerated response to injury and immobilization with sensory, motor, and autonomic features. Typically, patients present with pain, edema, and muscle wasting in an affected extremity.

Scintigraphic findings are variable depending on the stage of disease. Early disease (up to 5–6 months) usually shows increased blood flow. Later in the course of disease, blood flow may be normal or decreased. The classic pattern has been described as a unilateral increase in flow and blood pool activity with increased periarticular uptake on delayed images. This pattern is seen less than 50% of the time but provides the highest diagnostic accuracy. The periarticular uptake on delayed images is found in most cases (>95%), although specificity is lower if this finding is

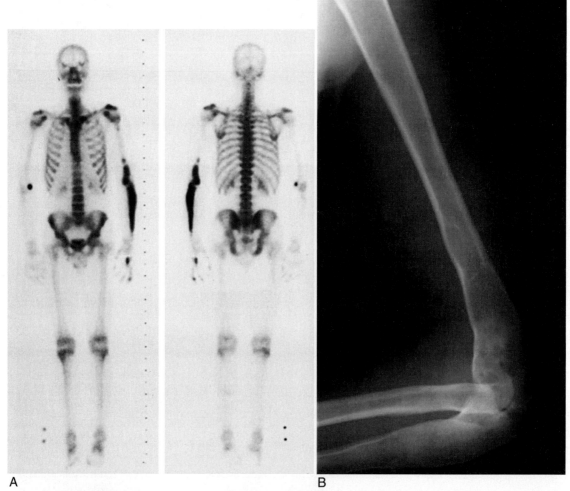

A   B

Figure 6-28   Fibrous dysplasia. **A,** Uptake is markedly increased in the distal humerus, most of the forearm, and focal areas in the hand. **B,** Corresponding radiograph of the left elbow reveals characteristic expansile lesions of fibrous dysplasia.

Box 6-10   Bone Dysplasias Associated with Increased Skeletal Tracer Uptake

Fibrous dysplasia
Osteogenesis imperfecta
Osteopetrosis
Progressive diaphyseal dysplasia (Engelmann's disease)
Hereditary multiple diaphyseal sclerosis (Ribbing's disease)
Melorheostosis

---

seen without the increased blood flow. Infection and arthritis could cause false positives. Some variants have been found, including cold or decreased uptake in some adults. Children often have normal or decreased uptake.

Stress Fractures

A significant change in activity level or a repetitive activity may lead to injury to the bone. The reaction to this injury is remodeling of the bone. Cortical bone may become weakened and buttressed by periosteal and endosteal new bone. The final result of imbalance between resorption and replacement is a stress fracture (Table 6-4). If the process causing injury is allowed to continue to the point of overt fracture, healing predictably takes several months or more, compared with the several weeks required for healing of an early stress reaction. Therefore, prompt diagnosis and appropriate change in activity is critical.

Skeletal scintigraphy is exquisitely sensitive to the remodeling process and typically shows abnormalities at least 1–2 weeks before the appearance of radiographic changes in stress fractures. The characteristic scinti-

Box 6-11   Metabolic Bone Disorders

OSTEOPOROSIS

Primary (Idiopathic)

Senile, postmenopausal

Secondary

Disuse	
Drugs	Corticosteroids, chemotherapy, anticonvulsants
Endocrine	Hyperthyroidism, primary hyperparathyroidism, Cushing's disease, hypogonadism

OSTEOMALACIA

Vitamin D	Vitamin D deficiency, hereditary disorders of vitamin D metabolism
Decreased calcium	Calcium malabsorption, inadequate intake, calcitonin secreting tumors
Phosphate loss	Renal tubular disease, hemodialysis, transplant
Other	Liver disease, phenytoin, prematurity

HYPERPARATHYROIDISM

Primary	Parathyroid adenoma, parathyroid hyperplasia
Secondary	Chronic renal insufficiency, phosphate metabolism abnormalities, parathyroid hyperplasia
Tertiary	Autonomous parathyroid glands from long standing secondary hyperparathyroidism

RENAL OSTEODYSTROPHY	Chronic renal failure
HYPOPARATHYROIDISM	Iatrogenic loss/damage parathyroid glands during thyroidectomy; pseudohypoparathyroidism genetic end-organ resistance

METAL TOXICITIES

Aluminum-induced bone disease

Fluorosis

Heavy metal poisoning

---

graphic appearance is that of intense uptake at the fracture site. The configuration is oval or fusiform with the long axis of increased uptake parallel to the axis of the bone (Fig. 6-38).

MRI is currently the modality most commonly used to evaluate stress fracture. It can provide additional information such as the status of soft tissues and tendons. MRI does not expose patients to ionizing radiation. MRI can identify marrow edema early in the stress response, but edema alone is nonspecific. MRI may be helpful by identifying a true fracture in an area of edema. Fractures are visualized as linear abnormalities on T_1 scans.

Spondylolysis occurs in the lumbar spine in the pars articularus. This is often seen due to repetitive trauma in young athletes. Most commonly the abnormality occurs at L4-5. In some instances, all examinations may be normal, including MRI and radiographs, but a SPECT study may reveal the pathology (Fig. 6-39).

Shin Splints

The term *shin splints* is applied generically to describe stress-related leg soreness. Patients complain of mild to moderate exercise-induced pain along the medial or posteromedial aspect of the tibia. In nuclear medicine, the term is now used to describe a specific combination of clinical and scintigraphic findings. Increased tracer uptake is seen on the scintigram, typically involving a large portion of the middle to distal tibia (Fig. 6-40). Most cases are bilateral although not necessarily symmetrical. The radionuclide uptake is superficial, only mild to moderate in intensity, and lacks a focal aspect seen with true stress fractures. Hyperemia is limited, unlike stress fractures which show intense hyperemia.

A phenomenon perhaps related to shin splints is *activity-induced enthesopathy*. The term simply refers to a disease process at the site of tendon or ligament attachment to bone. In athletes, repeated microtears with subsequent healing reaction can result in increased tracer uptake at corresponding locations. Osteitis pubis, plantar fasciitis, Achilles tendonitis, and some cases of pulled hamstring muscles are examples. A periosteal reaction develops at the site of stress, resulting in increased skeletal tracer localization.

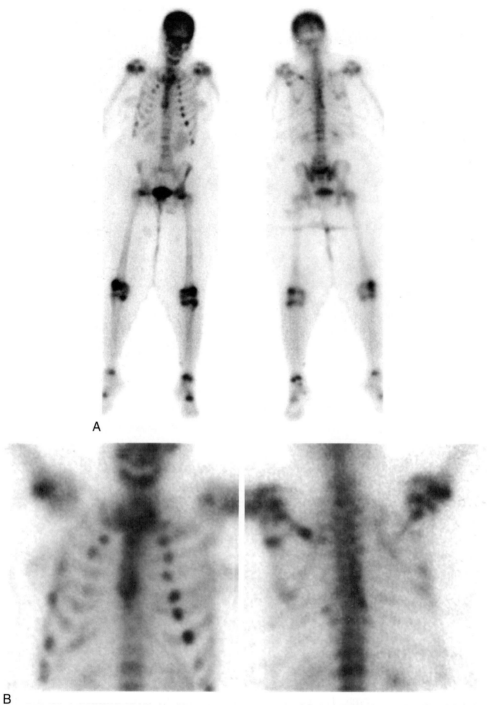

Figure 6-29   Renal osteodystrophy. Whole body (**A**) and spot images (**B**) of a patient with long-standing renal failure show classic skeletal changes of severe renal osteodystrophy. Abnormal activity is seen in the face and skull as well as the distal ends of the long bones. The rib tip activity has been called the rachitic "rosary bead" configuration. Focal uptake in the left scapula was a fracture although brown tumors can have a similar appearance.

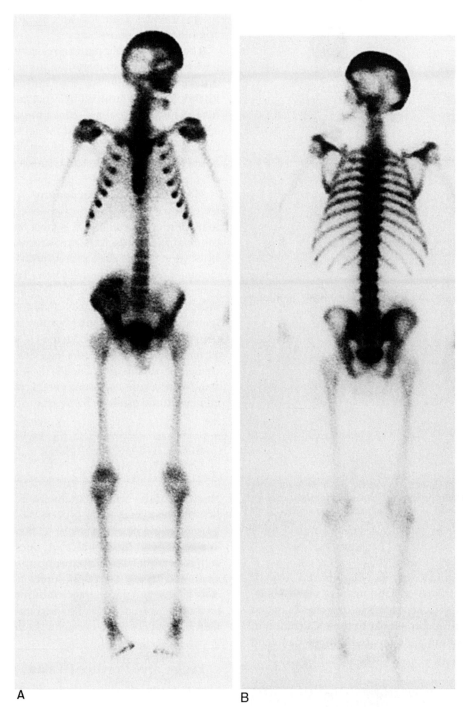

A   B

Figure 6-30   Renal osteodystrophy. **A–B,** The absence of soft tissue uptake is striking with an appearance similar to the "superscan" seen in metastatic disease. The prominent rib end activity may help differentiate the two etiologies. The native kidneys had failed, and a renal transplant is noted in the right iliac fossa.

Continued

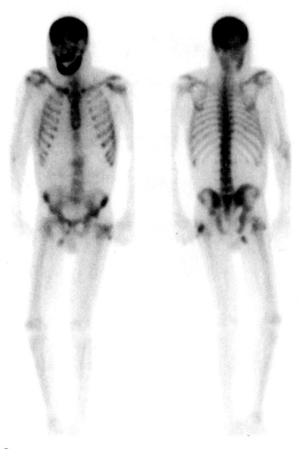

C

Figure 6-30, cont'd   **C,** Increased activity in the skull and sternum may be especially prominent. Note the increased axial skeletal uptake and paucity of soft tissue background activity.

Rhabdomyolysis

Another athletic injury that is seen in this day of marathons and triathlons is rhabdomyolysis (Fig. 6-41). The localization of skeletal tracers in exercise-damaged skeletal muscle is probably similar to the localization in damaged myocardium. Calcium buildup in damaged

---

Box 6-12   Distribution of Increased Skeletal Uptake in Hyperparathyroidism

Diffuse axial
Periarticular
Skull
Mandible, fascial bones
Costochondral junctions
Sternum
Lungs
Stomach

---

tissue provides a site for radionuclide deposition when combined with phosphate.

The scintigraphic pattern reflects the muscle groups undergoing injury. In marathon runners, the most striking uptake is usually in the muscles of the thigh. Rhabdomyolysis induced by renal failure is generally diffuse. The time course of scintigraphic abnormality appears to be similar to that for acute myocardial infarction. The greatest degree of uptake is seen at 24–48 hours following injury. The changes resolve by 1 week.

Heterotopic Bone Formation

Heterotopic bone formation can occur in the muscle due to numerous conditions. It is most often a direct result of trauma to the muscle in myositis ossificans (Fig. 6-42). However, it can also be a serious problem in paralyzed muscles and prolonged immobilization. The bone scan in these patients will reveal increased Tc-99m MDP deposition in the muscles on delayed images. Often, the blood flow and immediate blood pool images show more intense activity than the delayed images. Increased soft tissue uptake on a bone scan typically occurs long before any radiographic change. If patients are treated in these early stages, they may avoid more severe and lasting complications such as severely contracted and ossified muscles at the hips in paraplegia.

BONE INFARCTION AND OSTEONECROSIS

Necrosis of the bone has numerous causes (Box 6-13). Because this is an evolving process, the appearance on skeletal scintigraphy depends greatly on the time frame in which imaging is performed. With acute interruption of the blood supply, newly infarcted bone appears scintigraphically cold or photon-deficient. In the postinfarction or healing phase, osteogenesis and tracer uptake at the margin of the infarcted area are increased. Skeletal scintigrams can show intensely increased tracer uptake during the healing period.

Legg-Calvé-Perthes Disease

Legg-Calvé-Perthes disease most commonly affects children between the ages of 5–9 years with predominance in boys (4:1 to 5:1). It is a form of osteochondrosis and results in avascular necrosis of the capital femoral epiphysis. The mechanism of injury is unknown except that the vascular supply of the femoral head is thought to be especially vulnerable in the most commonly affected age group.

The best scintigraphic technique for detecting the abnormality in the femoral head is to use some form of magnification and to image in the frogleg lateral projection. Classically, early in the course of the disease before healing has occurred, a discrete photon-deficient area can be seen

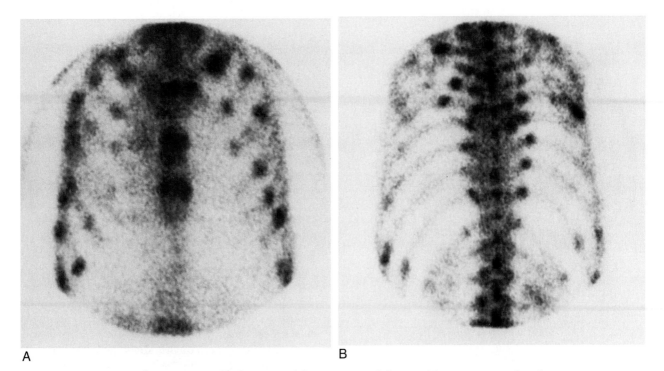

A   B

Figure 6-31   Osteomalacia. Anterior **(A)** and posterior **(B)** views. The patient was referred to rule out metastatic disease. The unusually large number of rib lesions raised the suspicion of metabolic bone disease rather than metastases.

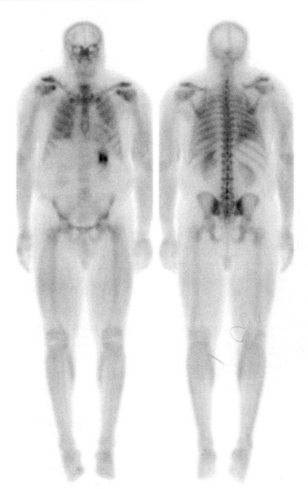

Figure 6-32   Hyperparathyroidism. Whole body views show diffusely increased uptake in the lungs and stomach.

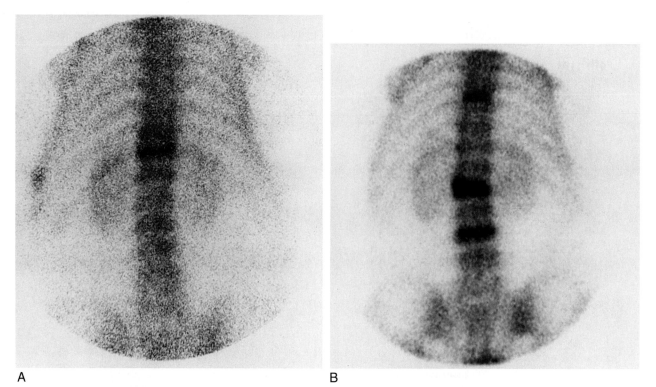

A B

Figure 6-33 Osteoporosis on surveillance images obtained several months apart. **A,** The initial study shows a single vertebral compression fracture caused by osteoporosis involving the lower thoracic spine. **B,** The subsequent study shows healing with normalization of uptake in the initial abnormality. Three new compression fractures are seen in the thoracic and lumbar spine.

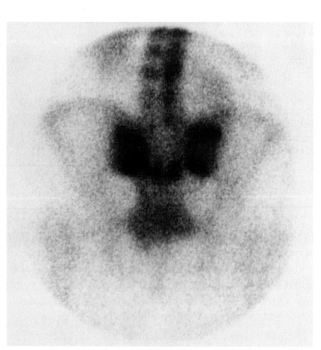

Figure 6-34 Sacral insufficiency fracture. Posterior spot view of a patient with osteoporosis. The patient has an H-type pattern with a horizontal band of increased uptake across the body of the sacrum and bilaterally increased uptake in the sacral alae.

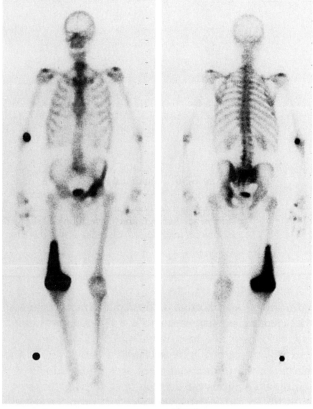

Figure 6-35 Monostotic Paget's disease involving the right distal femur. The uptake is extremely intense, with the appearance of bony expansion. The observation about expansion must be made with caution because of the extreme intensity of uptake and "blooming" of the recorded activity. Also note involvement of the ischium.

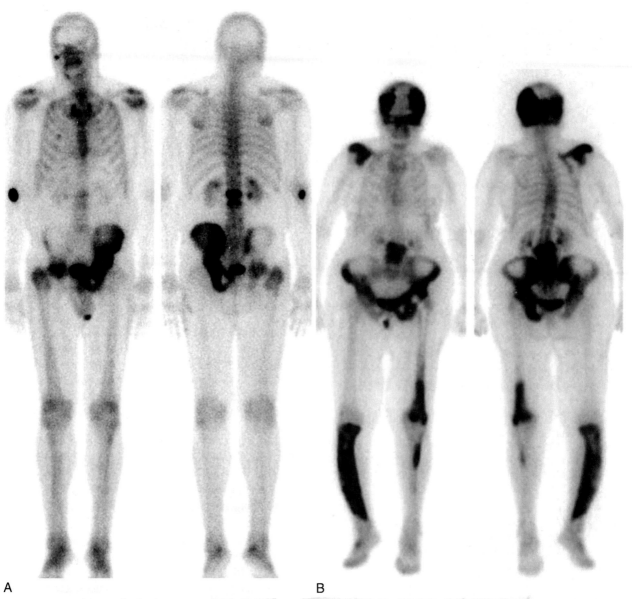

A   B

Figure 6-36   Multifocal Paget's disease. **A,** Abnormal uptake in the left hemipelvis, upper lumbar spine and, to a lesser extent, right hip in a patient with Paget's disease. When Paget's disease involves the axial bones, it must be differentiated from metastatic disease by the location and bone expansion. Radiographic correlation will show the typical coarsened trabeculae. **B,** When the sites are more numerous, the diagnosis is obvious based on the typical distribution of lesions.

in the upper outer portion of the capital femoral epiphysis with a lentiform configuration (Fig. 6-43). Areas of photon deficiency are well demonstrated by SPECT imaging.

As healing occurs, increased uptake is first seen at the margin of the photon-deficient area, and gradually the scintigram demonstrates filling in of activity. In severe cases, the femoral head never reverts to normal. Increased tracer uptake is seen for a prolonged period—many months or more.

Currently MRI is the imaging modality of choice for the evaluation of Legg-Calvé-Perthes disease, as well as other causes of osteonecrosis. Compared with nuclear scintigraphy, MRI has comparable or higher sensitivity and higher specificity. MRI also provides a range of additional information, including evaluation of articular cartilage, detection of acetabular labral tears, and visualization of metaphyseal cysts that are indicators of prognosis.

Steroid-Induced Osteonecrosis

Skeletal scintigraphy rarely shows photon deficient areas in steroid-induced osteonecrosis. The vast majority of

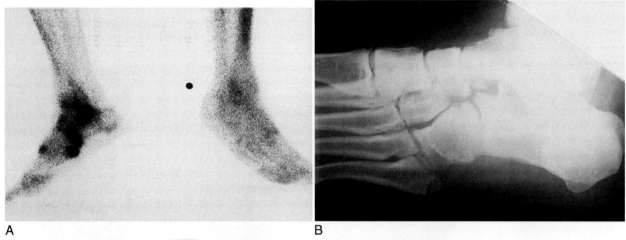

Figure 6-37 Trauma to the distal extremity. **A,** Skeletal scintigram of a patient who had sustained direct trauma to the right foot and ankle reveals multiple focal areas of abnormal tracer accumulation from fracture. **B,** The radiograph illustrates fractures of the base of the fifth metatarsal and lateral cuneiform.

Table 6-3 Skeletal Scintigraphy in Trauma: Time Course from Fracture to Return to Normal

Fracture type and site	Percent of normal	
Nonmanipulated Closed Fractures*	**1 year**	**3 years**
Vertebra	59	97
Long bone	64	95
Rib	79	100
All Fractures†	**<1 year**	**2–5 years**	**>5 years**
All sites	30	62	84

*Adapted from Matin P: The appearance of bone scans following fractures, including immediate and long term studies, *J Nucl Med* 20:1227-1231, 1979.
†Adapted from Kim HR, Thrall JH, Keyes JW Jr: Skeletal scintigraphy following incidental trauma, *Radiology* 130:447-451, 1979.

Table 6-4 Sequence of Findings in Stress Reaction

	Clinical findings	X-ray	Scintigram
Normal (resorption = replacement)	–	–	–
Accelerated remodeling (resorption > replacement)	+/–	–	+
Fatigue (resorption >> replacement)	+	+/–	+++
Exhaustion (resorption >>> replacement)	++	+	++++
Cortical fracture	++++	++++	++++

Adapted from Roub LW, et al: Bone stress: a radionuclide imaging perspective, *Radiology* 132:431-438, 1979.

cases show increased radiotracer uptake. Although the pathogenesis of steroid-induced osteonecrosis is still being debated, it is a chronic process manifested by microfractures and repair. The net effect most often seen scintigraphically is increased tracer localization.

Sickle Cell Anemia

Skeletal scintigrams in patients with sickle cell anemia have a number of characteristic features that suggest the diagnosis (Fig. 6-44). In the skull, the expanded marrow space results in bilaterally increased calvarial uptake of tracer. In the extremities, patients usually have greater relative uptake compared with the axial skeleton than is seen in normal subjects. This increased uptake may be related to the persistence of hematopoietic elements throughout the extremities, including the hands and feet, of patients with sickle cell anemia. As noted earlier, in normal adults the red marrow extends only to the proximal portions of the femurs and humeri. The overall skeleton-to-background ratio is usually good and is accentuated by the increased appendicular uptake.

In many patients with sickle cell anemia, the kidneys appear somewhat larger than normal, which may be related to a defect in the ability to concentrate urine. Avid accumulation of skeletal tracer is sometimes seen in the spleen, presumably because of prior splenic infarction and calcification (Fig. 6-45).

Infarctions in bone and bone marrow result in both acute and long-standing changes. If the involvement is primarily in the marrow space, the skeletal scintigram may not reveal the extent of the lesion as it does not involve the cortex where Tc-99m MDP binds. The image may be normal acutely. Within a few days as

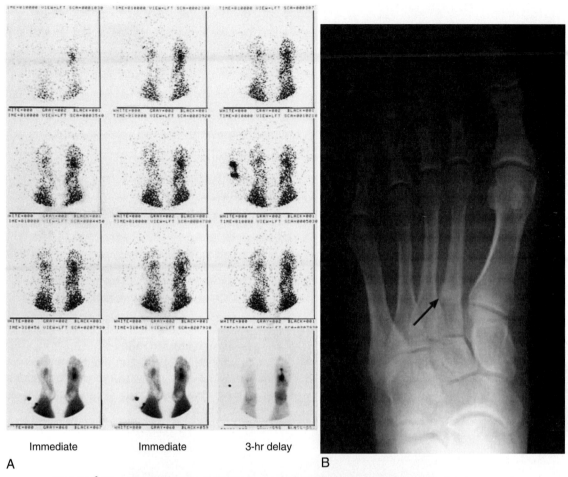

Immediate   Immediate   3-hr delay

A   B

Figure 6-38   Stress fracture. **A,** Three-phase skeletal scintigram of the feet in plantar view reveals marked early hyperemia to the left midfoot. The immediate views (*lower left and middle*) reveal increased uptake in the same area. The 3-hour delayed view shows marked focal uptake corresponding to the base and shaft of the second metatarsal, compatible with stress fracture. **B,** A radiograph performed later confirmed the fracture with callus formation (*arrow*) in the base of the second metatarsal.

healing begins, the scan typically demonstrates increased uptake.

MRI can demonstrate marrow infarctions immediately. Bone marrow scans using Tc-99m sulfur colloid are also sensitive and are positive immediately after the infarct (Fig. 6-46). Affected areas fail to accumulate tracer and are seen as cold or photon deficient. The presence of chronic marrow defects from prior bone marrow infarctions persist. Thus the significance of a photon-deficient area on marrow scanning is somewhat uncertain unless a recent baseline study is available for comparison. Here again, MRI has an advantage in distinguishing acute from chronic changes.

The correlation between the marrow scan and the bone scan is also important in the differentiation of acute osteomyelitis from infarct. If the marrow shows a defect in the region of increased bone scan activity, it is consistent with infarct. If the marrow shows no change, then

any increased activity on the bone scan in an acute situation is most likely osteomyelitis.

OSTEOMYELITIS

Acute hematogenous osteomyelitis typically begins by seeding of the infectious organism in the marrow space. The untreated process extends through Volkmann canals horizontally and in the Haversian canal system axially. The skeletal scintigram is almost invariably abnormal by the time clinical symptoms develop. Increased tracer uptake is the typical finding (Fig. 6-47). Numerous studies in the literature document the superior sensitivity of skeletal scintigraphy compared with conventional radiography in the diagnosis of acute hematogenous osteomyelitis.

In children, *Staphylococcus aureus* is the most common organism and is probably responsible for 50% or

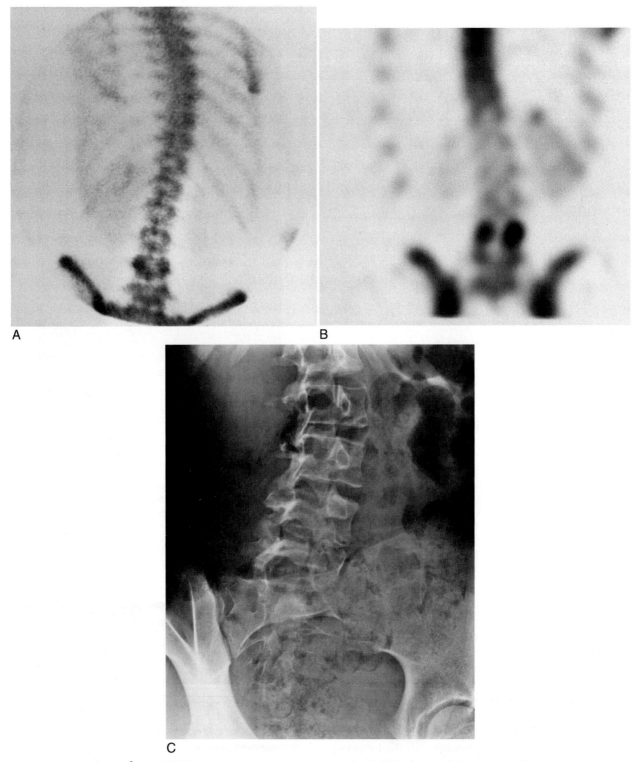

A

B

C

Figure 6-39   Spondylosis. **A,** Posterior scintigram from a child with low back pain after athletic injury. Uptake is bilaterally increased at L5. **B,** Corresponding coronal view from a SPECT study reveals a characteristic pattern for spondylolysis. **C,** Comparison radiograph reveals defect in the pars interarticularis corresponding to the area of abnormal uptake on the scintigram.

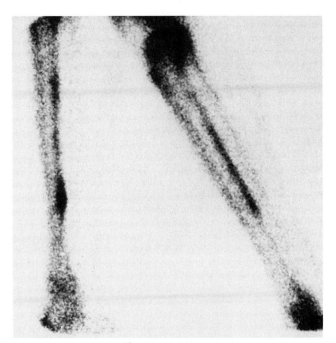

Figure 6-40 Shin splint. Lateral views of a patient demonstrating the classic finding of increased tracer uptake along the posterior and medial aspects of the tibia on the left. A similar pattern can be seen on the right, but with the addition of a focal area distally, which could indicate stress fracture.

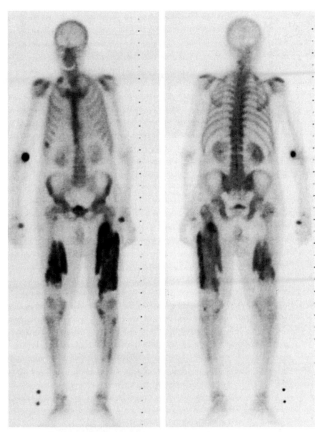

Figure 6-42 Myositis ossificans. Anterior and posterior whole body scintigrams with extensive myositis ossificans involvement.

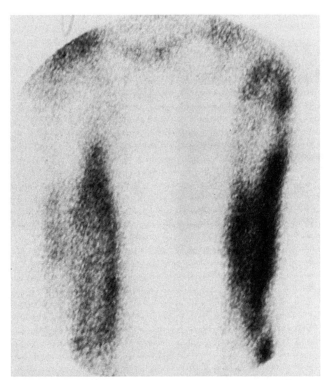

Figure 6-41 Rhabdomyolysis. Anterior view of the thighs in a patient who recently competed in a marathon. Bilateral soft tissue uptake is compatible with rhabdomyolysis.

Box 6-13 Etiologies of Aseptic Bone Necrosis

Trauma (accidental, iatrogenic)
Drug therapy (steroids)
Hypercoagulable states
Hemoglobinopathies (sickle cell disease and variants)
After radiation therapy (orthovoltage)
Caisson disease
Osteochondrosis (pediatric age group; Legg-Calvé-Perthes disease)
Polycythemia
Leukemia
Gaucher's disease
Alcoholism
Pancreatitis
Idiopathic

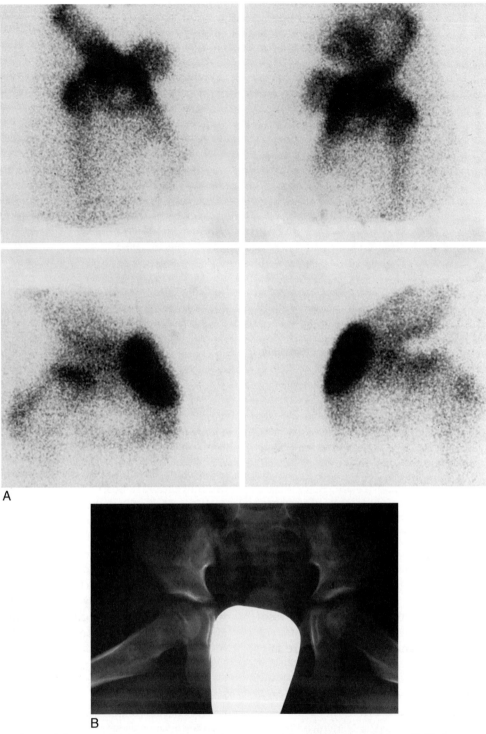

Figure 6-43   Legg-Calvé-Perthes disease. **A,** (*top row*). Scintigrams by standard parallel-hole collimator fail to reveal the abnormality Pinhole images of the same patient (*bottom row*) reveal the characteristic lentiform area of decreased uptake on the left. **B,** Corresponding radiograph done months later reveals deformity of the left femoral epiphysis with flattening, increased density, and increased distance between the epiphysis and the acetabulum.

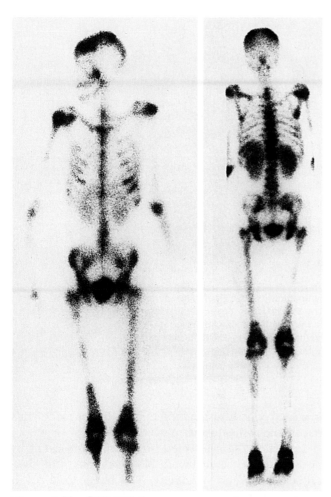

Figure 6-44   Sickle cell disease. Anterior and posterior whole body views. Calvarial uptake is increased with relative thinning at the midline. There is prominent skeleton to soft tissue uptake. The kidneys appear large, and the spleen shows intense uptake. Uptake in the knees and ankles is greater than expected for an adult subject. The photon-deficient areas in the right femur are due to bone and bone marrow infarction.

more of cases. The skeletal infection is commonly associated with some other staphylococcal infection, often of the skin. Enteric bacteria and *Streptococcus* are also important pathogens.

Osteomyelitis in adults may occur by hematogenous spread or by direct extension in an area of cellulitis. The foot is a common site of direct extension in diabetic patients, whereas the spine is commonly involved by the hematogenous route. In nondiabetic adults, the axial skeleton is more commonly involved than the appendicular skeleton (Fig. 6-48).

Osteomyelitis may involve any skeletal structure. When vertebrae are involved, the organisms may be carried through the perispinous venous plexus, producing involvement at multiple levels. When the vertebral endplates are involved, the infection may extend into the disc space causing diskitis. Diskitis is characterized by narrowing of the disc space and increased uptake in the adjacent vertebral bodies from osteomyelitis of the adjacent bone.

In some patients, especially children, increased pressure in the marrow space or thrombosis of blood vessels results in paradoxically decreased tracer uptake and a cold or photon-deficient lesion. False-negative scintigraphic studies are unusual but have been reported in infants under the age of 1 year. Other causes of false-negative examinations are imaging very early in the course of disease and failure to recognize the significance of photon-deficient areas.

For the diagnosis of osteomyelitis, MRI is typically performed with gadolinium enhancement. Again, MRI is very sensitive but is limited as a survey technique. If clinical findings point to a specific location, MRI is useful. When polyostotic disease is suspected or clinical findings are not well-localized, skeletal scintigraphy remains a useful survey technique. The characteristic appearance of osteomyelitis by gadolinium-enhanced MRI is an area of enhancement, whereas the centers of abscesses do not enhance. MRI is not as useful in evaluating the feet of diabetic patients because of changes such as Charcot's disease. The underlying changes and poor blood flow are nonspecific and make diagnosis difficult.

Scintigraphic Findings of Osteomyelitis

Dynamic (or three-phase) imaging is a special technique used in the differential diagnosis of cellulitis and osteomyelitis (*see* Box 6-2). This is an important differential diagnosis for diabetic patients who have a high incidence of both problems because of the therapeutic implications of prolonged treatment when osteomyelitis is diagnosed.

The key diagnostic criteria of osteomyelitis are shown in Box 6-14. Typical osteomyelitis appears positive on all three phases of the study. Early or arterial hyperemia with focally, and possibly diffusely, increased radiotracer uptake on blood pool images is seen. Progressive focal accumulation then occurs in the involved bone on delayed images (Fig. 6-49). Cellulitis, on the other hand, typically demonstrates delayed or venous phase hyperemia and increased blood pool images activity but no focally increased uptake in bone on delayed images (Fig. 6-50).

Although the technique has been shown useful in distinguishing cellulitis from osteomyelitis, bone scan is not specific. The same sequence of image findings seen in osteomyelitis can be seen in neuropathic joint disease, gout, fractures (including stress fractures), and rheumatoid arthritis, among other conditions (Box 6-15). Improved specificity can be achieved by comparing the three-phase bone scan to radiographs.

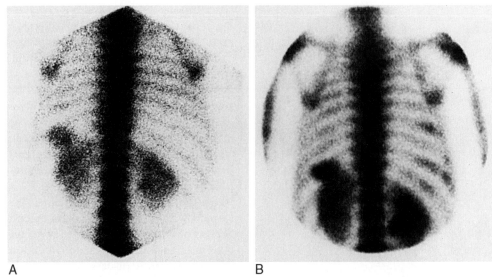

Figure 6-45 Sickle cell crisis. Posterior views with intensity set high obtained at the time of onset of acute chest pain (**A**) and several days later (**B**) from a patient with sickle cell anemia. The initial image reveals no abnormality in the ribs. The follow-up image demonstrates increased uptake, particularly in the right ribs, associated with healing of the infarctions. Note the uptake in the spleen on both images. Typically, once the spleen is visualized scintigraphically, it remains positive.

Prosthesis Evaluation

Numerous attempts have been made to use skeletal scintigraphy in the evaluation of patients after total joint replacement or implantation of other metallic prostheses. These patients often experience severe pain. The distinction between component loosening and infection is critical in guiding management.

The findings on skeletal scintigraphy are not specific enough for a reliable distinction between loosening of a prosthesis and infection (Fig. 6-51). Reactive bone around a loose prosthesis may be indistinguishable from increased tracer uptake resulting from osteomyelitis. In cases of a loose prosthesis, uptake is usually increased in the region of the greater and lesser trochanters and at the tip of the prosthesis. Loosening may also be seen as diffusely increased uptake around the acetabular component. This increased activity is presumably due to remodeling of bone in response to movement of the prosthesis. Some increased uptake is expected as a normal healing response for 1 year after placement of a cemented prosthesis and for 2–3 years after placement of a noncemented prosthesis. However, increased activity may persist indefinitely. Although seldom performed, a baseline study 6 months to 1 year following surgery is very useful for future comparison.

In osteomyelitis, activity is increased in the bone surrounding the prosthesis. However, a negative bone scan is useful because it helps rule out both osteomyelitis and prosthesis loosening. The differential diagnosis between loosened prosthesis and infection is better made with tracers such as radiolabeled white blood cells.

Detection of an infected prosthesis with In-111 or Tc-99m HMPAO-labeled white blood cells offers the highest sensitivity and specificity. This tracer localizes in areas of infection and not in areas of remodeling or reactive bone. Use of labeled white blood cells has three pitfalls. First, false-negative studies may occur in low-grade chronic osteomyelitis. Second, cellulitis can be difficult to distinguish from septic arthritis. Third, false-positive studies can result from normal radiolabeled white cell uptake in bone marrow around a prosthesis. The combination of white blood cell and sulfur colloid marrow scanning is combined to avoid this pitfall. Infection is diagnosed only in areas of radiolabeled white blood cell uptake that are negative for marrow activity.

BONE MARROW SCINTIGRAPHY

Bone marrow scintigraphy is not important in current practice but does have a small number of indications. The procedure is most commonly performed with Tc-99m sulfur colloid, which localizes in the reticuloendothelial elements of the red marrow.

In patients with sickle cell anemia, bone marrow imaging demonstrates the extent of marrow expansion into the extremities (*see* Fig. 6-46). In most normal subjects, the marrow is confined to the proximal thirds of the femurs and humeri. In patients with hemoglobinopathies,

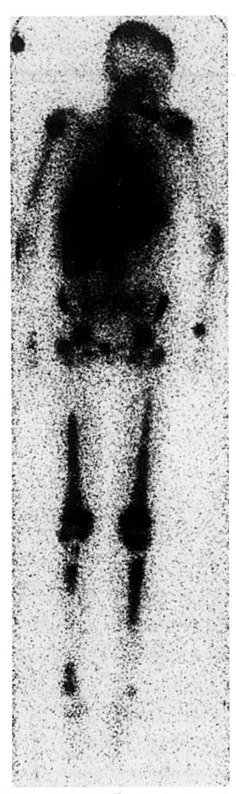

Figure 6-46   Sickle cell anemia: technetium-99m sulfur colloid bone marrow scan. The intensity has been set to maximize visualization of marrow. Note the intense uptake in the liver. The uptake in the bone marrow extends throughout the upper and lower extremities. The numerous focal defects indicate marrow infarctions. Based on one examination, new abnormalities cannot be distinguished from old ones.

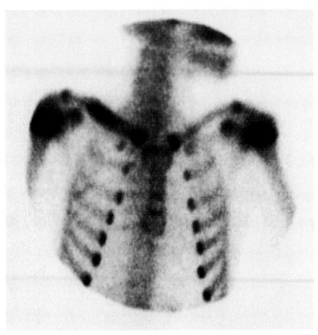

Figure 6-47   Osteomyelitis of the right clavicle. Anterior scintigram in a child show uptake on the right is markedly greater than in the left clavicle.

the marrow uptake is typically seen throughout the appendages. Marrow imaging is highly sensitive for detection of bone marrow infarction and can also define the extent of involvement. The major limitation is not being able to distinguish new from chronic infarctions. Moreover, areas involved by osteomyelitis demonstrate defects on marrow imaging, so the technique is not useful in distinguishing infarction from osteomyelitis. In current practice, marrow imaging is often used in conjunction with labeled white blood cells to diagnose osteomyelitis. As noted in the discussion of prosthesis evaluation, in marrow-bearing areas the combination of increased radio-labeled white blood cell uptake and absence of Tc-99m sulfur colloid uptake is specific for osteomyelitis.

BONE MINERAL MEASUREMENT

A number of methods have been developed for quantitative measurement of bone mineral mass. Until recently, all of the techniques were based on the absorption of photons in bone, the differential absorption in bone tissue versus soft tissue, and calibration of absorption percentage against calcium-containing reference standards. A number of ultrasound techniques, based on the rate of sound transmission through bone, are now available.

The simplest technique is single-photon absorptiometry (SPA). In this technique, a photon source (typically

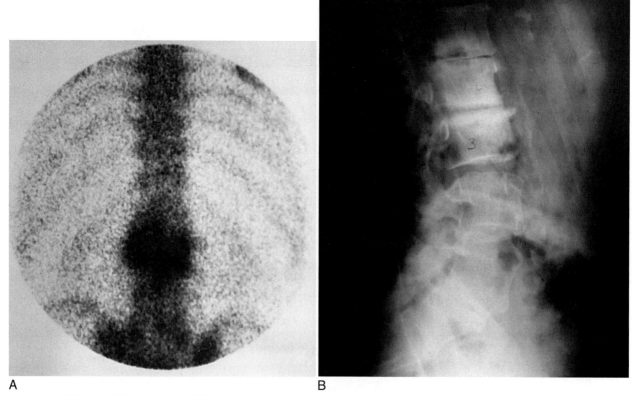

Figure 6-48   Osteomyelitis of the spine. **A,** Posterior spot view of an adult show intensely increased uptake in the midlumbar region, involving more than one vertebral level. **B,** Corresponding radiograph shows destructive and sclerotic changes involving the L2 vertebral body and adjacent portions of L1 and L3. The process has involved the intervertebral disks with loss of height in the disk space.

Box 6-14   Three-Phase Skeletal Scintigraphy: Interpretive Criteria

Osteomyelitis: *arterial* hyperemia, progressive focal skeletal uptake with relative soft tissue clearance; in children a focal cold area may be seen if osteomyelitis is associated with infarction

Cellulitis: *venous* (delayed) hyperemia, persistent soft tissue activity; no focal skeletal uptake (may have mild to moderate diffusely increased uptake)

Septic joint: periarticular increased activity on dynamic and blood pool phases that persists on delayed images; less commonly the joint structures appear cold if pressure in the joint causes decreased flow or infarction

---

iodine-125) is collimated and scanned across the radius or calcaneus or both. These sites are selected for the minimal soft tissue because correction for soft tissue attenuation is not possible in the SPA technique.

Dual-photon absorptiometry (DPA) again uses a collimated photon source that is scanned over the skeletal part of interest. It is a more flexible technique because the soft tissue attenuation can be corrected based on the differential absorption of the beam at different energies. In DPA, gadolinium-153 with photon energies of 40–100 keV is typically used. Areas frequently studied with DPA are the lumbar spine and both the neck and intertrochanteric region of the femur. The single- and dual-photon techniques have given way to x-ray-based approaches in current practice.

Bone densitometry measurements can also be made with either dedicated x-ray densitometer devices or special quantitative computed tomography (QCT) algorithms. Single- and dual-energy techniques have been described for both x-ray and QCT. The advantage of the x-ray technique is higher photon flux compared with SPA and DPA instruments. Radiation exposure is essentially identical for dual-energy x-ray densitometry and DPA. The most versatile and widely used technique in current practice is dual energy x-ray absorptiometry (DXA). DXA is the basis for the World Health Organization criteria for categorizing osteopenia and osteoporosis.

The main advantage of QCT is the ability to measure cortical and trabecular bone separately. Dual-energy

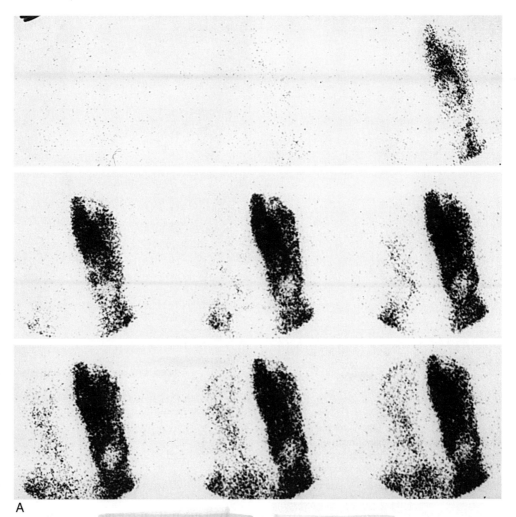

A

Figure 6-49   Osteomyelitis: three-phase study. **A,** Sequential dynamic images in a middle-aged man with diabetes and osteomyelitis. Note the intense arterial phase hyperemia.

Continued

QCT has the additional advantage over single-energy QCT of allowing correction for fat in the marrow space. Both techniques are quite flexible with respect to body part examined. QCT is an important research tool but is too expensive for population screening.

Several ultrasound devices are now approved by the U.S. Food and Drug Administration for measurement of bone mass. Sound is transmitted faster in dense bone than in osteopenic bone and the devices are calibrated against other methods to correlate with bone mass. Application of the technique is limited to peripheral structures such as the calcaneus. The low cost, small size, and ease of use of ultrasound devices make them attractive for population screening. However, current data indicate that spine measurements are necessary to follow the effects of therapy because the spine is the most sensitive structure for assessing response to drug treatment.

The main application of bone mineral measurements is to establish baseline diagnostic measurements in the evaluation of patients with suspected osteopenia and osteoporosis and to follow the course of therapy. Primary osteoporosis has been divided into two subtypes. Type I or postmenopausal osteoporosis is related to decreased estrogen secretion after menopause. Type II or senile osteoporosis is presumably due to age-related impaired bone metabolism. Risk factors for osteoporosis include female sex, Caucasian or Asian race, smoking, chronic alcohol intake, and a positive family history. Early menopause, long-term treatment with corticosteroids, and a number of nutritional disorders including malabsorption are also risk factors. Obesity is protective.

The World Health Organization has established a classification system for bone mass based on DXA

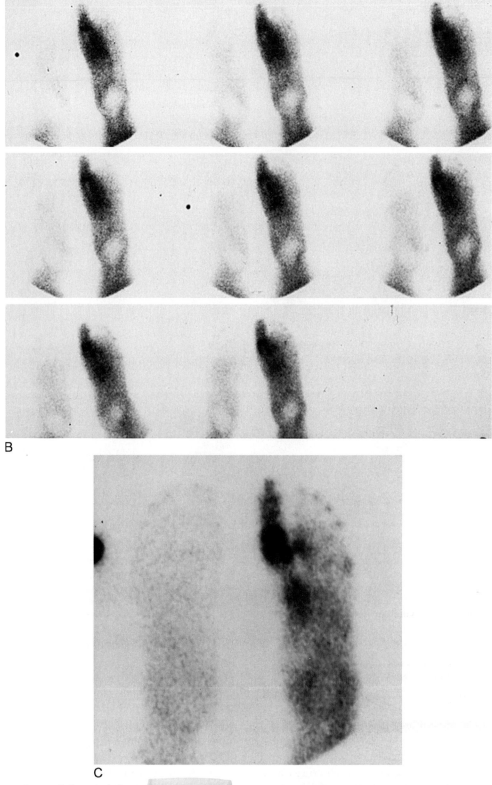

Figure 6-49, cont'd   **B,** Blood pool images already show localization in skeletal structures. **C,** Delayed static images reveal intense focal accumulation in multiple areas of the great toe and distal first and second metatarsals.

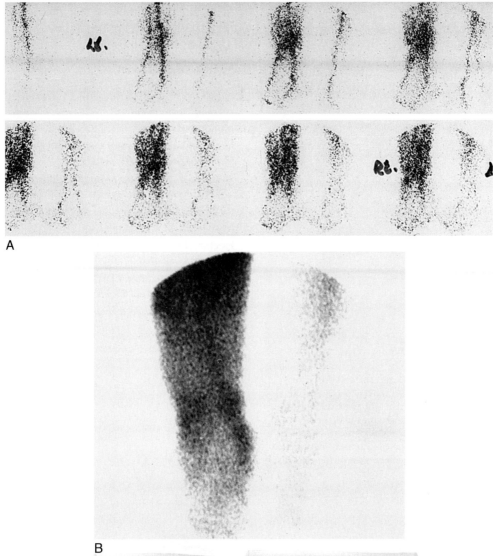

A

B

Figure 6-50   Cellulitis: three-phase study. **A,** Sequential images from the flow phase of a diabetic patient with cellulitis. The ankle region and the visualized portion of the leg show marked hyperemia. **B,** Follow-up blood pool images revealed diffusely increased activity in the areas corresponding to the hyperemia. No focal abnormality was demonstrated on follow-up late-phase imaging that would suggest osteomyelitis.

Box 6-15   Lesions That Can Mimic Osteomyelitis on Three-Phase Skeletal Scintigraphy

Osteoarthritis
Gout
Fracture
Stress fracture
Osteonecrosis (healing)
Charcot's joint
Osteotomy
Reflex sympathetic dystrophy syndrome

---

measurements of the spine and femoral neck. A measurement in an individual is compared with the mean and standard deviation (SD) for a young control population. A reading within 1 SD is considered normal. Osteopenia is taken as 1–2.5 SD below the control mean and osteoporosis is defined as 2.5 SD or more below the control mean. When the standard deviation is reported in this way, it is referred to as the *T score*.

The use of bone mineral density has been accelerated by the availability of new drugs such as alendronate, a bisphosphonate that localizes in bone and promotes mineralization. Estrogen is also widely used in postmenopausal women but is not uniformly well-tolerated,

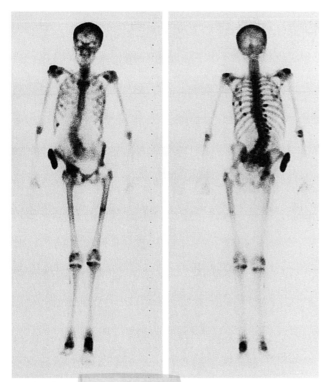

Figure 6-51   Loose hip prosthesis. Anterior and posterior whole body images in a patient with severe scoliosis and skeletal metastases from carcinoma of the breast. The patient has a loose left femoral prosthesis. Uptake is increased at the tip of the prosthesis and subtly increased in the region of the trochanters, especially the greater trochanter. Uptake is intensely increased in the right femoral head because of degenerative arthritic changes.

and concerns remain about its effects on other diseases such as breast cancer.

SUGGESTED READING

Collier BD, Fogelman I, Rosenthal L: *Skeletal nuclear medicine*. St Louis, Mosby, 1996.

Connolly LP, Strauss J, Conolly SA: Role of skeletal scintigraphy in evaluating sports injuries in adolescents and young adults. *Nucl Med Ann* 171-209, 2003.

Fournier RS, Holder LE: Reflex sympathetic dystrophy: diagnostic controversies. *Semin Nucl Med* 28:116-123, 1998.

Freeman LM, Blaufox MD: Metabolic bone disease. *Semin Nucl Med* 27:195-305, 1997.

Freeman LM, Blaufox MD: Orthopedic nuclear medicine (Part I). *Semin Nucl Med* 27:307-389, 1997.

Freeman LM, Blaufox MD: Orthopedic nuclear medicine (Part II). *Semin Nucl Med* 28:1-131, 1998.

Treves ST: *Pediatric nuclear medicine*. New York, Springer, 1998.

Nuclear medicine has played an important role in liver and spleen imaging for decades, although many of the radiopharmaceuticals, methodologies and indications have changed over time. Cholescintigraphy exemplifies the continued importance of functional and physiological imaging for diagnosis of a variety of hepatobiliary diseases, including acute cholecystitis, biliary obstruction, and biliary leak in an era with high quality and rapidly improving anatomic imaging modalities.

Various other functional scintigraphic liver and spleen imaging studies use radiopharmaceuticals with different physiological mechanisms of uptake and distribution (Table 7-1, Fig. 7-1). These include Tc-99m-labeled red blood cells for diagnosis of cavernous hemangioma and for functional splenic imaging, and Tc-99m MAA to assess

Table 7-1	Liver Radiopharmaceuticals and Clinical Indications	
Radiopharmaceutical	**Mechanism of uptake**	**Indication**
Tc-99m sulfur colloid	Kupffer cell uptake	Focal nodular hyperplasia
Tc-99m iminodiacetic acid (HIDA)	Hepatocyte uptake	Cholescintigraphy
Tc-99m red blood cells (RBCs)	RBC labeling/blood pool distribution	Cavernous hemangioma
Tc-99m macroaggregated albumin (MAA)	Blood flow, capillary blockage	Hepatic arterial perfusion
Xenon-133	Lipid soluble	Focal fatty tumor uptake
Gallium-67 citrate	Lactoferrin transport and iron binding	Tumor/abscess imaging
F-18 fluorodeoxyglucose (F-18 FDG)	Glucose metabolism	Tumor imaging

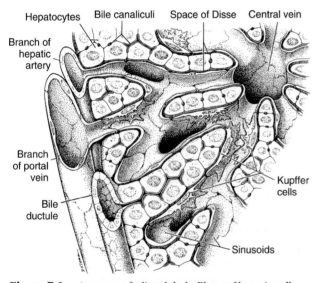

Figure 7-1 Anatomy of a liver lobule. Plates of hepatic cells (hepatocytes and Kupffer cells) are distributed radially around the central vein. Branches of the portal vein and hepatic artery located at the periphery of the lobule deliver blood to the sinusoids. Blood leaves through the central vein (proximal branch of hepatic veins). Peripherally located bile ducts drain bile canaliculi that course between hepatocytes.

hepatic intraarterial perfusion of tumors and liver to predict chemotherapeutic drug distribution and effectiveness. Technetium-99m sulfur colloid (Tc-99m SC) liver and spleen scintigraphy has a more limited role today than in the past, but important applications persist.

CHOLESCINTIGRAPHY

Cholescintigraphy with Tc-99m iminodiacetic acid (Tc-99m-IDA) analogs is indicated for diagnosis of various acute and chronic hepatobiliary diseases (Box 7-1). The most common indication is for the diagnosis of acute cholecystitis, but cholescintigraphy also often provides unique physiologic information on bile drainage in patients with suspected biliary obstruction and bile leakage. Dynamic cholescintigraphy is used to evaluate blood flow to the liver, hepatic extraction, biliary excretion, patency of the biliary tract, and gallbladder contraction, all providing important diagnostic information.

Radiopharmaceuticals

Iodine-131 rose bengal was introduced in 1955 as the first hepatobiliary imaging agent extracted by hepatocytes and cleared through the biliary tract. However, its suboptimal imaging characteristics and relatively high radiation dosimetry limited its clinical utility. I-123 labeled rose bengal was superior in both regards but never gained widespread use because of limited availability and, perhaps more importantly, the introduction in the 1970s of Tc-99m-IDA hepatobiliary imaging radiopharmaceuticals.

Tc-99m IDA Chemistry

Tc-99m labeled IDA radiopharmaceuticals were originally synthesized to be heart-imaging agents, based on the structural similarities between IDA and lidocaine molecules (Fig. 7-2). The high hepatic extraction of an early IDA compound (dimethyl IDA) prompted the acronym HIDA, for hepatobiliary IDA.

Box 7-1	Cholescintigraphy: Clinical Indications

Acute cholecystitis
Acute acalculous cholecystitis
Biliary obstruction
Postcholecystectomy syndrome
Sphincter of Oddi dysfunction
Biliary leak
Chronic acalculous cholecystitis
Biliary diversion procedure
Biliary stent
Focal nodular hyperplasia
Hepatocellular carcinoma
Enterogastric bile reflux
Biliary atresia

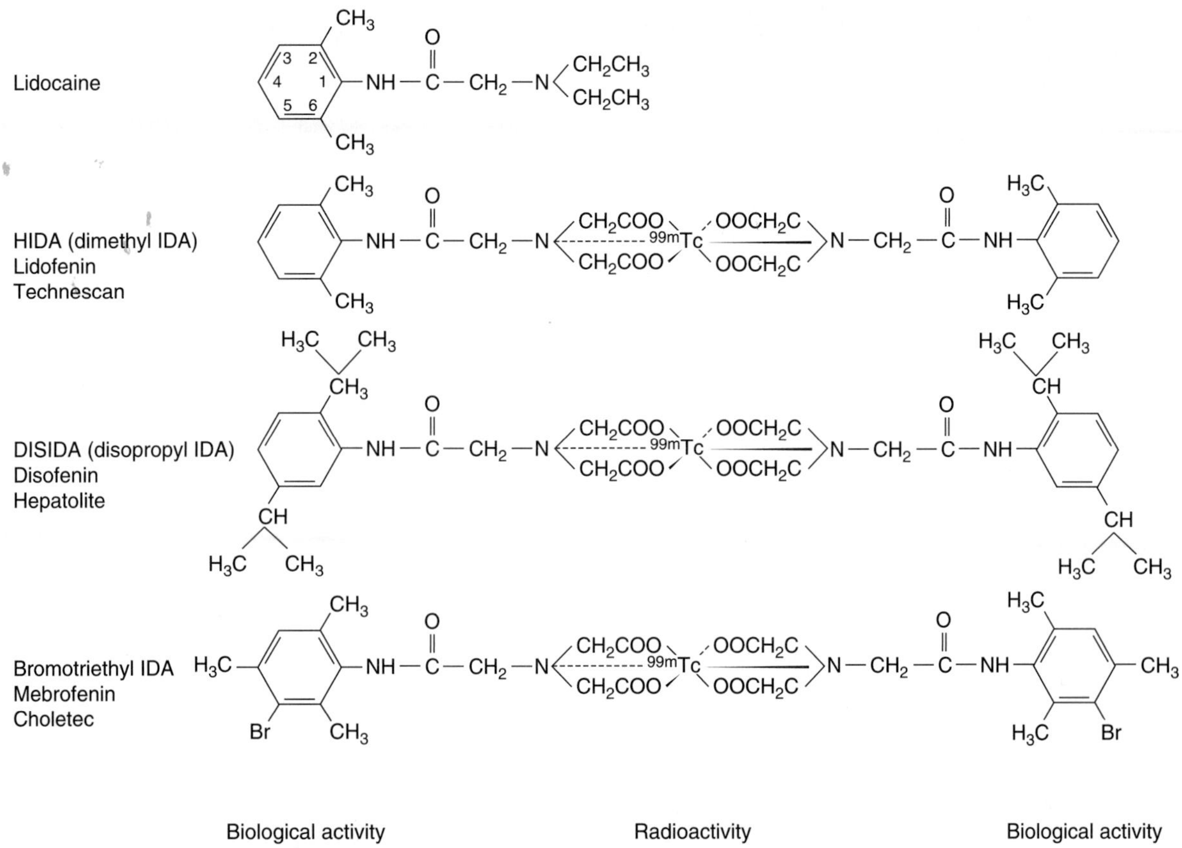

Figure 7-2 Chemical structure of Tc-99m IDA radiopharmaceuticals. Note similarity of Tc-99m aminoacetic acid analogs (Tc-99m IDAs) to lidocaine. Radioactivity is located centrally (Tc-99m), bridging two ligand molecules. Iminodiacetate (NCH$_2$COO) attaches to Tc-99m and the acetanilide analog (IDA) of lidocaine at the periphery carries the biological activity. Substitutions on aromatic rings differentiate the various Tc-99m IDAs and determine their pharmacokinetics.

Numerous Tc-99m IDA analogs were developed with different chemical substitutions around the aromatic ring (*see* Fig. 7-2). Subsequent analogs offered improvements in hepatocellular uptake and more rapid blood clearance. These analogs were known by many acronyms (e.g., BIDA, DIDA, EIDA, PIPIDA).

The U.S. Food and Drug Administration (FDA) has approved three Tc-99m IDA radiopharmaceuticals. The first agent approved was Tc-99m lidofenin (HIDA); however, it is no longer in clinical use. The two presently available radiopharmaceuticals are Tc-99m disofenin (DISIDA; Hepatolite, DuPont-Merck) and Tc-99m mebrofenin (BrIDA; Choletec, E.R. Squibb).

The IDA radiopharmaceuticals are organic anions that act as bifunctional chelates. The iminodiacetate (NCH$_2$COO) attaches at one end to the radiotracer (Tc-99m) and at the other end to an acetanilide analog of lidocaine, which determines the biological function (*see* Fig. 7-2). Relatively minor structural changes in the phenyl ring (N substitutions) result in significant alterations in the IDA pharmacokinetics (Table 7-2).

The final Tc-99m IDA complex exists as a dimer, with two molecules of the chelating agent (IDA) reacting with one atom of Tc-99m. This configuration, with Tc-99m serving as a bridging atom between the two ligand molecules, confers stability to the technetium complex and determines hepatobiliary excretion.

Kit Preparation

The Tc-99m IDA radiopharmaceuticals are available as kits that contain the IDA analog and stannous chloride in lyophilized form. The Tc-99m–IDA complex is formed by the simple addition of pertechnetate to the vial. The product is stable for at least 6 hours after reconstitution.

Mechanism of Uptake and Clearance

Tc-99m IDA radiopharmaceuticals have the same hepatocyte uptake, transport, and excretion pathways as bilirubin. After intravenous injection, Tc-99m IDA is tightly

Table 7-2	Normal Pharmacokinetics of Tc-99m Iminodiacetic Acid Analogs (IDAs)		
Agent	Hepatic uptake (%)	Clearance half-life (min)	2-hr Renal excretion (%)
Tc-99m lidofenin (HIDA)	84	42	>14
Tc-99m disofenin (DISIDA)	88	19	<9
Tc-99m mebrofenin (BrIDA)	98	17	<1

bound to protein in the blood, minimizing renal clearance. The radiotracer is transported into the hepatocyte by a high-capacity, carrier-mediated, anionic clearance mechanism. After hepatocellular uptake, the tracer is transported into bile canaliculi by an active membrane transport system. Tc-99m IDA compounds are stable in vivo and, in contrast to bilirubin, are excreted in the original radiochemical form without being conjugated or undergoing significant metabolism. Because they travel the same pathway as bilirubin, Tc-99m IDA agents are subject to competitive inhibition by high levels of serum bilirubin.

Pharmacokinetics

Once the Tc-99m IDA radiopharmaceutical is excreted from the hepatocytes and reaches the bile canaliculi, it follows the physiologic flow of bile. Approximately two-thirds of bile flow enters the gallbladder via the cystic duct and the remainder travels through the common duct and the sphincter of Oddi into the second portion of the duodenum (Fig. 7-3). The relative flow into each is determined by the patency of the biliary ducts, sphincter of Oddi tone, and intraluminal pressures.

With older Tc-99m IDA compounds (e.g., Tc-99m lidofenin [HIDA]), serum bilirubin levels greater than 5 mg/dl resulted in poor image quality. However, today's radiopharmaceuticals (Tc-99m disofenin and mebrofenin) provide diagnostic images with bilirubin levels as high as 20–30 mg/dl because of their higher extraction efficiency (*see* Table 7-2). Mebrofenin has somewhat greater hepatic uptake and resistance to displacement than disofenin and is preferable in patients with hepatic dysfunction.

Poor liver function causes altered biliary pharmacokinetics (i.e., delayed uptake and delayed clearance). The kidneys serve as an alternative route of excretion for IDA radiopharmaceuticals, normally excreting up to 10% of the dose (*see* Table 7-2) with a larger percent as hepatic function decreases.

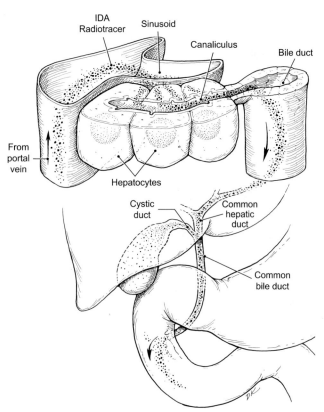

Figure 7-3 Physiology of bile flow and pharmacokinetics of Tc-99m IDA. Bilirubin is transported in the blood bound to albumin, extracted by the hepatocyte, secreted into the bile canaliculi, and cleared through the biliary tract into the bowel. Hepatic uptake and clearance of Tc-99m IDA is similar to bilirubin except that it is not conjugated or metabolized.

Dosimetry

Tc-99m disofenin and Tc-99m mebrofenin result in similar radiation absorbed dose to the patient. The highest estimated radiation dose (target organ) is usually to the large bowel, approximately 2 cGy (2 rads) (Table 7-3). The radiation dose to the gallbladder is variable, depending on whether the gallbladder fills, its ability to contract, and the length of time before it is stimulated to contract.

Patient History

The patient's clinical history should be reviewed carefully before initiating cholescintigraphy. The nuclear physician should know the answer to these questions: What is the clinical question being asked by the referring physician? Are the symptoms acute or chronic? When and what did the patient last eat? Has the patient received any drugs which could affect normal biliary physiology and thus interpretation of results? Has ultrasonography or other imaging been performed, and if so, what did it show? Has the patient had biliary surgery?

Table 7-3	Dosimetry for Tc-99m Iminodiacetic acid (IDA) Radiopharmaceuticals	
	cGy/185 MBq (rads/5 mCi)	
	Disofenin (Hepatolite)	**Mebrofenin (Choletec)**
Liver	0.19	0.24
Gallbladder	0.60	0.69
Large intestine	1.90	2.37
Urinary bladder	0.46	0.14
Ovaries	0.41	0.51
Testes	0.03	0.03
Marrow	0.14	0.17
Total body	0.08	0.10

If the patient has had a biliary diversion procedure, what is the anatomy? Are there any intra-abdominal tubes or drains? If so, where are they placed and which tubing drains each? Should they be open or clamped to answer the clinical diagnostic question?

Patient Preparation

The patent must not eat for 3–4 hours prior to starting the study to ensure that the gallbladder is not contracted, which would prevent radiotracer entry. It is important to know when the last meal was and if that meal contained enough fat to cause gallbladder contraction (>10 gm).

If the patient has been fasting for more than 24 hours, the gallbladder will likely be full of concentrated viscous bile which can also prevent radiotracer entry. The patient should receive cholecystokinin (CCK) prior to the study to empty the gallbladder. Tc-99m IDA must not be administered until at least 30 minutes after cessation of the CCK infusion to allow adequate time for gallbladder relaxation.

All morphine-related drugs must be withheld for approximately 6 hours prior to the study because they can cause a functional partial biliary obstruction that may be indistinguishable from a true obstruction. In urgent situations, naloxone (Narcan) has been used prior to the study to reverse the effect of opiate drugs.

Methodology

A standard protocol for cholescintigraphy is summarized in Box 7-2. An initial 60-second flow study (1–3 seconds/frame) is followed by 1-minute frames acquired for 59 minutes. Right lateral and left anterior oblique views are obtained at 60 minutes to aid in confirming or excluding gallbladder filling that may otherwise be difficult to ascertain because of duodenal activity. Delayed

Box 7-2	Cholescintigraphy: Protocol Summary

PATIENT PREPARATION

Nothing by mouth (NPO) for 4 hours before study. If fasting longer than 24 hours, infuse sincalide.

RADIOPHARMACEUTICAL

Tc-99m mebrofenin or Tc-99m disofenin, 5 mCi intravenous injection:

Adults: bilirubin   <2 mg/dl   5.0 mCi (185 MBq)
                2–10 mg/dl   7.5 mCi (278 MBq)
                >10 mg/dl   10.0 mCi (370 MBq)

Children: 200 μCi/kg (no less than 1 mCi or 35 MBq)

INSTRUMENTATION

Camera: large-field-of-view gamma camera
Collimator: low energy, all purpose, parallel hole
Window: 15% over 140-keV photopeak

PATIENT POSITIONING

Supine; upper abdomen in field of view.

COMPUTER SETUP

1-sec frames × 60, then 1-min frames × 60

IMAGING PROTOCOL

1. Inject Tc-99m IDA intravenously as a rapid infusion and start computer.
2. At 60 min, acquire right lateral and left anterior oblique images.
3. If the gallbladder has not filled and acute cholecystitis is suspected, inject morphine sulfate (MS) intravenously, 0.04 mg/kg over 1 min (if there is good biliary duct clearance and biliary-to-bowel transit).
   Acquire study for additional 30 minutes.
   Tc-99m IDA reinjection may be necessary if liver activity has washed out.
4. Perform delayed imaging at 2 to 4 hr if:
   a. MS is not administered and gallbladder has not filled.
   b. Other indications (e.g., hepatic insufficiency, partial common duct obstruction, suspected biliary leak).

imaging, morphine sulfate, and CCK are all optional maneuvers to be discussed.

Cholecystokinin

Physiology

CCK is a 33-amino acid polypeptide hormone with numerous physiological effects, most notably gallbladder contraction and relaxation of the sphincter of Oddi (Box 7-3). The C-terminal octapeptide of CCK is the physiologically active portion of the hormone. Sincalide (Kinevac, Squibb) is the only commercial synthetic form of CCK available in the United States. It is the C-terminal octapeptide.

Bile is normally stored and concentrated in the gallbladder. The bile is discharged into the intestines in response to gallbladder contraction and sphincter of Oddi relaxation. In the small bowel, bile acids play an important role in fat absorption.

The fat in an ingested meal stimulates CCK secretion from the mucosa of the proximal small bowel and its systemic release. The serum CCK level rises gradually and then plateaus (Fig. 7-4). The interaction of CCK with receptors in the gallbladder wall and sphincter of Oddi initiates gallbladder contraction and relaxation of the sphincter. The serum CCK remains elevated and the gallbladder stays contracted until the production of CCK declines after the meal has cleared from the stomach and proximal small bowel.

Sincalide

This synthetic commercially available analog of CCK is commonly used as a pharmacologic intervention in conjunction with cholescintigraphy. Many of the diagnostic indications are listed in Box 7-4.

Since the early days of oral cholecystography, both fatty meals and injectable CCK analogs have been used to evaluate gallbladder contraction. Although a fatty meal may be more physiological, this approach has disadvantages. It assumes normal gastric emptying, which can be quite variable between patients. Slow gastric emptying will result in a delay in endogenous stimulation of CCK. Also, the degree of gallbladder contraction depends on the fat content of the ingested meal.

Intravenous sincalide permits better standardization and reproducibility than a fatty meal. CCK analogs have been used with ultrasonography to evaluate gallbladder contraction. However, cholescintigraphy has proven more accurate and reproducible. Ultrasonography is operator-dependent and quantification assumes geometric assumptions of gallbladder shape. With cholescintigraphy, frequent image acquisition that does not require technologist interaction is routine and quantification of the gallbladder ejection fraction is volume-based (counts are proportional to volume) (Box 7-5).

Methodology

When administered during oral cholecystography in the 1970s, it was found that bolus infusions of CCK can cause spasm of the gallbladder neck in some patients and result in ineffective gallbladder contraction. Thus it became common practice in the 1980s with cholescintigraphy to infuse sincalide intravenously over at least 30 seconds,

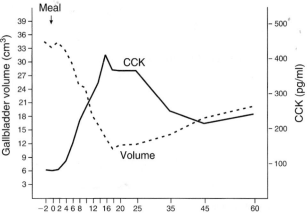

Figure 7-4   Physiology of gallbladder contraction. After ingestion of a fatty meal, serum cholecystokinin (CCK) rises to a peak between 15 and 30 minutes, depending on the type of meal and rate of gastric emptying. Gallbladder contraction begins before peak serum CCK. CCK continues to be released by the duodenum until food empties from the stomach and proximal bowel. The gallbladder remains contracted until serum CCK falls below contraction threshold. It then relaxes and ceases emptying.

Box 7-5 Cholecystokinin (Sincalide) Cholescintigraphy: Protocol

SINCALIDE ADMINISTRATION
Three validated methods with normal values

1. 60-min infusion: Set up computer acquisition for
   60 1-min frames (128 × 128).
   Infuse 0.01 μg/kg of sincalide over 60 min using
   infusion pump.
   Abnormal GBEF is <40% (Ziessman et al. 2001)
   or
2. 30-min infusion: Set up computer acquisition for 30
   1-min frames.
   Infuse 0.02 μg/kg of sincalide over 30 min using
   infusion pump.
   Abnormal GBEF is <30% (Ziessman et al. 1992)
   or
3. 45-min infusion: Set up computer acquisition for 60
   1-min frames
   Infuse sincalide at dose rate of 0.02 μg/kg/min for
   45 min using infusion pump
   Calculate GBEF at 60 min
   Abnormal GBEF is <40% (Yap et al. 1991)
   or

FATTY MEAL PROTOCOL

1. Set up computer for 60 1-min frames (128 × 128)
2. Ingest 240 ml (8 oz. can) of Ensure Plus (Abbot
   Laboratories)
3. Calculate GBEF at 60 min.
4. Abnormal GBEF is <33% (Ziessman et al. 2003)

COMPUTER PROCESSING GALLBLADDER EJECTION FRACTION (GBEF)

1. Select region of interest for the gallbladder and
   adjacent liver background.
2. Derive time-activity curve.
3. Calculate GBEF = maximum counts minus minimum
   counts divided by maximum counts, corrected for
   background.

usually 1–3 minutes. The administered dose has varied among all users from 0.01–0.04 μg/kg, although the most commonly used is 0.02 μg/kg.

Recent studies have shown that even 1–3 minute infusions of 0.01–0.02 μg/kg sincalide result in ineffective contraction of the gallbladder in up to one third of normal subjects (Table 7-4). However, slower infusions of 30–60 minutes result in good contraction in the same subjects. The explanation is thought to be that some persons have spasm of the neck of the gallbladder with similar to 1–3 minute infusions similar to that seen with a bolus infusion. The spasm is caused by the supraphysiological nature of the infusion rate (Fig. 7-5).

Normal values have never been established for the 3-minute infusion method. The value of 35% as abnormal was used for many years without substantiating normal data. Recent studies that have attempted to establish normal values have been unsuccessful because of the wide range of individual response to this dose rate. However, normal values have been established for 30-, 45-, and 60-minute infusions and this methodology is recommended (*see* Table 7-4). Protocols for these three methodologies are described (*see* Box 7-5).

Furthermore, approximately half of patients receiving a 1- to 3-minute infusion have abdominal cramping and nausea, which bears no relationship to whether or not the patient has hepatobiliary pathology but rather to the methodology of infusion. Adverse symptoms are not seen with slower infusions of 30–60 minutes.

When clinically indicated (*see* Box 7-4), sincalide can be infused twice in a patient study because of its short 2.5-minute half-life in serum. For example, sincalide may be given prior to cholescintigraphy for a patient fasting for more than 24 hours prior to the study followed by another infusion after the 60-minute study to evaluate gallbladder contraction. Caution is indicated in giving sincalide after a patient has received morphine

Table 7-4 Comparison of 3-Minute and 30- to 60-Minute Sincalide Infusion Methods

Gallbladder Ejection Fraction in Normal Subjects

Study	Dose	Infusion length	GBEF range (%)	False positives*	Normal values
Ziessman 1992	0.02 μg/kg	3 min	0-100	8/23 (35%)	>0%
Ziessman 2001	0.01 μg/kg	3 min	12-74	6/20 (30%)	>7%
Ziessman 1992	0.02 μg/kg	30 min	25-97	2/23 (9%)	>30%
Ziessman 2001	0.01 μg/kg	60 min	52-88	1/20 (5%)	>40%

*GBEF value <35%.

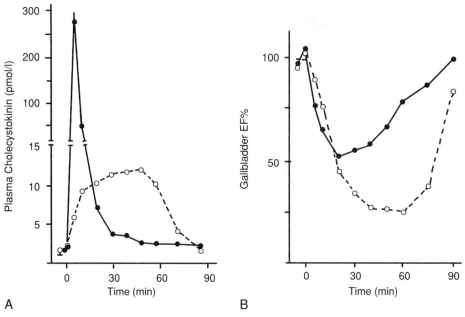

Figure 7-5   Response of serum CCK and gallbladder to one and 60 minute infusions of sincalide. **A,** With sincalide infusion of 60 minutes *(open circles)*, the plasma CCK pattern of increase and plateau is very similar to that seen with fatty meal ingestion *(see* Fig. 7-4). However, with a one minute infusion *(closed circles)*, serum CCK has a very rapid upslope and supraphysiological peak, with rapid return to baseline. **B,** Gallbladder contraction with a slow infusion *(open circles)* is both more prolonged and to a greater degree. (Modified from Hopman et al. *Br. Med J* 292: 375, 1986, with permission.)

sulfate because morphine's pharmacological effect of 4-6 hours may counteract the effect of sincalide.

When sincalide is given before cholescintigraphy, Tc-99m IDA should not be injected until 30 minutes after cessation of sincalide infusion to allow time for full gallbladder relaxation. When given prior to cholescintigraphy, sincalide may alter Tc-99m IDA pharmacokinetics, causing a delay in biliary-to-bowel transit, discussed in the *Biliary Obstruction* section.

When sincalide is not available, a fatty meal may be administered as an alternative. Normal values will vary depending on the amount of fat in the meal and the length of the study. Thus, a meal with an established protocol and validated normal values should be used *(see* Box 7-5).

Normal Cholescintigraphy

Blood Flow

Because of the liver's predominantly venous origin of blood flow (75% portal vein and 25% hepatic artery), the liver is not normally seen during the early arterial blood flow phase, but rather 6-8 seconds after flow to the spleen and kidneys (Fig. 7-6).

Early diffusely increased blood flow may be seen when there is arterialization of the liver's blood supply (e.g., with cirrhosis or generalized tumor involvement). Focally increased liver blood flow occurs with an intrahepatic malignant mass or abscess. Increased blood flow to the region of the gallbladder fossa can be seen with severe acute cholecystitis. Localized extrahepatic increased blood flow may suggest unexpected pathology.

Liver Morphology

During the early hepatic phase, prior to biliary secretion, liver size and the presence or absence of intrahepatic lesions can be assessed. Because the study is usually acquired dynamically only in the anterior view, this information is limited.

Hepatic Function

Liver function can be assessed visually by noting the rapidity of Tc-99m IDA extraction and clearance from blood pool. Blood pool in the heart should clear by 5-10

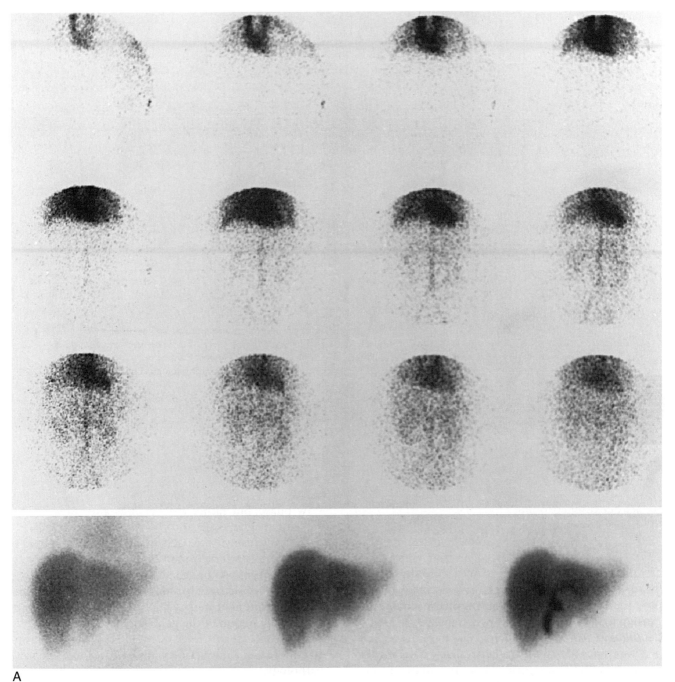

A

Figure 7-6   Normal technetium-99m IDA studies. **A,** *Top three rows,* Two-second blood flow images. Blood flow to the liver is delayed compared with the spleen and kidneys because of the liver's predominantly portal venous blood flow. *Bottom,* Heart blood pool seen on immediate image clears over next two frames at 5 and 10 minutes, consistent with good hepatic function.

Continued

minutes (*see* Fig. 7-6). Delayed blood pool and background clearance is seen with hepatic dysfunction (Fig. 7-7). Hepatic dysfunction may be *prehepatic* in origin (e.g., congestive heart failure), *hepatic* (e.g., hepatitis or cirrhosis), or *posthepatic* (e.g., late common duct obstruction).

Gallbladder Filling

The gallbladder normally begins to fill by 10 minutes and is usually filled by 30–40 minutes, although 60 minutes is the standard time interval defined as normal (*see* Fig. 7-6). The normal size and shape is quite variable.

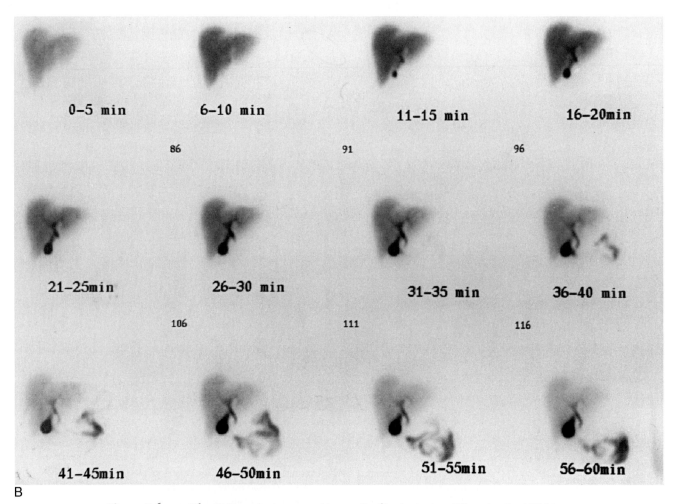

B

Figure 7-6, cont'd   **B,** Five-minute summed images for 60 minutes in a different patient. Right, left, and common hepatic ducts are seen by 15–20 minutes and common bile duct by 30 minutes. Biliary-to-bowel clearance is noted at 36 minutes. Gallbladder is visualized early.

Biliary Clearance

The smaller peripheral biliary ducts are not usually visualized unless enlarged. The left and right hepatic bile ducts, common hepatic duct, and common bile duct are usually seen, particularly with frequent image acquisition and computer cinematic display (*see* Fig. 7-6). The left hepatic ducts may be prominent because of the anterior position of the left lobe.

Although evidence of dilation can be seen on cholescintigraphy, duct size cannot be accurately determined. The strength of cholescintigraphy is that the functional patency of normal-sized or enlarged biliary ducts can be evaluated. The common bile duct is usually seen by 20 minutes and clears to less than 50% of peak activity by 60 minutes. Transit from the biliary ducts to the small intestine (biliary-to-bowel transit) normally occurs by 60 minutes.

Clinical Applications for Cholescintigraphy

Some of the more common clinical indications for cholescintigraphy will be discussed (*see* Box 7-1).

Acute Cholecystitis

The most frequent indication for Tc-99m IDA cholescintigraphy at most hospitals is to confirm or exclude clinically suspected acute cholecystitis.

Pathophysiology

Acute cholecystitis is usually initiated by obstruction of the cystic duct. An impacted calculus (stone) is the cause in over 95% of cases. Following obstruction, a progression of sequential histopathological inflammatory changes in the gallbladder wall ensues beginning with venous and lymphatic obstruction (Box 7-6), which results in edema followed by white blood cell infiltration, hemorrhage, ulceration, necrosis, and finally gangrene and perforation.

Clinical Presentation

Characteristic clinical symptoms are the acute onset of colicky right upper quadrant pain, nausea, and vomiting. Patients have leukocytosis but usually normal liver function tests. Even for patients with classic symptoms, typical physical findings, and suggestive laboratory values, a confirmatory imaging study is usually required prior to surgery.

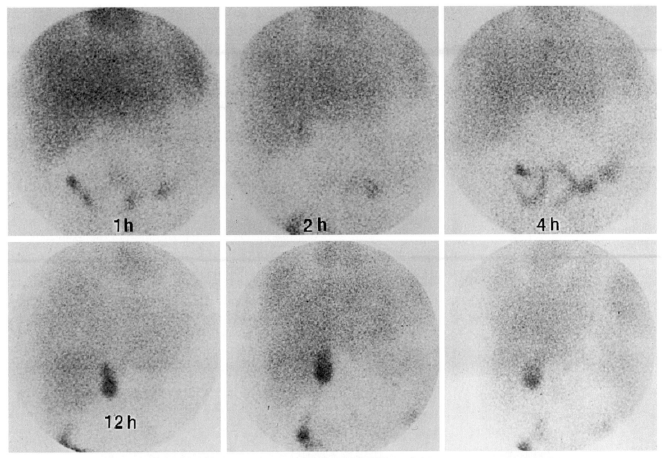

Figure 7-7 Delayed gallbladder visualization with severe hepatic insufficiency. Very slow blood pool clearance and poor liver-to-background ratio caused by liver dysfunction. Gallbladder is not visualized until 12 hours. Last two images are right and left anterior oblique views.

| Box 7-6 | **Pathophysiology of Acute Cholecystitis – Sequential Progression of Events** |

Cystic duct obstruction
Venous and lymphatic outflow obstruction
Mucosal edema and congestion
Neutrophilic leukocyte infiltration
Hemorrhage and necrosis
Gangrene
Perforation

Ultrasonography

An impacted stone in the cystic duct or neck of the gallbladder is diagnostic of acute cholecystitis; however, this is a rare finding with ultrasonography. Most patients with acute cholecystitis have cholelithiasis and ultrasonography has a high sensitivity for detection of gallbladder stones. However, this finding is not specific for acute cholecystitis. Asymptomatic gallstones are common and often not related to the cause of abdominal pain. Of patients presenting in the emergency room with acute abdominal pain who have gallstones on ultrasonography, less than half are ultimately diagnosed with acute cholecystitis.

Many of the ultrasonographic findings seen with acute cholecystitis are nonspecific. Thickening of the gallbladder wall and pericholecystic fluid occur with other acute and chronic diseases. Intramural lucency from edema is a more specific indicator of acute inflammation. The "sonographic Murphy's sign" (localized tenderness in the region of the gallbladder) in experienced hands is reported to be diagnostic. However, this observation is operator-dependent and not always reliable.

The combination of gallstones, intramural lucency, and the sonographic Murphy's sign makes the diagnosis of acute cholecystitis very likely. However, most patients with acute cholecystitis do not have all these findings. Investigations that have directly compared sonography with cholescintigraphy for the diagnosis of acute cholecystitis have found cholescintigraphy to be superior (Table 7-5).

An advantage of ultrasonography is that it can detect other findings and diseases that may be causing the patient's symptoms, such as common duct dilation

Table 7-5 Acute Cholecystitis: Accuracy of Cholescintigraphy and Ultrasonography

Study	n	Sensitivity/Specificity % Cholescin-tigraphy	Ultraso-nography
Stadalnik 1978	120	100 / 100	70 / 93
Weissmann 1979	90	98 / 100	
Freitas 1980	186	97 / 87	
Suarez 1980	62	98 / 100	
Szalabick 1980	271	100 / 98	
Weissmann 1981	296	95 / 99	
Zeman 1981	200	98 / 82	67 / 82
Worthen 1981	113	95 / 100	67 / 100
Mauro 1982	95	100 / 94	
Ralls 1982	59	86 / 84	86 / 90
Freitas 1982	195	98 / 90	60 / 81
Samuels 1983	194	97 / 93	97 / 64

caused by biliary obstruction, pancreatic and liver tumors, renal stones, pulmonary consolidation, and pleural effusion. Practically, cholescintigraphy and ultrasonography provide complementary information.

Cholescintigraphy

Cholescintigraphy is considered the study of choice to confirm the diagnosis of acute cholecystitis because it reveals the underlying pathophysiology (i.e., cystic duct obstruction, manifested by nonfilling of the gallbladder).

Scintigraphic Diagnosis Nonfilling of the gallbladder by 60 minutes after Tc-99m IDA injection is abnormal but not specific for acute cholecystitis (Fig. 7-8). Chronic cholecystitis is a common cause for nonvisualization at 60 minutes but the gallbladder fills on delayed imaging. Nonvisualization of the gallbladder by 3-4 hour delayed imaging is diagnostic of cystic duct obstruction and, in the appropriate clinical setting, acute cholecystitis. Morphine sulfate, discussed later, is now often used as an alternative to delayed imaging to confirm the diagnosis of acute cholecystitis (Fig. 7-9).

At times it may be difficult to differentiate gallbladder filling from activity in overlapping duodenum and

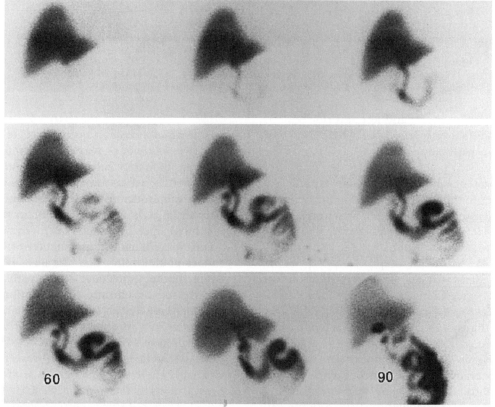

Figure 7-8 Delayed gallbladder visualization with chronic cholecystitis. At 60 minutes, the gallbladder is not definitely visualized. Focal activity is seen just lateral to the proximal common duct. However, the next image in the left anterior oblique view confirms that the focal activity is due to duodenal activity. Gallbladder visualization occurs at 90 minutes.

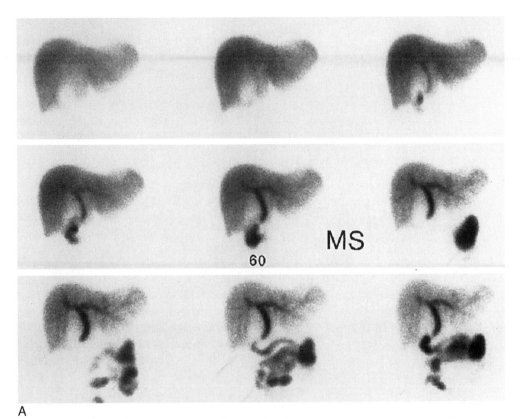

A

Figure 7-9   Morphine-augmented cholescintigraphy. **A,** Patient with clinically suspected acute cholecystitis. Tc-99m IDA images for 60 minutes show good visualization of common hepatic and common bile ducts, biliary clearance into the duodenum, but no gallbladder visualization. Morphine sulfate (MS) is given. The gallbladder is not visualized, confirming diagnosis of acute cholecystitis by 90 minutes.

Continued

common duct. Right lateral and left anterior oblique (LAO) views at 60 minutes can be very helpful to confirm or rule out gallbladder filling (Fig. 7-10). In the right lateral projection, the gallbladder lies anteriorly. In the LAO projection, the gallbladder, an anterior structure, moves to the patient's right and the common duct and duodenum, more posterior structures, move to the patient's left. Upright imaging and ingestion of water are techniques that can be used to clear duodenal activity.

Accuracy   Many studies have reported on the sensitivity and specificity of cholescintigraphy for making the diagnosis of acute cholecystitis (Table 7-5). More than two-thirds of these investigations reported the sensitivity to be greater than 95% and the specificity greater than 90%. Morphine-augmented cholescintigraphy has accuracy similar to the delayed imaging method (Table 7-6).

Although some false positives (nonfilling of the gallbladder in patients without acute cholecystitis) occur, the specificity can be maximized by anticipating situations associated with an increased incidence of a false-positive study (Box 7-7) and by using proper methodology.

The optimal time window for performing cholescintigraphy (i.e., after fasting for 3–4 hours but not more than 24 hours) has been discussed. Patients with hepatic insufficiency have delayed uptake and clearance of Tc-99m IDA, which may result in delayed and unpredictable gallbladder visualization because of the altered pharmacokinetics. Delayed imaging up to 24 hours may be necessary (*see* Fig. 7-7).

The most common cause for a false-positive study is chronic cholecystitis. Less than 1% of patients with chronic cholecystitis have a totally obstructed cystic duct caused by chronic inflammation. Another 5% have delayed gallbladder visualization because of partial cystic duct obstruction (*see* Fig 7-8). However, some will have a functional obstruction with nonfilling of the gallbladder caused by a noncontracting gallbladder full of viscous bile. Delayed imaging or morphine administration minimizes this potential cause for false-positive cholescintigraphy but does not eliminate it.

Another important group at increased risk for false-positive cholescintigraphy for acute cholecystitis is sick hospitalized patients with concurrent serious illness.

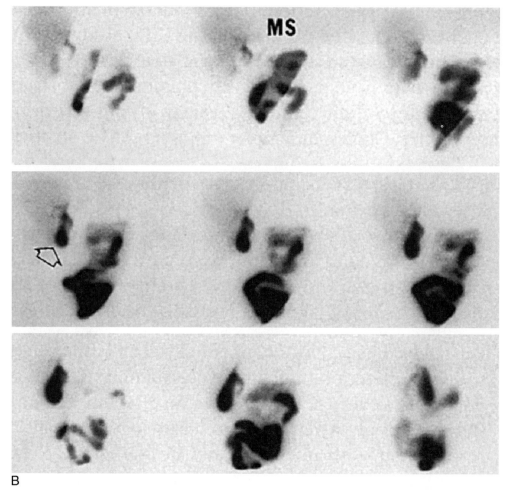

Figure 7-9, cont'd   **B,** A second patient shows no gallbladder filling at 60 minutes *(upper left),* so MS was given. Gallbladder filling begins within 5 minutes and is definite by 10 minutes *(arrowhead).* Acute cholecystitis is ruled out.

They often have had no oral intake for days or weeks and are receiving hyperalimentation (*see* Box 7-7).

False-negative studies (gallbladder filling in a patient with acute cholecystitis) are very uncommon. This can occur with incomplete obstruction of the cystic duct. Obstruction of the distal cystic duct can result in proximal dilation which might be misinterpreted as a small gallbladder, called the *cystic duct sign* or *nubbin sign.* As discussed later, acute acalculous cholecystitis has a higher false-negative rate than acute calculous cholecystitis. Very rarely, morphine administration may convert a true positive to a false negative in a patient with acute cholecystitis.

Morphine Augmentation   The 3- to 4-hour time period often required for cholescintigraphy using the delayed imaging method to diagnose acute cholecystitis is not optimal for an acutely ill patient, who requires prompt diagnosis and therapy. As an alternative to delayed imaging, morphine sulfate is now often routinely used to shorten the duration of cholescintigraphy.

Morphine sulfate increases intraluminal biliary pressure by constricting the sphincter of Oddi, which causes preferential flow of bile to and through the cystic duct, if it is patent. The dose of morphine required to constrict the sphincter of Oddi is less than that required for pain relief.

Morphine sulfate, 0.04 mg/kg, is infused intravenously when the gallbladder does not fill by 60 minutes. With cystic duct patency, the gallbladder will then begin to fill by 5–10 minutes after morphine infusion and filling will be complete by 20–30 minutes. Thus, the entire Tc-99m IDA study requires only 90 minutes (*see* Fig. 7-9).

Morphine should not be given if there are scintigraphic findings suggestive of biliary obstruction, such as poor clearance into the bowel (delayed biliary-to-bowel transit) and/or significant retention of radiotracer in biliary ducts (<50% clearance from peak). Intravenous morphine produces a functional partial common duct obstruction that cannot be differentiated on scintigraphy from a pathologic obstruction caused by stone or

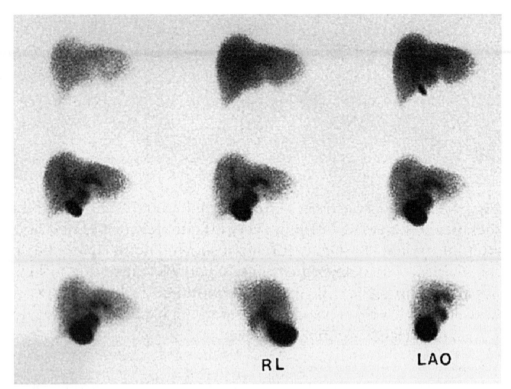

Figure 7-10   Differentiating gallbladder from common duct and duodenum. Separating the gallbladder from the common bile duct and duodenum is difficult *(middle row)* before obtaining right lateral (RL) and LAO views. The LAO view delineates the common bile duct, but no biliary-to-bowel clearance has occurred and therefore there is no duodenal activity. In the LAO view, the gallbladder moves to the right (anteriorly), and the common bile duct and duodenum move to the left (posteriorly).

Table 7-6	Accuracy of Morphine-Augmented Cholescintigraphy	
Study	**Sensitivity (%)**	**Specificity (%)**
Choy	96	100
Kim	100	100
Keslar	100	83
Vasquez	100	85
Fig	94	69*
Flancbaum	97	95
Fink-Bennett	95	96
Kistler	93	78*

*High percentage of patients with concurrent illness and chronic cholecystitis.

Box 7-7   Causes for False Positive Cholescintigraphy for Acute Cholecystitis

Fasting <4 hr
Fasting >24 hr
Concurrent severe illness
Chronic cholecystitis
Hepatic insufficiency
Hyperalimentation
Alcoholism (?)
Pancreatitis (?)

stricture. Thus, the diagnosis of biliary obstruction cannot be made once morphine is given. If biliary obstruction has not been excluded by 60 minutes, morphine should not be administered. Delayed images should then be obtained for up to 3–4 hours.

Rim Sign   Increased hepatic uptake adjacent to the gallbladder fossa (rim sign) is seen on cholescintigraphy in approximately 25–35% of patients with acute cholecystitis

(Fig. 7-11). It may be seen throughout the initial 60-minute study; however, it is easier to discern as Tc-99m IDA clears from normal hepatocytes in the rest of the liver.

The importance of the rim sign is twofold. First, it is a very specific scintigraphic finding for acute cholecystitis. This sign becomes diagnostically useful to confirm that a patient at increased risk for false-positive cholescintigraphy (*see* Box 7-7) (e.g., a sick hospitalized

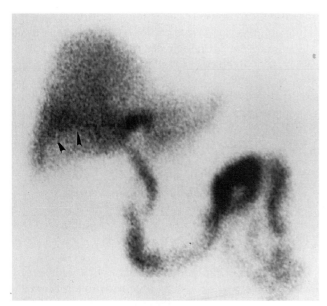

Figure 7-11 Rim sign. Increased liver uptake in the region of the gallbladder fossa. Normal biliary-to-bowel transit, but no gallbladder visualization at 60 minutes. Delayed imaging showed no gallbladder filling. The rim sign is specific for acute cholecystitis and is associated with increased complications.

patient with concurrent serious illness) does indeed have acute cholecystitis. The rim sign confirms that non-filling of the gallbladder is a true-positive, not a false-positive study.

Second, the rim sign identifies patients with acute cholecystitis who have more severe disease and are at increased risk for complications (e.g., gallbladder perforation and gangrene). Even if they do not have these complications, patients with the rim sign tend to be at a later stage of the pathophysiological spectrum of disease (e.g., hemorrhage and necrosis) rather than edema and white blood cell infiltration (*see* Box 7-6).

The pathophysiological mechanism for the rim sign is explained by severe local inflammation in the liver adjacent to the gallbladder. In severe acute cholecystitis, the gall-bladder inflammatory process may spread directly to the adjacent normal liver, which results in increased blood flow to that region. The high extraction efficiency of the liver for Tc-99m IDA results in local increased uptake compared to adjacent noninflamed liver. Regional delayed clearance may be secondary to inflammatory edema with obstruction of biliary canaliculi.

Acute Acalculous Cholecystitis

The acalculous form of cholecystitis is a life-threatening disease that occurs in seriously ill hospitalized patients, usually in the intensive care unit (Box 7-8). Because of its high mortality (30%) and morbidity (55%), early diagnosis is imperative. However, because of concomitant serious illness, diagnosis is often delayed.

Box 7-8 Clinical Conditions Associated with Acute Acalculous Cholecystitis

Postoperative
Multiple trauma
Extensive burns
Shock
Acquired immunodeficiency syndrome
Mechanical ventilation
Vasculitis
Multiple transfusions

As the name suggests, acute acalculous cholecystitis is acute cholecystitis without stones, either in the gall-bladder or obstructing the cystic duct. However, in the majority of cases, there is cystic duct obstruction. The obstruction is caused by inflammatory debris, inspissated bile, and/or local edema, perhaps aggravated by dehydration. However, there is a substantial minority of patients with acute acalculous cholecystitis who do not have cystic duct obstruction but rather have direct inflammation of the gallbladder wall as a result of systemic infection, ischemia, or toxemia.

There has long been a concern that the accuracy for cholescintigraphy for the acalculous variety of acute cholecystitis would be less than for acute calculous cholecystitis, particularly in those patients without cystic duct obstruction. False negative cholescintigraphy (gall-bladder filling) might occur because of the lack of cystic duct obstruction. Data over the years has been conflicting but does suggest a lower sensitivity for the diagnosis of acute acalculous cholecystitis compared to the calculous form of the disease (Table 7-7).

If a false-negative study (filling of the gallbladder) is suspected in a patient with a high clinical suspicion for acute acalculous cholecystitis, sincalide may be helpful. An acutely inflamed gallbladder would not be expected

Table 7-7 Acute Acalculous Cholecystitis: Accuracy of Cholescintigraphy

Study	n	Sensitivity (%)	Specificity (%)
Shuman 1984	19	68	
Weissmann 1983	15	93	
Mirvis 1986	19	90	61
Swayne 1986	49	93	
Ramanna 1984	11	100	
Flancbaum 1995	16	75	100
Prevot 1999	14	64	100
Mariat 2000	12	67	100

to contract normally. Thus, good contraction would exclude the disease. However, poor contraction is not specific. The patient may have an underlying chronic cholecystitis or be on drugs (Box 7-9) or have a disease process (Box 7-10) that inhibits gallbladder emptying. No adverse affects have been reported with the administration of sincalide to patients with suspected acute acalculous cholecystitis.

A radiolabeled leukocyte study could be used to confirm the diagnosis. In-111 leukocytes are preferable to Tc-99m HMPAO leukocytes because the latter radiopharmaceutical clears through the biliary tract. Early imaging at 1–2 hours before biliary clearance may obviate this problem. The disadvantage of In-111-leukocytes is the usual imaging time at 24 hours, although earlier imaging might be useful (e.g., at 4 hours). If positive, the diagnosis is confirmed; if negative, repeat imaging at 24 hours may be indicated.

Chronic Cholecystitis
Symptomatic chronic cholecystitis presents with recurrent colicky right upper quadrant pain. The clinical diag-

nosis is typically made by detection of gallstones on ultrasonography. Laparoscopic cholecystectomy is the usual treatment. Histopathologically, the gallbladder wall is infiltrated with chronic inflammatory cells and fibrotic. Routine 60-minute cholescintigraphy is usually normal. Less than 5% of patients have abnormal findings (e.g., nonfilling or more commonly delayed filling of the gallbladder) or delayed biliary-to-bowel transit. These findings are neither sensitive nor specific for chronic cholecystitis.

Cholelithiasis is common but often asymptomatic. Patients with asymptomatic gallstones usually have normal gallbladder contraction. However, patients with symptomatic chronic cholecystitis typically have poor gallbladder contraction, as demonstrated by a low gallbladder ejection fraction (GBEF) when stimulated with sincalide or a fatty meal. Thus, sincalide cholescintigraphy has been used to differentiate patients with symptomatic chronic cholecystitis from those with asymptomatic gallstones and chronic recurrent abdominal pain from other causes. However, the primary role of sincalide cholescintigraphy in chronic cholecystitis is to diagnose the acalculous form of chronic cholecystitis.

Chronic Acalculous Cholecystitis
The acalculous variety of chronic cholecystitis is uncommon, occurring in approximately 5% of patients with symptomatic chronic cholecystitis. It is clinically and histopathologically indistinguishable from chronic calculous cholecystitis, except for the lack of gallstones. Over the years, it has been referred to by various other names including acalculous biliary disease and cystic duct syndrome (Box 7-11). Because the symptoms may be similar to other disease processes, a noninvasive imaging method to preoperatively confirm the suspected diagnosis is desirable.

Numerous investigations between 1980 and 1990 reported that sincalide cholescintigraphy can confirm the diagnosis of chronic acalculous cholecystitis. Poor gallbladder contraction after sincalide infusion can

---

Box 7-9 Drugs Associated with Poor Gallbladder Contraction

Morphine
Atropine
Nifedipine (calcium channel blocking agent)
Indomethacin
Progesterone
Oral contraceptives
Octreotide
Theophylline
Benzodiazepine
Phentolamine (alpha-adrenergic blocking agent)

Box 7-10 Diseases Associated with Poor Gallbladder Contraction

Diabetes mellitus
Sickle cell disease
Irritable bowel syndrome
Truncal vagotomy
Pancreatic insufficiency
Crohn's disease
Celiac disease
Achalasia
Dyspeptic syndrome
Obesity
Cirrhosis
Pregnancy

Box 7-11 Synonyms for Recurrent Pain Syndromes of Biliary Origin

CHRONIC ACALCULOUS CHOLECYSTITIS

Acalculous biliary disease
Gallbladder spasm
Cystic duct syndrome

SPHINCTER OF ODDI DYSFUNCTION

Papillary stenosis
Biliary spasm
Biliary dyskinesia

preoperatively predict postcholecystectomy symptomatic relief and histopathological evidence of chronic cholecystitis (Fig. 7-12); a normal GBEF excludes the disease.

The most scientifically rigorous investigation is a prospective randomized study by Yap and colleagues. The investigation found the positive predictive value of sincalide cholescintigraphy is greater than 90%. Other studies have found similar results but were mostly retrospective. This is also the only clinical study that established its own normal values based on their slow method of infusion (*see* Box 7-5). The published studies that have confirmed a high accuracy for sincalide cholescintigraphy investigated a selected group of patients who have been extensively worked up to exclude other diseases and were followed for many months or years, thus allowing time for other diseases to present. Thus, the patients referred for sincalide cholescintigraphy had a relatively high likelihood of having chronic cholecystitis. Sincalide cholescintigraphy confirmed the clinically suspected diagnosis. The accuracy of this test in a group of patients with a lower likelihood of disease might not be expected to be as high.

Sincalide cholescintigraphy should be performed after an appropriate clinical workup. It is best done on an outpatient basis while the patient is asymptomatic and not acutely sick or hospitalized because other diseases and therapeutic drugs may adversely affect gallbladder function (*see* Boxes 7-11 and 7-12).

Normal (or abnormal) values for GBEF depend on the method of infusing sincalide. Normal values have not been established for a 3-minute infusion. That method should not be used. For a 30-minute infusion, less than 30% is abnormal; for a 45–60 minute infusion, less than 40% is abnormal (*see* Box 7-5 and Table 7-4).

A persistent misconception is that reproduction of the patient's pain with CCK infusion is diagnostic of chronic acalculous cholecystitis. CCK has a variety of effects on the gastrointestinal tract (*see* Box 7-3), one being that it stimulates intestinal motility, which can cause cramping pain. The pain of patients with irritable bowel syndrome can be aggravated by CCK infusion. Up to 50% of normal controls receiving sincalide over 1–3 minutes complain of abdominal cramps. However, those receiving the same total dose over at least 30 minutes do not experience pain, whether or not they have chronic cholecystitis.

Box 7-12   Sequential Pathophysiology of High-Grade Biliary Obstruction

1. Complete or near complete biliary obstruction
2. Increased intrabiliary pressure
3. Decreased bile flow
4. Ductal dilation
5. Biliary cirrhosis

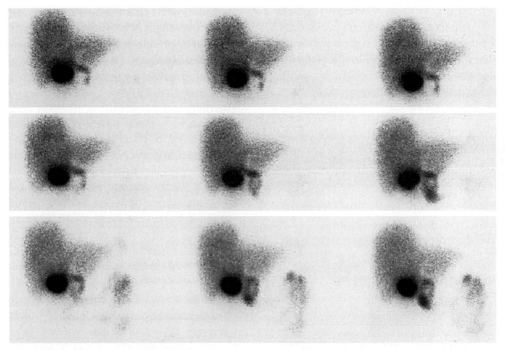

Figure 7-12   Chronic acalculous cholecystitis. Extremely poor contraction of the gallbladder is evident after sincalide infusion (GBEF, 20%). Biliary-to-bowel transit is delayed, a nonspecific finding that may be seen with chronic cholecystitis.

Biliary Duct Obstruction

Obstruction of the bile ducts is often suspected clinically by the patient's symptoms and elevated serum liver function tests (e.g., direct serum bilirubin, alkaline phosphatase) and confirmed by anatomical imaging methods (e.g., ultrasonography and magnetic resonance cholangiopancreatography [MRCP]). Dilation of biliary ducts is diagnostic of obstruction in patients who have not had prior obstruction or biliary surgery.

However, biliary obstruction may occur in the absence of hyperbilirubinemia or jaundice, which is usually a late manifestation. Obstruction does not always result in dilation of the bile ducts. Furthermore, dilation can occur in the absence of obstruction. In these latter two situations, cholescintigraphy can play a particularly important diagnostic role.

Cancerous and noncancerous causes of biliary tract obstruction usually present differently (Table 7-8). Malignancy (e.g., pancreatic or biliary duct cancer) typically causes high-grade obstruction with painless jaundice, whereas choledocholithiasis usually produces either severe acute pain with complete obstruction or intermittent pain of low-grade obstruction. Pancreatitis tends to cause only mild partial obstruction. High-grade biliary obstruction may present with Charcot's triad of fever, chills, and hyperbilirubinemia.

High-Grade Biliary Obstruction

Pathophysiology   The sequence of pathophysiological events in high-grade obstruction progresses in a predictable manner (Box 7-12), although the time course may vary depending on the rapidity of onset, the degree of obstruction, and its etiology. High-grade obstruction causes increased intraductal pressure. The resulting backpressure markedly reduces bile flow and causes biliary duct dilation. With persistence of obstruction, there is increased hepatocellular permeability and ultimately hepatocellular damage culminating in biliary cirrhosis.

Table 7-8 Biliary Obstruction: Clinical Presentations	
Degree of Obstruction	**Usual Etiology**
High-grade—complete obstruction	
Painless jaundice	Malignancy
Acute severe abdominal pain	Choledocholithiasis
Charcot's Triad (fever, chills, hyperbilirubinemia)	Biliary obstruction
Low-grade—partial obstruction	
Recurrent biliary colic	Choledocholithiasis
No jaundice or liver function abnormalities	Choledocholithiasis

Hyperbilirubinemia is a late manifestation of obstruction. Elevation of the serum alkaline phosphatase occurs earlier in the natural history and is more specific. Ductal dilation, the anatomical imaging sine qua non of biliary obstruction, may not become evident until 24–72 hours after the initiating event. Cholescintigraphy can confirm the diagnosis before dilation occurs by depicting the physiology, a reduction in bile flow (Fig. 7-13).

Partial Biliary Obstruction

The pathophysiology of partial obstruction is less well understood. Ducts often do not dilate with low-grade or intermittent biliary obstruction, probably because of the lower intraductal pressure and the intermittent nature of the process. The etiology is usually choledocholithiasis. In some cases, ductal dilation may be restricted by edema and scarring.

Noninvasive Imaging   Oftentimes the imaging diagnosis of partial biliary obstruction is made with ultrasonography and MRCP. However, in patients without jaundice, anatomical imaging may be unrewarding. In these cases, cholescintigraphy can help determine the need for a more invasive workup, such as endoscopic retrograde cholangiopancreatography (ERCP) or percutaneous cholangiography.

Ultrasonography   The diagnosis of obstruction is made by noting dilation of the biliary tree. Dilation is most common with long-standing obstruction, particularly when secondary to malignant etiologies. Although the degree of dilation is not directly proportional to the serum bilirubin, the largest, most dilated ducts tend to occur in deeply jaundiced patients. An obstructing mass may be detected with ultrasonography. Biliary duct stones are rarely seen.

Magnetic Resonance Cholangiopancreatography   MRCP is now widely used for diagnosis of biliary obstruction. The rapid T2-weighted scans viewed in the coronal plane mimic the appearance of contrast cholangiography. It is superior to ultrasonography for detecting stones too small to result in ductal dilatation. Its diagnostic accuracy for detection of a variety of benign and malignant processes approaches ERCP or percutaneous transhepatic cholangiography. However, it is still an anatomic imaging methodology and cannot evaluate bile flow.

Discordance between anatomical imaging and functional imaging with cholescintigraphy is not uncommon in high-grade or low-grade obstruction. For example, ductal dilation may not be seen, whereas cholescintigraphy demonstrates abnormal delayed bile flow. Functional abnormalities may precede morphologically evident disease. In other patients with dilated ducts from prior exploration or chronic passage of stones, cholescintigraphy may show normal bile flow and no obstruction.

Cholescintigraphy   Cholescintigraphy is particularly useful in those patients with suspected biliary obstruction who have normal-sized biliary ducts or in patients

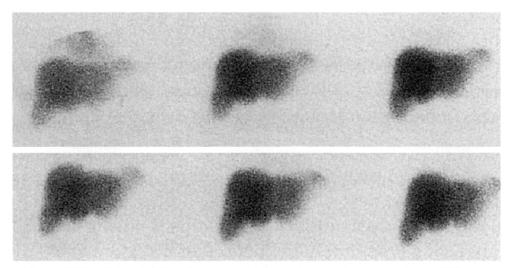

Figure 7-13   High-grade biliary obstruction. Good hepatic uptake, but no secretion into biliary ducts or gallbladder. The elevated backpressure prevents tracer from entering the biliary system.

who have had prior biliary obstruction and have persistently dilated ducts. The scintigraphic pattern of complete or high-grade obstruction of recent onset is an "Aunt Minnie," that is, good hepatic extraction and uptake of Tc-99m IDA but no excretion into the biliary tree (persistent hepatogram) (*see* Fig. 7-13). With complete obstruction, delayed imaging for up to 24 hours may show no change. With less complete but high-grade obstruction, there can be slow excretion into biliary ducts on delayed imaging at 2–24 hours.

The longer the obstruction goes on, the more likely there will be associated evidence of hepatic dysfunction (delayed hepatic uptake, prolonged blood pool), which can make differentiation of primary common bile duct obstruction from parenchymal dysfunction more difficult.

With partial common duct obstruction, the scintigraphic findings are quite different than those seen with high-grade obstruction (Fig. 7-14). Prompt hepatic uptake and secretion into biliary ducts is typically seen. The two most important cholescintigraphic findings are delayed transit into the bowel (delayed biliary-to-bowel transit) and delayed clearance of radiotracer from biliary ducts (Box 7-13).

However, delayed biliary-to-bowel transit is not a sensitive indicator of obstruction (Box 7-14). Up to 50% of patients with partial obstruction have biliary-to-bowel transit by 60 minutes. Therefore, it is particularly important to judge whether there has been good clearance of bile tracer from the biliary ducts by 60 minutes. Generally, at least 50% clearance from peak is expected. If not, delayed imaging at 2 hours, or alternatively, sincalide infusion can be given. Subsequent biliary-to-bowel transit rules out obstruction. Segmental obstruction will show similar scintigraphic findings as described, but in a regional liver pattern.

Less common and specific findings include filling defects within distal biliary ducts. This finding is most likely to be detected on the cinematic display as biliary duct filling begins. Persistent ductal segmental narrowing with proximal retention of activity is strongly suggestive of partial obstruction. However, these findings are really anatomical, and the real value of cholescintigraphy is the ability to analyze biliary physiology. Thus, significant retention of Tc-99m IDA within biliary ducts at 60 minutes, with or without biliary-to-bowel transit, should raise the suspicion of partial obstruction.

In patients who have had previous obstruction or biliary tract surgery, biliary ducts often remain permanently dilated. Thus, anatomical imaging methods of evaluation are not helpful. In patients who have recurrent symptoms, cholescintigraphy can differentiate obstructive from nonobstructive dilation. With nonobstructed dilation, there should be good ductal clearance and normal biliary-to-bowel transit.

Delayed biliary-to-bowel transit has various causes other than partial biliary obstruction (Box 7-14). Delayed transit is seen in patients who have received sincalide prior to the study for the purpose of emptying the gallbladder (Fig. 7-15). As the prokinetic effect of sincalide dissipates, the gallbladder relaxes. The resulting negative intraluminal gallbladder pressure causes bile to flow preferentially towards the gallbladder rather than through the common duct and sphincter of Oddi.

Morphine-related drugs can produce a functional obstruction with delayed biliary duct clearance and biliary-to-bowel transit. Delayed transit may also be seen in some patients with chronic cholecystitis. Finally, one report found that 20% of patients without biliary disease may have delayed biliary-to-bowel transit, sometimes referred to as a hypertonic sphincter of Oddi (Fig. 7-16).

Functional causes of delayed biliary-to-bowel transit can be confirmed by having the patient change position,

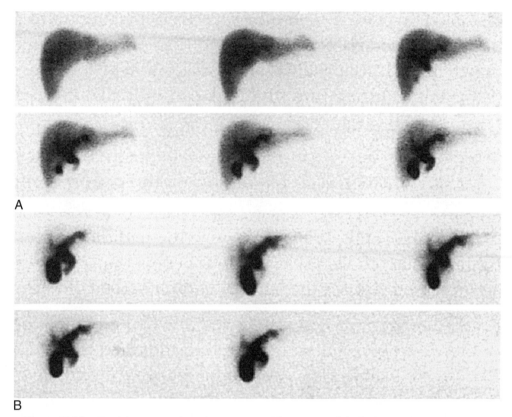

A

B

Figure 7-14 Partial common duct obstruction. **A,** The common bile duct appears increasingly prominent. Refluxed bile is seen in the left hepatic duct. No biliary-to-bowel transit occurs by 60 minutes. **B,** Sincalide infusion with sequential images. No gallbladder contraction and minimal biliary-to-bowel transit occur. The pattern is consistent with partial common duct obstruction.

walk around, and by obtaining delayed images at 2 hours. With obstruction, there would be persistent retention of activity within biliary ducts. Alternatively, sincalide can be given. The use of sincalide is a more reproducible method. In either case, persistent pooling in the biliary ducts (particularly in the common duct) after sincalide infusion is consistent with partial obstruction, whereas clearance rules out obstruction.

Accuracy For high-grade obstruction, the sensitivity for diagnosis approaches 100% and the specificity is greater than 95%. Rarely, cholestatic jaundice (e.g., drug-induced [erythromycin, chlorpromazine]), may have similar findings. For low-grade or intermittent obstruction, the sensitivity and specificity have been reported to be 95% and 85%, respectively.

Summary Noninvasive anatomic imaging procedures such as ultrasound and CT are the initial screening procedures in patients with surgical jaundice. MRCP has become an important anatomic diagnostic method. However, jaundice occurs relatively late in the natural history of obstruction. Scintigraphy is useful in patients whose symptoms are suggestive of obstruction but who are not jaundiced and have minimal liver function abnormalities. Scintigraphy may show low-grade

---

Box 7-13 Scintigraphic Diagnosis of Partial Biliary Obstruction

Delayed biliary-to-bowel transit beyond 60 minutes
Poor biliary duct clearance at 60 minutes
No further biliary duct clearance on delayed imaging at 120 minutes
No biliary duct clearance with sincalide administration between 60 and 120 minutes

---

Box 7-14 Causes of Delayed Biliary-to-bowel Transit

Biliary obstruction
Sincalide administration prior to cholescintigraphy
Opiate drugs
Chronic cholecystitis
Normal variation (hypertonic sphincter of Oddi)

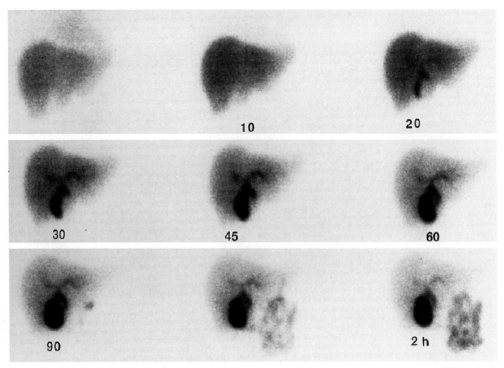

Figure 7-15   Delayed biliary-to-bowel transit due to sincalide pretreatment. Gallbladder fills by 30 minutes, common duct is seen at 60 minutes, but no bowel clearance is seen. Delayed images show intestinal clearance starting at 90 minutes and decreased activity in the common duct by 2 hours.

obstruction or segmental intrahepatic obstruction. Cholescintigraphy is also useful in distinguishing abdominal pain caused by acute cholecystitis from that secondary to biliary obstruction. It may diagnose the presence of both problems. Patients who have had prior obstruction or common duct exploration and persistently dilated atonic biliary ducts are prime candidates for cholescintigraphy.

Choledochal Cyst

A choledochal cyst is a congenital dilation of the biliary system. It is not a true cyst but rather a saccular or fusiform biliary duct dilation. Often it involves the common hepatic and common bile duct but it may occur anywhere within the biliary system, usually extrahepatic but rarely intrahepatic (Caroli's disease), and it may be multifocal (Fig. 7-17).

A choledochal cyst usually presents clinically in young children as biliary obstruction, pancreatitis, or cholangitis. However, they may be asymptomatic and found incidentally. On rare occasion, they will first present in adulthood. Ultrasonography or CT may reveal a cystic structure but often cannot ascertain whether the structure connects with the biliary tract.

Cholescintigraphy can confirm that the cystic structure connects to the biliary system. Tc-99m IDA tracer will fill the choledochal cyst and often have very prolonged reten-

tion within it, depending on its size and the degree of obstruction. Delayed images are often required (Fig. 7-18).

Biliary Atresia

This neonatal disease of unknown etiology is characterized by inflammatory sclerosis and obliteration of extrahepatic and intrahepatic bile ducts. Untreated, it leads to cirrhosis and death within the first years of life. Treatment involves surgery, a palliative hepatic portoenterostomy (Kasai procedure) performed in the neonatal period and subsequent liver transplantation.

Biliary atresia must be differentiated from neonatal hepatitis and cholestasis. Clinical features of biliary atresia include jaundice after full-term birth that lasts longer than 2 weeks, hepatomegaly, and hyperbilirubinemia. Early diagnosis of biliary atresia is critical because surgery must be performed within the first 60 days of life before irreversible liver failure ensues.

Infants with idiopathic neonatal hepatitis or cholestasis are often preterm and/or small for gestational age. The most common causes include Alagille syndrome (arteriohepatic dysplasia), progressive familial intrahepatic cholestasis, alpha-1 antitrypsin deficiency, and cystic fibrosis.

Cholescintigraphy has long been used to help differentiate biliary atresia from other causes of neonatal jaundice. The congenitally atretic bile ducts produce a picture

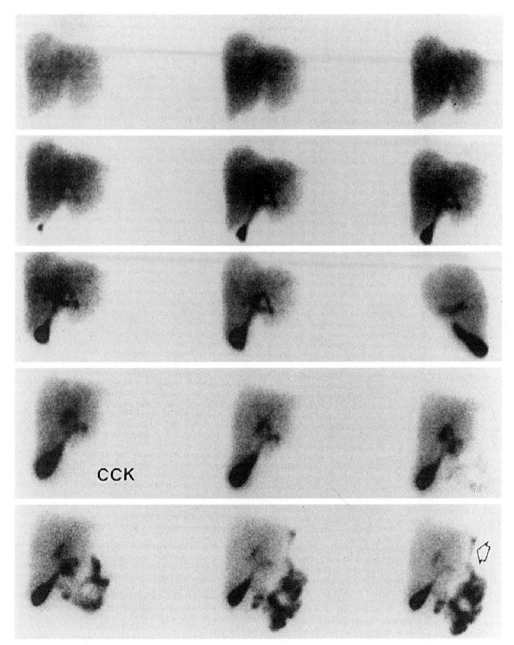

Figure 7-16 Delayed biliary-to-bowel transit in normal subject. *Top three rows,* Sequential images acquired over 60 minutes. Gallbladder fills. Biliary ducts are visualized, but no biliary-to-bowel transit is seen at 60 minutes. *Lower two rows,* Sincalide is infused over 30 minutes. Gallbladder contracts (GBEF, 51%), and biliary-to-bowel transit is seen due to concomitant relaxation of sphincter of Oddi. *Arrowhead,* Mild gastric reflux. This is a normal subject with a hypertonic sphincter of Oddi.

of high-grade obstruction (Fig. 7-19). Patients should be pretreated with phenobarbital (5 mg/kg/day for 5 days) before cholescintigraphy to maximize sensitivity for detection. The drug activates liver excretory enzymes. Ideally, the serum phenobarbital level should be checked prior to the study to ensure a therapeutic serum level of the drug.

The usual administered dose of Tc-99m IDA is 200 µCi/kg with 1 mCi being the minimal dose because 24-hour images are required. No biliary clearance into the bowel by 24 hours is consistent with biliary atresia. Patients with nonobstructive causes of neonatal jaundice usually have biliary clearance into the bowel during the first 24 hours after injection of Tc-99m IDA. False-positive

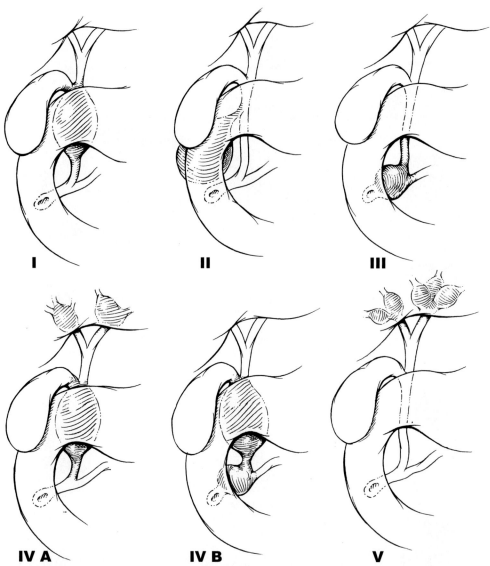

Figure 7-17   Schematic drawings of various types of choledochal cysts. Type I: Cystic dilation of an extrahepatic duct (most common); Type II: sac or diverticulum opening from the common bile duct; Type III: choledochocele, located within the duodenal wall; Type IV A: involving intrahepatic and extrahepatic biliary ducts; Type IV B dilatation of multiple segments confined to extrahepatic biliary ducts; Type V: multiple intrahepatic ducts (Caroli's disease).

studies (no biliary-to-bowel clearance) occasionally occur in patients with severe forms of parenchymal liver disease. When the clinical diagnosis is uncertain, a repeat study may be indicated.

Postoperative Biliary Tract

Cholescintigraphy provides diagnostic information in postoperative patients with suspected complications from biliary tract surgery (e.g., laparoscopic or open cholecystectomy, biliary duct surgery, gallstone lithotripsy, and biliary enteric anastomoses). Cholescintigraphy can be used in the differential diagnosis of the postcholecystectomy syndrome. Posttherapeutic evaluation with Tc-99m IDA can be useful in patients treated for obstruction with

papillotomy/sphincterotomy or biliary stents (i.e., to confirm patency or diagnose restenosis) (Fig. 7-20).

Postcholecystectomy Pain Syndrome

Recurrent abdominal pain of hepatobiliary origin after cholecystectomy may be caused by a retained or recurrent biliary duct stone, postoperative inflammatory stricture, or sphincter of Oddi dysfunction (*see* Box 7-15). Rarely, a cystic duct remnant acts like a small gallbladder and produces symptoms identical to those of acute or chronic cholecystitis.

Partial Biliary Obstruction

Partial biliary obstruction caused by retained or recurrent common duct stones and inflammatory fibrosis are the most common causes of postcholecystectomy

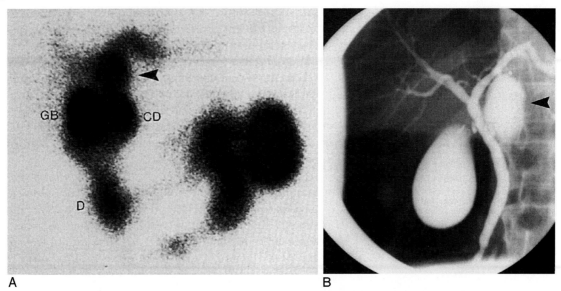

A   B

Figure 7-18   Choledochal cyst. 25-year-old with abdominal pain. Sonography noted a cystic structure adjacent to the common hepatic duct; however, a definite connection to the biliary system could not be ascertained. **A,** Tc-99 IDA images acquired at 90 minutes after the liver had cleared show filling of choledochal cyst in the region of the common hepatic duct (*arrowhead*). *CD,* Common duct; *GB,* gallbladder, *D,* duodenum. **B,** Cholangiogram confirmed the diagnosis.

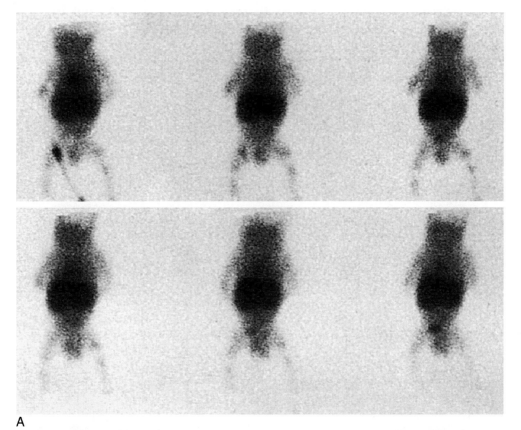

A

Figure 7-19   Biliary atresia. Four-week-old child. Serum phenobarbital level was in therapeutic range. **A,** Images every 10 minutes for 1 hour after injection of Tc-99m mebrofenin shows no biliary-to-bowel transit.

Continued

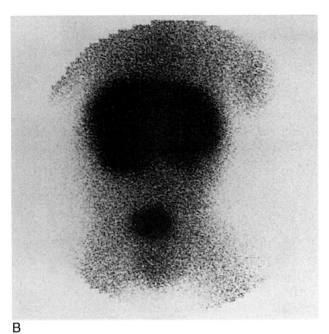

B

Figure 7-19, cont'd   **B,** Images at 4 (not shown) and 24 hours show no bowel activity, only renal clearance into the bladder. Surgery confirmed biliary atresia.

syndrome. The scintigraphic findings described for partial common duct obstruction apply, that is, delayed biliary-to-bowel-transit and delayed clearance of biliary ducts (Fig. 7-21). Because the gallbladder is not present to act as a pressure release reservoir for bile, ductal dynamics directly predict the adequacy of biliary drainage. Diagnostic scintigraphic findings are those of

persistent activity within the common duct and delayed biliary-to-bowel transit.

Sphincter of Oddi Dysfunction

Sphincter of Oddi dysfunction (SOD) is a partial biliary obstruction at the level of the sphincter of Oddi, not caused by stones or stricture. It occurs in up to 14% of postcholecystectomy patients and presents as intermittent abdominal pain and transient liver function abnormalities. Therapy is often sphincterotomy for a fixed *(papillary stenosis)*, whereas a functional and reversible obstruction *(biliary dyskinesia)* may respond to drugs (e.g., nifedipine) and sphincter toxins (e.g., Botox).

ERCP has been used to exclude a stone or fibrosis as the cause for the partial biliary obstruction. Delayed drainage of contrast material beyond 45 minutes seen during ERCP is consistent with the diagnosis but nonspecific. MRCP has largely replaced ERCP. Sphincter of Oddi manometry is the gold standard used by gastroenterologists. An elevated sphincter pressure (>40 mm Hg) is considered diagnostic. However, this technique is invasive, not widely available, technically difficult, and prone to interpretative errors. Further-more, medications given during ERCP can affect the results, reproducibility is a concern, and pancreatitis a serious complication. Thus a noninvasive alternative would be preferable.

Cholescintigraphy permits physiological assessment of duct drainage. Because this entity is a partial biliary obstruction. Scintigraphic findings are delayed biliary duct clearance at 60 minutes and no further clearance between 1–2 hours. Early studies suggested that image analysis is diagnostic in the majority of cases.

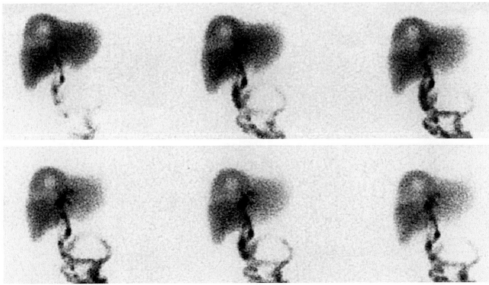

Figure 7-20   Patent biliary stent. Common duct stent was placed to relieve obstruction from a malignant tumor. Tc-99m IDA study confirms patency of the stent. Note the hepatic mass in the liver dome.

Box 7-15   Causes of Postcholecystectomy Pain Syndrome

Retained or recurrent choledocholithiasis
Inflammatory stricture
Sphincter of Oddi dysfunction
Nonhepatobiliary origin
Cystic duct remnant (obstrmucted or inflamed)

Various quantitative methods have been used to further improve on image analysis (e.g., bile duct $t_{1/2}$, percent emptying at specific time intervals). Results have been mixed. Sincalide has been advocated as a pharmacologic intervention to improve diagnostic accuracy by increasing bile flow (*see* Box 7-3) and stressing the capacity of the biliary ducts, thus revealing more subtle abnormalities that might not otherwise be seen. The reported accuracy of the various methodologies has varied with no general consensus on the best method. One technique that incorporates image analysis and semiquantitative parameters using sincalide infusion is described (Box 7-16, Fig. 7-22).

It is stated that a characteristic finding of SOD is a paradoxical response of the sphincter of Oddi to CCK (e.g., contraction rather than relaxation) and that this finding might be used diagnostically to confirm the disease. However, this paradoxical response was initially described in animal studies administering CCK as a bolus. It was occasionally reported at manometry in clinical studies but again the drug was given as a rapid infusion. It has never been shown that when given at physiological dose rates a paradoxical response of the sphincter of Oddi actually occurs.

Biliary Leaks

In most cases, bile leaks occur after cholecystectomy or other biliary tract surgery. Sometimes obstruction can be the cause. The laparoscopic method has become the procedure of choice for elective cholecystectomy, however, it is associated with a somewhat higher rate of bile duct injury than open cholecystectomy.

Although ultrasonography and CT can detect fluid collections, the type and origin of the collection is often uncertain. Cholescintigraphy can determine whether the fluid collection is of biliary origin rather than due to ascites, hypoproteinemia, or other causes. With cholescintigraphy, the approximate location and rate of biliary leakage can be estimated. This information is important prognostically. Slow bile leaks usually resolve spontaneously with conservative therapy; however, more rapid leaks require surgical correction.

Before percutaneous drainage of a biloma, cholescintigraphy can help ensure that central biliary obstruction is not present. With obstruction, it is unlikely that bile leakage can be effectively treated by percutaneous drainage without addressing the underlying cause of obstruction. Follow-up cholescintigraphy can be used to confirm resolution or persistence of the leakage.

Scintigraphically, bile leakage often manifests initially as a progressively increasing collection of radiotracer in the region of the gallbladder fossa or hepatic hilum. The activity may progressively spread into the subdiaphragmatic space, over the dome of the liver, into the colonic

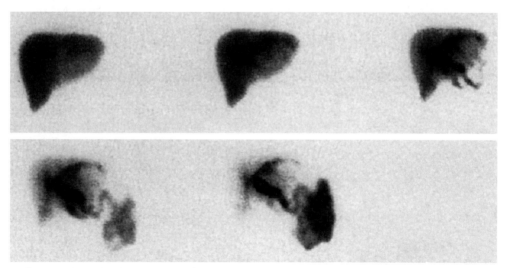

Figure 7-21   Biliary stricture causing partial obstruction. Images acquired at 5, 10, 20, 40, and 60 minutes. Common hepatic and bile ducts are dilated above an abrupt distal cutoff; however, there is normal biliary-to-bowel transit. The patient had a prior cholecystectomy.

Box 7-16   Sphincter of Oddi Dysfunction Protocol—Sincalide and Semiquantitative Score

PREPARATION

Fasting for 2 hr prior to study

COMPUTER SETUP

1-min frames × 60

IMAGING PROTOCOL

1. Infuse sincalide 0.02 μg/kg × 10 min (altered from original protocol that was 3-min infusion)
2. 15 min after sincalide infusion, inject 5 mCi Tc-99m mebrofenin or disofenin intravenously.

COMPUTER PROCESSING ANALYSIS

1. Draw regions of interest around liver and common duct and derive time-activity curves.
2. Use image analysis in conjunction with time-activity curves.
3. Time-activity curves will help determine time to hepatic peak and % CBD emptying.

SCINTIGRAPHIC SCORING

	Score
1. Peak liver uptake	
a. Less than 10 min	0
b. 10 min or greater	1
2. Time of biliary visualization	
a. Less than 15 min	0
b. Greater than 15 min	1
3. Prominence of biliary tract	
a. Not prominent	0
b. Prominence of major extrahepatic ducts	1
c. Prominence of major intrahepatic ducts	2
4. Bowel visualization	
a. Less than 15 min	0
b. 15–30 min	1
c. Greater than 30 min	2
5. CBD emptying	
a. More than 50%	0
b. Less than 50%	1
c. No change	2
d. Increasing activity	3
6. CBD-to-liver intensity ratio	
a. CBD $_{60\,min}$ $\leq$ liver $_{60\,min}$	0
b. CBD $_{60\,min}$ > liver $_{60\,min}$ but less than liver $_{15\,min}$	1
c. CBD $_{60\,min}$ higher than liver $_{60\,min}$ and equal to liver $_{15\,min}$	2
d. CBD $_{60\,min}$ higher than both liver $_{60\,min}$ and liver $_{15\,min}$	3

TOTAL SCORE

Score of >5 is consistent with sphincter of Oddi dysfunction (Sostre et al. 1992). CBD, common bile duct.

gutters, or manifest as free bile in the abdomen (Figs. 7-23 and 7-24). Positioning the patient on their right side allows the radiotracer to pool in the gutter. Delayed imaging may be required to detect a small or slow leak. Patient repositioning can help confirm its presence (e.g., lateral decubitus views). Peritoneal tubing, drains, and collection bags may exhibit accumulation and should be imaged as well.

Biliary Diversion Surgery

Biliary enteric bypass procedures are created in patients for a wide range of benign and malignant diseases associated with biliary obstruction. Complications are not uncommon.

Ultrasonography has imaging limitations in the presence of gas in the anastomotic bowel segment or refluxed biliary air following surgery. Two thirds of attempts are reported as indeterminate. Biliary dilation may be present in over 20% of patients even though obstruction has been adequately relieved by surgery. It may not be possible to reach the biliary tract using ERCP if a long Roux-en-Y loop has been created as part of the anastomosis. MRCP has high accuracy in visualizing the postoperative stricture and detecting obstruction when new dilation is present. However, cholescintigraphy is the only noninvasive method that can distinguish obstructed dilated ducts from those that are chronically dilated but not obstructed.

Scintigraphy is well-suited to diagnose bile leakage, functional patency of the anastomosis, or recurrent obstruction. It is important to be aware of the postoperative anatomy of the patient being imaged. Although biliary scintigraphy is useful in a variety of anastomoses (choledochoduodenostomy, cholecystoduodenostomy, and cholecystojejunostomy), it is particularly valuable in patients with choledochojejunostomy or intrahepatic cholangiojejunostomy. Choledochojejunostomy is a direct anastomosis of the extrahepatic portion of the common bile or common hepatic duct to a Roux-en-Y jejunal loop. The intrahepatic cholangiojejunostomy requires direct anastomosis between small bowel and intrahepatic ducts.

With scintigraphy, intestinal excretion by 1 hour with or without ductal dilatation is consistent with functionally patent. Intestinal excretion greater than 1 hour is suggestive of partial obstruction. However, retention of activity in bile ducts is a more reliable indicator. Persistent or worsening biliary duct retention between 1 and 2 hours is fairly specific for obstruction. Stasis with minimal intestinal excretion and pooling in the region of the biliary enteric anastomosis may be seen at 1 hour. This may be positional and can be confirmed and resolved by imaging the patient upright. Persistent nonvisualization of the biliary system and intestine suggests complete biliary duct obstruction.

Other Gastrointestinal Surgical Anastomoses

Cholescintigraphy can provide functional information about other surgical procedures involving the gastrointestinal tract (e.g., Billroth I and II, Whipple resection). In

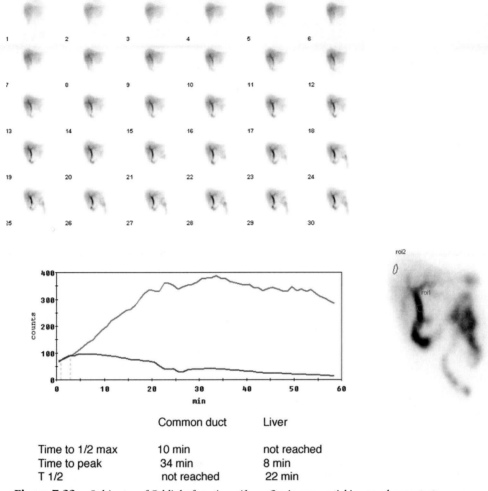

Figure 7-22   Sphincter of Oddi dysfunction. *Above,* 2-min sequential images demonstrate delayed clearance from the common duct. *Right,* Regions-of-interest are draw for the common duct and liver. *Below,* Time-activity curves of the common duct and liver. This patient had a scintigraphic score of 7, positive for sphincter of Oddi dysfunction. See Box 7-16 for scoring method.

Billroth II anastomoses, Tc-99m IDA can evaluate afferent loop patency. The afferent loop should fill readily in an antegrade direction from the common duct. There is normally progressive accumulation of activity within the loop which becomes abnormal when the filling persists for more than 2 hours.

Liver Transplants

The major role for cholescintigraphy is to aid in the detection of the postoperative complications of bile leaks and obstruction. The findings of rejection on cholescintigraphy are nonspecific signs of liver dysfunction. Liver biopsy is necessary to make the diagnosis.

Trauma

Posttraumatic problems that must be clinically differentiated include hepatic laceration, hematoma, bile duct transection, extrahepatic biliary leakage, intrahepatic biloma formation, and perforation of the gallbladder. CT and ultrasonography can diagnose liver parenchymal injury. Only biliary scintigraphy can demonstrate communication between the biliary tree and space-occupying lesions that represent biloma formation.

Bile leakage is common after penetrating and blunt trauma. It may initially be occult and detected only after clinical deterioration or discharge of bilious material from surgical bed drains. Cholescintigraphy can be used to differentiate between rapid and slow bile leakage, which can help the surgeon decide whether intervention or watchful waiting is indicated and assess resolution of leakage in patients treated conservatively.

Primary Benign and Malignant Tumors

Liver tumors that contain hepatocytes would be expected to take up Tc-99m IDA, thus cholescintigraphy can be helpful in the differential diagnosis of primary benign and malignant hepatic tumors (e.g., focal nodular hyperplasia, hepatic adenoma, and hepatocellular carcinoma) (Table 7-9).

Focal Nodular Hyperplasia and Hepatic Adenoma

The natural history and therapy of these two benign

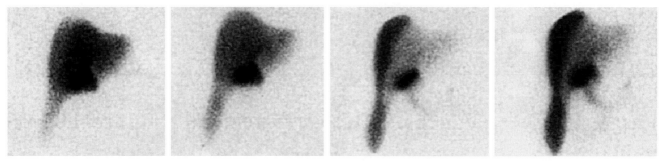

Figure 7-23 Post-cholecystectomy biliary leak. CT scan 4 days after surgery showed intraabdominal fluid. HIDA study, ordered to determine if the fluid collection was of biliary origin, confirms a biliary leak. Sequential images are from 60 minutes *(left)* to 6 hours *(right)* after injection. Bile extravasates into the portal region, over the liver dome, and into the colic gutter.

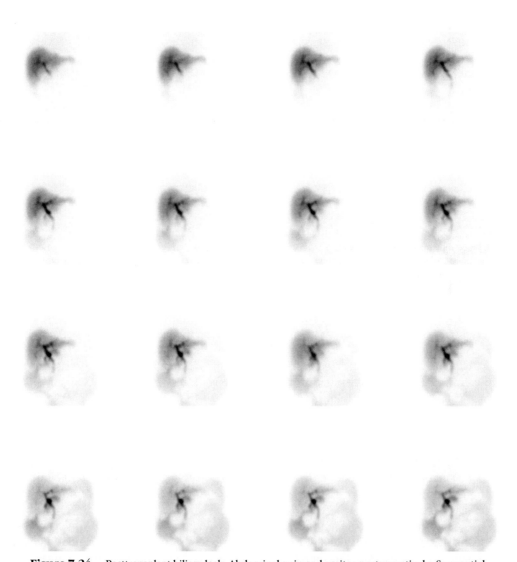

Figure 7-24 Posttransplant biliary leak. Abdominal pain and ascites postoperatively. Sequential images show prompt intraperitoneal leak emanating from the region of the extrahepatic biliary ducts. At surgery, an occluded biliary stent was found with active bile leakage.

Table 7-9   Differential Diagnosis of Primary Hepatic Tumors with Technetium-99m HIDA

Lesion	Flow	Uptake	Clearance
Focal nodular hyperplasia	Increased	Immediate	Delayed
Hepatic adenoma	Normal	None	—
Hepatocellular carcinoma	Increased	Delayed	Delayed

tumors are quite different. Focal nodular hyperplasia is usually asymptomatic, often discovered incidentally, and requires no specific therapy, whereas hepatic adenomas are often symptomatic and may cause serious hemorrhage that can be life-threatening. Adenomas have a strong association with oral contraceptives; focal nodular hyperplasia does not.

Focal nodular hyperplasia contains all hepatic cell types (i.e., hepatocytes, Kupffer cells, and bile canaliculi). Characteristic findings seen with cholescintigraphy are increased blood flow, prompt hepatic uptake, but delayed clearance (Fig. 7-25). This characteristic pattern is seen in more than 90% of patients with focal nodular hyperplasia. Poor clearance presumably is caused by abnormal biliary canaliculi. The overall accuracy is higher than the traditional Tc-99m sulfur colloid method used to diagnose focal nodular hyperplasia, which shows uptake in about two-thirds of patients (see section on *Focal Nodular Hyperplasia Under Tc-99m Sulfur Colloid*). Hepatic adenomas consist exclusively of hepatocytes; therefore it is surprising and not understood why it rarely exhibits uptake on cholescintigraphy.

Hepatocellular Carcinoma Tc-99m IDA cholescintigraphy also demonstrates characteristic findings for hepatocellular carcinoma (hepatoma). The malignant hepatocytes are hypofunctional compared to normal liver. During the first hour of cholescintigraphy, no uptake within the lesion (cold defect) is seen. Delayed imaging at 2–4 hours often shows "filling in," or continuing uptake within the tumor and concomitant clearing of adjacent normal liver (Fig. 7-26). This pattern is very specific for hepatoma. However, poorly differentiated hepatomas may not fill in on delayed imaging. Tc-99m IDA uptake may be seen at sites of distant hepatocellular metastases (e.g., lung).

Enterogastric Bile Reflux

Alkaline gastritis occurs secondary to enterogastric reflux, seen most commonly after gastric resection surgery. Symptoms are similar to those of acid-related

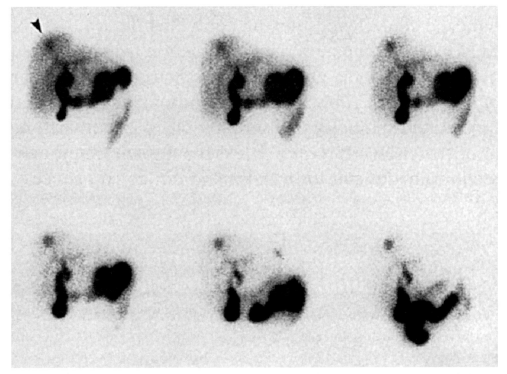

Figure 7-25   Focal nodular hyperplasia. Sequential images every 5 minutes show early uptake by tumor in the dome of the liver *(arrowhead)* that persists throughout the 60-minute study as the normal liver clears the tracer. Focal uptake persisted on delayed images acquired at 3 hours.

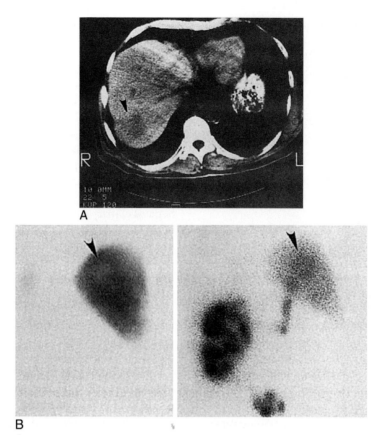

Figure 7-26   Hepatocellular carcinoma. **A,** CT shows a large mass in the posterior aspect of the right lobe *(arrowhead).* **B,** *Left,* Tc-99m HIDA posterior view acquired at 5 minutes shows a cold defect in the same mass as seen on CT *(arrowhead). Right,* Posterior view. Two-hour HIDA images show increased uptake within the lesion *(arrowhead)* and good washout of the remainder of the liver. Surgery confirmed hepatocellular carcinoma.

disease. Cholescintigraphy can demonstrate the bile reflux (Fig. 7-27). Some bile reflux is not uncommonly seen in normal subjects on routine cholescintigraphy, particularly if morphine sulfate or CCK has been administered. However, the greater the quantity and the more persistent the reflux, the more likely that the reflux is related to the patient's symptoms. Quantitative methods for estimating the amount of reflux have been described.

TC-99M RED BLOOD CELL LIVER SCINTIGRAPHY

Cavernous hemangiomas are the most common benign tumor of the liver and the second most common hepatic tumor, exceeded in incidence only by liver metastases.

Liver hemangiomas are usually asymptomatic. They are discovered incidentally on CT or ultrasonography during the clinical workup or staging of a patient with a known primary malignancy or during evaluation of unrelated abdominal symptoms or disease. They require no specific therapy but must be differentiated from other, more serious liver tumors.

Pathology

Cavernous hemangiomas of the liver have abnormally dilated, endothelium-lined vascular channels of varying sizes separated by fibrous septa. Histopathologically, they are not related to capillary hemangiomas, angiodysplasia, or infantile hemangioendotheliomas. Ten percent of these cavernous hemangiomas are multiple. Lesions larger than 4 cm are often called giant cavernous hemangiomas.

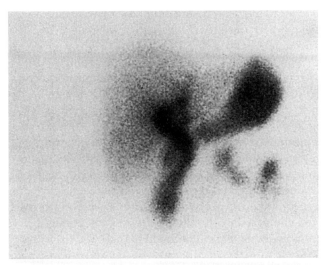

Figure 7-27   Enterogastric reflux. Sixty minutes after injection of Tc-99m IDA, reflux of labeled bile into the stomach is seen. Bile gastritis was confirmed at endoscopy.

Diagnostic Imaging

Noninvasive diagnosis of cavernous hemangioma of the liver is important because it can obviate the need for biopsy, which on occasion can result in hemorrhage-associated morbidity and even mortality.

Ultrasonography

The typical sonographic pattern for hemangioma (i.e., a homogeneous, hyperechoic mass with well-defined margins and posterior acoustical enhancement) is neither sensitive nor specific for the diagnosis of cavernous hemangioma.

Computed Tomography

Strict CT criteria for hemangioma include relative hypoattenuation before intravenous contrast injection, early peripheral enhancement during the rapid bolus dynamic phase, progressive opacification toward the center of the lesion, and complete isodense fill-in, usually by 30 minutes after contrast administration. Frequently, not all criteria are satisfied. When these criteria are used to maximize specificity, the sensitivity of CT is only 55%; less strict criteria result in a high false-positive rate. Accuracy is even poorer with multiple hemangiomas.

Magnetic Resonance Imaging

Cavernous hemangiomas have a characteristic appearance on MRI, with high signal intensity on T2-weighted spin-echo images (light bulb sign). Gadolinium contrast shows findings similar to those seen with CT with contrast. Although MRI is much more accurate than CT, various benign and malignant tumors may give false-positive results. MRI is par-

ticularly helpful in the diagnosis of small lesions and those adjacent to major vessels or vascular organs.

Tc-99m-Labeled Red Blood Cell (Tc-99m RBC) Scintigraphy

With modern multiheaded SPECT cameras, the radionuclide imaging technique has good sensitivity and an exceedingly low false positive rate. Although not as sensitive for detection of small hemangiomas as MRI, it is more specific

Radiopharmaceutical

Labeling the patient's erythrocytes with Tc-99m pertechnetate is done by the same methodology as discussed in Chapter 11 in the section on *Gastrointestinal Bleeding, Radiolabeling with Tc-99m RBCs* (*see* Box 7-9). The in vitro kit method is now the preferred approach because of its high labeling efficiency and ease of preparation.

Mechanism of Localization and Pharmacokinetics

After injection, the Tc-99m-labeled red blood cells (RBCs) are distributed within the blood pool of the liver. The labeled cells require time to exchange and equilibrate within the large, relatively stagnant, nonlabeled blood pool of the hemangioma (Fig. 7-28). This equilibration time varies from 30–120 minutes. Thus, early images will typically show the cavernous hemangioma to be cold but delayed images will demonstrate increased uptake.

Dosimetry

The total body radiation absorbed dose is approximately 0.4 cGy (rads). The target organ is the heart

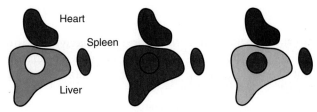

Figure 7-28   Tc-99m erythrocyte pharmacokinetics in liver hemangioma. *Left,* Immediately after injection the hemangioma is "cold." Blood pool activity within the liver is greater than activity within the hemangioma. Time is required for the radiolabeled RBCs to equilibrate with the unlabeled RBCs in the blood pool volume of the hemangioma. *Middle,* As the Tc-99m-labeled RBCs increasingly enter the hemangioma and mix with the unlabeled cells, activity in the hemangioma becomes equal to normal liver. *Right,* When fully equilibrated (60–120 minutes), activity within the hemangioma exceeds that in the surrounding liver and is equal to activity in the heart and spleen.

wall, which receives 1.2 cGy (rads), followed by the spleen and kidney (Table 7-10). The bladder dose depends on the method of labeling and the degree of free Tc-99m pertechnetate.

Methodology

A combined three-phase planar and single-photon emission computed tomography (SPECT) technique is used (Box 7-17). SPECT is mandatory for state-of-the-art Tc-99m RBC hepatic scintigraphy. Planar flow and early blood pool images are not necessary for diagnosis, although they show characteristic findings.

Image Interpretation

Image interpretation should be performed with CT or ultrasonography available for direct anatomical correlation to ensure proper identification of the abnormality in question.

Normal Hepatic Vascular Anatomy

The liver has a complex vascular system (Figs. 7-1 and 7-29). It receives approximately two-thirds of its blood supply from the portal vein and only one third from the hepatic artery. The sinusoids act as the capillary bed for the liver cells. Blood leaves the liver through the hepatic veins, which then empty into the inferior vena cava. The caudate lobe is an exception in that it also has a direct connection with the vena cava. Much of this normal vascular anatomy of the liver is seen with Tc-99m-labeled RBCs (Figs. 7-30 to 7-34).

Normal Distribution

Organs with the highest activity per pixel are the heart and spleen, followed by the kidney. The normal liver has much less blood pool activity. The aorta, inferior vena cava, and occasionally the portal vein can be seen with

Table 7-10	Dosimetry for In Vitro Tc-99m Red Blood Cell Scintigraphy	
Target	**Rads/25 mCi (cGy/925 MBq)**	**Rad/mCi**
Heart wall	1.350	0.054
Bladder wall	1.275	0.051
Spleen	1.025	0.041
Blood	0.875	0.035
Liver	0.650	0.026
Kidneys	0.625	0.025
Ovaries	0.425	0.017
Testes	0.175	0.007
Total body	0.375	0.015

Box 7-17 Tc-99m Red Blood Cell Liver Hemangioma Scintigraphy: Protocol Summary

PATIENT PREPARATION

None

RADIOPHARMACEUTICAL

Tc-99m pertechnetate, 25 mCi, labeled to RBCs (in vitro kit method)

Inject intravenously; bolus injection for flow images

INSTRUMENTATION

Camera: large-field-of-view gamma with SPECT capability

Energy window: 15% centered over 140-keV photopeak

Collimator: low energy, high resolution, parallel hole

IMAGE ACQUISITION

Planar Imaging

1. Blood flow: 1-sec frames for 60 sec on computer and 2-sec film images.
2. Immediate images: acquire 750k–1000k count planar image in same projection and other views as necessary to best visualize lesion(s).
3. Delayed images: acquire 750k–1000k count planar static images 1–2 hr after injection in multiple projections (anterior, posterior, lateral, and oblique views).

Single-Photon Emission Computed Tomography

1. Position patient supine on imaging table. Raise patient's arms above head.
2. Center liver in field of view.
3. Rotate camera head around patient to ensure that camera does not come in contact with patient. Liver should remain completely in field of view during test rotation.

SPECT Camera Setup

Window	15% window centered over 140-keV Tc-99m photopeak
Setup	Step and shoot
Collimator(s)	High or ultrahigh resolution

Computer Setup

Acquisition Parameters	
Patient orientation	Supine
Rotation	Clockwise
Matrix	128 × 128 word mode
Image/arc combination	128 images/360°
Time/frame	10 sec/stop
Reconstruction Parameters	
Filters	Manufacturer specific Personal preference
Attenuation correction	Yes
Reformatting	Transverse, sagittal, coronal

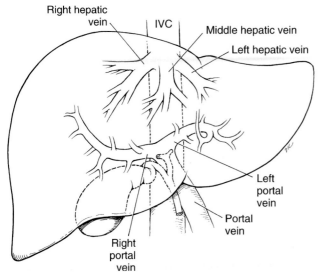

Figure 7-29 Vascular anatomy of the liver. Blood supply to the liver is predominantly from the portal vein (75%) and to a lesser extent from the hepatic artery (25%). Both enter the liver in the portal area. Hepatic artery and its branches are not shown here. Portal vein divides into right and left branches and then subdivides. Smaller branches with hepatic artery branches and canaliculi define the periphery of lobules (*see* Fig. 7-1). Hepatic veins originate at lobule center (central veins), feeding into right, middle, and left hepatic veins, which drain into the inferior vena cava *(IVC)*.

planar imaging. Portal branching vessels and hepatic veins can be seen with SPECT.

Diagnostic Criteria

With planar imaging, the arterial blood flow to a hemangioma is usually normal. Immediate blood pool images typically have decreased uptake within the hemangioma compared with adjacent liver, although early increased uptake is occasionally seen (Figs. 7-31 and 7-32).

On 1- to 2-hour delayed imaging, hemangiomas have increased activity compared with adjacent liver. The uptake is usually equal to that of the blood pool of the heart and spleen. Giant cavernous hemangiomas often show heterogeneity of uptake on delayed images, with areas of decreased as well as increased uptake (*see* Fig. 7-31). These cold regions, often located centrally, are caused by thrombosis, necrosis, and fibrosis. Benign and malignant liver tumors, abscesses, cirrhotic nodules, and cysts have decreased activity compared to normal liver (*see* Fig. 7-30).

Accuracy

Tc-99m RBC scintigraphy has a very high positive predictive value, approaching 100%, so a positive test is likely to be a true positive. After more than three decades of clinical use, very few false-positive studies have been reported,

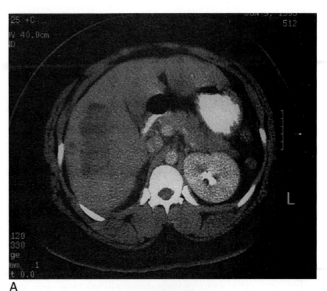

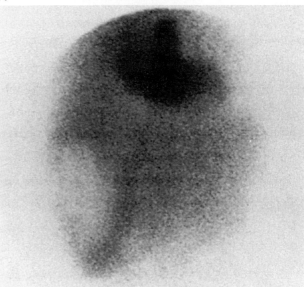

B

Figure 7-30 Negative Tc-99m RBC study for hemangioma. **A,** CT scan shows a large lesion in right lobe of the liver. **B,** Planar Tc-99m RBC scan is cold in the same region and negative for hemangioma. Metastatic colon cancer was diagnosed.

and it is considerably more specific than CT. Although a few large hepatomas have been misinterpreted as hemangiomas, most hepatomas are negative on scintigraphy. A large series of moderately sized hepatomas found no false positives. Angiosarcomas are extremely rare but are a reported cause of false positives. A few other carcinomas have been reported to be positive, usually because they produce local obstruction of sinusoids. Although extensive fibrosis or thrombosis may rarely result in a false-negative study, areas of increased uptake are usually also seen.

The diagnostic sensitivity of Tc-99m RBC imaging depends primarily on lesion size and the camera system

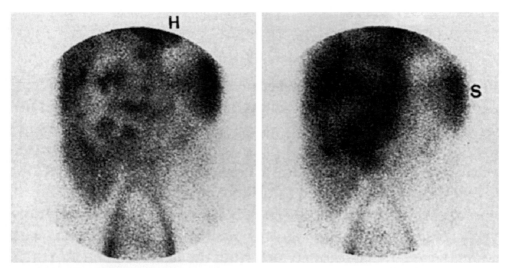

Figure 7-31   Giant cavernous hemangioma. *Left,* Immediate postinjection image shows a large, relatively photopenic area involving most of the left lobe and a large portion of the right lobe. Some focal areas of increased uptake are seen. *Right,* Delayed 1-hour image shows filling of the initial cold area and increased uptake throughout this large hemangioma that is equal to the heart *(H)* and spleen *(S).*

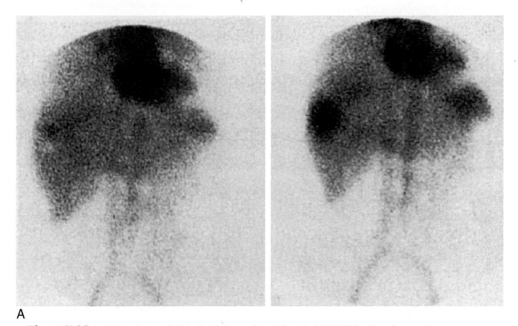

Figure 7-32   Comparison of planar, single-, and multiheaded SPECT for liver hemangioma. **A,** Planar study. *Left,* Immediate postinjection image shows photopenic region in superolateral portion of the right lobe with small area of increased uptake. *Right,* Delayed image at 60 minutes shows complete filling in, diagnostic of hemangioma.

Continued

used. SPECT is superior to planar imaging because of its improved contrast resolution (Figs. 7-32 to 7-35). SPECT is especially useful for the detection of small hemangiomas, those located centrally in the liver, multiple hemangiomas (*see* Figs. 7-32 and 7-35), and those adjacent to the heart, kidney, and spleen (*see* Fig. 7-34). In seven comparison studies performed between 1987 and 1991, the mean overall sensitivity for planar imaging was 55% and for SPECT was 88% (Table 7-11).

Lesion size and location are critical determinants of detectability (Table 7-12). Generally, planar imaging can demonstrate hemangiomas down to about 3 cm in size. Single-headed SPECT has good sensitivity for hemangiomas 2 cm and larger, whereas multiheaded

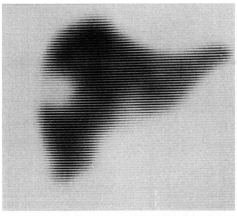

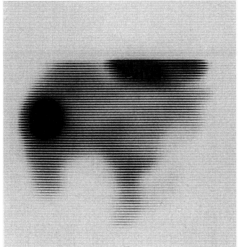

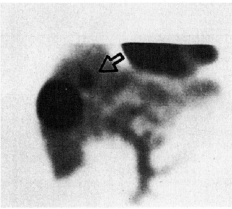

B

Figure 7-32, cont'd   B, SPECT coronal sections. *Top,* Single-headed Tc-99m sulfur colloid SPECT coronal section with well-defined cold defect. *Middle,* Single-headed camera with comparable Tc-99m RBC coronal section shows increased uptake in lesion, consistent with hemangioma. Although contrast resolution is improved with SPECT, there is no diagnostic advantage over planar imaging. *Bottom,* Triple-headed SPECT shows the hemangioma, as well as another small hemangioma immediately adjacent *(arrow)* not seen with single-headed SPECT. The small hemangioma measured 0.9 cm on CT.

SPECT can detect almost all hemangiomas greater than 1.4 cm and may show lesions as small as 0.5 cm, although the sensitivity for detection is reduced (*see* Table 7-9). With multiheaded SPECT, the increased sensitivity is achieved by using ultra-high-resolution collimators (*see* Fig. 7-30).

TC-99M SULFUR COLLOID LIVER-SPLEEN IMAGING

Tc-99m sulfur colloid (SC) was introduced in 1963 and was the standard clinical method for liver-spleen imaging until the advent of CT. Although not a frequently requested study today, there are still occasional clinical indications.

Mechanism of Localization and Pharmacokinetics

After intravenous injection, Tc-99m SC colloid particles 0.1–1.0 μm in size are extracted from the blood by reticuloendothelial cells, the Kupfer cells of the liver (85%), macrophages of the spleen (10%), and bone marrow (5%). Tc-99m SC has a single-pass liver extraction efficiency of 95% and a blood clearance half-life of 2–3 minutes. Uptake is complete by 15 minutes. After phagocytosis, the Tc-99m SC particles are fixed intracellularly.

Other factors besides extraction efficiency influence the distribution of colloid particles (e.g., blood flow, particle size, and disease states). Increased blood flow to a region of the liver increases the local regional delivery and extraction of colloid. Larger colloid particles increase the proportion that will be taken up by the liver. Conversely, smaller particles will increase distribution to bone marrow.

Kupffer cells are distributed throughout the liver (*see* Fig. 7-1) but make up less than 10% of liver cell mass. Most liver diseases affect hepatocytes and Kupffer cells similarly. Disease results in local, diffuse, or heterogeneously decreased uptake because of destruction or displacement of normal liver.

With severe diffuse liver disease, a generalized reduction in hepatic extraction and increased distribution to the spleen and bone marrow (colloid shift) occurs. With splenomegaly or immunologically active states, increased splenic uptake can be seen.

Preparation

Tc-99m SC is available in kit form and requires 15 minutes to prepare. Acid is added to a mixture of Tc-99m pertechnetate and sodium thiosulfate, which is heated in

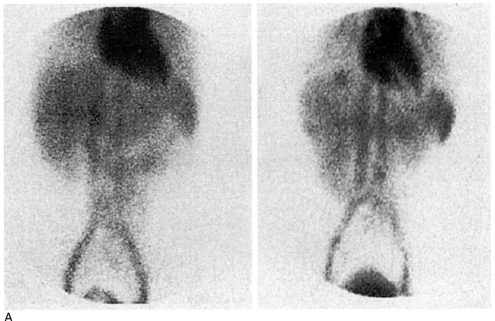

A

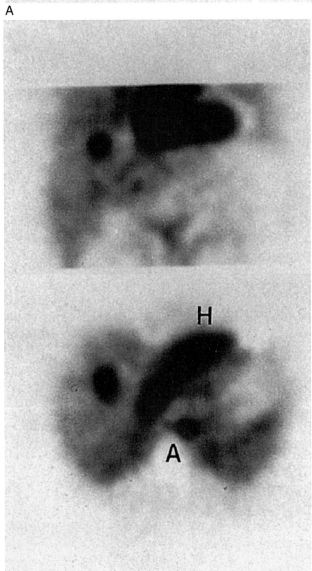

B

Figure 7-33   Improved visualization of small hemangioma with SPECT. **A,** *Left,* Immediate postinjection planar image shows neither decreased nor increased uptake, probably because of small lesion size. *Right,* After 1.5-hour delay, planar study shows mildly increased focal uptake in the liver dome. If lesion had been more central, it may not have been seen due to overlying activity. **B,** SPECT coronal *(top)* and transverse *(bottom)* sections are strongly positive for hemangioma with high target-to-background ratio. Note the heart *(H)* and aorta *(A)*.

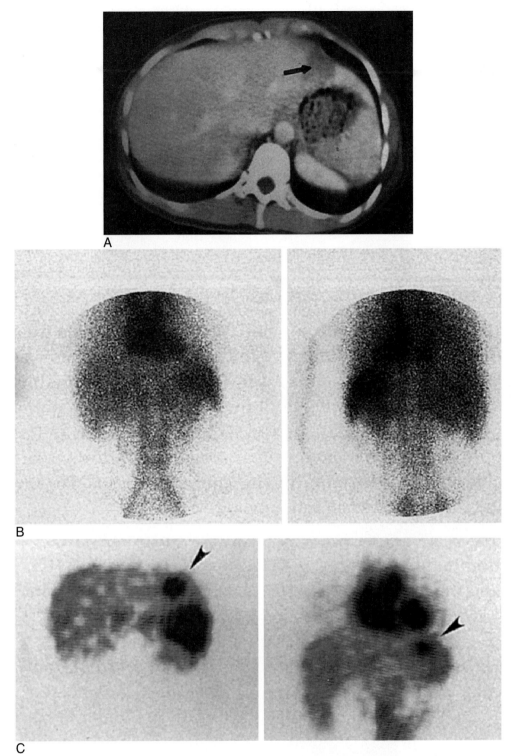

Figure 7-34   Negative planar but positive SPECT hemangioma study. **A,** Liver CT scan shows lesion of uncertain etiology in the left lobe *(arrow).* **B,** Planar anterior *(left)* and posterior *(right)* Tc-99m RBC study is negative, probably because of proximity of lesion to hot spleen. Oblique views were not helpful. **C,** SPECT study performed with an old single-headed camera clearly detects the hemangioma *(arrowheads)* adjacent to the spleen and the heart's left ventricle in coronal *(right)* and transverse *(left)* slices.

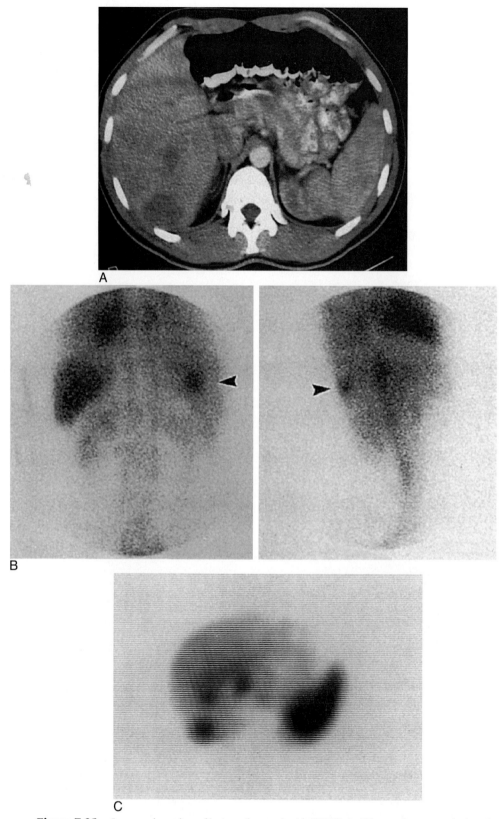

Figure 7-35   Increased number of lesions detected with SPECT. **A**, CT scan shows two lesions in middle and posterior aspect of the right lobe. **B**, Only the larger and more posterior lesion is positive on planar imaging *(arrowheads)*. **C**, Both lesions are seen with SPECT. The inferior vena cava and aorta are medial to the hemangiomas.

a water bath (95–100°F) for 5–10 minutes. Labeling efficiency is greater than 99%.

Dosimetry

Estimated radiation dose from Tc-99m sulfur colloid is 1.7 cGy (rads) to the liver and 1.1 cGy (rads) to the spleen. (Table 7-13).

Clinical Applications

The clinical role today for Tc-99m SC is limited to situations in which it can add functional information not available from the usual anatomical imaging methods or used as a template for correlating imaging findings with another radionuclide study and for splenic imaging.

Methodology

No patient preparation is required. Imaging can start within 20 minutes after radiopharmaceutical injection. SPECT should be routine (Box 7-18). When acquired, planar images are obtained in multiple views.

Table 7-11	Planar Imaging vs. SPECT for Tc-99m RBC Detection of Hemangioma	

| | Sensitivity (%) | |
Study	Planar	SPECT
Tumah 1987	43	100
Malik 1987	77	100
Brodski 1987	44	78
Itenzo 1988	88	100
Brunetti 1988	69	100
Kudo 1989*	42	74
Ziessman 1991*	30	71
Overall	55	88

*Lower sensitivity in later years is caused by the larger number of small lesions.

Table 7-12	Sensitivity for Hemangioma Detection by Lesion Size with Multiheaded SPECT

Lesion (cm)	Sensitivity (%)
>1.4	100
>1.3	91
1.0–2.0	65
0.9–1.3	33
0.5–0.9	20

Table 7-13	Technetium-99m Sulfur Colloid: Radiation Dosimetry

| | Rads/5 mCi (cGy/185 MBq) | |
Organ	Normal	Diffuse parenchymal disease
Liver	1.7	0.8
Spleen	1.1	2.1
Bone marrow	0.14	0.4
Testes	0.006	0.016
Ovaries	0.028	0.06
Total body	0.095	0.09

Box 7-18	Tc-99m SC Liver-Spleen Scintigraphy: Protocol Summary

PATIENT PREPARATION

Study should not be performed immediately after a barium contrast study since attenuation artifacts may result.

CONTRAINDICATION

None

RADIOPHARMACEUTICAL

Planar imaging: 4 mCi (148 MBq)
SPECT: 6 mCi (296 MBq)
Pediatric patients: 30–50 μg/kg (minimal dose, 300 μCi)

INSTRUMENTATION

Camera: large-field-of-view gamma
Window: 15% over 140-keV photopeak
Collimator: parallel hole, low energy, high resolution

IMAGING PROTOCOL

1. Inject technetium-99m sulfur colloid intravenously.
2. Commence imaging 20 min after injection.

Planar Imaging

500k–1000k count images in multiple projections (ant., upright and supine, supine with costal marker, post., right and left lateral, ant. and post. oblique).
Upright imaging is preferable when possible to minimize respiratory excursion, a cause of image degradation.

SPECT

Acquisition protocol similar to that for technetium-99m RBC liver scintigraphy (*see* Box 7-17)

Image Interpretation

Interpretation of Tc-99m SC liver-spleen scans requires an appreciation of the normal variability of liver anatomy, the effect of extrinsic liver compression by normal and abnormal structures, and common artifacts (Figs. 7-36 to 7-39). Planar imaging with multiple views has been used successfully for many years. However, SPECT improves lesion detection because of its improved contrast resolution (Figs. 7-40 and 7-41).

Abnormal scintigraphic findings include hepatomegaly, heterogeneity of distribution, splenomegaly, colloid shift, and focal defects. Hepatomegaly is a non-specific finding that suggests hepatic dysfunction or an infiltrating process (Box 7-19). Hepatomegaly and heterogeneity of uptake may be the only findings in early lung and breast cancer because these liver metastases are small and diffusely infiltrating (Fig. 7-42). Colon cancer metastases to the liver are usually larger and focal at clinical presentation.

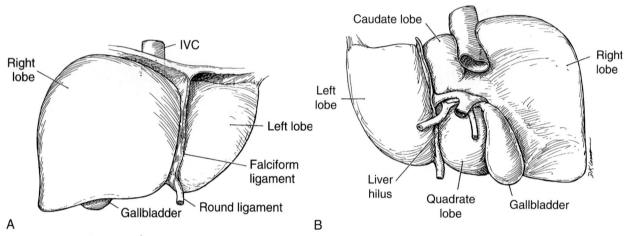

Figure 7-36   Normal anatomy of liver. **A,** Anterior view. *IVC,* Inferior vena cava. **B,** Posterior view.

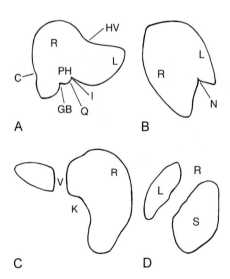

Figure 7-37   Normal anatomical landmarks and interpretative pitfalls for Tc-99m SC liver scintigraphy. **A,** Anterior. **B,** Right lateral. **C,** Posterior. **D,** Left lateral. *C,* Costal rib indentation; *GB,* gallbladder fossa; *HV,* notch from hepatic veins; *I,* incisura umbilicus (ligamentum teres); *K,* kidney impression; *L,* left lobe; *N,* notch between right and left lobes; *PH,* porta hepatis; *Q,* quadrate lobe; *R,* right lobe; *V,* vertebral spine attenuation; *S,* spleen.

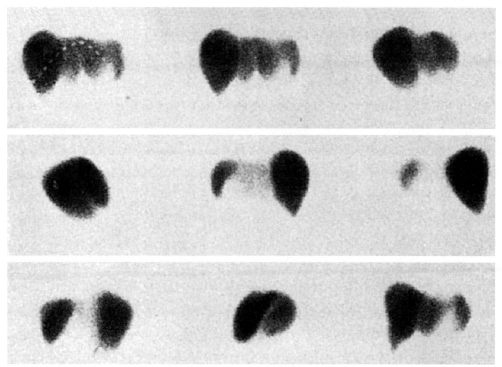

Figure 7-38   Normal Tc-99m sulfur colloid liver-spleen scan. Two anterior views, with cold line marker along costal margin in supine position *(top left)* and without marker in upright position *(top middle)*. In sequence, remaining images are right anterior oblique, right lateral, posterior, right posterior oblique (shallow), left posterior oblique, left lateral, and left anterior oblique.

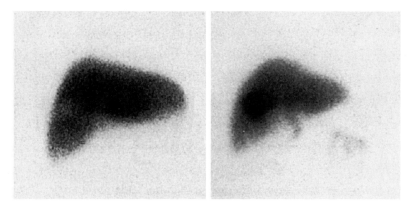

Figure 7-39   Liver photopenic defect caused by intrahepatic gallbladder. *Left,* Anterior Tc-99m sulfur colloid (SC) liver image with photopenic defect in lateral aspect of mid-right lobe. *Right,* Tc-99m IDA study performed immediately after sulfur colloid study showed gallbladder filling of the Tc-99m SC defect.

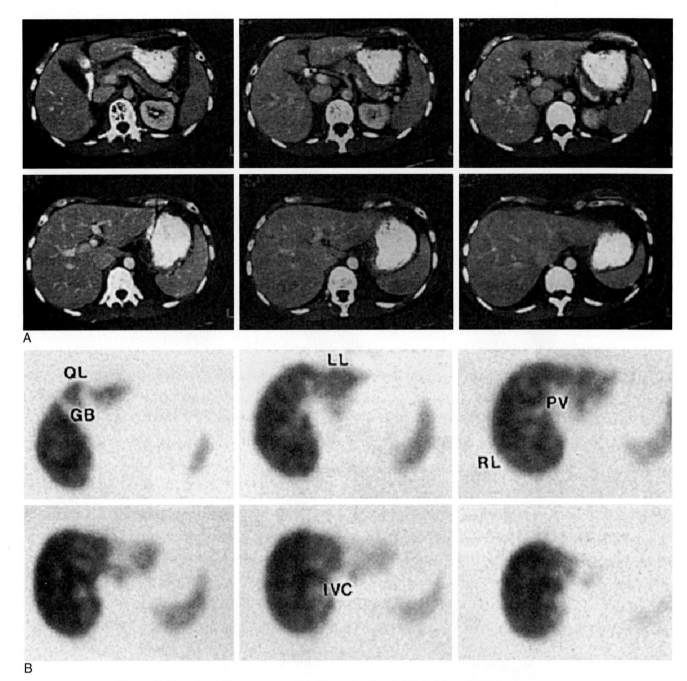

Figure 7-40   Normal liver anatomy: SPECT correlated with CT. **A,** Selected CT transverse sections. **B,** Corresponding SPECT slices. *GB,* Gallbladder fossa; *QL,* quadrate lobe; *PV,* portal vein bifurcation; *IVC,* inferior vena cava; *RL,* right lobe; *LL,* left lobe.

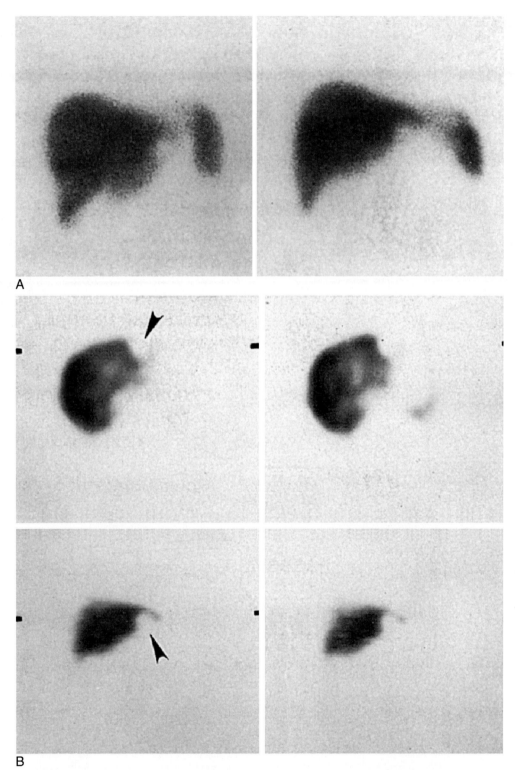

Figure 7-41   Improved lesion detectability with SPECT. Patient with malignant melanoma referred for Tc-99m SC study to rule out hepatic metastases. **A,** Anterior planar images in upright *(left)* and supine *(right)* views. Questionable defect at medial inferior aspect of the left lobe was thought to be a normal variation. **B,** Selected SPECT short-axis *(top two)* and coronal *(bottom two)* sections demonstrate well-defined lesion in anterior aspect of the left lobe *(arrowheads)*.

Box 7-19 Causes of Hepatomegaly

Infiltrative: fatty metamorphosis, alcoholic liver disease,
  amyloidosis, Gaucher's disease, Wilson's disease,
  granulomatous involvement
Congestive: heart failure, hepatic vein thrombosis
Neoplastic: primary and secondary tumors
Infectious: hepatitis, sepsis, malaria
Inflammatory: drugs (e.g., methyldopa, isoniazid)
Miscellaneous: cystic disease

Various methods have been used to estimate liver and spleen size. Estimates can be made using cobalt hot markers or lead cold markers at 1- to 2-cm increments. Generally, the normal liver's longest vertical and midclavicular line dimensions are 17 and 15 cm, respectively. Spleen size greater than 14 cm in its longest axis or greater than 110 cm^2 using two perpendicular dimensions is enlarged.

With proper intensity settings, bone marrow uptake is usually not perceptible. Splenic uptake on the posterior view is normally equal to or less than that of the liver. Colloid shift (increased splenic uptake) is seen with a variety of hepatic diseases (Figs. 7-43 and 7-44). Quantitative spleen-to-liver count ratios greater than 1.5 are abnormal.

Lung radiocolloid uptake is relatively uncommon. Causes include improper labeling with excessive aluminum causing large-particle clumping and various pathophysiological processes (e.g., severe liver dysfunction) (see Fig. 7-44). The lung uptake is probably the result of activation of normal lung macrophages and stimulation of RES cell migration from other parts of the body to the lung.

Liver

Decreased Uptake

Most benign and malignant lesions of the liver produce "cold" or "photopenic" defects on Tc-99m SC liver imaging (Box 7-20; see Figs. 7-41 and 7-42). Radiation therapy produces characteristic rectangular port-shaped hepatic defect. Diffusely decreased uptake is usually caused by hepatocellular disease, although early infiltrating tumor involvement appears similar.

Ancillary radionuclide tests have been used in conjunction with Tc-99m SC to add specificity to the scintigraphic diagnosis (e.g., In-111 leukocytes for infection and Tc-99m RBCs for hemangioma). Xenon-133,

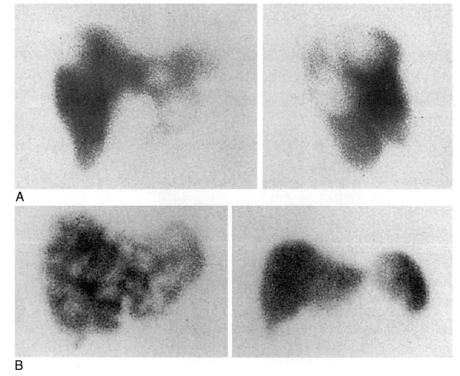

Figure 7-42   Colon cancer metastases on Tc-99m sulfur colloid (SC) study. **A,** Anterior and right lateral views show large metastases in the right and left lobes. **B,** Good response to chemotherapy. Extensive liver metastases on initial Tc-99m SC study *(left)* and definite response to therapy seen on follow-up 4 months later *(right)*.

a fat-soluble agent, exhibits increased uptake in focal fatty tumors and in generalized fatty metamorphosis of the liver.

Increased Uptake

Increased hepatic uptake on Tc-99m SC imaging is uncommon but quite characteristic for specific diagnoses (Box 7-21).

Superior Vena Cava Obstruction Collateral thoracic and abdominal wall vessels communicate with the recanalized umbilical vein delivering Tc-99m SC via the left portal vein to a small volume of tissue, usually in the region of the quadrate lobe, producing a "hot spot" (Fig. 7-45). This collateral blood flow has a relatively increased concentration of colloid compared with blood delivered to the bulk of the liver after systemic mixing. Injection in the lower extremity rather than the upper extremity results in a normal scan.

Focal Nodular Hyperplasia Focal nodular hyperplasia may have increased uptake because of both the

vascular nature of this benign tumor and the increased density of functioning Kupffer cells (Fig. 7-46). Focal nodular hyperplasia can often be confirmed with Tc-99m SC. Because this tumor has hepatocytes, bile ducts, and Kupffer cells, normal or increased colloid uptake is seen in two thirds of patients. One third appears cold for uncertain reasons. Hepatic adenoma (hepatocytes only) is always cold.

Budd-Chiari Syndrome Budd-Chiari syndrome (hepatic vein thrombosis) often has relatively more uptake in the caudate lobe than the remainder of the liver (Fig. 7-47). The impaired venous drainage of the majority of the liver results in poor hepatic function. The caudate lobe retains good function as a result of its direct venous drainage into the inferior vena cava.

Alcoholic Liver Disease

Many diseases affect the liver diffusely (Boxes 7-19 and 7-22). Alcoholic liver disease is the most common cause seen in fatty infiltration, acute alcoholic hepatitis, and

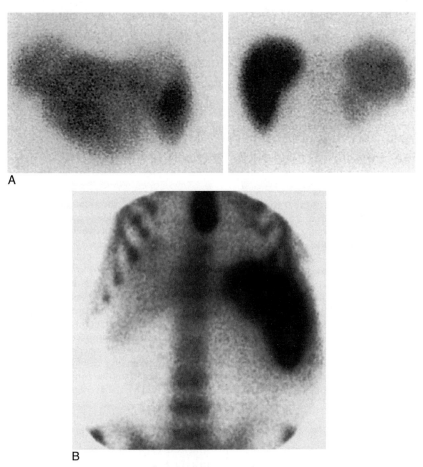

Figure 7-43 Hepatic parenchymal disease on Tc-99m SC study. **A,** Hyperpigmentation and biopsy-proven hemochromatosis in 52-year-old man. Anterior *(left)* and posterior *(right)* views show small right lobe, hypertrophied left lobe, large spleen, and colloid shift. **B,** Severe cirrhosis. Anterior view shows very small liver with poor uptake, enlarged spleen, and prominent colloid shift to the marrow and spleen.

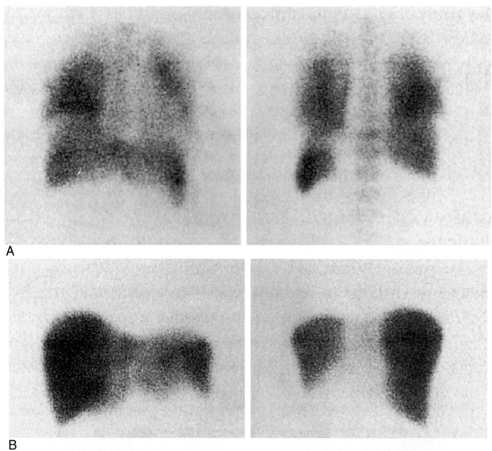

Figure 7-44 Tc-99m SC lung uptake due to fatty metamorphosis of the liver of pregnancy. **A,** During the patient's acute illness the liver-spleen scan showed increased lung uptake, colloid shift to the marrow and spleen, and inhomogeneous liver uptake. **B,** Follow-up study after patient clinically recovered. Tc-99m SC liver-spleen scan returned to normal.

Box 7-20   Causes of Focal Liver Defects
Cyst
Benign and malignant tumors
Dilated bile ducts
Abscess
Hematoma
Laceration
Localized hepatitis
Radiation therapy
Infarction
Cirrhosis (pseudotumors)
Fatty infiltration

Box 7-21   Causes of Increased Focal Uptake on Tc-99m SC Imaging
Superior vena cava syndrome (arm injection)
Inferior vena cava obstruction (leg injection)
Focal nodular hyperplasia
Budd-Chiari syndrome*
Cirrhosis (regenerating nodule)*

*Increased uptake relative to adjacent tissue, not absolute increased uptake.

cirrhosis. All may manifest as hepatomegaly; heterogenous uptake and colloid shift (*see* Fig. 7-43). The resulting scan pattern is related to the degree of pathology and the presence or absence of portal hypertension. With increasing severity, the liver, particularly the right lobe, shrinks; the left lobe compensates with hypertrophy and colloid redistribution becomes more marked (*see* Fig. 7-43). Splenomegaly with increased uptake occurs with portal hypertension.

Accuracy
Cold liver lesions can be detected on planar imaging if they are larger than 2–3 cm and on SPECT if larger than

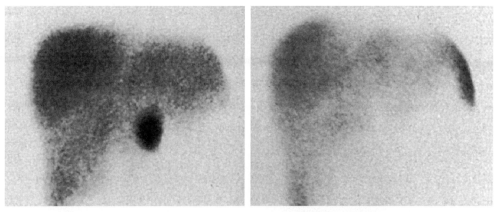

Figure 7-45   Superior vena cava syndrome. *Left,* Hot spot in region of quadrate lobe on Tc-99m sulfur colloid liver spleen scan in patient with lung cancer and superior vena cava obstruction. Radiotracer was injected in the arm. *Right,* Repeat study in same patient with radiotracer injected in lower extremity. No hot spot is seen.

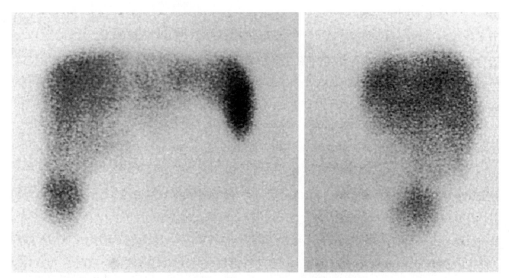

Figure 7-46   Focal nodular hyperplasia. Anterior *(left)* and right lateral *(right)* views show increased uptake in lesion at inferior tip of right lobe of liver. Angiography confirmed the diagnosis of focal nodular hyperplasia.

1.5-2 cm. Superficial lesions are more easily detected than deep ones.

SPECT aids in detecting smaller and more central lesions because of its improved contrast resolution. Multiheaded SPECT cameras using ultra-high-resolution collimators can provide resolution in the range of 1-1.2 cm.

Based on combined data from multiple studies, the sensitivity for detecting metastatic liver disease with planar Tc-99m SC imaging is 81% and the specificity is 90%. SPECT improves sensitivity by 10% but retains specificity.

SPLEEN SCINTIGRAPHY

The spleen serves as a reservoir for formed blood elements, as a site for clearance of microorganisms and particle trapping, as a potential site of hematopoiesis during bone marrow failure, and as a source of humor or cellular

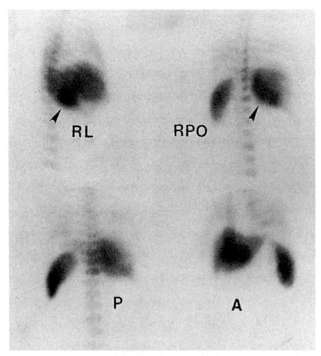

Figure 7-47 Budd-Chiari syndrome. Relatively increased uptake of Tc-99m sulfur colloid in region of caudate lobe *(arrowheads)* in patient with hepatic vein thrombosis. Images were acquired in the right lateral *(RL),* right posterior oblique *(RPO),* posterior *(P),* and anterior *(A)* projections. Note increased marrow uptake.

Box 7-22	**Causes of Liver Heterogeneity of Tc-99m SC Uptake**

Metastases (infiltrative, early)
Lymphoma, leukemia
Hepatitis
Fatty metamorphosis
Chronic passive congestion
Parenchymal liver diseases
Cirrhosis

response to foreign antigens. It plays a role in leukocyte production, contributes to platelet processing, and has immunological functions. Thus the spleen can be visualized by various radiopharmaceuticals with different mechanisms of uptake, such as Tc-99m SC (RES function),

In-111 leukocytes (leukocyte migration), Tc-99m erythrocytes (erythrocyte distribution), and damaged RBC imaging (sequestration).

Radionuclide splenic imaging is used to detect splenic infarcts (Fig. 7-48), postoperative splenic remnants, accessory spleens, splenosis, and polysplenia-asplenia syndromes (Fig. 7-49, *A*). Although Tc-99m SC scintigraphy can often make these diagnoses, liver uptake may obscure adjacent splenic uptake. In addition, the tip of the left lobe often migrates into the splenic bed after splenectomy. Direct CT correlation with the questionable mass/splenic remnant can aid in diagnosis. Imaging with heat or chemically damaged Tc-99m erythrocytes

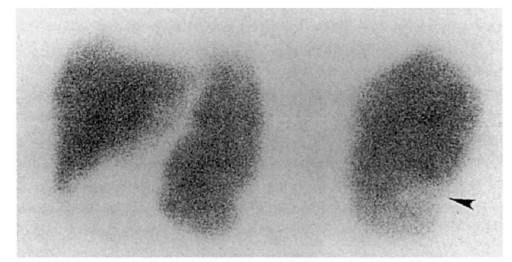

Figure 7-48 Splenic infarct. *Right,* Large, wedge-shaped defect *(arrowhead)* of the spleen in patient with massive splenomegaly and myeloid metaplasia on Tc-99m sulfur colloid study. *Left,* Smaller defects can also be seen on anterior view.

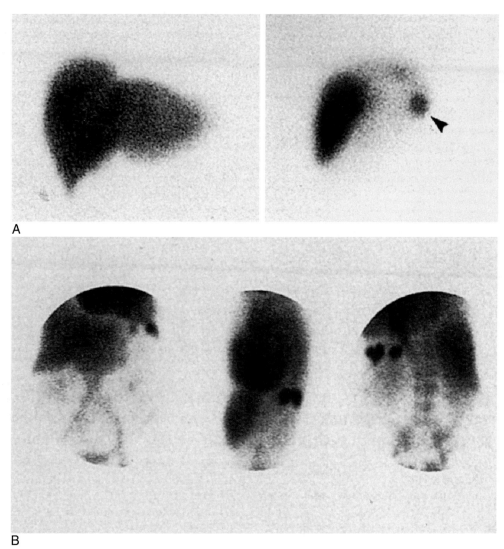

Figure 7-49 Splenic remnant and splenosis. **A,** Tc-99m SC with splenic remnant postsplenectomy best seen in the left lateral view *(arrowhead).* **B,** Splenosis, or autotransplantation of splenic tissue seen after splenic trauma. Damaged Tc-99m-labeled red blood cell study shows splenic tissue in left upper quadrant. *Left to right,* Anterior, left lateral, and posterior views.

can provide excellent splenic images with less liver up-take (Fig. 7-49, *B*).

Nonvisualization of the spleen may result from congenital absence or from acquired *functional asplenia* caused by interruption of the blood supply (splenic artery occlusion) or secondary to RES dysfunction (sickle cell crisis). Functional asplenia may be irreversible (Thorotrast irradiation, chemotherapy, amyloid) or reversible (sickle cell crisis). With sickle cell disease, discordance is seen between RES phagocytic function and other splenic functions.

TC-99M MAA HEPATIC ARTERIAL PERFUSION SCINTIGRAPHY

Oncologists have used regional intra-arterial chemotherapy to treat primary and metastatic cancer since the 1960s. Enthusiasm for this form of chemotherapy has varied over the years, waxing with the introduction of new technology that makes administration of the chemotherapy easier, safer, and potentially more effective and waning after disenchantment with the overall results in light of the technical difficulties and expense.

The advantage of a selective intraarterial approach to chemotherapy is based on the differential blood flow to tumor and normal liver. As tumor in the liver grows, it derives most of its blood supply from the hepatic artery, whereas normal liver cells are supplied predominantly by the portal circulation. Intraarterial chemotherapy delivers the drug preferentially to the tumor, minimizing exposure to normal liver and to drug-sensitive, dose-limiting tissues such as gastrointestinal epithelium and bone marrow, often the source of side effects from conventional intravenous chemotherapy.

Successful application of intraarterial chemotherapy requires that the drug be reliably and safely delivered to the tumor. After initial arteriographic assessment of the vascular supply of the tumor and liver, a therapeutic catheter is inserted either: (1) percutaneously, using a transfemoral or transaxillary approach and attached to an external infusion pump, or (2) surgically, connected to a subcutaneously implanted, constant-infusion pump (Fig. 7-50). Confirmation is needed to ensure that the perfusion distribution from the catheter truly encompasses the entire tumor without perfusion of other visceral organs (Figs. 7-51 to 7-55).

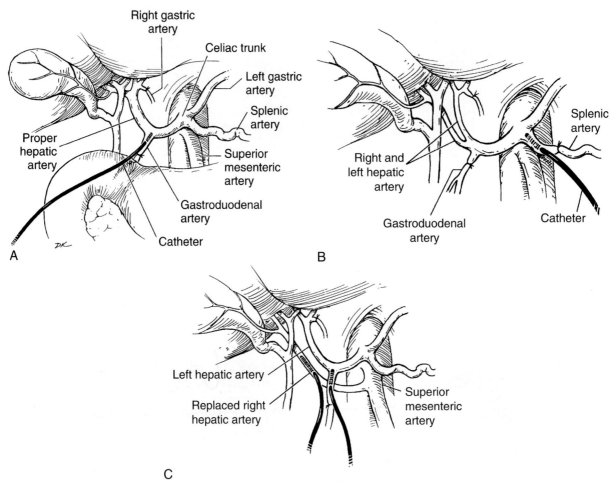

Figure 7-50 Surgical placement of intraarterial catheters. **A,** Standard anatomy. Gastroduodenal artery is ligated and catheter placed at junction of gastroduodenal and common hepatic arteries. Right gastric artery is ligated. **B,** Trifurcation. Right and left hepatic arteries originate too close to gastroduodenal artery to allow equal distribution to all areas of the liver. In this normal variation, gastroduodenal and right gastric arteries are ligated. Splenic artery is ligated and catheter is positioned at junction of splenic artery and celiac axis. **C,** Replaced right hepatic artery originating from superior mesenteric artery requires use of two catheters. Similarly, patient with left hepatic artery arising from left gastric artery requires two catheters.

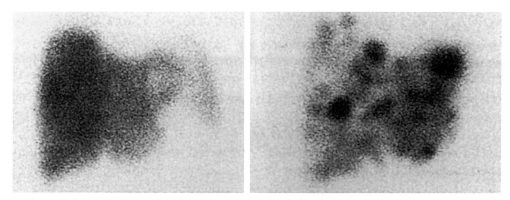

Figure 7-51   Comparison of Tc-99m macroaggregated albumin (MAA) with Tc-99m sulfur colloid. Patient with colon cancer and liver metastases. *Left,* Tc-99m sulfur colloid study shows multiple lesions involving right and left lobes. *Right,* Tc-99m MAA study shows solid tumor nodules involving both lobes of liver in pattern similar to defects seen on Tc-99m SC. Distribution of perfusion is good. No extrahepatic perfusion.

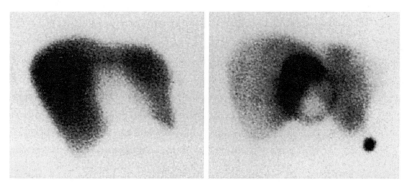

Figure 7-52   Tc-99m MAA hyperperfusion of peripheral rim of tumor. *Left,* Tc-99m sulfur colloid shows large tumor defect in midportion of the liver. *Right,* Tc-99m MAA study shows hyperperfusion of the periphery of the large tumor mass with a large, cold, necrotic center.

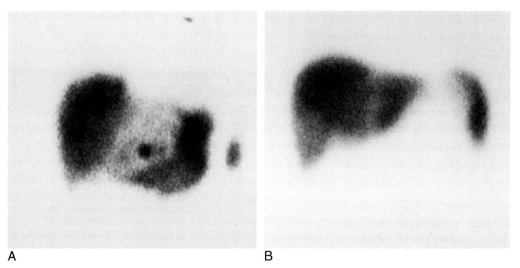

A   B

Figure 7-53   Extrahepatic perfusion. **A,** Poor perfusion to the left lobe and extrahepatic perfusion to the stomach. Focal hot spot is caused by partial catheter thrombosis. **B,** With catheter replaced, entire liver is well-perfused, although some extrahepatic perfusion to spleen is present.

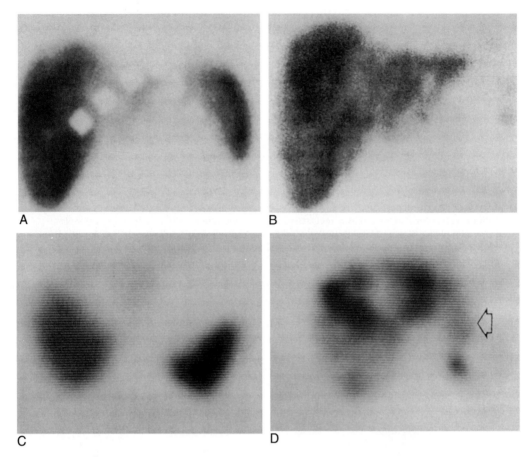

Figure 7-54 Extrahepatic perfusion: utility of SPECT. **A,** Tc-99m sulfur colloid (SC) planar study shows the left lobe replaced by tumor (cold markers overlie left lobe). **B,** Tc-99m macroaggregated albumin (MAA) planar study shows perfusion of the left lobe tumor without definite gastric perfusion. There is a suggestion of splenic perfusion, and activity adjacent to the left lobe could be gastric perfusion. **C,** Tc-99m SC SPECT transverse image shows a large tumor defect in the left lobe. **D,** Tc-99m MAA SPECT study shows hyperperfusion of the periphery of the large tumor nodule, which is cold centrally. Gastric perfusion is seen on the transverse SPECT slice *(arrowhead)*. Splenic perfusion was seen on other sections not shown here.

Although angiography is needed before initial catheter placement, it is not a good indicator of blood flow at the capillary level. The high flow rates required for good contrast angiography often do not reflect the actual perfusion pattern that occurs with the slower infusion rates used in chemotherapy delivery systems. A high-pressure contrast bolus may result in streaming, reflux, or retrograde flow. Contrast angiography cannot be performed through the small-bore, surgically placed catheters, which deliver chemotherapy at a rate of 1–5 ml/day.

Incorrect positioning of the intraarterial catheter results in inadequate perfusion of the tumor-involved liver and can cause extrahepatic perfusion to the stomach, pancreas, spleen, and bowel *(see* Fig. 7-53). This can be caused by difficulties in catheter placement due to normal vascular anatomical variation. Even if the catheter is properly placed initially, catheter movement,

occlusion, or arterial thrombosis may produce a change from the initial perfusion pattern. Tc-99m macroaggregated albumin (MAA) hepatic arterial scintigraphy reliably estimates the adequacy of blood flow to the tumor and determines the presence or absence of extrahepatic perfusion, a frequent cause of gastrointestinal and systemic toxicity.

Hepatic arterial perfusion scintigraphy is also used to quantify lung shunting (prior to using therapeutic Y-90 radiolabeled microspheres [Therasphere and SIR-Sphere]) to ensure minimal radiation to the lungs.

Mechanism of Localization and Pharmacokinetics

Tc-99m MAA particles are larger than capillary size (range, 10–90 μm; mean, 30–50 μm). When infused into

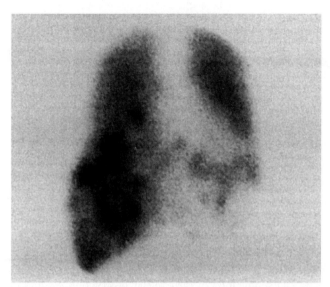

Figure 7-55   Lung uptake of Tc-99m macroaggregated albumin. Quantitation revealed 40% arteriovenous shunting.

the hepatic artery, they distribute according to blood flow and are trapped on first pass in the arteriolar-capillary bed of the liver. The irregularly shaped and malleable particles occlude a small percentage of the liver capillary bed, break down into smaller particles (effective liver half-life of 4 hours), and are eventually taken up by macrophages or cleared through the kidney.

Extrahepatic perfusion is seen on Tc-99m MAA perfusion imaging as uptake in abdominal visceral organs, including the stomach, spleen, and bowel (*see* Figs. 7-53 and 7-54). Although a small amount of arteriovenous shunting is common (1–7%), shunting of 10–40% is possible (*see* Fig. 7-55). Shunting results in less perfusion of the tumor, increased systemic exposure, and increased potential for side effects.

The typical pattern of tumor perfusion on Tc-99m MAA studies is greater uptake in the tumors compared with normal liver (tumor:nontumor uptake ratio of 3:1). Small tumor nodules show uniform uptake (*see* Fig. 7-51), whereas larger tumors often have increased uptake at the periphery of the tumor and relatively decreased uptake centrally because of necrosis (*see* Fig. 7-52). Selective hepatic angiography has demonstrated that most cancers are hypervascular, particularly at the periphery of the tumor, where active growth occurs (neovascularity). This increased tumor/nontumor flow ratio is a major advantage of the intraarterial technique.

Methodology

The method of Tc-99m MAA administration depends on the type of intraarterial catheter and whether it is placed percutaneously or surgically (Box 7-23).

Box 7-23   Tc-99m Macroaggregated Albumin Hepatic Arterial Scintigraphy: Protocol Summary

PATIENT PREPARATION

None

INSTRUMENTATION

Camera: large-field-of-view gamma
Collimator: low energy, all purpose, parallel hole
Energy window: 15% centered over 140-keV
    photopeak

RADIOPHARMACEUTICAL

Tc-99m MAA, 1–4 mCi (37–148 MBq) for planar imaging
    and 5–6 mCi (185–222 MBq) for SPECT
Infuse in small volume (0.5–1 ml) through an
    intraarterial catheter

METHOD OF ADMINISTRATION
Surgically Implanted Infusion Pump and Catheter

Insert 22-gauge 1-inch Huber needle into infusion pump
    side port.
After ascertaining free flow, infuse Tc-99m MAA slowly
    over 1 to 2 min and flush with 10 ml of saline.
Before removing needle, inject 5 ml of heparin
    (10 units/ml).

**Percutaneously Placed Catheter and External Infusion
Pump**

Place three-way stopcock as close as possible to the site
    of catheter entry.
With patient positioned under the camera so that
    entering flow can be monitored, gently flush catheter
    with 10–20 ml of normal saline.
Infuse Tc-99m MAA in 0.2-ml volume via the three-way
    stopcock.
Increase the external pump flow rate to 200 ml/hr.
Monitor progress of radioactive injectant on the
    persistence scope. As bolus approaches the liver,
    decrease flow rate of the pump to rate at which
    chemotherapy is to be delivered, generally 10–20
    ml/hr.

IMAGING PROTOCOL

Acquire images with the patient lying on the table
    supine.
Acquire 500k-count anterior image, then posterior, right
    and left lateral, and anterior chest views for equal
    time.
If extrahepatic gastric perfusion is suspected, 4 g of
    sodium bicarbonate–citric acid–simethicone
    effervescent granules should be given in 100 ml of
    water by mouth. The patient must be encouraged not
    to belch. Repeat anterior and left lateral images.
SPECT option: technique similar to Tc-99m sulfur colloid
    SPECT.

Clinical Applications

The Tc-99m MAA hepatic arterial perfusion study is often performed after initial catheter placement and before subsequent courses of chemotherapy, particularly if the patient has symptoms suggestive of gastrointestinal toxicity. Effectiveness of intraarterial chemotherapy is maximized if the entire tumor-involved liver is perfused and side effects are minimized if there is no extrahepatic perfusion or AV shunting to the lung.

Symptoms (e.g., pain, nausea, vomiting) caused by tumor involvement may be difficult to differentiate from those caused by extrahepatic perfusion of the stomach and bowel. The importance of extrahepatic perfusion is the high associated incidence of adverse symptoms (70% vs. 20% in patients without extrahepatic perfusion), including nausea, vomiting, gastritis, ulceration, and hemorrhage.

Image Interpretation

Hepatic uptake is typically inhomogeneous. Tumor nodules have increased uptake compared with surrounding normal liver. Multiple planar views (right lateral, anterior, posterior, left lateral) or SPECT can determine the perfusion distribution. Comparison with a recent CT can be helpful.

Arteriovenous shunting is noted as lung uptake (*see* Fig. 7-55). Tc-99m-MAA particles shunted through the tumor bypass the liver capillary bed and are trapped in the lung. Lung shunting gives an estimate of the percentage of drug not delivered to the tumor that may result in systemic exposure and toxicity.

SUGGESTED READING

Choy D, Shi EC, McLean RG, et al: Cholescintigraphy in acute cholecystitis: use of intravenous morphine. *Radiology* 151: 203-207, 1984.

Fig LM, Stewart RE, Wahl RL: Morphine-augmented hepatobiliary scintigraphy in the severely ill: caution is in order. *Radiology* 175: 473-476, 1990.

Freitas JE, Coleman RE, Nagle CE, et al: Influence of scan and pathologic criteria on the specificity of cholescintigraphy. *J Nucl Med* 24: 867-879, 1983.

Sostre S, Kaloo AN, Spiegler EJ, et al: A noninvasive test of sphincter of Oddi dysfunction in postcholecystectomy patients: the scintigraphic score. *J Nucl Med* 33: 1216-1222, 1992.

Weissmann HS, Freeman LM: The biliary tract. In *Freeman and Johnson's clinical radionuclide imaging*. Freeman LM, Ed. New York, Grune & Stratton, 1984.

Yap L, Wycherley AG, Morphett AD, Toouli J: Acalculous biliary pain: cholecystectomy alleviates symptoms in patients with abnormal cholescintigraphy. *Gastroenterology* 101: 786-793, 1991.

Zeman RK, Lee C, Stahl RS, et al: Ultrasonography and hepatobiliary scintigraphy in the assessment of biliary-enteric anastomoses. *Radiology* 145: 109-115, 1982.

Zeman RK, Lee C, Jaffe MH, Burrell MI: Hepatobiliary scintigraphy and sonography in early biliary obstruction. *Radiology* 153: 793-798, 1984.

Ziessman HA, Zeman RK, Akin EA: Cholescintigraphy: Correlation with other hepatobiliary imaging modalities. In *Diagnostic Nuclear Medicine,* 4th ed. Philadelphia, Lippincott Williams & Wilkins, 2003.

Ziessman HA, Silverman PM, Patterson J, et al: Improved detection of small cavernous hemangiomas of the liver with high-resolution three-headed SPECT. *J Nucl Med* 32: 2086-2091, 1991.

Ziessman HA, Fahey FN, Hixson DJ: Calculation of a gallbladder ejection fraction: advantage of continuous sincalide infusion over the 3-minute method. *J Nucl Med* 33: 537-541, 1992.

Ziessman HA, Muenz LR, Agarwal AK, ZaZa A: Normal values for sincalide cholescintigraphy: comparison of two methods. *Radiology*; 221: 404-410, 2001.

Ziessman HA, Thrall JH, Yang PJ, et al: Hepatic arterial perfusion scintigraphy with Tc-99m MAA. *Radiology* 152: 167-172, 1984.

Ziessman HA: Acute cholecystitis, biliary obstruction, and biliary leakage. *Sem Nucl Med* 33: 279-296, 2003.

Ziessman HA, Jones DA, Muenz LR, Agarval AK: Cholecystokinin cholescintigraphy: methodology and normal values using a lactose-free fatty-meal food supplement. *J Nucl Med* 33: 1263-1266, 2003.

Genitourinary System

Early renal radionuclide studies in the 1950s did not image the kidneys but used external gamma probes to generate time-activity clearance histograms. Probe studies subsequently gave way to gamma camera imaging. Because of advancements in magnetic resonance imaging (MRI), computed tomography (CT), and ultrasound, nuclear medicine techniques are mostly utilized for functional renal imaging and quantification, often providing information not possible with the anatomic or structural modalities. Some examples include: evaluation of blood flow and viability, differentiation of obstructive and nonobstructive hydronephrosis, confirming urinary leaks, and diagnosing acute pyelonephritis.

Other indications for renal scintigraphy (Box 8-1) include evaluation of viability, infection, and masses difficult to assess by other methods such as ultrasound. The ability to quantify function by effective renal plasma flow and glomerular filtration rate can provide a better measure of functional status than standard laboratory tests such as creatinine clearance. For each different diagnostic problem, different radiopharmaceuticals have been developed (Table 8-1). This chapter concentrates on agents that have been used clinically.

Table 8-1 Historical Perspective on Radionuclides for Renal Function Evaluation

Year	Radiopharmaceutical	Method
1952	I-131 Iopax	Urine counting
1956	I-131 Diodrast	Renogram
1960	I-131 hippuran	Renogram
1968	I-131 hippuran	Lasix renography
1968	Hg-203 chloride	Individual renal function
1969	Tc-99m gluconate	Renal scan
1970	Tc-99m DTPA	Renal scan, GFR
1971	I-131 hippuran	Single-sample ERPF
1974	Tc-99m DMSA	Renal scan
1984	I-131 hippuran	Captopril renography
1986	Tc-99m MAG3	Renal scan

RENAL ANATOMY AND FUNCTION

The kidneys are responsible for regulating water and electrolyte balance, excreting waste, secreting hormones (renin, erythropoietin), and activating vitamin D. They lie in the posterior abdomen at the level of the first to third lumber vertebra. The right kidney often lies slightly inferior to the left. The outer cortex contains the glomeruli and proximal convoluted tubules. The renal pyramids consisting of the collecting tubules and the loops of Henle make up the medulla. At the apex of the pyramids, papillae drain into the renal calyces. Cortical tissues between the pyramids are known as the columns of Bertin (Fig. 8-1, A).

The renal artery supplies the blood flow to the kidney. End arterioles lead to tufts of capillaries forming glomeruli in the renal cortex (Fig. 8-1, B). The most proximal end of the renal tubule, Bowman's capsule, surrounds the glomerulus. Each kidney contains more than 1 million of these basic functional units of the kidney, the nephron.

Normally, the kidneys receive 20% of cardiac output with renal plasma flow (RPF) averaging 600 ml/min. The kidneys clear the plasma and body of waste products. The clearance, or rate of disappearance, of a substance can be measured as:

$$\text{Clearance (ml/min)} = \frac{\text{urine concentration (mg/ml)} \times \text{urine flow (ml/min)}}{\text{plasma concentration (mg/ml)}}$$

Plasma clearance occurs by glomerular filtration and tubular secretion (Fig. 8-2). If an agent undergoes 100% first pass extraction, then it can be used to measure RPF. However, because extraction of agents used to measure renal function are less than 100%, the term *effective renal plasma flow* (ERPF) is used to describe the measurement.

Approximately 20% of RPF (120 ml/min) is filtered through the semipermeable membrane of the glomerulus. A pressure gradient created by the RPF and resistance in the vessel drives filtration from the vascular space into the renal tubules. Larger material such as protein-bound compounds will not be filtered, whereas small molecules with a polar charge will be filtered. The resulting ultrafiltrate consists of water and crystalloids but no colloids or cells. The molecule inulin is considered the gold standard for glomerular filtration measurement.

The remaining plasma moves into the efferent arteriole where active secretion occurs at the tubular epithelial cells. Molecules that could not be filtered may be cleared into the tubular lumen by active tubular secretion. Overall, tubular secretion accounts for 80% of renal plasma clearance. Paraaminohippurate (PAH) is the classic method for measuring ERPF because its high extraction mirrors the distribution of RPF: 20% of PAH is cleared by glomerular filtration and 80% is secreted into the renal tubules. PAH is actively secreted by anionic transporters on the proximal convoluted tubular cell membranes. It is not metabolized or retained in the kidney and is not highly protein-bound, so plasma extraction is high. However, PAH does have some plasma protein binding, and clearance is roughly 85–95%.

When urine passes along the tubule, essential substances such as glucose, amino acids, and sodium are conserved. The filtrate is concentrated as 65% of the water filtered at the glomerulus undergoes reabsorption in the proximal convoluted tubule. Active sodium pumping in the loop of Henle sets up an osmotic gradient allowing water to passively diffuse back into the interstitium. The remaining concentrated urine passes down the renal tubule, through the papillae of the medullary pyramids into the calyces. The calyces empty into the renal pelvis, and urine passes down the ureter into the bladder.

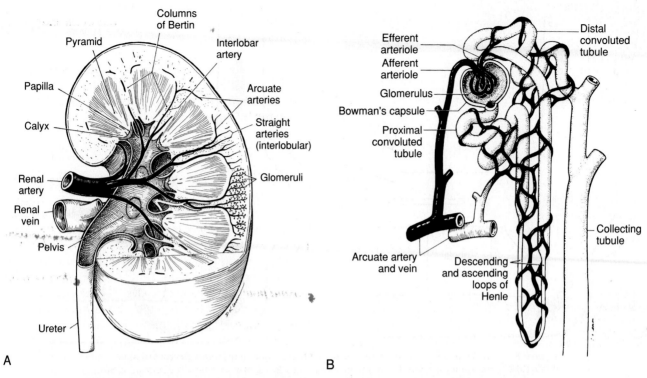

Figure 8-1   Renal anatomy. **A,** The outer layer or cortex is made up of glomeruli and proximal collecting tubules. The inner layer, or medulla, contains pyramids, made up of distal tubules and loops of Henle. The tubules converge at the papillae, which empty into calyces. The columns of Bertin, between the pyramids, are also cortical tissue. The renal artery and vein enter and leave at the hilus. The interlobar branches of the renal artery divide and become the arcuate arteries, which give rise to the straight arteries, from which arise the afferent arterioles that feed the glomerular tuft. **B,** The nephron consists of afferent vessels leading to the tuft of capillaries in the glomerulus, the glomerulus itself, and efferent vessels. Bowman's capsule surrounds the glomerulus and connects to the proximal and distal renal tubules and loops of Henle.

RENAL RADIOPHARMACEUTICALS

Renal radiopharmaceuticals are classified by their uptake and clearance mechanisms as agents for glomerular filtration, tubular secretion, or cortical binding (Table 8-2). The first step in image interpretation is understanding uptake physiology (Fig. 8-3). Renal radiopharmaceuticals are divided into those measuring glomerular filtration (Box 8-2), tubular secretion (Box 8-3), and cortical binding. The most important renal agents clinically are Tc-99m diethylenetriamine pentaacetic acid (Tc-99m DTPA), I-131 hippuran (I-131 OIH), Tc-99m mercaptylacetyltriglycine (Tc-99m MAG3), Tc-99m glucoheptonate (Tc-99m GH), and Tc-99m dimercaptosuccinic acid (Tc-99m DMSA).

Iodine-131 Orthoiodohippurate

I-131 OIH has long been a valuable tool for evaluating renal function. Although it has now been replaced in clinical use, it remains the foundation for discussion of other renal radiopharmaceuticals (Fig. 8-4). As a radiopharmaceutical chemically and pharmacokinetically similar to PAH, I-131 OIH is cleared by tubular secretion (80%) and by glomerular filtration (20%). The first pass extraction is high, roughly 85%. Therefore, hippuran accurately measures ERPF. The high level of clearance made I-131 OIH useful for imaging azotemic patients.

Chemistry and Radiolabeling

Hippuran can be radiolabeled with either I-131 or I-123 through an exchange reaction. Stabilizing and buffering agents are added for pH adjustments. The bond tends to degrade with time. Storage should be at 4°C or less, protected from light.

Pharmacokinetics

With normal renal function, peak renal concentration is reached within 2-4 minutes of intravenous injection. Subsequent visualization in the collecting system and bladder is faster than with Tc-99m DTPA. The time it takes for the activity to be cleared can be described in terms of the time

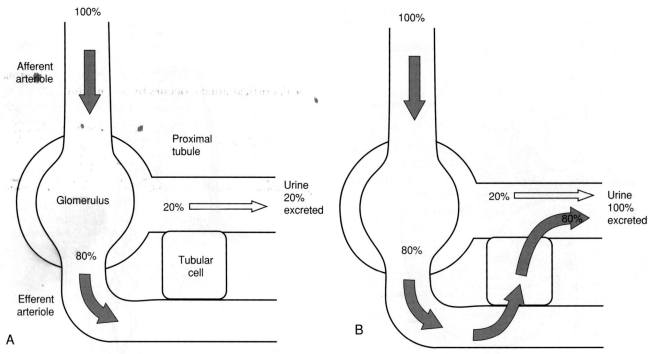

Figure 8-2   Renal plasma flow and function. **A,** Glomerular filtration. Twenty percent of renal blood flow to the kidney is filtered through the glomerulus. **B,** Tubular secretion. The remaining 80% of renal plasma flow is secreted into the proximal tubules from the peritubular space.

Table 8-2	Mechanism of Uptake for Renal Scintigraphy Agents

Uptake	Agent
Glomerular filtration (100%)	Tc-99m DTPA
Tubular (100%)	Tc-99m MAG3
Tubular (80%) and glomerular (20%)	I-131 and I-123 hippuran
Cortical binding (40%)	Tc-99m DMSA
Glomerular filtration (80%) and cortical binding (20%)	Tc-99m Glucoheptonate

required to clear 50% of the activity after reaching the peak cortical activity. This clearance half-time, or T₁/₂, for I-131 OIH is normally 10-15 minutes with 98% of the dose cleared from plasma within 24 hours.

Special Considerations
The long half life (8.08 days) and beta-radiation of the I-131 label necessitate a low administered dose of 200-400 uCi (7.4-14.8 MBq). This dose limit and the high-energy gamma photon (364 keV) contribute to poor spatial resolution and an inability to do dynamic arterial perfusion imaging. The dose to the thyroid from unlabeled radioiodine can be reduced by pretreatment

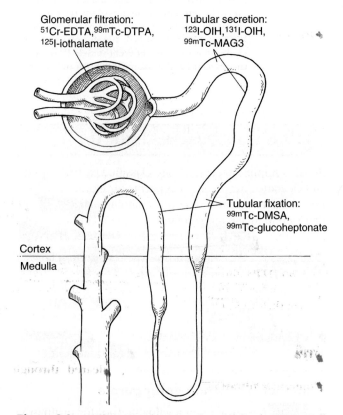

Figure 8-3   Different mechanisms of renal radiopharmaceutical uptake and excretion. These include glomerular filtration, tubular secretion, and cortical tubular binding.

Box 8-2 Agents Used for Glomerular Filtration

C-14 or H-3 inulin
I-125 diatrizoate
I-125 iothalamate
Co-57 vitamin B12
Cr-51 EDTA
In-111 DTPA
Yb-169 DTPA
Tc-99m DTPA

Box 8-3 Renal Tubular Radiopharmaceuticals Used to Quantify Effective Renal Plasma Flow

H-2 or C-14 paraaminohippurate (PAH)
I-125, I-131 iodopyracet
I-125, I-123, or I-131 orthoiodohippurate (OIH)
Tc-99m mercaptoacetyltriglycine (MAG3)

with thyroid blocking agents like supersaturated potassium iodide (SSKI). The United States Pharmacopeia (USP) mandates there be less than 3% free radioiodine. It was thought that the limitations created by the I-131 label would be overcome by utilizing I-123. Although theoretically a better label, there were logistical problems concerning timely distribution of I-123. Also, surprisingly high dosimetry limited the administered dose to 3 mCi, which resulted in poor flow studies. However, I-131 OIH has been replaced by technetium-99m labeled MAG3 and I-131 OIH is no longer available commercially.

Tc-99m Diethylenetriamine Pentaacetic Acid

The physical characteristics of the technetium label of Tc-99m DTPA allow dynamic arterial perfusion studies and much better discrimination of cortex and collecting system than I-131 OIH.

Chemistry and Radiolabeling

DTPA is a heavy metal chelator used for treatment of poisoning. Like other chelators, it is cleared through glomerular filtration. Tc-99m DTPA is convenient and inexpensive to prepare. A simple kit is available containing stannous tin as a reducing agent. The reduced technetium-99m forms a powerful chelating bond with the DTPA. Contaminants such as hydrolyzed and oxidized

technetium-99m (free pertechnetate) can be readily identified by chromatography.

Pharmacokinetics

Following intravenous injection of Tc-99m DTPA, normal peak cortical uptake occurs by 3–4 minutes. By 5 minutes, the collecting system is seen; the bladder is typically visualized by 10–15 minutes. The $T_{1/2}$ peak, or the time it takes for one-half of the maximal cortical activity to clear, is normally 15–20 minutes for Tc-99m DTPA.

Tc-99m DTPA is essentially completely filtered at the glomerulus with no tubular secretion or reabsorption. Because only 20% of renal function is the result of glomerular filtration, the first-pass extraction of a glomerular filtration agent is less than agents cleared by tubular secretion. In practice, normal first-pass Tc-99m DTPA extraction is less than the 20% of RPF due to factors such as the level of protein binding. The extraction fraction is only 40–50% that of Tc-99m MAG3 and is even lower compared to I-131 OIH. The lower extraction efficiency becomes clinically significant in patients with abnormal renal function or obstruction. In such cases, target-to-background ratios may be so poor that no diagnostic information is gained. At many sites, Tc-99m DTPA use is reserved for glomerular filtration rate (GFR) calculations, whereas blood flow and routine functional assessments are done with Tc-99m MAG3.

The rate of Tc-99m DTPA clearance depends on the amount of impurities in the preparation which bind to protein in the body. This leads to underestimation of GFR. Different preparations of Tc-99m DTPA may show highly variable protein binding that should be controlled. Although Tc-99m DTPA generally underestimates GFR, it is adequate for clinical use if the level of protein binding is minimized.

Tc-99m Mercaptoacetyltriglycine

Currently, Tc-99m MAG3 is the most commonly used renal radiopharmaceutical. It is cleared almost entirely by tubular secretion. The extraction efficiency is considerably higher than filtration agents. This results in better performance when function is compromised. The improved counting statistics of Tc-99m MAG3 over I-131 OIH permit blood flow imaging. In addition, the high-count time–activity curves and images are far superior with lower radiation dosimetry (Fig. 8-5). Tc-99m MAG3 images show significant anatomic detail while assessing function (Fig. 8-6).

Radiolabeling

Tc-99m MAG3 is available in kit form. Labeling involves the addition of sodium pertechnetate to a reaction vial. A unique feature of the Tc-99m MAG3 labeling process is that a small amount of air is added to the reaction vial to consume excess stannous ion for increased stability. Radiolabeling efficiency is 95% or greater.

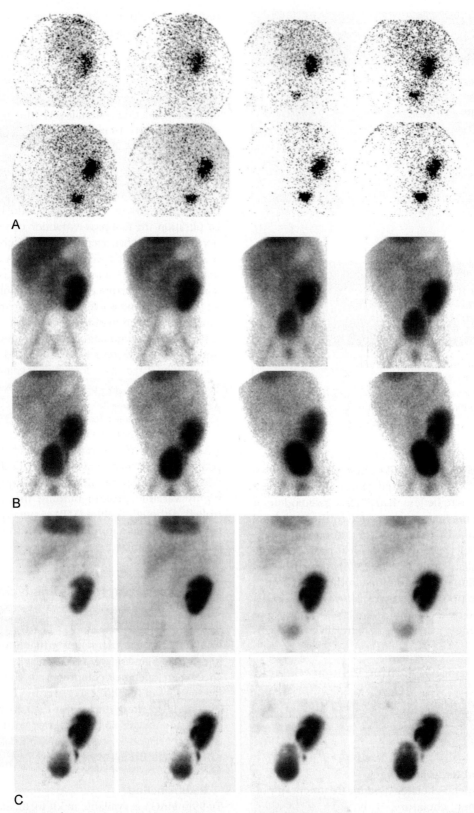

Figure 8-4   Radiopharmaceutical comparison in a renal transplant patient. **A,** I-131 hippuran provides excellent functional information but has poor image quality compared to technetium agents. **B,** Tc-99m DTPA image from the same day shows higher resolution. **C,** Tc-99m MAG3 done 30 hours later reveals the highest level of detail as well as an improved target to background ratio compared to DTPA.

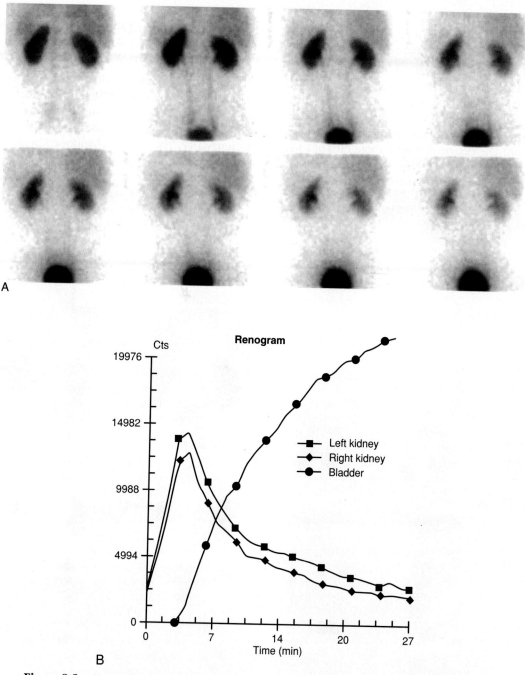

Figure 8-5   Normal Tc-99m MAG3. **A,** Normal dynamic functional images with prompt symmetric radiotracer uptake and rapid clearance over the study. **B,** Normal time–activity curves with a steep uptake slope, distinct peak, and rapid clearance confirming image analysis.

Pharmacokinetics

Because Tc-99m MAG3 is protein-bound and not filtered, it is exclusively cleared from the kidney by tubular secretion. It has a much higher first-pass extraction than a glomerular filtration agent like Tc-99m DTPA. Plasma protein binding is 97% for Tc-99m MAG3 as opposed to 70% for I-131 OIH. This binding keeps Tc-99m MAG3 in the vascular space, improving renal target-to-background ratios but slowing renal extraction. The clearance is only about 60% of I-131 OIH. The alternative route of Tc-99m MAG3 excretion is via the hepatobiliary route. Liver activity and biliary tract clearance are frequently noted. The normal time to peak activity is 3–5 minutes. Normal clearance and half-peak values are similar to other agents described.

Cortical Binding Radiopharmaceuticals: Technetium-99m Dimercaptosuccinic Acid and Technetium-99m Glucoheptonate

Renal cortical imaging evaluates viability, infection, and structural abnormalities difficult to assess by ultrasound and CT. The original cortical imaging agents used a diuretic, chlormerodrin, labeled with mercury-203 and mercury-197. These were abandoned in favor of Tc-99m DMSA (a chelating agent) and Tc-99m GH (a former conventional brain scan agent). Tc-99m DMSA is the better agent for evaluating the renal cortex (Figs. 8-7 and 8-8).

The rapid transit of most renal radiopharmaceuticals (Tc-99m DTPA, I-131 OIH, and Tc-99m MAG3) does not

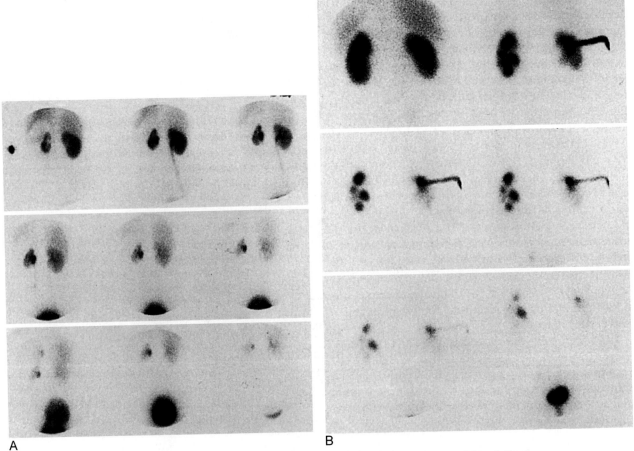

A

B

Figure 8-6 Abnormal Tc-99m MAG3 examples revealing anatomic and functional data. **A,** Small scarred left kidney secondary to vesicoureteral reflux contributing 15% to overall function. Good cortical clearance is seen. **B,** Obstruction of right kidney secondary to cervical carcinoma. A nephrostomy tube is draining well and bilateral function is good. Prominent left pelvis and calyces mostly clear by the end of the study; this study shows hydronephrosis but no significant obstruction. The last image was taken with the bladder in view.

Continued

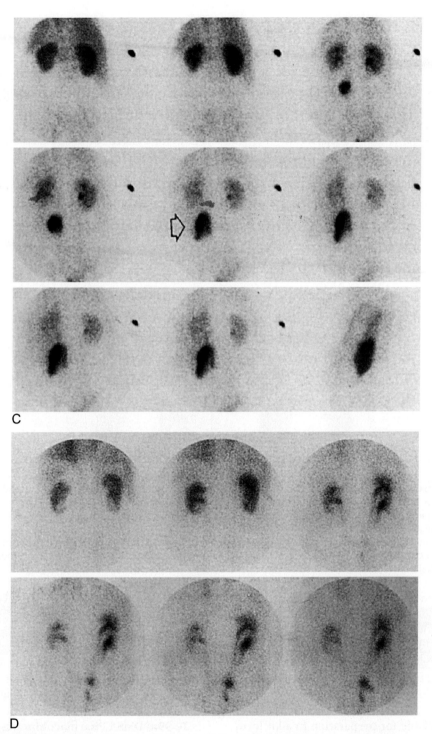

Figure 8-6, cont'd   C, Ureteral leak *(arrow)* detected on sequential images in a postoperative patient. **D,** Duplicated right collecting system, a congenital abnormality associated with lower pole reflux and upper pole obstruction.

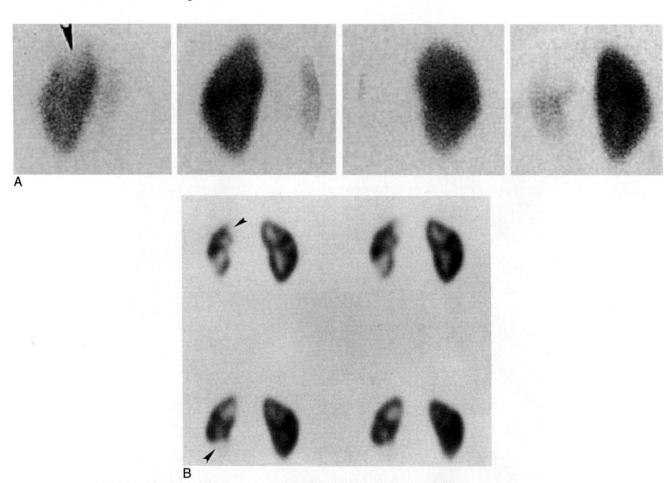

Figure 8-7 Tc-99m DMSA planar and SPECT studies in two patients with cortical scars caused by reflux. **A,** Planar images were acquired using a pinhole collimator. *Left to right,* Left posterior oblique (LPO), posterior (left kidney), posterior (right kidney), and right posterior oblique views. Cortical defect in the left superior pole *(arrowhead)* is best seen on the LPO view. **B,** High-resolution SPECT. Sequential 3.5-mm coronal sections show a cortical defect in the right upper pole and a larger defect in the right lower pole *(arrowheads)*. Note a distinct separation of cortex from medulla and collecting system with SPECT.

allow high-resolution imaging of the cortex. On the other hand, the stable cortical uptake of Tc-99m DMSA and Tc-99m GH produces high-quality images using either pinhole imaging or single-photon emission computed tomography (SPECT). Delayed imaging results in high target-to-background ratios and good resolutions.

Radiolabeling

Both agents are available for preparation in a kit form using Tc-99m pertechnetate reduced by stannous ion. The introduction of air can lead to degradation of the label and lead to increased background activity, including in the liver. Tc-99m DMSA radiolabeling produces multiple forms of the Tc-99m DMSA complex which may vary slightly in their clearance.

Tc-99m GH Pharmacokinetics

Approximately 80% of the injected dose of Tc-99m GH is cleared into the urine, with approximately 15–20% of the dose fixed in the proximal cortical tubules. Imaging is done

in two stages. Dynamic assessment of flow and function is obtained in the first 25–30 minutes after injection. An imaging sequence similar to Tc-99m DTPA or Tc-99m MAG3 is used. Following dynamic imaging, delayed static images are performed. Renal uptake depends on RPF and renal tubular function. An alternative route of excretion may occur through the liver and gallbladder filling may occur.

Tc-99m DMSA Pharmacokinetics

The mechanism of Tc-99m DMSA renal uptake and clearance is not entirely understood. Roughly 40% of the injected dose localizes in the cortex, predominantly in the proximal tubules. Imaging is generally done after a 2- to 3-hour delay to allow time for uptake and slow background clearance. In cases of decreased renal function, further delay may be needed. The low level of urinary excretion (approximately 25% of the dose) is not adequate for assessment of the collecting system and lower urinary tract.

Diseases affecting the proximal tubules, such as renal tubular acidosis and Fanconi's syndrome, inhibit Tc-99m

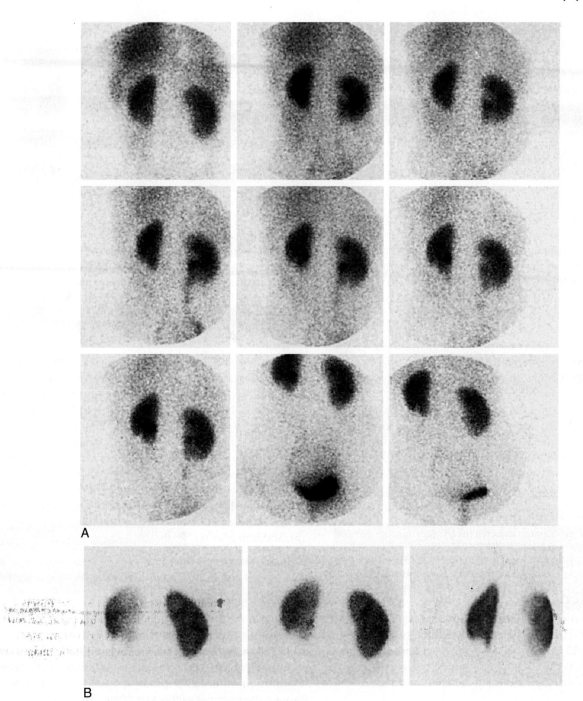

Figure 8-8   Tc-99m glucoheptonate imaging in a patient with vesicoureteral reflux, posterior views. **A,** Dynamic planar study. **B,** Delayed cortical imaging. Both phases show a cortical defect in the left lower pole. Delayed images acquired with a pinhole collimator which improved resolution. *Left to right:* Right posterior oblique, posterior, and left posterior oblique views.

DMSA uptake. Nephrotoxic drugs including gentamicin and cis-platinum also inhibit uptake. In cases where serum creatinine is significantly elevated, target-to-background ratios may be so poor that no useful diagnostic information can be gained.

Tc-99m DMSA is preferred over Tc-99m GH because its greater cortical uptake results in superior image resolution. Therefore, Tc-99m GH is currently rarely used. However, Tc-99m GH may be useful in patients with renal tubular acidosis because Tc-99m GH uptake is not affected, unlike with Tc-99m DMSA.

Dosimetry

Although the radiation dose to the patient from renal radiopharmaceuticals is low when renal function is normal, the absorbed dose rises significantly in the obstructed kidney or when renal function fails. Dosimetry of the important renal radiopharmaceuticals is listed in Table 8-3.

DYNAMIC RENAL IMAGING TECHNIQUES

Renal protocols must be tailored for specific clinical applications. This section provides a basic approach to these techniques and modifications. The protocols outline current use of the major clinical radiopharmaceuticals.

Dynamic Renography

Dynamic functional studies are generally acquired in two parts. The renal blood flow is assessed in the first pass of the radiopharmaceutical bolus to the kidney. Then over the following 25–30 minutes, uptake and clearance assess function.

Similar protocols can be used for the dynamic functional agents Tc-99m DTPA, Tc-99m GH, and Tc-99m MAG3 (Box 8-4). I-131 OIH count rates are insufficient for blood flow studies as the amount of administered activity is limited due to the higher absorbed radiation doses.

Method

Patient Preparation

Patients should be well-hydrated before the study. Dehydration does not affect blood flow, radiopharmaceutical uptake, or functional calculations (ERPF or GFR). However, excretion and washout can be delayed by dehydration, simulating obstruction.

It is important to document all medications the patient has taken that may affect the study, such as diuretics and blood pressure medicines. Any known anatomic anomalies and prior interventions are important factors to consider in positioning and image interpretation.

Patient Positioning

A supine position is preferred as kidneys are frequently mobile (or "ptotic") and can move to the anterior pelvis when patients are upright. Patients are placed so that the kidneys are closest to the camera, with the camera posterior for normal native kidneys and anterior for transplants, pelvic kidneys and horseshoe kidneys.

Dose

The dose of radiopharmaceutical varies with the agent. Typical doses are listed in the protocol boxes. In the past, higher doses of Tc-99m MAG3 up to 10–15 mCi were given, but as little as 3–6 mCi (111–222 MBq) is actually needed in adults. Although nomograms are available for calculating pediatric doses based on body surface area, Webster's rule is generally helpful: [age + 1]/ [age + 7] × adult dose.

Image Acquisition

Following a bolus injection of radiopharmaceutical, the image acquisition begins when activity is about to enter the abdominal aorta. Images are acquired at a rate of 1–3 seconds per frame for 60 seconds to assess renal perfusion. Then images are obtained at 60 seconds per frame for 25–30 minutes to evaluate parenchymal radiotracer uptake and clearance.

Computer Processing of Renal Studies

The uptake and clearance of radiopharmaceuticals is a dynamic process. Mentally integrating all the information in the many images of a renal scan is challeng-

Table 8-3   Radiation Dosimetry for Renal Radiopharmaceuticals in rad/mCi (cGy/MBq)

Organ	I-123 OIH	I-131 OIH	Tc-99m DTPA	Tc-99m MAG3	Tc-99m DMSA	Tc-99m GH
Bladder	0.95	5.167	0.27	0.6	0.07	0.28
Kidneys	0.05	0.167	0.09	0.0175	0.63	0.17
Ovaries	0.05	0.1	0.016	0.0325	0.013	0.016
Testes	0.03	0.067	0.01	0.02	0.007	0.01
Whole body	0.02	0.03	0.006	0.01	0.015	0.0075

Box 8-4   Protocol Summary for Dynamic Renal Scintigraphy

PATIENT PREPARATION
Hydration

Adults: drink 300–500 ml of water
Children: Intravenous hydration 10–15 ml/kg over 30 min; <1 year use dextrose 5% in 0.45% normal saline, >1 year of age D5 in 0.45% normal saline
Patient must void before starting study

RADIOPHARMACEUTICAL
Tc-99m DTPA

Adults: 15 mCi (555 MBq)
Children: 200 UCi/kg (2 mCi minimum, 10mCi maximum)

Tc-99m GH

Adults: 20 mCi (740 MBq)
Children: same as for Tc-99m DTPA

Tc-99m MAG3

Adults: 3–5 mCi (110–185 MBq)
Children: 100 UCi/kg (1 mCi minimum to 5 mCi maximum)

INSTRUMENTATION

Camera: large field of view gamma
Collimator: low energy, parallel hole
Photopeak: 15–20% window centered over 140 keV

PATIENT POSITION

Routine renal imaging: supine, posterior
Renal transplant: patient supine, camera anterior over allograft

COMPUTER ACQUISITION

Blood flow: 1- to 2-sec frames for 60 sec
Dynamic: 30-sec frames for 25 min
Pre-void image 500k count
Postvoid image

PROCESSING

Draw computer region of interest around kidneys and for background area
Generate time-activity curves for 60-sec flow phase and for 25-min dynamic study

---

ing, even for experienced clinicians. Computer-generated time-activity curves (TAC) provide a dynamic visual presentation of changes in activity over the course of the study. Usually separate TACs are drawn for the blood flow and dynamic function portions of the study.

Perfusion Time–Activity Curve
The first-pass perfusion TAC shows the blood flow to each kidney compared with arterial flow. A region of interest is drawn around each kidney and the closest major artery (aorta for native kidneys, iliac artery for transplanted kidneys) on the initial 60-second portion of the study. Although absolute flow (measured in milliliters per kilogram per minute) cannot be calculated with the radiotracers discussed, relative flow can be visualized or calculated using the upslope of the perfusion curve. A ratio of the activity compared to the aorta or K/A ratio can help follow changes in perfusion.

Dynamic Renal Function Time-Activity Curve
Evaluation of dynamic cortical function is done with a renal region of interest (ROI) corrected for background activity (Fig. 8-9). The selection of kidney ROI depends on the information needed. Whole kidney ROIs can be used for cortical function if the collecting system clears promptly. When a whole kidney ROI is used in a patient with retained activity in the collecting system, clearance will appear delayed on the time-activity curve (TAC). In cases of hydronephrosis and obstruction, a 2-pixel wide peripheral cortical ROI excluding collecting system is best, although some overlap with calyces is inevitable.

Various methods of background correction have been employed. A 2-pixel wide region of interest is drawn. It may be placed beneath the kidneys, around the kidneys, or in a crescent configuration. Because the kidneys overlap the liver and spleen, most background correction methods include some liver and spleen in the background ROI. Background correction is less critical in delayed images, such as those obtained with Tc-99m DMSA, because of the high target-to-background ratio on these delayed images.

At any point in time, the renogram represents a summation of uptake and excretion. Three phases are normally seen in the TACs. These include blood flow, cortical uptake, and clearance phases (Fig. 8-10). The TAC must be interpreted in conjunction with the images as the curves may be affected by many factors, such as retained activity in hydronephrosis, which can alter the slope. Any technical error or discrepancy between the appearance of the curve and the images must be reconciled.

Semiquantitative Assessment of Renal Function
Numerous values can be derived from the time-activity curves. These include time to peak activity, uptake slope, rate of clearance, and percent clearance at 20 minutes. The most commonly used parameters reflecting clearance are the 20/peak ratio and the 20/3 ratio. The 20/peak is the ratio of cortical activity at 20 minutes to the amount of peak activity. The 20/3 ratio is calculated by dividing the amount of activity at 20 minutes by the activity at 3 minutes.

Differential Function
Differential or split function is a universally performed calculation. A whole kidney ROI is needed so that no cortex is excluded. The ROI is related to generate a TAC

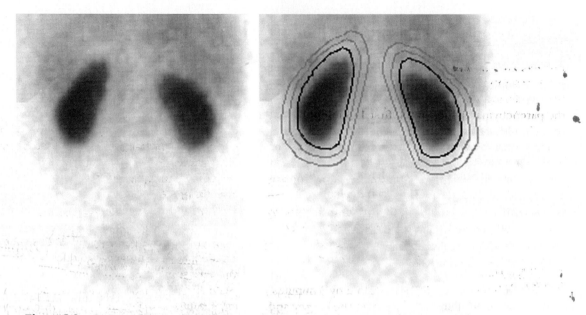

Figure 8-9 Regions of interest (ROI) for time–activity curves. *Left,* An image at 3 minutes with peak cortical activity is chosen for the ROIs. *Right,* Regions of interest are drawn for the kidney *(dark lines)* and for background correction *(gray lines)*.

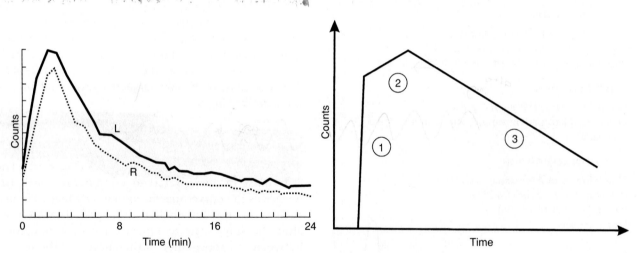

Figure 8-10 Normal renogram can be divided into phases. *1,* Initial blood flow (30–60 seconds). *2,* Cortical uptake phase (normally 1–3 minutes). *3,* Clearance phase representing cortical excretion and collecting stem clearance.

representing the amount of activity in each kidney during the peak nephrogram phase. Values are selected in the range of 1–3 minutes after injection (after the blood flow phase and before the excretory phase). The actual counts in each kidney are expressed as a fraction of 100% total function. Normally, the relative contribution for each kidney lies between 45–55%. This value does not indicate if the overall or global renal function is normal or abnormal. A calculation of GFR or ERPF can be done as a separate study to quantify actual function.

Interpretation
Flow Phase

Blood flow to the kidneys is normally seen within 2–5 seconds of abdominal aorta visualization. It is important to assess the quality of the injection bolus, as delayed renal visualization may be artifactual due to suboptimal injection technique. If the slope of the arterial time–activity curve is not steep or if activity visibly persists in the heart and lungs, the injection may have been too strung out. Any asymmetry in tracer activity suggests abnormal perfusion to the side of decreased or delayed activity. A smaller or scarred kidney will have less flow due to a decrease in parenchymal tissue volume (Fig. 8-11).

Cortical Function Phase

Like the nephrogram phase of an intravenous pyelogram (IVP), normal kidneys accumulate radiopharmaceutical in the parenchymal tissues in the first 1–3 minutes. The cortex should appear homogeneous. The calyces and renal pelvis are either not seen in this initial phase or appear relatively photopenic. If decreased function is present on one side, the rate of uptake and function are often delayed on that side relative to the better functioning kidney. This produces a "flip-flop" pattern; the poorly functioning side initially has lower uptake but the cortical activity on later images is higher than the better functioning side, which has already excreted the radiotracer.

Clearance Phase

The calyces and pelvis usually begin filling by 3 minutes. Over the next 10–15 minutes, activity in the kidney and collecting system decreases. With good function, most of the radiotracer clears into the bladder by the end of the study. In some healthy subjects, pooling of activity in the dependent calyces can result in focal hot spots. Lack of clearance or overlap of pelvocalyceal structures on the cortex suggests hydronephrosis. Because areas with increased activity appear larger, caution must be taken in diagnosing hydronephrosis on scintigraphic studies.

The normal ureter may or may not be seen. Prolonged, unchanging, or increasing activity suggests dilatation. Because peristalsis and urine flow rates cause such variable visualization, care must be taken in diagnosing reflux into the ureters when activity remains in the kidney. On these studies, indirect determination of reflux can be done when ureteral activity persists after the kidneys have cleared. However, reflux is best detected on a direct vesicoureterogram (VCUG) with activity introduced directly into the bladder via a catheter.

The bladder is normally well seen. Prevoid and postvoid bladder images evaluate emptying and postvoid residual. A distended bladder can cause an obstructed pattern. In a patient with neurogenic bladder or outlet obstruction, the renal scan is best performed with a urinary catheter in place. In infants and small children, the bladder may appear quite large and higher in position than might be expected when looking at the outline of the child's body.

Clinical Applications of Renal Scintigraphy

The clinical uses of renal scintigraphy are numerous. Renal imaging can assess blood flow, relative size, and

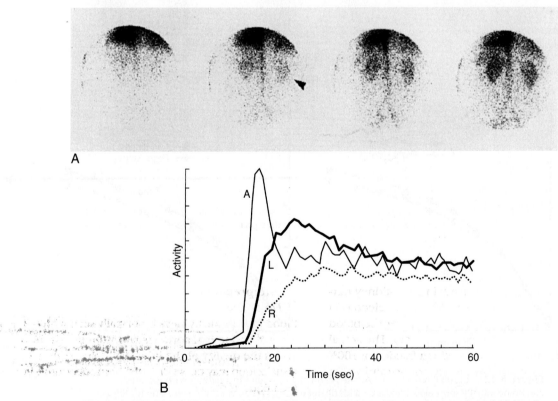

Figure 8-11   Renal blood flow analysis. **A,** Sequential 2-second frames show moderately delayed and decreased blood flow to the right kidney *(arrowhead).* **B,** Sixty-second time activity curves confirm the imaging findings. Initial upslope of the right kidney *(R)* is delayed compared with the aorta *(A)* and left kidney *(L).*

functional parameters. Although functional abnormalities can be seen in acute and chronic renal failure, the pattern is not specific for the etiology (Fig. 8-12). Abnormal blood flow can be seen with renal artery stenosis, thrombosis, avulsion, venous thrombosis, and infarction. Static cortical imaging is most often done to evaluate pyelonephritis and some possible masses.

Renovascular Hypertension

More than 90% of patients with hypertension have no identifiable cause ("essential hypertension"). Renovascular hypertension (RVH) accounts for a significant proportion of those patients with trea causes for their elevated blood pressure. Although the prevalence of renovascular hypertension is less than 1% in nonselected patients, 15-45% of patients referred to specialty centers for refractory hypertension have RVH.

The two main causes of RVH are atherosclerosis and fibromuscular dysplasia. Not all cases of renal artery stenosis cause functional renovascular hypertension. Almost half of normotensive patients over the age of 60 years have atherosclerotic lesions in their renal vessels.

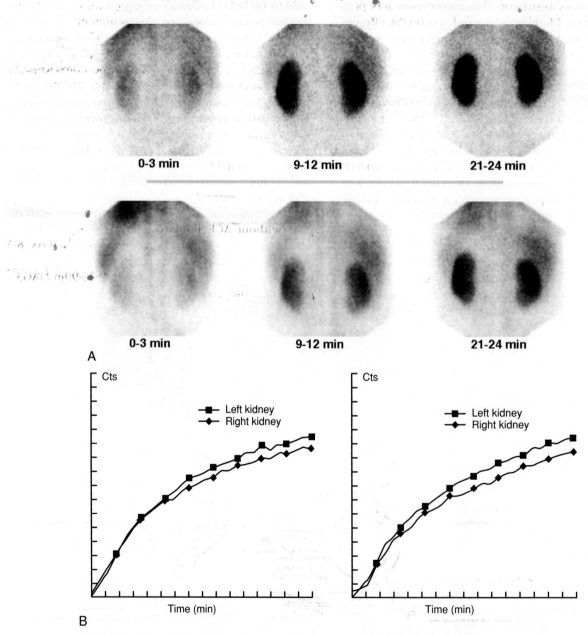

Figure 8-12   Chronic renal failure. **A,** The Tc-9m MAG3 studies in a patient with elevated creatinine initially show slow clearance with bilateral cortical retention *(top row).* The findings are not specific for the cause of dysfunction. A follow-up study done 6 months later shows no change and cardiovascular disease was the assumed etiology of the chronic failure *(bottom row).* **B,** The time–activity curves show slight worsening between the two studies, that is, a slower rising curve.

In addition, many hypertensive patients have renal artery stenosis unrelated to their blood pressure, showing no response to angioplasty or stenting of the stenosis.

When an arterial lesion causes significant vascular stenosis in the renal artery or one of its major branches, glomerular perfusion pressure drops, causing glomerular filtration to fall. The kidney responds by releasing the hormone renin from the juxtaglomerular apparatus. Renin converts angiotensinogen made in the liver to angiotensin I. In the lungs, angiotensin I is converted by angiotensin converting enzyme (ACE) to vasoactive angiotensin II, which acts as a powerful vasoconstrictor. This constriction acts peripherally to raise blood pressure and acts on the efferent arterioles of the glomerulus to raise filtration pressure, thus maintaining GFR. (Fig. 8-13).

If renal blood flow remains low, the kidney will become scarred and contracted with time. If RVH is present, early intervention decreases arteriolar damage and glomerulosclerosis. This increases the chance for a cure. It is therefore critical to identify patients who would benefit from invasive therapy such as angioplasty, arterial stenting, or surgery. However, physical exam and lab tests are generally nonspecific. It is not practical or desirable to subject all suspicious patients to invasive angiography. It is not practical or desirable to subject all suspicious patients to invasive angiography.

Noninvasive imaging tests play an important role in evaluation of the kidneys. However, IVP has false-positive and false-negative rates of approximately 25% for the detection of RVH. Conventional radionuclide studies using Tc-99m DTPA and Tc-99m MAG3 have sensitivity and specificity similar to IVP. Abnormal function is nonspecific and can be seen in other disease states. CT angiography and MR angiography are able to identify arterial stenosis noninvasively, but do not take into account the functional effects of any anatomic lesion.

The development of ACE inhibition renography using captopril (Capoten) led to a sensitive, noninvasive functional method for diagnosing renovascular hypertension. ACE inhibitors work by blocking the conversion of angiotensin I to angiotensin II (Fig. 8-14). This causes GFR to fall in RVH patients relying on the compensatory mechanism to maintain perfusion pressure. Functional changes can be seen on scintigrams and renograms.

Indication

ACE inhibition renography should be considered for patients at moderate- to high-risk for renovascular hypertension. This includes patients with severe hypertension, hypertension resistant to medical therapy, abrupt or recent onset, onset under the age of 30 or over the age of 55 years, abdominal or flank bruits, unexplained azotemia, worsening renal function during ACE inhibitor therapy, and occlusive disease in other beds.

Imaging Protocol

Two radionuclide studies are performed: one with and one without ACE inhibitor. An example of an ACE inhibitor renography protocol is listed in Box 8-5. Radiopharmaceuticals that have been used include I-131 OIH and Tc-99m DTPA, but now Tc-99m MAG3 is most commonly used. It is possible to perform both studies

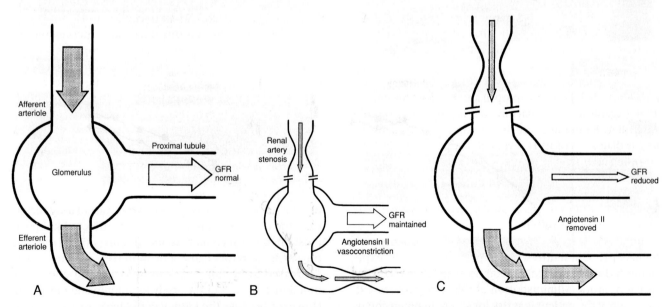

Figure 8-13   Pathophysiology of renin-dependent renovascular disease: pharmacological effect of captopril. **A,** Normal glomerular filtration rate *(GFR).* **B,** Renovascular hypertension. Because of reduced renal plasma flow, filtration pressure and GFR fall. Increased renin and resulting angiotensin II produces vasoconstriction of the efferent glomerular arterioles, raising glomerular pressure and maintaining GFR. **C,** Captopril blocks the normal compensatory mechanism and GFR falls.

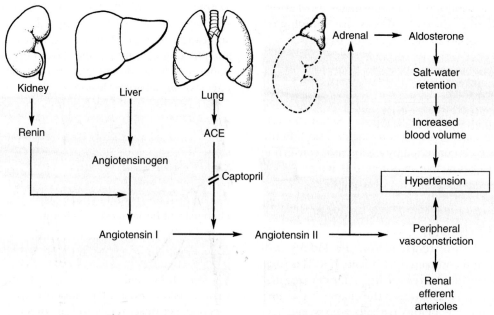

Figure 8-14 Renin-angiotensin-aldosterone physiology and site of angiotensin-converting enzyme (ACE) inhibitor (captopril). See text for detail.

using a 1-day protocol. The 1-day protocol involves first doing a baseline exam using a low-dose of 1 mCi (37 MBq) of Tc-99m MAG3 radiopharmaceutical followed by a post-ACE inhibitor study using 5-10 mCi of Tc-99m MAG3 (185-370 MBq).

Alternatively, the two studies are performed on separate days with 3-5 mCi of Tc-99m MAG3 (111-185 MBq). A baseline study is only done in those patients with an abnormal ACE inhibitor study. The radiotracer should be allowed to clear and decay, so at least 24 hours between the studies is needed.

Patient preparation involves discontinuing all ACE inhibitors (2-3 days for captopril and 5-7 days for longer-acting agents such as enalapril and lisinopril) before the study. If ACE inhibitors are not discontinued the sensitivity for diagnosis of RVH is reduced approximately 15%. Stopping angiotensin receptor blockers and halting calcium channel blockers should also be considered. Diuretics should be stopped to prevent a dehydrated condition. Otherwise, most antihypertensives have little or no effect on the results.

Intravenous access should be obtained as patients with renin-dependent renovascular hypertension usually experience a drop in systemic blood pressure after receiving ACE inhibitors. Administration of fluids may be critical, especially if the patient is at risk for severe hypotension or has cardiovascular risk factors such as recent myocardial infarction or carotid/coronary artery disease.

The loop diuretic furosemide (Lasix) is frequently administered simultaneously with the radiopharmaceuti-

cal. This ensures clearance of the collecting system, which might otherwise affect visual and quantitative interpretation. Furosemide acts on Henley's loop distal to where Tc-99m MAG3 is secreted. Therefore, furosemide does not affect the cortical retention or clearance of Tc-99m MAG3.

Captopril (25-50 mg) is crushed and dissolved in water. A 1-hour delay is then necessary to allow absorption to occur. Although this delay adds inconvenience and variable absorption may occur, captopril is still frequently used. Alternatively, the ACE inhibitor enalapril (Vasotec), given intravenously at 40 ug/kg up to 2.5 mg over 3-5 minutes, can shorten the time before imaging to 15 minutes and ensures that consistent ACE inhibitor levels are achieved. A baseline blood pressure should be recorded. Serial blood pressure measurements should be taken and the patient should be carefully monitored for hypotension through the end of imaging.

Image Interpretation

In patients with renin-dependent renovascular hypertension, the decreased blood flow to the affected kidney is most often *not* seen on baseline or conventional renography. ACE inhibitors cause a drop in GFR, which leads to decreased urine flow that can be visualized during the functional portion of the study as a diminished function. However, because the kidney could have abnormal function due to numerous etiologies, a baseline study is done. In patients with renovascular hypertension, function generally improves in the absence of ACE inhibitors. In normal patients and in those with renal disease due to other

Box 8-5   Angiotensin-Converting Enzyme (Captopril) Renography Protocol Summary

PATIENT PREPARATION

Liquids only 4 hours before the study

Hydration: 7 ml/kg water 30–60 minutes before the study or intravenous hydration 10 ml/kg (maximum 500 ml) half-normal saline over 1 hour. Keep vein open during study in case of hypotension.

Discontinue certain medications: ACE inhibitors (3 days short-acting, 5–7 days longer-acting agent), angiotensin receptor blockers; consider stopping calcium channel blockers and diuretics

RADIOPHARMACEUTICAL TC-99M MAG3

2-day protocol: 3–6 mCi (111–222 MBq)

1-day protocol: use 1–2 mCi (37–74 MBq) for baseline then 5–10 mCi (185–376 MBq) ACE inhibitor study

IMAGING PROCEDURE

1. Check baseline blood pressure
2. Administer ACE inhibitor

    Captopril: adults, 25–50 mg (dissolve in water) orally 1 hour before study; children, 0.5 mg/kg (maximum 25 mg)

    Enalapril 40 µg/kg (maximum 2.5 mg) intravenously infused over 3–5 minutes
3. Monitor and record blood pressure every 15 minutes for oral medication and every 5 min for IV enalapril. A large drop in pressure may require fluids intravenously
4. Administer 20–40 mg furosemide intravenously at the time of injection
5. Inject radiopharmaceutical 60 minutes after oral captopril or 15 minutes after enalapril
6. Imaging protocol is similar to dynamic renography (see Box 8-4)

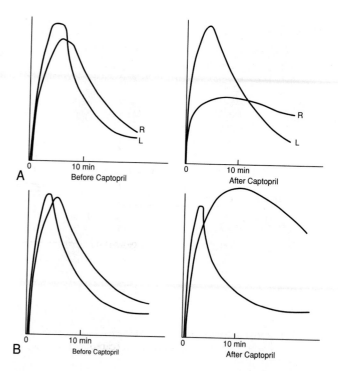

Figure 8-15   Renovascular hypertension. **A,** A comparison of Tc-99m DTPA and Tc-99m MAG3 curves. *Left,* Baseline DTPA study shows normal function bilaterally. *Right,* After captopril, peak and overall renal function falls on one side from the drop in GFR. **B,** The baseline MAG3 study is unremarkable (*left*) but ACE inhibitor study shows the effect on renal function as cortical retention (*right*).

etiologies (such as chronic scarring from pyelonephritis), function does not improve on a baseline study compared to the ACE inhibitor examination.

In general, the diagnostic pattern seen will depend on the type of radiopharmaceutical used (Fig. 8-15). If the glomerular agent Tc-99m DTPA is used, the ACE-inhibitor–induced drop in GFR leads to a marked drop in radiotracer filtration and uptake. The most common pattern is an overall drop in function seen as slower uptake and a lower peak (Fig. 8-16). A tubular-secretion agent such as Tc-99m MAG3 does not usually show the same decrease in uptake; tubular uptake and secretion are not affected by GFR changes from the ACE inhibitor. The decreased urine flow causes delayed Tc-99m MAG3 washout and the primary finding will be cortical retention (Fig. 8-17).

If bilateral cortical retention is seen, the finding is likely artifact and not bilateral renal artery stenosis. Among patients with bilateral cortical retention sent to arteriogram, roughly two-thirds had no significant stenosis. Dehydration or hypotension are often the cause (Fig. 8-18).

When looking at the TAC patterns, the degree of change is significant. As seen in Fig. 8-19, several response patterns are possible after ACE inhibitor imaging. It is critical to look at the degree of change from baseline. The pattern may change from a normal baseline to mildly-reduced or markedly-reduced function. A kidney with decreased function may progress to worsening grades of function. The greater the change, the more likely significant renal artery stenosis is present causing renovascular hypertension.

Quantitation can aid in assessing functional change seen on the images. With Tc-99m DTPA, a 10% decrease in relative function (differential function or split renal function) or a decrease in absolute function (calculated GFR) greater than 10% is considered "high probability" or positive; a change of 5–9% is intermediate or borderline in significance. Although a change in relative (differential) cortical function may not be seen with Tc-99m MAG3, if a change of 10% or greater occurs, it is considered "high probability." Although no change will be seen

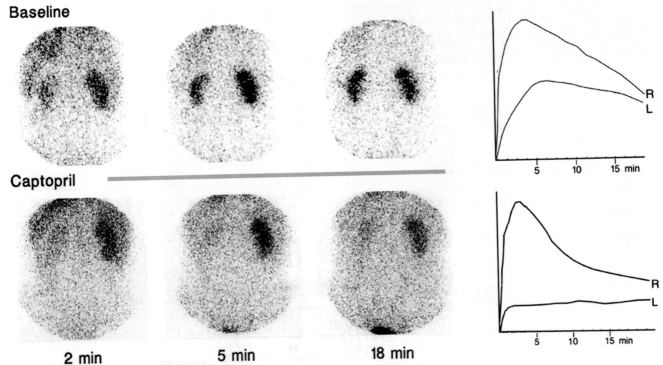

Baseline

Captopril

2 min   5 min   18 min

Figure 8-16   Effects of renovascular hypertension on Tc-99m DTPA. *Top*, The baseline study shows mildly decreased function on the left. *Bottom*, Exam after captopril reveals severe deterioration on the left kidney with diminished peak and overall function.

in RPF or ERPF calculated with Tc-99m MAG3, the cortical retention will be reflected in an increased 20/peak or 20/3 ratios. An increased time to peak (T_{max} or T_{peak}).

The kidney must function well enough to actually show a change in function when ACE inhibitors are given. Therefore, a small shrunken kidney or one with poor baseline function can be difficult to interpret. In general, ACE inhibitor renography is accurate when the serum creatinine is normal or only mildly elevated (creatinine <1.7 mg/dL).

If the protocol has been properly followed, sensitivity and specificity of ACE inhibitor renography have been reported to be approximately 90% and 95%, respectively. However, the sensitivity and specificity are lower in patients with elevated creatinine. False positives are rare but have been reported in patients on calcium channel blockers.

Reporting

If the ACE inhibitor study is normal, the study should be read as "low probability" of a renin-dependent renovascular hypertension. This means the posttest chance of renovascular hypertension is less than 10%. In general no additional workup is needed. If the 2-day protocol was used, the patient need not return for a baseline

study. An "intermediate probability" should be reported in patients with an abnormal baseline study who show no change after ACE inhibitors. Patients in this group would include those with ischemic nephropathy (who often have a unilateral small kidney), bilateral cortical retention and those showing only small changes in function. If these patients were considered as positives, the sensitivity of the exam would remain high but the specificity for RVH would be lowered to 50–75%.

A "high probability" (Box 8-6) result indicates a greater than 90% chance of RVH, and indicates these patients are highly likely to improve with angioplasty or surgery. These high-probability exams occur when function markedly worsens on the ACE inhibitor challenge when compared to the baseline study. Again, in a positive study, Tc-99m MAG3 will show worsening as marked cortical retention, whereas Tc-99m DTPA will show a fall in peak function and a decrease in relative function or GFR.

Urinary Tract Obstruction

Uncorrected urinary obstruction can lead to recurrent infection, diminished function, progressive loss of nephrons, and parenchymal atrophy. When the upper urinary tract is obstructed, there is backpressure from the

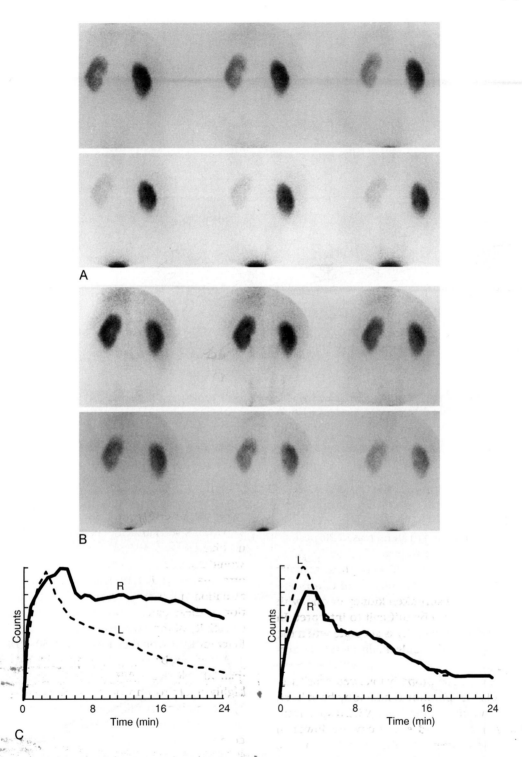

Figure 8-17   Positive captopril study with Tc-99m MAG3. **A,** The captopril study was performed first. Note prompt symmetrical initial uptake. Over time the left kidney washes out normally, but the right shows almost all activity remaining in the cortex. **B,** Following captopril, the scan shows marked cortical retention in the abnormal right kidney. **C,** *Left:* captopril, *right:* no captopril. The pattern is confirmed on the time–activity curves and is "high probability" for RAS as a cause for renovascular hypertension.

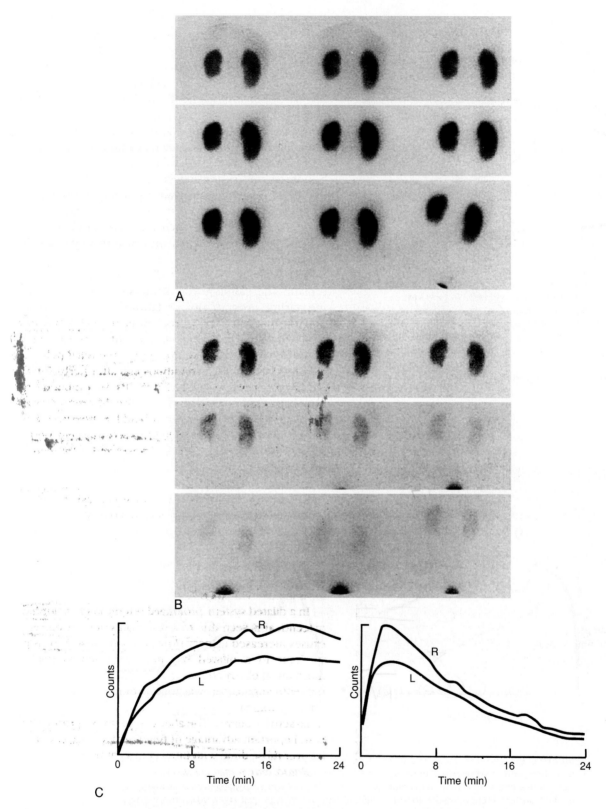

Figure 8-18   Bilateral cortical retention from dehydration. **A,** Captopril-stimulated study with Tc-99m MAG3. There is bilateral cortical retention and minimal urinary bladder clearance over 30 minutes. **B,** Baseline study without captopril shows normal cortical function and good clearance into the bladder. **C,** *Left,* captopril; *right,* baseline time–activity curves confirm the impression that bilateral renal artery stenosis may be present. The arteriogram on this patient was normal. Further investigation revealed the patient had abstained from food and drink for nearly 12 hours before captopril study but was hydrated for the subsequent baseline exam, and the resulting dehydration was presumed to cause the false-positive imaging pattern.

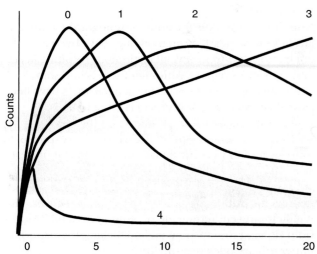

Figure 8-19   Renogram pattern changes with ACE inhibitors. The possible patterns after captopril with progressive worsening of function (0–4). Normal TAC curves (grade 0) have low probability of RVH. As curve grade (1–4) worsens from the normal baseline, the likelihood of RVH increases. Grade 1: Peak mildly delayed but greater than 5 min and with delayed excretion. Grade 2: Very delayed uptake but some washout. Grade 3: Extremely delayed uptake with no washout. Grade 4: Complete renal failure where blood pool moves through the kidney without an extraction phase.

Box 8-6   Positive ACE Inhibitor Renography Results

TC-99M DTPA

Primary positive finding:
　　Overall drop in function
Quantitation changes:
　　>10% decrease in GFR
　　>10% decrease in differential function
Other findings:
　　Delayed time to peak
　　Increased cortical retention

TC-99M MAG3

Primary positive finding:
　　cortical retention
Other findings:
　　Delayed time to peak
　　Decreased differential function less common

---

pelvis onto the tubules and vessels. Within hours of onset, renal blood flow, glomerular filtration, and renal output are decreased. If a high-grade obstruction is corrected promptly, function can recover fully; however, if left uncorrected for over a week, only partial recovery is expected. Therefore, a screening test that could noninvasively diagnose significant obstruction is very important.

Ultrasonography is a sensitive method of identifying a dilated collecting system but can not reliably determine if this is due to significant mechanical obstruction or merely nonobstructive hydronephrosis (such as from reflux, primary megaureter, or a previous obstruction which has been relieved). Contrast studies such as IVP and conventional radionuclide renography show overlapping findings that overlap between obstructed and nonobstructed systems: delayed filling, dilatation, and decreased washout. Retrograde pyelography, endoscopy and noncontrast CT scans can often identify the etiology of an obstructed system (such as a ureteral calculus) but do not provide functional information important in management.

The Whitaker test, first described in the 1970s, remains the standard for diagnosing obstruction by measuring pressure-flow relationships in the renal pelvis. This is an invasive technique involving bladder catheterization and inserting a needle into the renal pelvis under fluoroscopy. Pressure in the renal pelvis is measured under basal conditions and after perfusion of a dilute contrast solution (Fig. 8-20). In a dilated but nonobstructed collecting system, the differential pressure between the kidney and bladder measures less than 10–12 cm of water. In an obstructed system, perfusion pressure exceeds 15 cm of water and is frequently much higher.

Diuretic Renography

Diuretic renography is an excellent, noninvasive method for evaluating patients with suspected obstruction. Serial diuretic renography can be performed to determine the significance of a partial obstruction. It is also possible to assess effectiveness of stenting or surgical correction of an obstruction. A list of conditions that this test is used for is included in Box 8-7.

In a dilated system, prolonged retention of radiopharmaceutical is seen due to a reservoir effect. A diuretic causes increased urinary flow and will cause a prompt washout in a dilated but nonobstructed system. If mechanical obstruction is present, the narrowed lumen prevents augmented washout; prolonged retention of tracer proximal is seen and can be quantified on the time–activity curves. The ability to perform quantitation is an important advantage of functional radiotracer studies over those done with intravenous contrast dye.

Radiopharmaceuticals

The original agent used for diuretic renography was I-131 OIH. When renal function is normal, Tc-99m DTPA can be used successfully but should not be used in patients with azotemia. Tc-99m MAG3 has become the agent of choice because of its excellent quality images and high clearance rate, even in patients with renal insufficiency or immaturity.

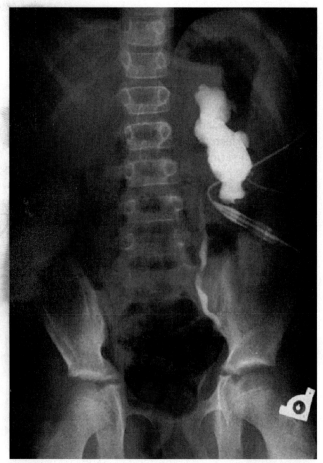

Figure 8-20 Whitaker test. Dilute contrast solution is infused into a dilated renal pelvis at the rate of 10 ml/min. Pressure measurements are obtained to evaluate for suspected obstruction.

Methods

Numerous protocols for diuretic renography exist, and attempts to standardize methodology have been made by comparing data from several institutions resulting in several consensus papers. Although there is still some variability among institutions, many general areas have been agreed on. An example protocol is listed in Box 8-8.

Patient Preparation Patients must be well-hydrated so fluid is available for mobilization in response to diuresis and to prevent dehydration from the diuresis. The bladder should be catheterized in children and infants, in those who can not void voluntarily, and when neurogenic bladder or outlet obstruction is present. This will help prevent retrograde pressure from a full bladder from slowing the washout and mimicking the pattern of upper urinary track obstruction.

Diuretic Administration Furosemide is a loop diuretic that inhibits sodium and chloride reabsorption, markedly increasing urine flow in normal patients. The injection is given slowly over 1-2 minutes with an onset

---

Box 8-7 Urological Conditions Studied by Diuresis Renography

Ureteropelvic junction obstruction
Megaureter: obstructive, nonobstructive, refluxing
Horseshoe kidney
Polycystic kidney
Prune-belly syndrome
Ectopic ureterocele
Urethral valves
Postoperative states
Pyeloplasty
Ureteral reimplantation
Urinary diversion
Renal transplant ureteral obstruction
Obstructing pelvic mass
Ileal loop diversion

Box 8-8 Diuretic Renography Protocol Summary

PATIENT PREPARATION

Hydration as described in dynamic renography protocol
Place Foley catheter in children; consider in adults
If not catheterized, bladder emptying must be complete before diuretic injection and after 20-min study.

FUROSEMIDE DOSE

Children: 1 mg/kg to maximum 40 mg (may require more in severe azotemia)
Adults: base dose on creatinine level

Serum Creatinine (mg/dl)	Creatinine Clearance (ml)	Furosemide Dose (mg)
1.0	100	20
1.5	75	40
2.0	50	60
3.0	30	80

IMAGING PROCEDURE

Inject Tc-99m MAG 3-6 mG (111-222 MBq)
Acquire study for 20 minutes
Slowly infuse furosemide intravenously over 60 sec
Obtain pre-void and postvoid image in uncatheterized patients

IMAGE PROCESSING

On computer, draw ROI around entire kidney and pelvis
Generate time-activity curves
Calculate a half-emptying time or fitted half-time

of action within 30–60 seconds and a maximal effect seen at 15 minutes. The reported diuretic administration times have varied with injection times at 20 minutes after the radiopharmaceutical (F+20), at the same time as the radiopharmaceutical (F+0), and 15 minutes before the study (F−15). A commonly used method is the F+20 furosemide protocol.

Interpretation

In a normal, nondilated kidney, the TAC rapidly reaches a sharp peak and spontaneously clears rapidly. Furosemide diuresis accelerates the rate of radiotracer washout in a normal kidney. If an ROI is placed over the ureter, a transient spike after diuretic injection indicates passage of a bolus of accumulated activity from the renal pelvis.

A dilated but nonobstructed system may initially look like a normal kidney with a steep TAC uptake slope. However, a sharp peak is not seen and, as the dilated system fills, the TAC may show continued accumulation or a plateau 20–30 minutes after tracer injection. After furosemide infusion, a nonobstructed hydronephrotic kidney clears promptly due to increased urine flow (Fig. 8-21). An obstructed system, on the other hand, will not respond to the diuretic challenge; activity will continue to accumulate or sometimes stays at a plateau (Fig. 8-22).

The distinction between obstruction and nonobstructed hydronephrosis decreases as the collecting system volume becomes larger. In very distended systems, delayed washout may be seen whether obstruction is present or not. An "indeterminate" pattern of clearance is seen with little change on the images and the TAC (Fig. 8-23, *D*). This pattern can be explained by the formula: $T_t = V/F$, where V is the volume of the system, F is the flow rate, and T_t is the transit time through the system. According to this formula, as the volume increases, the transit time lengthens.

If renal function is very impaired, diuretic response to lasix may be markedly diminished, leading to prolonged washout even if no obstruction is present. In patients with azotemia, an increased Lasix dose or the F−15 diuretic infusion may be used. However, even with additional modifications, it may not be possible to induce sufficient diuresis to exclude obstruction in a poorly functioning kidney (Fig. 8-24).

At times, it is useful to quantitate collecting system clearance half-time or washout half-time ($T_{1/2}$). Numerous methods for calculating the $T_{1/2}$ have been described. The activity can be measured when the diuretic is given; then the length of time it takes to reach half that level can be used. As this does not account for the delay in furosemide effect, a more precise method might be to fit a curve to the steepest portion of the washout time–activity curve. In general, a $T_{1/2}$ less than 10–15 minutes indicates no obstruction is present, whereas values greater than 20 minutes are considered obstructed. Values between 15–20 minutes fall in a gray zone or indeterminate range.

Serial studies may be used to monitor patients with partial obstruction, with previously treated obstruction, or who are at risk for worsening obstruction. Some situations where this might be needed include cervical carcinoma and known partial ureteropelvic junction obstruction. Also, patients at high risk for functional deterioration from reflux, such as ileal loop diversions of the ureters, may be followed with interval studies. Periodic diuresis renography can help determine at what point aggressive intervention is needed.

Pitfalls and Limitations

An indeterminate diuretic renogram is neither positive nor negative and does not rule out obstruction. The Whitaker test had a similar category. Some nonobstructed patients with very hydronephrotic kidney collecting systems will have an indeterminate response because of the reservoir effect.

A limited response to furosemide may also be seen in infants. Because neonates have functionally immature kidneys, the lasix renogram may appear falsely obstructed. A follow-up study may be helpful in patients diagnosed with neonatal hydronephrosis. In general, surgeons prefer to perform surgery when the infant is larger and the genitourinary tract more mature.

Renal insufficiency poses another problem. A flat response may be seen with diuretics because function is inadequate for effective diuresis. A larger dose of lasix or administering the Lasix well before the exam begins (F−15 minutes) can be helpful sometimes. However, serum creatinine may remain normal if impairment is unilateral. Although serum creatinine is not a reliable indicator of the level of functional impairment, radionuclide calculation of GFR and ERPF are useful. Generally, function must not be less than 15% of normal. If the GFR on the affected side is less than 15 ml/min, diuretic renography is unreliable.

Other problems may affect interpretation. The effect of a full or neurogenic bladder must always be considered. A repeat exam after bladder catheterization may be helpful. Certain conditions, such as a pelvic kidney or low-lying renal transplant that may remain overlapped with the bladder, limit interpretation.

Renal Transplant Evaluation

Renal transplantation is a well-established surgical procedure (Fig. 8-25). Scintigraphy can assess many complications including acute rejection, acute tubular necrosis (or more properly termed, vasomotor nephropathy), vascular problems, and obstruction. Many radionuclide methods have been used to evaluate the renal allograft function and identify acute rejection (including gallium-67, labeled leukocytes, and platelets), but these have lacked specificity. Conventional renal scintigraphy has been widely used to evaluate function. Although the number of these examinations has decreased because many kidneys are

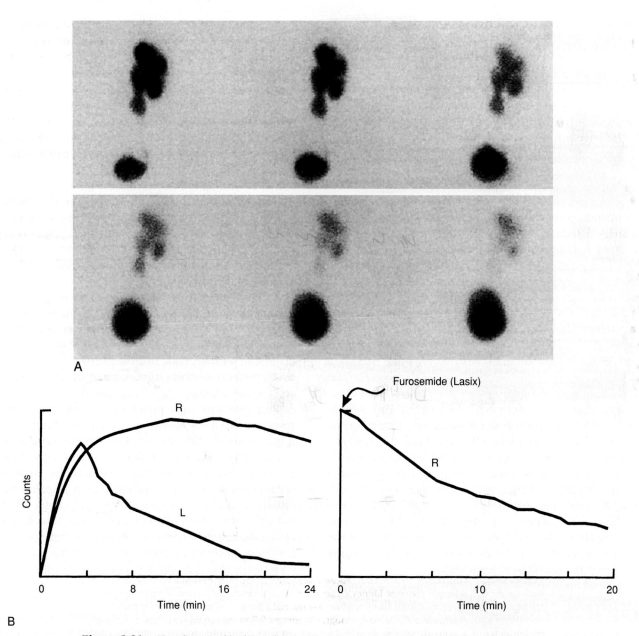

Figure 8-21   Nonobstructed hydronephrosis. Diuretic renogram of a patient with surgically treated vesicoureteral obstruction of the right kidney. **A,** Postfurosemide images show that the retained activity responds promptly to the diuretic with almost complete clearance. **B,** Time-activity curve promptly declines with Lasix, signifying no obstruction.

now evaluated by ultrasound and biopsy, radionuclide evaluation remains an important screening tool.

Kidneys for transplantation come from three sources: a deceased donor (cadaveric kidney), a living related donor, or a living unrelated donor. All potential donors are carefully screened with immunological matching and undergo functional and anatomic evaluation. Although cadaveric kidneys are carefully screened and transported, allografts from living donors generally have the best prognosis. One-year allograft survival rates are 90–94% for living related donor kidneys and 88–90% for cadaveric transplants.

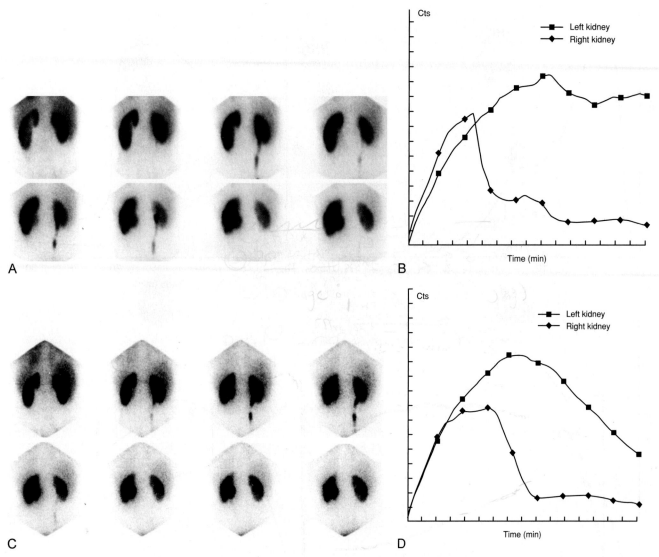

Figure 8-22   Obstructed hydronephrosis. **A,** Progressive filling of an enlarged collecting system is seen on the left, whereas the right kidney clears normally following Lasix administration at 10 minutes. **B,** Time–activity curves show washout on the right but no overall clearance on the left consistent with obstruction. **C,** Diuretic renography images following surgical correction of the left ureteropelvic junction obstruction show in the same patient hydronephrosis but improved clearance. **D,** Postoperative TACs confirm that no significant obstruction remains on the left.

The development of improved immunosuppressive drug therapy has been critical in the marked increase in allograft survival in recent years. These drugs act largely by suppressing the CD4 T-cell activity. Glucocorticoid steroids remain essential in the treatment and prevention of rejection. Now most regimens use triple-therapy, which include not only glucocorticoids and calcineurin inhibitors (tacrolimus or less often cyclosporin) but also an antiproliferative agent (such as azathioprine) that prevents mitosis and nonspecifically suppresses lymphocyte proliferation. Due to the increased risk of acute rejection in the immediate posttransplant period, anti-interleukin (IL)-2 monoclonal antibodies may also be given. T-cell specific monoclonal antibody muromonab-CD3 (OKT3), as

well as numerous other new and investigational agents, may be used to prevent and treat acute rejection. However, it is critical to determine precisely when these agents are needed and how to monitor patients due to potential serious acute and long-term side effects of these medications.

Multiple problems may be present in a patient who has undergone renal transplantation. A list of commonly encountered complications is provided in Table 8-4. These include vascular problems, rejection, leaks, and ureteral obstruction from extrinsic impression or effects of implantation. Rejection is commonly described in terms of the time frame in which it occurs: hyperacute, accelerated acute, acute, and chronic. Interpretation depends a great deal on the length of time from transplantation as well as

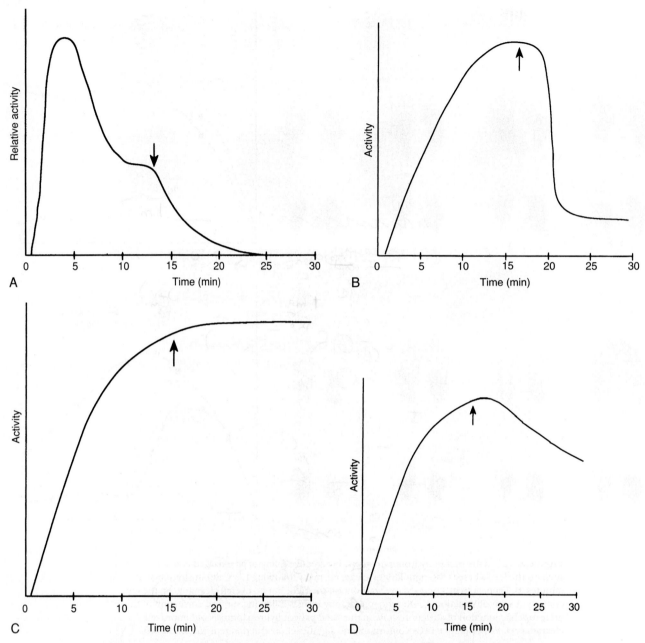

Figure 8-23   Diuresis renography time–activity curves (TACs). In these examples, Lasix is given at peak collecting system filling *(arrows)*. **A,** Normal kidney response to diuretic. The short plateau before further emptying represents diuretic-induced flow just before rapid clearance. **B,** Dilated nonobstructed kidney. The slowly rising curve represents progressive pelvocaliceal filling. With diuretic *(arrow),* rapid clearance occurs. **C,** Obstructed kidney. The diuretic has no effect on the abnormal TAC. **D,** Indeterminate response. Following diuretic, very slow partial clearance is seen. This can be the result of an extremely distended system but obstruction is not excluded.

the type of transplant. A baseline study is very useful in predicting long-term allograft function and assessing acute complications.

Medical Complications

Vasomotor Nephropathy or Ischemic Nephropathy   A common early complication of the transplanted kidney is vasomotor nephropathy (also properly called ischemic nephropathy or delayed graft function).

Although this is still sometimes commonly referred to as acute tubular necrosis (ATN), this terminology is not an entirely correct description. ATN is just one possible component of the process and there may be little if any destruction of the tubular elements. Vasomotor nephropathy is actually an ischemic response damaging the kidney at some point prior to completing transplantation. The functional impact ranges from a mild, rapidly

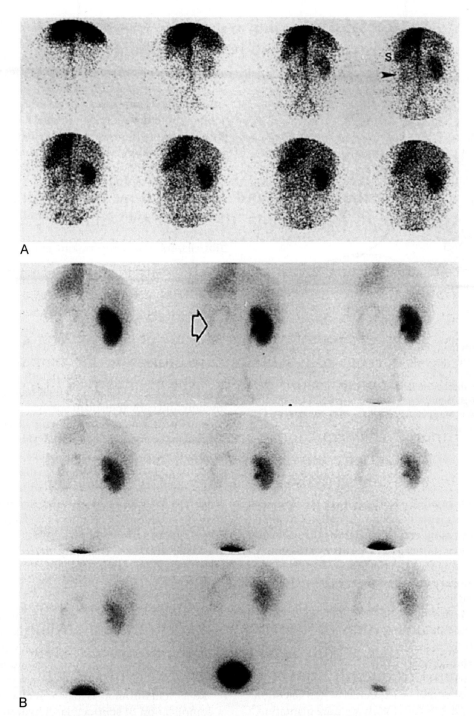

Figure 8-24   High-grade vesicoureteral junction obstruction secondary to tumor. **A,** Flow study shows very decreased perfusion to the left kidney *(arrowhead)*. **B,** Dynamic sequential images at 5-minute intervals show only a thin rim of cortex with poor uptake *(open arrowhead)* and a large photopenic collecting system consistent with hydronephrosis. Diuresis renography would not be useful as no tracer enters the collecting system.

resolving disorder to a slower recovery or total anuria (nonoliguric ATN). The severity of damage increases if the time between the donor's death and transplantation is prolonged. Vasomotor nephropathy is most common in cadaveric kidneys, occurring up to 50% of the time. However, it can be seen in grafts from living donors (5%),

especially if the surgery was complicated. Therefore, the renal function will be impaired at the time of transplant and should recover spontaneously beginning after transplantation and continuing over 1–2 weeks (Fig. 8-26).

Hyperacute Rejection   Careful HLA immunologic matching has eliminated hyperacute rejection. This is

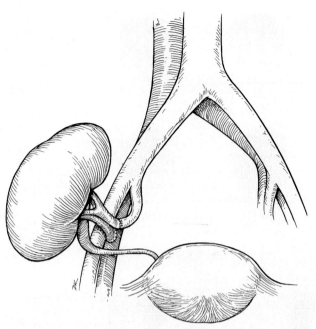

Figure 8-25   Renal transplant surgery. For technical reasons, the initial allograft is usually placed in the right iliac fossa. The vessels are attached end to end for the artery and side to side for the vein. The ureter is usually directly implanted into the recipient's bladder. After an initial failure, a second graft is usually placed in the left. If a pancreas is transplanted simultaneously, the pancreas is usually placed on the right.

the result of preformed antibodies in the recipient's circulation from a major histocompatibility or blood group mismatch causing renal vasculature thrombosis. The classic story is of the surgeon witnessing the kidney turning blue in the operating room after performing the vascular anastamosis. When this occurs, the allograft cannot be salvaged.

Accelerated Acute Rejection   Accelerated acute rejection is also uncommon but occurs in patients with antibodies already in their system, as in sensitization from pregnancy or from multiple blood transfusions. The patient presents with clinical signs of acute rejection at an earlier time than would be expected. When rejection develops in the first 3–5 days following transplantation, accelerated acute rejection should be suspected. Unlike hyperacute rejection, accelerated rejection often responds to therapy.

Acute Rejection   Acute rejection (AR) is a relatively frequent transplant complication. Although it can occur at any time, AR does not typically occur until at least 5–7 days after transplantation and is most common in the first 3 months. Typically, the patient becomes desensitized to the allograft over time, and AR is rarely seen after 1 year in a patient taking appropriate immunosuppressive therapy.

AR may be caused by two immunologic pathways: T cells or humoral antibodies. With either of these immunological mechanisms, the scintigraphic pattern is similar. Allograft vasculature is affected unlike with vasomotor nephropathy (Figs. 8-27 and 8-28). Arteritis, microinfarcts, and hemorrhage occur in the parenchyma along with lymphocytic infiltration. Clinically, it is common for the patient to be febrile and the allograft to be swollen and painful. Laboratory values include rising creatinine and an elevated sedimentation rate.

Chronic Allograft Nephropathy   Previously referred to as chronic rejection, chronic renal allograft nephropathy (CR) is a cumulative, delayed, and irreversible process. Vascular constriction, chronic fibrosis, tubular atrophy, and glomerulosclerosis from immunologic and nonhumoral etiologies occur. Over months to years, this fibrosis causes cortical loss and decreased function. Dilatation of the collecting system may occur as the cortex thins. Risk factors for early development (less than 1 year) include damage from early ischemic injury (severe ATN), prior severe rejection, subclinical rejection, and long-term calcineurin-inhibitor therapy. There is no effective therapy available for CR and it is now the leading cause of graft failure given improved therapy and early transplant survival.

Immunosuppressive Drug Toxicity   Another important cause of allograft dysfunction is drug nephrotoxicity of therapeutic drugs. Renal allograft drug toxicity was classically described in relation to cyclosporin and was often related to high levels of the drug and early administration. Currently, cyclosporine toxicity is seldom seen. It has been largely replaced with other agents and, when prescribed, the lower levels of the drug are safer. It is important to remember that similar changes can be seen with other antirejection agents.

Surgical Complications

Vascular Occlusion   Arterial thrombosis is a rare postoperative complication of transplantation, occurring in less than 1% of patients. It is usually related to kinking or difficulty performing the anastamosis with a short donor artery. No flow or function is seen in this situation.

Renal vein thrombosis may be seen in native kidneys as a complication of septicemia, dehydration, or nephrotic syndrome. These patients can be managed most often medically and function may recover. In the transplanted kidney, renal vein thrombosis can occur as a postoperative complication or related to autoimmune problems. The thrombus leads to infarct and hemorrhage. However, unlike the native kidney, there are no venous collaterals to drain the kidney and the effect is often severe with loss of the allograft.

Arterial Stenosis   Postoperative renal artery stenosis should be suspected in patients who develop hypertension following transplantation surgery. Stenosis may

Table 8-4   Complications after Renal Transplantation

Complication	Usual time of occurrence postoperatively	Comments
PRESURGICAL INSULT		
Vasomotor nephropathy (ATN) resolution	Minutes to hours	Cadaveric transplants; semicaler spontaneous
AUTOIMMUNE: REJECTION		
Hyperacute rejection	Minutes to hours	Preformed antibodies irreversible
Accelerated rejection	1–5 days	History of prior transplant or transfusion
Acute rejection	After 5 days, most common during first 3 months	Cell mediated, responsive to treatment
Chronic allograft nephropathy (chronic rejection)	Months to years	Humoral, irreversible, inevitable
Cyclosporin toxicity	Months	Reversible with drug withdrawal
SURGICAL		
Urine leak/urinoma	Days or weeks	
Hematoma	First few days	
Infection	First few days	
Lymphocele	2–4 months	
VASCULAR		
Renal artery stenosis	After first month	
Vascular occlusion		
Infarcts		
Renal		
Obstruction (extrinsic mass, stricture or calculi)	Days, months, years	
Vesicoureteroreflux		

occur in up to 10% of patients. Although the anastomotic site is the most common site, stenosis in other locations (including the iliac artery) must be considered. The imaging protocol is similar to the renovascular hypertension work up for native kidneys described in Box 8-6. The only difference is the anterior positioning of the camera over the allograft. Interpretation criteria are the same as for native kidneys.

Urinary Leak   Necrosis of the ureteral anastomosis in the immediate postoperative period can result in urinary leakage. Although other imaging modalities, such as ultrasound, can identify fluid in the pelvis, nuclear medicine techniques are better able to specifically identify the source.

Ureteral Obstruction   Although uncommon, ureteral obstruction may be caused by kinking of the ureter, extrinsic mass compression (e.g., hematoma, lymphocele), intraluminal obstruction (from blood clot or calculus), or periureteral fibrosis. Some degree of collecting system dilatation without significant mechanical obstruction is often seen from postoperative hematomas and seromas. Hydronephrosis from obstruction must be differentiated from dilatation caused by reflux. This can be done with diuretic renography. Ureteral obstruction often resolves spontaneously.

Lymphoceles   Because the transplanted kidney has no lymphatic connections, lymphoceles can form in the transplant bed. This may occur in up to 10% of transplants and is seen typically 2–3 months posttransplant. These are only clinically important if they impinge on ureter or vasculature.

Methods

Renal allograft evaluation is performed using the dynamic scintigraphy protocol with Tc-99m MAG3 listed in Box 8-4, with the exception of positioning. The patient is imaged anteriorly with the camera centered over the allograft in the lower pelvis. It is useful to include at least some of the native kidneys in the field of view as they may contribute to overall function. Some portion of the bladder should be seen, and the entire bladder is included on prevoid and postvoid images.

Numerous semiquantitative and quantitative methods have been described. ERPF, GFR and Tc-99m MAG3 clearance are all good indices of renal function. More commonly, semiquantitative techniques such as the 20/3 ratio described in the dynamic renography section are used as

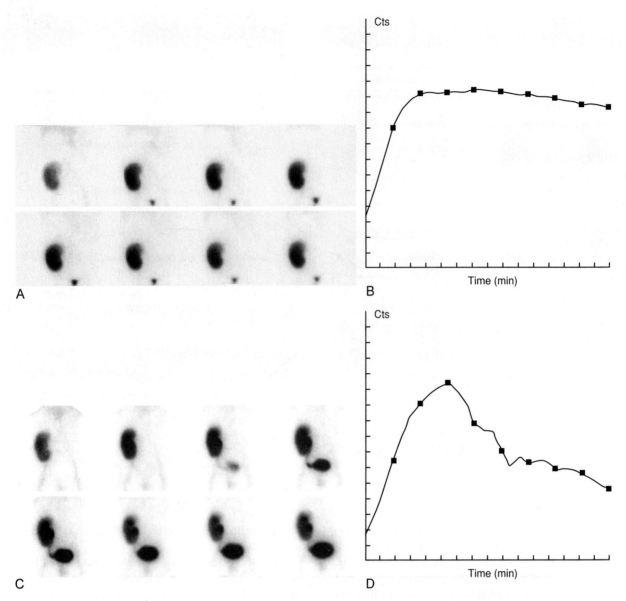

Figure 8-26 Vasomotor nephropathy (ATN). **A,** Baseline images obtained 24 hours after transplantation reveal prompt uptake but significant cortical retention. **B,** Baseline TAC shows a steep upslope which goes against vascular involvement and poor overall clearance confirming the diagnosis of vasomotor nephropathy. **C,** A follow-up exam shows resolution of the abnormal findings and relatively good function, which is confirmed on the TAC curves in **D**.

a measure of radiopharmaceutical transit and cortical retention.

In general, a study should be done within a day or two of transplantation to obtain a picture of the baseline level of function. This baseline is critical in accurately assessing any problems that occur later and improves detection of subtle abnormalities. The protocol can be modified to answer any question that arises. If concern for renal artery stenosis exists, the ACE inhibitor protocol is used. The diuretic renography protocol can be followed when hydronephrosis develops or obstruction is suspected. Delayed images over the course of 1–2 hours can help clarify the etiology of fluid collections and assess possible urine leaks.

Interpretation

Because the medical and surgical complications described previously occur at certain times, renal transplant scintigrams must be interpreted with the age of the transplant as well as the clinical context (including physical symptoms, laboratory values, and current medications) in mind. The type of allograft (cadaveric or living related donor transplant) is especially important and needs to be considered when evaluating vasomotor nephropathy or the expected level of renal function.

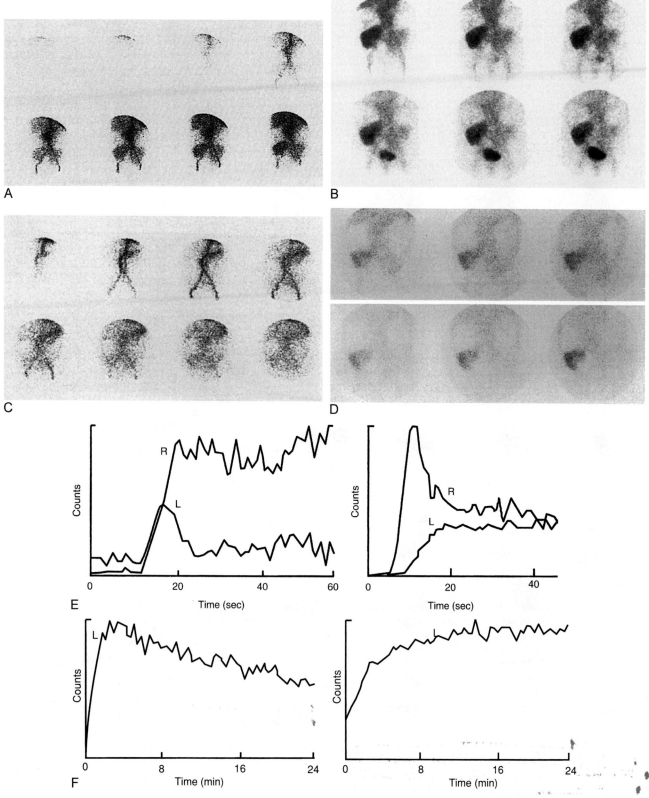

Figure 8-27 Acute allograft rejection. Tc-99m MAG3 images of a right iliac fossa cadaveric transplant. Good baseline blood flow **(A)** and good function **(B)** are seen at the end of first week. Two days later, the patient developed fever, allograft tenderness and elevated serum creatinine. Repeat blood flow is diminished **(C)** and functional images show cortical retention **(D)**. These findings are consistent with acute rejection. **E,** Perfusion time activity curves show initial good blood flow *(left)* which falls on the follow up study *(right)* due to acute rejection. **F,** The TACs over the 25-minute study show adequate baseline function *(left)* and that deteriorates at the time of rejection *(right)*.

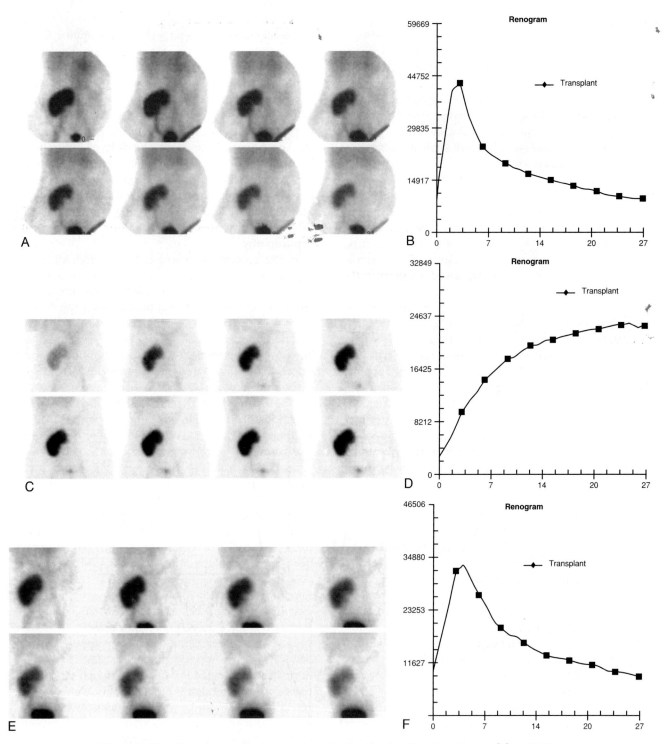

Figure 8-28   Time course of acute transplant rejection. Baseline functional images (**A**) and TACs (**B**) are unremarkable. Two months later, images show delayed uptake and cortical retention (**C**). This is confirmed on the TAC (**D**). Function improves with immunosuppressive therapy on the follow-up scan (**E**) and time–activity curve (**F**) 1 week later.

A baseline study is essential in the immediate postoperative period to be able to interpret any abnormality seen. During the perfusion phase, the transplanted kidney normally becomes the "hottest" structure within 2–4 seconds of appearance of activity in the adjacent iliac artery following a good bolus of radiopharmaceutical. The images and functional time–activity curves normally show a prompt peak and rapid clearance. The expected level of perfusion and function will typically diminish over the years as discussed later.

A living related donor allograft will usually function better and clear radiotracer more rapidly than a cadaveric allograft. Therefore, "normal" function is somewhat relative. Because the level of function will vary from kidney to kidney as well as over time, a baseline study done in the first 24–48 hours is extremely helpful. If rejection is suspected later, it may not be diagnosed properly without the baseline comparison.

In vasomotor nephropathy, scintigraphic images show normal perfusion but poor function with delayed cortical clearance and decreased urine excretion (see Fig. 8-26). Vasomotor nephropathy is seen on the baseline study done in the first 24–48 hours following surgery, most often in a cadaveric allograft, and resolves over 1–3 weeks. Although the degree of impairment varies, no urine output is seen in severe cases. Severe cortical retention or function that does not rapidly improve on serial studies has strong negative prognostic implications with few such kidneys surviving over 6 months. Because it usually resolves spontaneously, it is suspicious if function does not improve or if it worsens. There may be a new ischemic or nephrotoxic insult or, most likely, acute rejection may be developing.

Nephrotoxic effects of immunosuppressive therapy may demonstrate a pattern of prompt uptake and delayed clearance similar to vasomotor nephropathy. This used to be frequently seen due to cyclosporine toxicity and can still occur, although it may be due to other agents given the currently used low cyclosporin doses. The time frame of the exam allows these two processes to be differentiated. Vasomotor nephropathy is seen immediately whereas time is required for nephrotoxicity or true ATN to occur.

If hyperacute rejection was ever to be imaged, there would be essentially no perfusion and a photopenic area would be seen where the kidney should be on subsequent functional images. This pattern of absent flow and function can be seen occasionally, but it is due to severe vascular compromise such as renal artery thrombosis or renal vein thrombosis (Fig. 8-29, *A*). It should be noted that renal vein thrombosis in a transplanted kidney appears differently from the usual appearance in native kidneys (Fig. 8-29, *B*). Native kidneys can rely on venous collaterals until function often recovers, but these collaterals are absent in a transplanted kidney.

The classic dynamic imaging pattern of acute rejection is decreased perfusion with delayed uptake. Tc-99m MAG3 will also show cortical retention. Because AR affects small renal parenchymal vessels, the allograft may show diminished blood flow on the perfusion portion of the exam. Because dynamic perfusion imaging is difficult to do, it is sometimes necessary to assess perfusion based on the early portion of the TAC for the entire functional part of the study. The delayed radiopharmaceutical uptake is seen with a shallow upward slope of the TAC and an early patchy image. The kidney shows a prolonged parenchymal transit with cortical retention (*see* Figs. 8-27 and 8-28) and may appear enlarged. Table 8-5 compares acute rejection and vasomotor nephropathy.

In the immediate postoperative period, AR may be superimposed on a patient with previously identified vasomotor nephropathy. In these cases, the cortical retention of vasomotor nephropathy on the baseline exam does not resolve as expected or shows worsening function on serial exams. Obviously, this means a baseline study is extremely helpful. Although the uptake slope of the functional curve is usually normal with vasomotor nephropathy and more shallow with AR, it may be technically difficult to differentiate the two complications on the basis of differences in perfusion. In addition, both conditions show cortical retention on the renogram. However, the later time course of AR compared with vasomotor nephropathy will allow them to be differentiated if a baseline study has been done. Of course, other problems such as infection, renal artery or vein thrombosis, and leak must be excluded.

In CR, the blood flow and function images may initially appear normal. Often, the changes of CR may only be revealed through quantitative means such as ERPF and GFR measurement. Quantitation will show decreased function with a downward trend over time on serial examinations (Fig. 8-29). As the CR worsens, parenchymal retention is seen, although this is in a poorly functioning kidney with all functional parameters appearing abnormal. The cortex appears patchy and less intense than normal and clearance is delayed. Although mild to moderate cortical retention is often seen in CR, more marked retention is likely due to another process. When a scan is ordered in a kidney older than 1–2 years, it is important to remember that AR seldom occurs if the patient is adequately immunosuppressed. Usually, significant cortical retention is a sign of true ATN.

The nephrotoxic effect of immunosuppressive therapy such as cyclosporine A has a similar appearance to AR. The functional portion of the study shows slow uptake, cortical retention, and decreased function. A biopsy may be needed to differentiate changes from drug toxicity and other chronic allograft diseases from AR or ATN, especially when blood levels of the drug are not elevated.

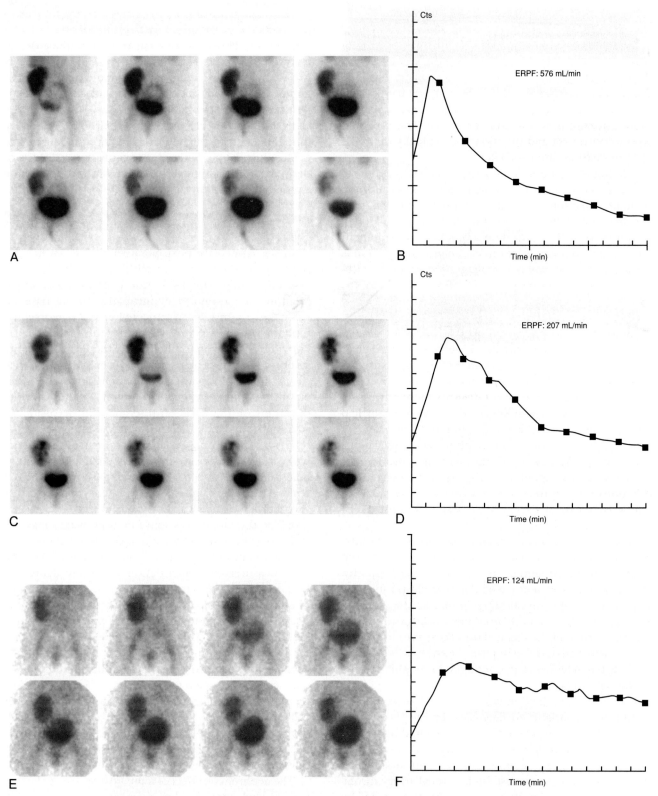

Figure 8-29 Chronic renal allograft nephropathy (formerly called chronic rejection). Baseline scan (**A**) and baseline time-activity curve (**B**) 24 hours after transplantation reveal good uptake and clearance. Note the presence of a Foley catheter draining the bladder and some function in native kidneys at the top edge of the image. Images done over 1 year later are unremarkable (**C**), although some decline is suggested on the time-activity curve (**D**). A steady decline in ERPF is characteristic and often the only way to diagnose the early stages of disease. Four months later as creatinine continued to rise, the scan shows a visible decline in function (**E**), also seen on the curve (**F**).

Table 8-5   Comparison of Acute Rejection and Vasomotor Nephropathy

	Baseline scan	Follow-up scan	Perfusion	Renal transit time
Acute rejection	Normal	Worsens	↓	↑
Vasomotor nephropathy (ATN)	Abnormal	Improves	Normal	↑

Although vascular complications are rare, they must be suspected in the anuric patient. Renal artery occlusion leads to absent perfusion and a photopenic defect on the functional portion of scintigraphy. Although renal vein thrombosis in native kidneys has a variable appearance depending on severity and stage of resolution, the classic appearance is of an enlarged kidney with intense cortical retention initially; deteriorating function and a patchy nephrogram are possible later. In a transplanted kidney, there are no venous collaterals to drain the kidney so the impact is more severe, causing

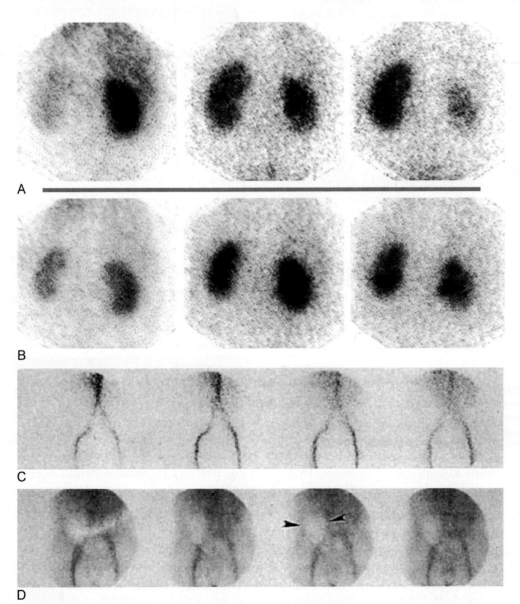

Figure 8-30   Renal vein thrombosis. **A,** Renal vein thrombosis in a native kidney. The I-131 01H scan reveals poor uptake and delayed clearance in the left native kidney which improves on a follow-up scan 4 months later. **B,** Images from a renal allograft with renal vein thrombosis. The radionuclide angiogram demonstrates no perfusion to the transplanted kidney. **C,** Dynamic images acquired immediately after the flow study and sequentially every 5 minutes show a photopenic defect *(arrowheads)* resulting from nonviable allograft causing attenuation but having no uptake **(D).**

the kidney to have a similar appearance to renal artery occlusion.

A postoperative leak may occur at the anastomotic site or due to rupture of an obstructed allograft. A progressive accumulation of activity outside of the urinary tract may be seen on dynamic scintigraphic images. A slow leak may be seen as a photopenic defect from a nonradiolabeled urinoma (Fig. 8-31). If Tc-99m DTPA is being used, delayed imaging at 2 hours or later may be needed to detect increasing activity in this fluid collection. Delayed images with Tc-99m MAG3 may be misinterpreted as showing a leak due to the normal bowel activity appearance over time. Other fluid collections such as lymphoceles and hematomas may be noted as fixed pararenal, photon-deficient areas.

An obstructed allograft may present with hydronephrosis or diminished urine output. Diuretic renography can be useful in evaluating suspected obstruction in a similar manner as in native kidneys. It is important that no AR is present and that function is adequate to respond to the diuretic (ERPF >75 ml/min).

MEASURING RENAL FUNCTION: ERPF AND GFR

Clinical assessment of renal function using blood urea nitrogen (BUN) and serum creatinine is a relatively crude process, as a significant decrease in function must occur before changes in BUN and creatinine are seen. Also, changes in metabolism and diet, differences in muscle mass, and certain medications can affect creatinine levels. Occasionally, creatinine clearance is measured and is more accurate. However, the 24-hour urine collection makes it difficult to use.

In the laboratory, accurate quantification of GFR and ERPF is possible with substances that are not radioactive. Because it is freely filtered at the glomerulus but is neither secreted at the tubules nor reabsorbed, the molecule inulin is the model for GFR measurement. If a substance has complete first-pass extraction through the kidney, it can measure RPF. Approximately 90% of PAH is extracted and has been used to estimate RPF; however, as it is incompletely cleared, the term ERPF is used. Inulin and PAH are technically demanding to use, requiring continuous infusion to achieve a steady state; its clearance is then measured through multiple blood and urine samples.

Nuclear medicine techniques have evolved utilizing analogs of inulin and PAH. Different combinations of plasma sampling and imaging techniques are available. These nuclear medicine techniques provide simple and accurate methods to quantify function.

Effective Renal Plasma Flow

The radiolabeled forms of hippuric acid, I-131 OIH and I-123 OIH, have been used to quantify ERPF. The urinary clearance of I-131 OIH is approximately 85% of PAH. The difference is attributed to higher plasma protein binding and differences in tubular transport. Currently, Tc-99m MAG3 has replaced the hippuran agents in clinical use. Because Tc-99m MAG3 does not undergo glomerular filtration and has a slightly lower level of tubular secretion, it has a reported roughly 60% that of hippuran. However, extensive studies have been done that prove ERPF values obtained with Tc-99m MAG3 are accurate once corrected for the different extraction fraction.

Although the most precise ERPF techniques involve multiple blood samples, researchers have studied clearance patterns to determine the best times for sampling so that single blood sample protocols can be done. By waiting for a time point when the radiopharmaceutical has fully distributed in the body and blood pool, any decrease in activity should reflect renal clearance. A blood sample at 44 minutes has shown to be reproducible within 19 ml/min.

Glomerular Filtration Rate

Many radiopharmaceutical analogs of inulin have been used to evaluate glomerular filtration. Tc-99m DTPA and I-125 iothalamate (Glofil) are available in the United States for calculating GFR. In the past, variable protein binding levels due to impurities in Tc-99m DTPA led to inaccuracies in GFR calculations. With careful monitoring to ensure a low level of protein binding near 1%, Tc-99m DTPA is an excellent radiopharmaceutical for GFR measurement.

Cr-51 EDTA is widely utilized for GFR evaluation in many countries but is not available in the United States. The long half-life (27.7 days) and high-energy gamma emissions (320 keV) necessitate a low dose not suitable for gamma-camera imaging. However, delayed scintillation well counter measurements can be done accurately, adding to convenience. It closely approximates inulin clearance without the protein binding problem that can occur when using DTPA.

Like ERPF determinations, multiple blood sample techniques were first used to calculate GFR. Single- and two-blood sample techniques were then developed. The single-blood sample technique is reliable and most widely used. However, although the single-sample technique is the most practical, the blood sampling must be done much later than with ERPF, most commonly at 3 hours, making it much less convenient.

Normal GFR values are approximately 100 ml/min for adults. The results are accurate unless function is markedly diminished (GFR <30 ml/min). In infants, renal function reaches adult levels by 2 years of age. Pediatric GFR values should be corrected for body surface area.

Camera Technique

Often, an imaging department is not set up to perform the scintillation counting and wet lab work needed to calculate GFR and ERPF using blood sampling techniques. Camera based methods require no blood sampling and only a few minutes of imaging time (Fig. 8-32).

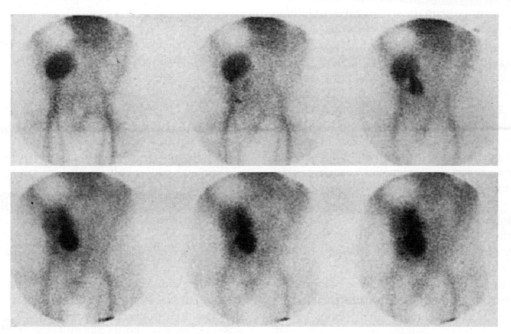

Figure 8-31   Postoperative urinary leak. Rapid leakage resulted from disrupted surgical anastomosis. Note accumulation of radiotracer just inferior to the transplant but superior and lateral to the bladder.   No bladder filling is seen.

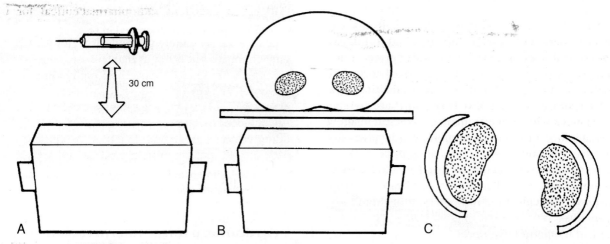

Figure 8-32   Gamma camera technique for quantitation of glomerular filtration (GFR). **A,** One-minute image of the Tc-99m DTPA syringe acquired before and after injection, 30-cm distance from the center of the collimator. **B,** After injection, 15-sec/frame images are acquired for a total of 6 minutes. **C,** Kidney and background regions are selected on the images to obtain counts. After correcting for background and attenuation, the net renal cortical uptake as a percentage of the total injected dose is determined.

Precise adherence to protocol is necessary for these techniques, and they are more prone to error than the blood sampling methods.

In order to perform a camera-based GFR calculation, a small known dose of Tc-99m DTPA is counted a set distance from the camera face to determine the count rate before injecting it into the patient. The actual administered dose is then corrected for the postinjection residual in the syringe and serves as a standard. If the dose is too large, it may overwhelm the counting capabilities of the system and lost counts would affect accuracy, causing overestimation of GFR.

After injection, images are acquired for 6 minutes. ROIs are drawn around the kidneys and the counts are background subtracted. Attenuation of the photons caused by varying renal depth is corrected using formuli based on patient weight and height. The fraction of the standard taken up by the kidneys in the 1–2.5 minute or 2–3 minute frames is correlated with the GFR measured by one of the accepted standard methods (such as multiple blood sample, single blood sample, or less accurately by creatinine clearance). A similar camera based approach can be used for ERPF calculation.

It should be noted that any method for measuring function may not be "accurate" measurements of function, but they are proven to be precise. Because these results are highly reproducible in any one patient, patients can be followed over time using this method.

RENAL CORTICAL IMAGING

It is often difficult clinically to distinguish upper urinary tract infections (UTI) from lower tract UTI. However, the long-term complications and therapeutic implications of renal parenchymal infection are very different from those of lower urinary tract disease. Infection and reflux can lead to cortical scarring, renal failure, and hypertension.

In most instances today, lesions of the renal cortex are evaluated with the structural imaging modalities ultrasound, CT, and sometimes MRI. However, there are specific instances when nuclear medicine cortical imaging adds vital information. Most commonly this involves suspected pyelonephritis in the pediatric patient. Occasionally, cortical scintigraphy is used to differentiate a prominent column of Bertin seen on ultrasound from a true mass. Although either Tc-99m DMSA or Tc-99m glucoheptonate could be used, Tc-99m DMSA is preferred because of its superior resolution.

Acute Pyelonephritis

Acute pyelonephritis usually results from reflux of infected urine. The clinical diagnosis of acute pyelonephri-

tis based on fever, flank pain, and positive urine cultures is unreliable and especially difficult in infants. Therefore, recurrent infections often occur and lead to significant damage and scarring. This process is a significant cause of long-term morbidity, causing hypertension and chronic renal failure. The need for a noninvasive test to diagnose acute pyelonephritis is clear.

Originally, contrast IVP was used. However, IVP was found to be insensitive, in addition to the risk associated with intravenous contrast. CT can often identify the inflammatory change in the kidney, as can radiolabeled white blood cells and gallium-67 citrate. However, these tests are not suitable for frequent use, especially in children. Ultrasound is widely used to assess the kidney and is generally considered an essential part of the pyelonephritis workup. However, sonography is relatively insensitive to the inflammatory changes of acute pyelonephritis, as well as the residual cortical defects and scars. Reported ultrasound sensitivities range from 24–40% for pyelonephritis and are approximately 65% for the detection of scars.

Cortical scintigraphy with Tc-99m DMSA is significantly more sensitive then sonography. Sensitivities for acute pyelonephritis are difficult to determine as Tc-99m DMSA itself is considered the gold standard. Most frequently, cortical scanning is done in children with acute pyelonephritis. It may also be performed as part of the workup of patients with vesicoureteral reflux who have no evidence of active pyelonephritis.

Method

With Tc-99m DMSA, dynamic imaging is not performed because background clearance is slow and only a small percentage of the radiotracer is cleared by the kidney. Only delayed cortical planar or SPECT imaging is acquired. An example protocol is discussed in Box 8-9.

Planar imaging usually requires at least both posterior and posterior oblique views. A pinhole collimator or converging collimator provides magnification and improved resolution. High-resolution SPECT affords excellent resolution, although a multiple head camera with high resolution collimators is preferable. In addition, children may require sedation for SPECT as they must be completely still for the entire acquisition. With Tc-99m GH, similar delayed-imaging protocols are used, although dynamic imaging can be acquired first.

Cortical Scan Image Interpretation

The normal Tc-99m DMSA scan should show a homogeneous distribution throughout the renal cortex. The shape of the kidney is variable, as is the thickness of the cortex. The upper poles may often appear less intense due to splenic impression on the cortex, fetal lobulation, and

Box 8-9 Renal Cortical Imaging Protocol Summary

RADIOPHARMACEUTICAL

Tc-99m DMSA: adult, 5 mCi (185 MBq); child, 50 mg/kg (minimum dose of 600 uCi)

Tc-99m GH: adult 15–20 mCi (555–740 MBq); child, 200 mCi/kg

INSTRUMENTATION

Planar camera: large-field-of-view gamma camera, parallel-hole collimator for differential calculation. Pinhole collimator for cortical images. Converging collimator may be used for adults.

SPECT: dual- or triple-head preferred

IMAGING PROCEDURE

Patient should void before starting

Inject radiopharmaceutical intravenously

Image at 2 hours after injection.

Acquire parallel collimator images for 500k on anterior and posterior views for differential calculation.

Pinhole images acquire for 100k counts per view. Position patient so each kidney is imaged separately, but the camera is same distance from patient.

Quantify function as geometric mean (square root of the product of anterior and posterior counts)

SPECT

Camera: dual-head or triple-headed with low-energy ultra-high resolution collimator

Matrix: 128 × 128

Zoom: as needed

Orbit: noncircular body contour, rotate 180 degrees, step and shoot 40 views/head, 3 degrees/stop, 40-sec/stop

Reconstruction: 64 × 64 Hamming filter with high cutoff

Smoothing kernel

Attenuation correction

---

attenuation from liver and spleen. The central collecting system and medullary regions are photon deficient as Tc-99m DMSA tubular binding occurs in the cortex. The columns of Bertin will show radiopharmaceutical uptake and may appear quite prominent. In a study performed to differentiate prominent column of Bertin from true mass, the Tc-99m DMSA scan will show radiotracer uptake in a column of Bertin but not in a mass caused by tumor.

Areas of cortical tubular dysfunction from infection or scar present as cortical defects. This may be caused by localized mass effect and edema from the inflammatory process, as well as by actual tubular dysfunction and ischemia. A tumor will also present as a defect because cortical scanning is not specific. Therefore, comparison with ultrasound is advisable.

Infection may present as a focal ill-defined lesion or as a multifocal process (Fig. 8.33). A diffuse decrease in activity may also be seen; if it occurs without volume loss, it would suggest a diffuse inflammatory process. Scars would be expected to have localized, sharp margins and may occur in a small kidney with associated cortical loss. However, it is extremely difficult to tell an area of acute inflammation from a scar without serial images, particularly in patients with clinically silent infections.

In the workup of acute abnormalities due to acute pyelonephritis, serial scans may also be useful to assess the extent of recovery. In general, it is advisable to wait 6 months from the acute infection to allow recovery. The acute inflammatory changes in pyelonephritis will usually resolve over time (nearly 40%) or significantly improve (44%). Any defect persisting after 6 months should be considered a chronic scar.

Multiheaded SPECT is more sensitive than planar techniques for detection of small defects because of its better contrast resolution. However, specificity may be somewhat lower because some apparent cortical defects actually may be caused by normal variations such as fetal lobulation and splenic impression. Experience with either technique can give excellent clinical results.

Clinical Applications

Radionuclide Cystography

Radionuclide cystography was introduced in the late 1950s to diagnose vesicoureteral reflux (VUR) and is widely accepted as the technique of choice for the evaluation and follow-up of children with UTIs and reflux. The radionuclide method is more sensitive than contrast-enhanced cystography for detecting reflux and results in considerably less radiation exposure to the patient. In many centers, contrast-voiding urethrocystography is reserved for the initial workup of male patients to exclude an anatomical cause for reflux, such as posterior urethral valves.

Vesicoureteral Reflux

Untreated reflux and infection are associated with subsequent renal damage, scarring, hypertension, and chronic renal failure. VUR occurs in approximately 1–2% of the pediatric population. In patients with acute pyelonephritis, VUR is present in approximately 40% of patients. In untreated patients, VUR is responsible for 5–40% of end-stage renal disease in patients under 16 years of age and 5–20% of adults less than 50 years old.

VUR is caused by a failure of the ureterovesical valve. The normal ureter passes obliquely through the bladder wall and submucosa to its opening at the trigone. As urine fills the bladder, the valve passively closes, preventing reflux. If the intramural ureteral length is too short in relation to its diameter or if the course is too direct, the valve will not close completely and reflux results. As

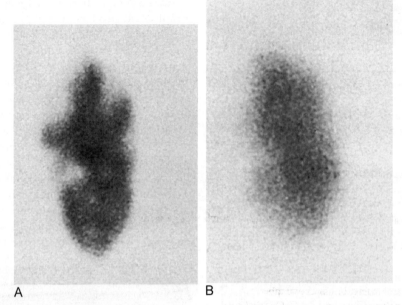

A   B

Figure 8-33   Acute pyelonephritis. Tc-99m DMSA study in an 11-year-old child using a pinhole collimator. **A,** Multiple cortical defects are seen, particularly in the upper pole. **B,** Follow-up study obtained 6 months later, after appropriate antibiotic therapy, shows resolution of most defects.

a child grows, the ureter usually grows in length more than in diameter, resulting in decreased reflux and eventual resolution in 80% of patients. Spontaneous resolution by 2–3 years of age is seen in 40–60% of VUR diagnosed prenatally. Even among patients with severe reflux, resolution occurs spontaneously in 20% within 5 years.

Renal damage is more likely in patients with severe rather than mild or moderate grades of reflux. Reflux by itself is not pathological; that is, sterile low-pressure reflux does not cause renal injury. The intrarenal reflux of infected urine is required for damage to develop. In patients without reflux, pyelonephritis has been presumed to be secondary to etiologies such as fimbriated bacteria, which can climb the ureter.

Antibiotic therapy is the first line of defense. Renal scaring has been decreased from 35–60% in untreated patients down to 10% with therapy. The goal of therapy is to prevent infection of the kidney until reflux resolves spontaneously. However, antibiotics do not completely protect the kidney from infection and scar. Therefore, patients must be carefully monitored, and serial Tc-99m DMSA scans may be helpful.

VCUG screening is recommended for siblings of patients with reflux. It must be remembered that reflux and pyelonephritis may be clinically silent. These siblings are at an increased risk of approximately 40% for VUR.

Methodology

Indirect radionuclide cystography can be performed as part of routine dynamic renal scintigraphy done with Tc-99m DTPA or Tc-99m MAG3. The child is asked to not void until the bladder is maximally distended. When the bladder is as full as can be tolerated, a pre-voiding image is obtained. Then dynamic images are acquired during voiding. A postvoid image is obtained once voiding is done. Although this test has an advantage because the bladder is not catheterized, upper-tract stasis often poses a problem for interpretation. In addition, the indirect method cannot detect the reflux that occurs during bladder filling (20%).

Direct radionuclide cystography is the most commonly used method for diagnosing reflux. It is done as a three-phase process with continuous imaging during bladder filling, micturition, and after voiding. Besides diagnosing reflux, this procedure can quantitate postvoid bladder residuals.

The protocol for radionuclide retrograde cystography and residual bladder volume calculation is listed in Box 8-10. The high sensitivity depends on rapid and continuous imaging. Tc-99m sulfur colloid and Tc-99m DTPA are the radiopharmaceuticals most commonly used. Tc-99m pertechnetate may be absorbed through the bladder, particularly if the bladder is inflamed. A solution of 1 mCi of radiotracer in 500 ml normal saline provides sufficient concentration.

Dosimetry

The absorbed radiation dose is quite low. A list is provided in Table 8-6. From 50–200 times less radiation is

Box 8-10   Radionuclide Retrograde Cystography Protocol Summary

RADIOPHARMACEUTICAL

Tc-99m sulfur colloid, 1 mCi (37 MBq)

PATIENT PREPARATION

Insert Foley aseptically, inflate balloon, tape to secure
Use clean weighed diaper for infants

POSITION

Patient supine with bladder and kidneys in field of view. Camera under table.

INSTRUMENTATION

Camera: single-head, large FOV, collimator: converging for newborns <1 yr; all-purpose otherwise.
Computer: 64 × 64 word matrix
Filling phase: 10-sec frame for 60 sec; pre-void 30-sec; voiding 2-sec/frame for 120 sec; postvoid 30-sec

IMAGING PROCEDURE

Hang 500-ml bag of normal saline 25 cm above table.
Inject radiotracer into tubing connected to bladder catheter
Filling phase: fill bladder to maximal capacity (age 2+) × 30 = volume instill (ml)
Fill until drip slows or voids around catheter

VOIDING PHASE

Place camera perpendicular to table
Place patient sitting on bedpan with back against camera (infants remain supine and void into diaper)
Deflate Foley balloon, have patient void
Measure urine volume (or weigh diaper to determine output)

INTERPRETATION

Total bladder volume residual postvoid volume and bladder volume at initiation of reflux can be measured.

$$\text{Residual bladder volume (ml)} = \frac{\text{Voided volume (ml)} \times \text{Residual counts/min}}{\text{Maximal counts/min} - \text{Residual counts/min}}$$

delivered to the gonads from the radionuclide method than with contrast cystography.

Image Interpretation

In a normal study, no radiotracer is seen in the ureters or kidneys. Any reflux is abnormal and readily detected by the presence of activity above the bladder (Fig. 8-34). Reflux grades have been described for radiographic contrast studies (Fig. 8-35). In this system, criteria used include the level reflux reaches, the dilatation of the renal pelvis, and ureteral dilation and tortuosity. However, anatomic resolution is much lower with scintigraphic methods and calyceal morphology is not well defined.

A radionuclide grading system would report activity confined to the ureter grade I reflux, similar to the radiographic grade I. A scintigraphic grade II would include reflux to the renal pelvis and corresponds to the x-ray cystography grades II and III. If a diffusely dilated system is seen on the scintigrams, it corresponds to grades IV-V seen with contrast cystography.

Radionuclide cystography is more sensitive than the radiographic contrast technique. The radionuclide technique permits detection of reflux volumes on the order of 1 ml. In one study comparing the two techniques, 17% of reflux events were seen only on the radionuclide exam. Although radionuclide voiding cystography can miss low level I reflux due to the adjacent bladder activity, it is generally accepted that level I reflux is of little consequence. If a study is negative but clinical suspicion

Table 8-6   Radiation Dosimetry for Tc-99m Retrograde Cystography

Organ	mrads/mCi *or* cGy/37 MBq
Bladder	18–27
Ovaries	1–2
Testes	<1–2
Kidneys	0.02–0.4

is high, refilling the bladder will improve sensitivity. This is not routinely done, however.

SCROTAL SCINTIGRAPHY

It has been possible to scintigraphically evaluate blood flow to the acutely painful scrotum since the early 1970s. Although scrotal scintigraphy is a very sensitive and specific tool for the differentiation of acute testicular torsion from acute inflammatory causes, it is now of historical interest. Ultrasound is clearly the method of choice for evaluation of the painless scrotal mass.

Testicular viability after torsion of the spermatic cord depends on the length of time between the onset of pain and surgical correction. Atrophy may occur after as little as 4–6 hours after onset and is inevitable by 10 hours after torsion. Therefore, testicular torsion is a sur-

gical emergency. Scintigraphy can confirm the clinically suspected diagnosis of torsion and direct the patient to surgery while preventing unnecessary exploration of patients with epididymitis as a cause for the pain.

Radiopharmaceutical

Tc-99m pertechnetate is the radiopharmaceutical used for testicular scanning. It serves as a blood flow and blood pool (soft tissue extracellular space) marker. Tc-99m pertechnetate is rapidly available from a molybdenum generator and requires no time to perform labeling.

Methodology

Patient preparation involves giving an oral thyroid-blocking medication such as potassium perchlorate. This will

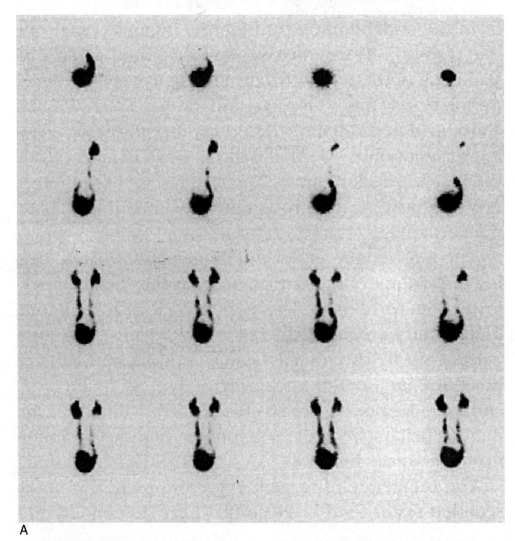

A

Figure 8-34   Vesicoureteral reflux. **A,** During the filling phase, reflux is seen first on the right, then bilaterally in **B**. On voiding, the left side clears better than the right. Reflux is seen in the renal pelvic region bilaterally from grade II-III reflux.

Continued

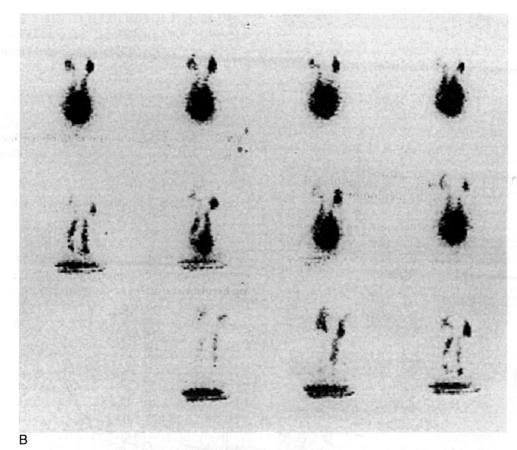

B

Figure 8-34, cont'd.

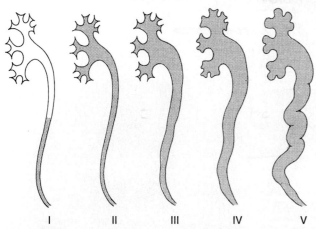

Figure 8-35   Vesicoureteral grading system (International Reflux Study Committee). *I,* Ureteral reflux only. *II,* Reflux into ureter, pelvis, and calyces without dilatation. *III,* Mild to moderate dilatation/tortuosity of ureter and calyceal dilatation. *IV,* Moderate dilatation and tortuosity of ureter and moderate dilation of the renal pelvis. The angles of the fornices obliterated but the papillary impressions maintained. *V,* Gross dilation and tortuosity of the ureter and gross dilation of the renal pelvis and calyces. Papillary impressions no longer visible in most calyces.

reduce radiotracer thyroid uptake normally seen with this agent. However, scanning should not be delayed for this medication. Rapid imaging is essential, and the entire exam should only take 15-20 minutes.

Correct positioning is extremely important. A marker should be placed on the thigh of the symptomatic side to ensure the correct side is identified. The testicles may be supported in a scrotal sling with the penis taped out of the field of view. A rubberized lead marker can be placed behind the testes to decrease background activity from the thighs. A lead strip marker may be placed on the median raphe on later delayed images to better separate right and left testes, as they are often asymmetric in size and rotated.

Image Interpretation

Normal Pattern

On flow images, the iliac arteries should be seen simultaneously and should appear symmetric. Because flow to the testicles through the spermatic cord and testicular artery is relatively low, only a low-grade diffuse activity may be seen without clear-cut visualization of the spermatic cord vessels. The static soft tissue phase images show low-grade symmetric activity, usually somewhat less than the thigh.

Bladder activity accumulating over time and penile blood flow can lead to difficulties with interpretation if care is not taken. The later images are better saved for marker placement rather than for interpretation.

Acute Testicular Torsion

The scintigraphic findings in acute testicular torsion depend on the time that has elapsed since the acute event. In early torsion, within a few hours of onset, flow images may show no significant asymmetry, although occasionally a "nubbin sign" may be seen from activity in a small portion of the obstructed proximal spermatic vessels. The soft tissue phase images decreased activity may be seen in the region of the involved testicle (Fig. 8-36).

Delayed Torsion

Later in the course of torsion, beyond the point when testicular salvage might occur, the image findings change dramatically. This stage has been described as "missed torsion," although the term *delayed torsion* is preferred. A halo of increased activity develops from hyperemia to the dartos through the pudendal arterial supply to the scrotum. The testicle itself appears as a central area of photon deficiency (Fig. 8-37). Over time the halo effect becomes more prominent, resulting in a "donut sign." The donut sign pattern is not specific and is seen in testicular abscess.

Acute Epididymitis

Bacterial epididymitis and epididymoorchitis usually occur in late adolescence and early adulthood coincident with the onset of sexual activity. The scintigraphic findings are dramatically different from acute or delayed torsion. The early dynamic phase shows markedly increased activity in the spermatic cord vessels, and increased activity is also seen on the delayed soft tissue images (Fig. 8-38). Therefore, it must be remembered that inflammation and infection produce hyperemia seen as asymmetric blood flow and soft tissue uptake.

Torsion of the Testicular Appendage

Torsion of one of the testicular appendages is common from 7-14 years of age. Although painful, it is not serious and resolves spontaneously. Management is conservative and nonsurgical. On physical exam, a "blue-dot" sign may be seen on transillumination and a nodule may be palpable. Radionuclide studies may be normal or may show focal low-grade increased activity at the site of inflammation.

Other Disorders

Scrotal scintigraphy is not recommended for the assessment of abscess, varicoceles, hydroceles, or testicular masses. These are better assessed by ultrasound. Reactive hydroceles are often present on scrotal scintigrams and present as crescent shaped areas of decreased activity. Varicoceles may show dramatically increased

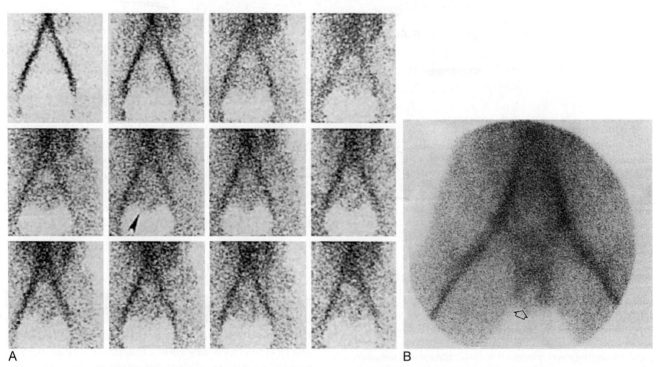

A   B

Figure 8-36   Acute testicular torsion. **A,** Minimal asymmetry *(arrowhead)* is seen on flow images (often no flow changes are seen). **B,** Blood pool images show decreased activity on the right *(open arrowhead)* from acute testicular torsion.

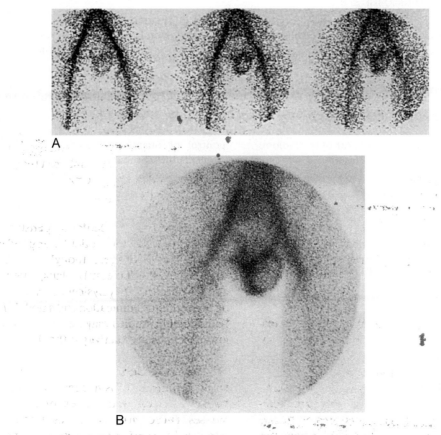

Figure 8-37 Delayed testicular torsion in a patient with pain for over 24 hours. **A,** Two-second frames show increased flow to the painful left scrotum. **B,** Blood pool images show a halo pattern on the left consistent with delayed torsion. The testicle was not viable at surgery.

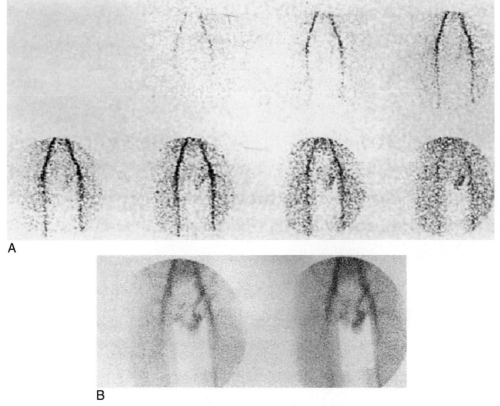

Figure 8-38 Acute epididymitis in a patient with acute pain in the left testicle. **A,** Increased flow is seen to the lateral left scrotum. **B,** Blood-pool images have a similar pattern consistent with epididymitis. The symptoms resolved over the course of a week on antibiotics.

activity late in the venous structures. An abscess will show intensely increased flow and a "donut sign" not unlike a missed torsion.

SUGGESTED READING

Blaufox MD, Aurell M, Bubeck B, et al: Report of the radionuclides in nephrology committee on renal clearance. *J Nucl Med* 37: 1883-1890, 1996.

Dubovsky EV, Russell CD, Bischof-Delaloye A, et al: Report of the radionuclides in nephrology committee for evaluation of transplanted kidney (review of techniques). *Semin Nucl Med*, 175-188, 1999.

Gates GF: Glomerular filtration rate: estimation from fractional renal accumulation of Tc-99m DTPA (stannous). *AJR* 138: 565-570, 1982.

O'Reilly P, Aurell M, Britton KE, et al: Consensus on diuretic renography for investigating the dilated upper urinary tract. *J Nucl Med* 37: 1872-1876, 1996.

Pieppsz A, Blaufox MD, Gordon I, et al: Consensus on renal cortical scintigraphy in children with urinary tract infection. *Semin Nucl Med*, 160-174, 1999.

Prigent A, Cosgriff P, Gates GF, et al: Consensus report on quality control of quantitative measurements of renal function obtained from the renogram: International Committee from the scientific committee of radionuclides in nephrology. *Semin Nucl Med*, 146-159, 1999.

Russell CD, Dubovsky EV: Reproducibility of single-sample clearance of Tc-99m-mercaptoacetyltriglycine and I-131-orthoiodohippurate. *J Nucl Med* 40: 1122-1124, 1999.

Taylor A, Nally J, Aurell M, et al: Consensus report on ACE inhibitor renography for detecting renovascular hypertension. *J Nucl Med* 37: 1876-1882, 1996.

There are numerous radiopharmaceuticals available for tumor imaging. Many of these are not specific for any particular tumor. Rather, they involve organ-specific radiotracer binding. For example, a bone scan detects the secondary bone remodeling caused by metastasis. Other radiopharmaceuticals target a specific aspect of a tumor such as a receptor or an antibody directed against a tumor antigen. The type of localization for several radiopharmaceuticals is listed in Box 9-1.

Box 9-1 Overview of Tumor-Imaging Radiopharmaceuticals

ORGAN-SPECIFIC
Cold Spot Imaging

Thyroid imaging: Iodine-123, Technetium-99m pertechnetate
Liver imaging: Technetium-99m sulfur colloid

Hot Spot Imaging

Brain scans: Technetium-99m DTPA, Technetium-99m glucoheptonate
Bone imaging: Technetium-99m MDP, Technetium-99m HDP

NONSPECIFIC

Gallium-67 citrate
Thallium-201 chloride
Technetium-99m sestamibi
Technetium-99m tetrofosmin
Fluorine-18 fluorodeoxyglucose (FDG)

TUMOR-TYPE SPECIFIC

Iodine-131: papillary-follicular thyroid cancer
Iodine-131 MIBG: neural crest tumors (adrenal medulla tumor imaging)
Iodine-131 NP-59: adrenal cortical tumor imaging
Technetium-99m HIDA: hepatocyte origin tumors
Radiolabeled monoclonal antibodies against tumor surface antigens
    Indium-111 OncoScint: colorectal and ovarian cancer
    Technetium-99m CEA-SCAN: colorectal cancer
    Indium-111 ProstaScint: prostate cancer
    Technetium-99m Verluma: small cell carcinoma of the lung
Radiolabeled peptides
    Indium-111 OctreoScan: somatostatin receptor imaging of neuroendocrine tumors
    Tc-99m NeoTect: somatostatin receptor imaging of lung carcinoma

This chapter discusses tumor-imaging radiopharmaceuticals not covered in other chapters (Table 9-1). Some of these are nonspecific tumor-imaging agents such as gallium-67 (Ga-67), thallium-201 (Tl-201), Tc-99m sestamibi (MIBI), and Tc-99m tetrofosmin. Another nonspecific imaging agent, F-18 fluorodeoxyglucose (F-18 FDG), is covered separately in Chapter 10.

Among the agents with specific tumor uptake, the radiotracer may bind to a cell membrane receptor or to a surface antigen. The receptor binding of indium-111 (In-111) OctreoScan is based on its similarity to the peptide hormone somatostatin. Monoclonal antibody binding to specific tumor surface antigens is found in agents such as In-111 OncoScint (colorectal and ovarian cancer), Tc-99m CEA-Scan (colorectal cancer), In-111 ProstaScint (prostate cancer), Tc-99m Verluma (small cell lung carcinoma), and In-111 Zevalin or I-131 Bexxar (lymphoma).

Two topics related to tumors will be discussed: palliation of metastatic bone pain with bone-seeking radiopharmaceuticals and lymphoscintigraphy. Sentinel lymph node detection has become an important tool in the management of melanoma and breast cancer.

GALLIUM-67 TUMOR IMAGING

Gallium-67 (Ga-67) was initially evaluated as a bone-imaging agent. However, it gained widespread use as a tumor imaging agent (Fig. 9-1). In 1969, Ga-67 was first used clinically for the detection of Hodgkin's disease. Subsequently, Ga-67 showed a high degree of sensitivity for non-Hodgkin's lymphoma, metastatic melanoma, and hepatocellular carcinoma. Although Ga-67 is taken up by numerous other tumors (such as those of lung, head and neck, and soft tissue sarcomas), its clinical role in these diseases has been limited.

The evaluation of Hodgkin's and non-Hodgkin's lymphoma has been the most common clinical use for Ga-67 use. For years, Ga-67 and computed tomography (CT) were used together in the staging, restaging, and post-therapy monitoring of lymphoma. Over time, CT became the primary staging modality, although Ga-67 provided superior results for restaging and therapy response questions. Currently, the role of Ga-67 is increasingly limited in the evaluation of lymphoma as the use of F-18 FDG positron emission tomography (PET) in lymphoma expands.

Chemistry and Physics

Ga-67 does not have optimal physical characteristics for scintigraphic imaging. It decays by electron capture and emits several gamma rays: 93, 185, 288, and 394 keV (approximately 100, 200, 300, and 400 keV). Usually, the lower three peaks are used for imaging because of their higher abundance. Neither the high- nor low-energy photons are well-suited for gamma camera imaging. The low-level photons are subject to a higher scatter fraction and the high-energy photons penetrate the collimator septa, which degrades image quality.

Pharmacokinetics

Gallium is a group III element in the periodic table (Fig. 1-1) with a biological behavior similar to iron. The biodistribution in the body is complex. As an iron analog, it is

Table 9-1 Physical Characteristics of Tumor-Imaging Radionuclides

Radionuclide	Chemical or pharmaceutical	Physical half-life (hr)	Principal mode of decay	Photopeaks		Dose in mCi (MBq)
				keV	Percent abundance	
Gallium-67	Citrate	78	Electron capture	93	41	10 (370)
				185	23	
				300	18	
				394	4	
Thallium-201	Chloride	73	Electron capture	69–83	94	3 (111)
Tc-99m	Sestamibi	6	Isomeric transition	140	88	25 (925)
	Tetrofosmin					25 (925)
	CEA-SCAN					30 (1110)
In-111	Pentetreotide (OctreoScan)	67	Electron capture	173	90	6 (222)
	OncoScint			247	94	5 (185)
	ProstaScint					5 (185)

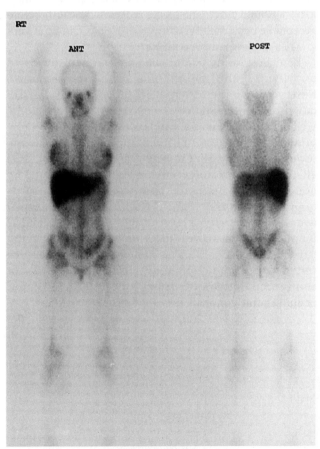

Figure 9-1   Normal gallium-67 distribution. Whole body scan of a 50-year-old woman obtained 72 hours after injection. Highest uptake is normally seen in the liver, followed by bone and marrow. Uptake is seen in the colon, lacrimal glands, nasopharyngeal region, and breast.

transported in the blood by iron transport proteins, especially transferrin. The kidney excretes 15–25% of the administrated dose within the first 24 hours. From that point on, however, the bowel is the major route of excretion. Total body clearance is slow, with a biological half-life of 25 days. Two days after injection, about 75% of the administered dose remains in the body.

The pharmacokinetics and distribution of Ga-67 citrate are not optimal from an imaging standpoint. It has slow background clearance, so imaging is usually delayed until 48 or 72 hours after injection. The considerable uptake normally seen in liver, bone, and bone marrow makes tumor detection difficult in or near these organs. The excretion into bowel and the slow large-bowel clearance create problems detecting abdominal tumor uptake. The use of laxatives and further delayed imaging up to 7 days may help overcome this problem.

Ga-67 biodistribution and uptake can be altered by a number of substances (Box 9-2). The effects are largely seen in the bone marrow, liver, and kidneys. Elevated serum iron from multiple transfusions or iron dextran administration competes with Ga-67 for transferrin binding sites. Chemotherapy and radiation therapy also commonly change the normal pattern of activity. For example, vincristine administered within 24 hours of Ga-67 injection can depress liver uptake, whereas interstitial nephritis from chemotherapy increases renal uptake. The MRI contrast agent gadolinium may cause decreased tumor uptake. These changes are reversible. The effects of chemotherapy, for example, usually resolve 4–6 weeks after the end of treatment (Fig. 9-2).

Box 9-2   Factors Altering Ga-67 Biodistribution

INCREASED RENAL UPTAKE

Chemotherapy
Iron overload: multiple transfusions, iron dextran
Renal disease: ATN, acute renal failure
Infiltrative processes: leukemia, lymphoma, amyloidosis
CHF

DECREASED HEPATIC UPTAKE

Chemotherapy
Iron overload
Liver failure

DIFFUSELY INCREASED OSSEOUS UPTAKE

Chemotherapy
Iron overload
Chronic anemia
Gadolinium contrast
Leukemia
Elevated serum aluminum

Tumor localization of Ga-67 relates to increased iron uptake and binding in cancer cells. An adequate blood supply is necessary for tracer delivery and increased vascular permeability plays a role in accumulation. Uptake appears to predominantly rely on Ga-67 binding to transferrin receptors on tumor cell membranes. Once inside the cell, the radiopharmaceutical binds to intracellular proteins and localizes in the lysosomes. Transferrin receptor levels drop after therapy, leading to decreased Ga-67 accumulation. Other methods of localization may be important. For example, binding to lactoferrin may also be important in certain tumors such as Burkitt's lymphoma and Hodgkin's disease.

Dosimetry

With a typical adult dose of 10 mCi, the large intestine receives the highest radiation, about 9 rads (9 cGy). The spleen and bone marrow receive 5–6 rads (5–6 cGy), and the liver receives 4.6 rads (4.6 cGy). Dosimetry information is listed in Table 9-2. It should be noted that Ga-67 is excreted in the breast milk.

Methodology

Advancements in instrumentation and technique have resulted in marked improvements in image quality and tumor detectability compared to the early years of Ga-67 imaging. Some of these advances include improved gamma camera resolution, multiheaded detectors, improved computers, multichannel acquisition, and single photon emission computed tomography (SPECT).

Although 3-5 mCi (111–185 MBq) of Ga-67 is used for imaging inflammatory processes, 8–10 mCi (260–370 MBq) is used for tumor imaging. The higher administered dose results in a greater count rate. This allows for delayed imaging with increased target-to-background ratios and high-quality planar and SPECT images. Delayed imaging is needed for bowel activity clearance and increased tumor-to-background ratio. The higher radiation dose is therefore acceptable because it improves tumor detectability at very low risk in these cancer patients.

Bowel cleansing before imaging has been advocated to minimize the impact of slow bowel clearance. However, this is controversial. Laxatives may lead to irritation and increased bowel activity. Patients should be well hydrated and do not need to fast.

Although the exact protocol varies between laboratories, planar and SPECT images are typically obtained 48–72 hours after injection. SPECT images should be done routinely for the chest and abdomen. This improves sensitivity and localization of abnormal lymph-node activity. Planar images can be obtained as long as 7–10 days after injection and SPECT imaging can be done at 5–6 days. Detection of mediastinal tumors may require oblique views if SPECT is not employed. Box 9-3 describes a typical Ga-67 tumor imaging protocol.

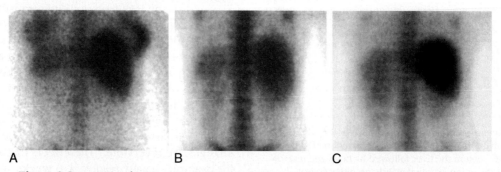

A   B   C

Figure 9-2   Gallium-67 altered biodistribution. **A,** Posterior view of the lumbar spine in a patient with lymphoma initially shows normal bone marrow activity. **B,** Following chemotherapy, the marrow activity increases, becoming isointense to liver. **C,** One year later, the biodistribution has normalized with activity much decreased.

Table 9-2 Radiation Absorbed Dose for Common Tumor-Imaging Radiopharmaceuticals in rads/mCi (cGy/3.7 MBq)

Organ	Ga-67	Tl-201	Tc-99m MIBI	Tc-99m tetrofosmin
Kidney	0.41	**1.2**	0.067	0.47
Thyroid		0.5		0.02
Heart wall		0.5	0.017	0.017
Liver	0.46	0.6	0.02	0.017
Spleen	0.53			
Bone marrow	**0.58**			
Bone	0.44			
Gallbladder			0.067	**0.2**
Testes	0.2	0.5	0.01	0.13
Ovaries	0.3	0.5	0.05	0.04
Urinary bladder			0.07	0.07
Large intestine	0.9	0.4	**0.2**	0.1
Breasts			0.007	0.013
Total body	0.26	0.23	0.2	0.02

Target organ in boldface type.

Because chemotherapy and radiation therapy before Ga-67 imaging can result in altered biodistribution, Ga-67 injection should be postponed at least 3 weeks following chemotherapy. If Ga-67 imaging is needed sooner, such as re-evaluation as required before the next 2-week cycle of chemotherapy, Ga-67 injection should be injected at least 1 week after prior treatment and 48 hours before the next therapy.

Image Interpretation

Soft tissue background activity can be high, but depends a great deal on body habitus. Delayed imaging at 48–72 hours is routine because time is needed for the high background activity to decrease. Ga-67 uptake is normally seen in the liver, spleen, salivary glands, bone marrow, and lacrimal glands (Fig. 9-1). The liver has the highest uptake of Ga-67, followed by bone, marrow, and then spleen. The kidneys have intense uptake for the first 24–48 hours after injection.

Box 9-3 Gallium-67 Citrate Tumor Imaging: Protocol Summary

PATIENT PREPARATION

Optional bowel preparation

RADIOPHARMACEUTICAL DOSE

Adult dose: 10 mCi (370 MBq)
Pediatric dose: 75–100 µCi/kg (minimum 500 µCi)

INSTRUMENTATION

Camera: Large field of view; dual-headed camera preferable
Collimator: Medium-energy parallel hole
Photopeaks: 20% windows around 93, 184, and 296 keV
Computer acquisition matrix: 128 × 128 byte mode

PROCEDURE

Whole body images initially at 48–72 hr and at 5–10 days as needed
SPECT of chest, abdomen, or both at 48–72 hr and delayed SPECT as needed up to 5–6 days
1. Inject Ga-67 intravenously.
2. Planar imaging: For dual-headed camera, simultaneous anterior and posterior whole body scanning mode requires 30-40 min. For single-headed camera, obtain 500k spot images of anterior chest and equal time for posterior chest, anterior and posterior abdomen, pelvis, and anterior head. Regions of special interest require 1000k. Image axillae with arms elevated.
3. SPECT:

Camera	Single-headed	Dual-headed
Collimator:	Medium energy	Two medium energy
Rotation:	360°	
Patient:	Supine	Supine
Computer acquisition parameters:	64 × 64 matrix 128 images/360° arc 20 sec/image	128 × 128 matrix 120 images/360°, 60 stops/head 40 sec/stop at 46 hr
Processing:	Filtered back-projection or iterative reconstruction	
	Attenuation correction:	Attenuation correction:
	Chest: no	Chest: no
	Abdomen: yes	Abdomen: yes

Renal uptake should decrease over time and appear only faintly by 48–72 hours.

Large bowel clearance is variable and can pose interpretive problems. It may be difficult to differentiate tumor from normal bowel. In addition, tumor may be masked by high levels of bowel uptake. Further delayed imaging may help clarify problems. Abdominal tumor activity remains fixed as the bowel activity.

Uptake is variable in the salivary and lacrimal glands as well as in the nasal mucosa. Lacrimal gland uptake is due to lactoferrin binding. Uptake in the parotid and lacrimal glands, the "panda sign," suggests Sjögren's syndrome or sarcoidosis (*see* Fig. 12-4). Radiation therapy for head and neck cancer may cause increased salivary uptake that can persist for years.

Female breast uptake varies with hormonal status (Fig. 9-3) and is particularly high with postpartum lactation. Oblique, lateral, and SPECT images can separate breast parenchyma from intrathoracic processes. Axillary lymph node activity may be missed due to overlapping tissues if the patient is not imaged with the arms up (Fig. 9-4).

Although any intense or asymmetrical nodal uptake is abnormal, faint hilar uptake may be seen normally and is common after chemotherapy. Hilar and mediastinal uptake can be caused by inflammatory processes such as granulomatous disease. If Ga-67 uptake is seen on a pretreatment scan but correlative CT reveals no abnormality, the uptake is not likely to be of any clinical significance.

Ga-67 accumulates at sites of recent trauma, surgery, or infection. Correlation with physical exam and history is very important. Postoperative sites may have increased activity for 2–3 weeks. Infectious etiologies such as pneumonia must be considered when abnormal Ga-67 accumulation is seen.

Multiple factors affect the ability of Ga-67 to detect a tumor. First, tumor histology plays a key role. The sensitivity of Ga-67 in several tumor types is listed in Table 9-3. Within a tumor type, high-grade tumors are more likely to accumulate Ga-67 than low-grade tumors. Lesion size is another important factor. Tumors less than 2 cm in diameter are not reliably detected with conventional planar imaging. In addition, very large masses such as those larger than 5 cm may be poorly visualized because of tumor necrosis. SPECT imaging improves detection of smaller lesions (Fig. 9-5). Because of its improved contrast resolution, lesions on the order of 1–1.5 cm can be visualized. The sensitivity of SPECT for tumor detection is 85–96% compared with 69% with planar imaging.

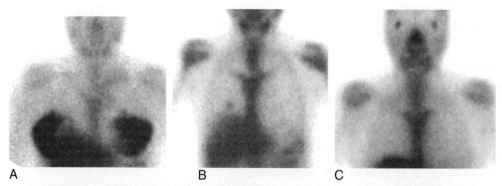

Figure 9-3   Variable Ga-67 uptake in the female breast. **A,** The female patient with Hodgkin's disease shown in Fig. 9-2 had intense breast activity on the initial scan. This was attributed to breast feeding which had been recently terminated. **B,** The activity resolved on a scan performed 6 months later. An underlying nodule was revealed in the right chest. **C,** The nodule resolved after the completion of chemotherapy.

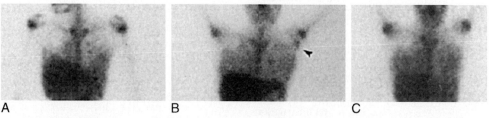

Figure 9-4   Axillary node uptake of gallium-67. **A–B,** Initial study reveals left axillary uptake (*arrowhead*) only when the arms are elevated. **C,** A follow-up study 3 months later shows resolution of the nodal involvement.

Table 9-3 Sensitivity of Gallium-67 for Tumor Detection

Tumor	Sensitivity (%)	Clinical utility
Hodgkin's disease	>90	+++
Non-Hodgkin's lymphoma	85	+++
Hepatocellular carcinoma	90	+++
Soft tissue sarcomas	93	+++
Melanoma	82	++
Lung cancer	85	++
Head and neck tumors	75	++
Abdominal and pelvic tumors	55	+

Table 9-4 Hodgkin's Disease Versus Non-Hodgkin's Lymphoma

	Hodgkin's disease	Non-Hodgkin's lymphoma
Cellular derivation	Unresolved Reed-Sternberg	90% B-cell 10% T-cell
SITE OF DISEASE		
Localized	Common	Uncommon
Nodal spread	Contiguous	Not continuous
Extranodal	Uncommon	Common
Mediastinal	Common	Uncommon
Abdominal	Uncommon	Common
Bone marrow	Uncommon	Common
Systemic symptoms	Uncommon	Common
Curability	>75%	<25%

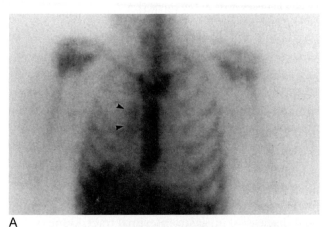

A

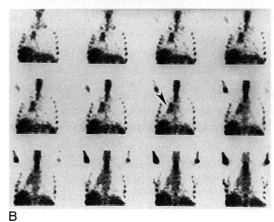

B

Figure 9-5   Gallium-67 thoracic SPECT. A 35-year-old man with Hodgkin's disease. **A,** Anterior planar chest image shows low-intensity uptake in the right hilum (*arrowheads*). **B,** SPECT shows definite hilar uptake (*arrowhead*) on sequential coronal chest sections owing to the improved contrast resolution of SPECT.

Clinical Applications

Hodgkin's Disease and Non-Hodgkin's Lymphoma

Hodgkin's disease (HD) and non-Hodgkin's lymphoma (NHL) differ clinically and pathologically (Table 9-4).

Initially, HD is usually seen as localized nodal disease in the neck or supraclavicular area (Fig. 9-6). Tumor involvement in the chest occurs in almost two-thirds of patients. Orderly spread to contiguous lymph nodes is typical. The Rye classification system describes four histological subtypes (Table 9-5). However, the stage of disease is the main factor in determining prognosis, not the histology. The Ann Arbor staging system is described in Box 9-4. Ga-67 has long played an important role in HD because staging is so critical.

NHL is a typically multicentric disease (Fig. 9-7) and 80% of patients have abdominal presentations involving mesenteric and retroperitoneal nodes (Fig. 9-8). Roughly 25% of patients with NHL will have extranodal sites and 45% will demonstrate intrathoracic tumor. The histologic cell type of the tumor is highly predictive of survival. Therefore, unlike HD where tumor stage is most important, tumor histology largely determines patient prognosis in NHL (Box 9-5).

Aggressive combination chemotherapy, with or without radiation therapy, can cure or produce long-term remission in a large percentage of patients with HD as well as many with high- and intermediate-grade NHL. Coincidentally, these are the same tumor types which typically accumulate Ga-67. Sensitivity for low-grade tumors, on the other hand, is poor. Low-grade tumors generally have an indolent clinical course. Ultimately, these patients relapse, transform to a higher-grade tumor, and cannot be cured.

Accuracy

Much of the data cited in the literature are older and do not reflect several factors that improved Ga-67 sensitivity. For example, lower-dose regimens (3–5 mCi) were used that are now reserved for inflammatory processes. In addition, camera technology and the

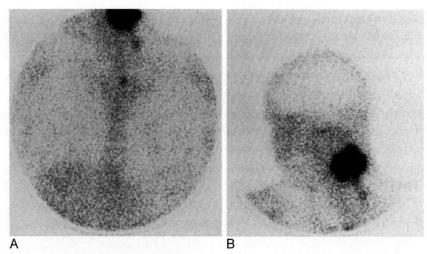

Figure 9-6   Hodgkin's disease in a 25-year-old man with a left neck mass. **A,** Left lateral view shows a large region of gallium-67 uptake in left side of the neck with a small nodal focus just inferior to it. **B,** Anterior view. Small focus can be seen inferior to mass on left side of neck. There is also focal uptake in the mediastinum (proven with SPECT).

Table 9-5 Rye Classification of Hodgkin's Disease		
Histological subgroup	Incidence (%)	Prognosis
Lymphocyte predominant	2–10	Excellent
Nodular sclerosis	40–80	Very good
Mixed cellularity	20–40	Good
Lymphocyte depleted	2–15	Poor

widespread use of SPECT have improved results. HD is generally detected with a sensitivity of 90–95% and specificity approaching 100%. Sensitivity for NHL is slightly lower at 85–90%, but specificity is similar to that with HD. Sensitivity is much lower for low-grade tumors, which are detected with Ga-67 only about half of the time.

Ga-67 Lymphoma Staging, Restaging, and Response to Therapy

CT is the primary modality for initial lymphoma staging with Ga-67 playing a much smaller role. However, it should be noted that Ga-67 is highly sensitive and the information it reveals often compliments the CT. In the past, Ga-67 scans helped clinicians determine that staging laparotomy was not necessary for HD. One problem with Ga-67 staging in lymphoma is that it often does not add information to the CT due to lower sensitivity in low-grade tumors and in extranodal disease (skin, gastrointestinal tract, kidneys, and testis).

Currently, Ga-67 is most often used to assess response to therapy. It is essential that a pretreatment scan is obtained to determine if the tumor is Ga-67 avid. Until recently, Ga-67 imaging was done at the end of a therapy cycle (Fig. 9-9). Ga-67 can accurately stratify patients into high-risk and low-risk prognostic groups in this process. Any patient with persistent disease has a very poor prognosis. At times, these restaging scans reveal new sites of disease as well (Fig. 9-10).

Ga-67 scans done early in the course of therapy, sometimes after a single cycle of chemotherapy or in midcycle, allow an even better assessment of prognosis than

Box 9-4 Ann Arbor Staging System for Hodgkin's Disease	
STAGE I	Involvement of single lymph node region or single extralymphatic site
STAGE II	Involvement of two or more lymph node regions on the same side of diaphragm; can also include localized involvement of extralymphatic site
STAGE III	Involvement of lymph node regions or extra lymphatic sites on both sides of diaphragm
STAGE IV	Disseminated involvement of one or more extralymphatic organs with or without lymph node involvement

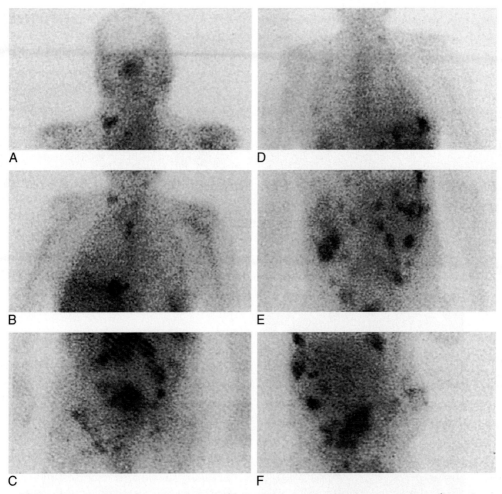

Figure 9-7   Non-Hodgkin's lymphoma. A 67-year-old man with multiple sites of gallium-67 uptake by tumor both above and below the diaphragm. **A–C,** Anterior spot views of the head, chest, and abdomen and pelvis, respectively. **D–F,** Posterior views of the chest and abdomen and right lateral view of the abdomen and pelvis, respectively.

images from the end of therapy. Patients with little response early in therapy have a lower survival rate with more frequent relapse than an early responder. One hypothesis for this finding is that cells resistant to first-line therapy are seen on these early scans. If imaging is delayed until after therapy is completed, the resistant cells may be present but not abundant enough to visualize. These cells are more likely to cause a recurrence than cells completely killed early in therapy. Not only does early imaging appear to be more accurate than scanning at the end of the chemotherapy cycle, but it is also a better predictor of survival than other factors such as tumor stage or CT appearance. Early modification of treatment protocol may benefit the high-risk patient.

Residual Mass

Another common use for Ga-67 is evaluation of a mass persisting on CT after therapy. Because CT images the size and shape of a mass rather than viability, CT cannot differentiate between viable tissue and fibrotic scar. Residual radiographic abnormalities are seen in 64–83% of patients with mediastinal disease and 30–50% of those with abdominal disease. In the mediastinum, it has been reported that Ga-67 has a sensitivity of 96% and a specificity of 80% for residual active tumor. CT, on the other hand, was 68% sensitive and only 60% specific for tumor.

Malignant Melanoma

Most malignant melanomas and metastases are gallium avid. Ga-67 has been used to detect metastases and determine response to chemotherapy or immunotherapy. The overall sensitivity and specificity for detecting metastasis are reported to be 82% and 99%, respectively. F-18 FDG PET is currently playing an increasing role in clinical care for melanoma.

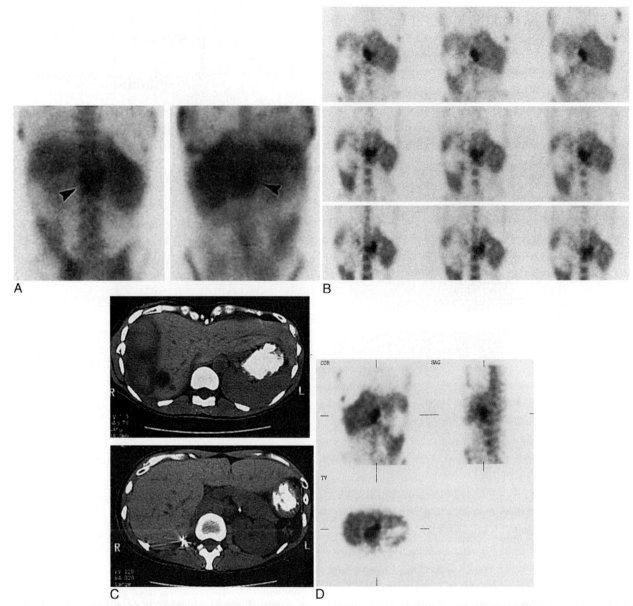

Figure 9-8 Gallium-67 abdominal SPECT. A 26-year-old woman with non-Hodgkin's lymphoma. **A,** The anterior (*right*) and posterior (*left*) planar images suggest uptake in the spine or prevertebral region (*arrowheads*). **B,** High-contrast SPECT sequential coronal views clearly confirm prevertebral periaortic node involvement. A defect is seen in the right lobe of the liver from a subcapsular hematoma as a complication of liver biopsy. **C,** Computed tomography. *Left:* Superior cut shows the large hematoma. *Right:* The tumor mass is anterior to the spine in a lower cut. **D,** Three-view SPECT display shows the tumor to be anterior to the spine, perhaps best seen in the sagittal view.

Hepatocellular Carcinoma

Although hepatocellular carcinoma is most often seen on CT as a single mass in the liver, it is frequently multifocal in patients with cirrhosis and hepatitis C. Because most hepatomas are gallium avid, Ga-67 has been used to differentiate hepatoma from a regenerating nodule ("pseudotumor") on CT (Fig. 9-11).

Lung Cancer

Overall, the sensitivity of Ga-67 for lung cancer has been reported to be 85–90%. However, gallium scanning is very limited in its ability to stage patients and determine operability. F-18 FDG PET has taken over this role. Uncommonly, Ga-67 has been used to determine the extent of pleural-based mesotheliomas and to help

Box 9-5   Revised European-American Lymphoma (REAL) Classification

B-CELL NEOPLASMS

Precursor B-cell neoplasm: B-cell lymphoblastic lymphoma

Peripheral B-cell neoplasms
  Chronic lymphoma or leukemia
  Mantle cell lymphoma
  Follicular lymphoma
  Marginal cell lymphoma
  Hairy cell leukemia
  Plasma cell myeloma
  Diffuse large B-cell lymphoma
  Burkitt's lymphoma

T-CELL AND NATURAL KILLER CELL NEOPLASMS

Precursor T-cell neoplasm: T-cell lymphoblastic leukemia/lymphoma

Peripheral T-cell and natural killer-cell neoplasms
  Chronic lymphoma or leukemia
  Large lymphocyte leukemia
  Mycosis fungoides
  Peripheral T-cell lymphomas
  Angiocentric lymphoma
  Intestinal T-cell lymphoma

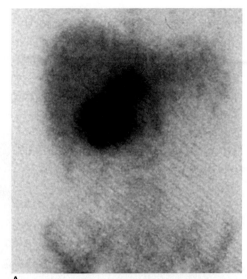

A

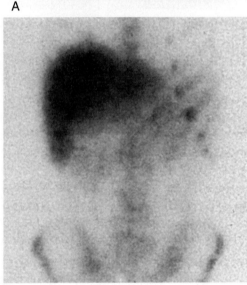

B

Figure 9-9   Non-Hodgkin's lymphoma: response to therapy. Resolution of gallium-67 uptake after appropriate therapy in a patient with non-Hodgkin's lymphoma. **A,** A large portal hepatic mass is seen before therapy. **B,** After therapy a residual mass was seen on computed tomography. No Ga-67 uptake is detected, although a photopenic mass effect appears to be present just below the liver because of residual nonviable tumor seen as a mass on CT.

differentiate malignant mesothelioma from benign pleural thickening.

Head and Neck Cancer

Varying results have been reported for Ga-67 in head and neck tumors. Sensitivity for tumor detection ranges from 56–86%. MRI and CT are the primary modalities for diagnosis. The prognosis is poor for patients with gallium avid residual masses after treatment. However, PET is better able to stage and restage head and neck cancer.

Abdominal and Pelvic Tumors

Ga-67 has been used successfully for the detection of draining nodal metastasis in testicular cancer. Uptake depends somewhat on histological subtype: 74% sensitive for metastatic embryonal cell carcinoma, 57% for metastatic seminoma, and 25% for testicular carcinoma.

Sensitivity of Ga-67 is generally poor for other tumors in the abdomen and pelvis. Reported sensitivities are: esophageal cancer, 41%; gastric tumors, 47%; colon cancer, 25%; pancreatic tumors, 15%. Similar low sensitivities have been reported for gynecologic tumors.

Soft Tissue Sarcomas

Most soft tissue sarcomas will accumulate Ga-67. An overall sensitivity of 93% has been reported for primary lesions, local recurrence, and metastatic disease. Liposarcoma, usually a low-grade tumor, has a high false-negative rate. A Ga-67 positive site that resolves after therapy is indicative of a favorable response.

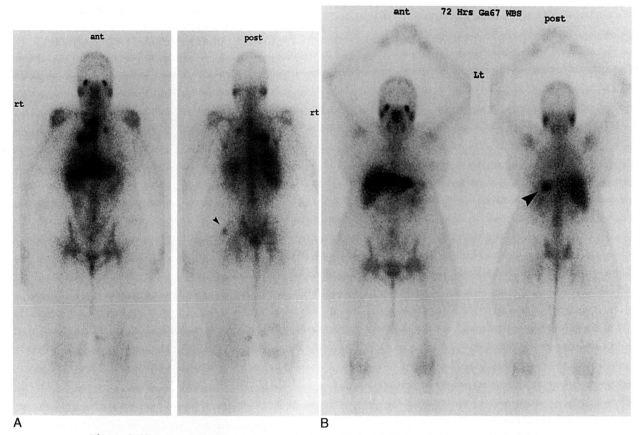

Figure 9-10   Hodgkin's disease: response to chemotherapy. A 30-year-old woman with nodular sclerosing Hodgkin's disease. **A,** Whole body gallium-67 scan shows multiple sites of tumor in the right perihilar and peritracheal regions, anterior mediastinum, and right and left lungs. Note uptake in the left buttock at the site of injection (*small arrowhead*). **B,** Follow-up scan after a course of chemotherapy shows resolution of Ga-67 uptake in the chest. New uptake in the stomach is secondary to gastritis, best seen in posterior view (*large arrowhead*). Gastric localization was confirmed by SPECT.

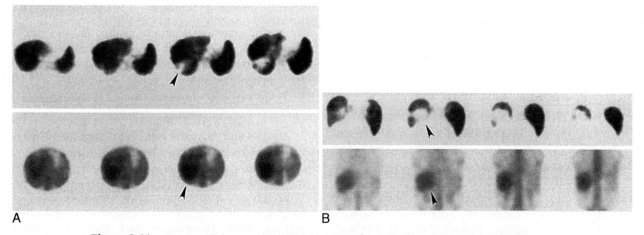

Figure 9-11   Hepatocellular carcinoma: SPECT gallium-67 and Tc-99m sulfur colloid. Transaxial **(A)** and coronal **(B)** SPECT slices.   SPECT was performed with an aging single-headed rotating gamma camera. The Tc-99m sulfur colloid liver spleen slices (*top*) show a large defect (*arrowheads*) in the posterior aspect of the right lobe. In comparable sections, the Ga-67 study (*bottom*) shows increased uptake (*arrowheads*) in the same area, consistent with the suspected tumor.

THALLIUM-201, TECHNETIUM-99M SESTAMIBI, AND TECHNETIUM-99M TETROFOSMIN TUMOR IMAGING

Myocardial perfusion agents, thallium-201 chloride (Tl-201), Tc-99m sestamibi (Tc-99m MIBI), and Tc-99m tetrofosmin are taken up in a large number of benign and malignant tumors. This section will briefly describe these agents and some possible applications. The use of Tl-201 for the detection of brain tumors is discussed in Chapter 13. The role of Tc-99m sestamibi in parathyroid adenoma diagnosis is covered in Chapter 5.

Radiopharmaceuticals

Thallium-201 Chloride

Chemistry and Physics

Tl-201 is a group IIIA metal in the periodic table (*see* Fig. 1-1) It decays by electron capture, emitting characteristic x-rays ranging from 69–83 keV (94% abundant) and two gamma rays, 167 keV (10% abundant) and

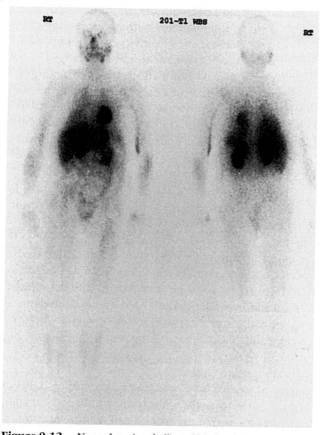

Figure 9-12   Normal resting thallium-201 distribution. Imaging started 15 minutes after injection show prominent uptake in the kidneys, heart, liver, and to a lesser extent, the bowel. Normally, the thyroid would be prominently seen. This patient has undergone total thyroidectomy for thyroid cancer. Adherence of Tl-201 to the arm vein on the side of the intravenous injection is common.

135 keV (3% abundant) with a physical half-life of 73 hours (Table 9-1).

Pharmacokinetics and Normal Distribution

After intravenous injection, Tl-201 is distributed throughout the body in proportion to regional blood flow (Fig. 9-12). The heart receives 3–5% of the administered dose, the liver receives 15%, and the kidneys receive 3.5%. Cardiac uptake is maximal at 10 minutes and peak uptake is probably similar for most tumors. Biological clearance is primarily via the kidneys and, to a much lesser extent, through the intestines. Total-body clearance is slow, with a 40-hour biological clearance.

Multiple factors play a role in the uptake of Tl-201 by tumors (Box 9-6). Blood flow is critical for radiotracer delivery. Tl-201 is then handled by cells as an analog of potassium. Tumor accumulation largely depends on the sodium-potassium ATPase pumping system on the cell membrane. It remains free in the cytosol with minimal localization in the nucleus or mitochondria.

Technetium-99m Sestamibi

Tc-99m MIBI (Cardiolite, marketed as Miraluma for breast tumor imaging by Dupont Pharmaceuticals) is a lipophilic cationic complex (methoxy-isobutyl-isonitrile). The technetium radiolabel provides superior images compared with Tl-201.

Pharmacokinetics and Normal Distribution

Compared with Tl-201, Tc-99m MIBI has less cardiac uptake (2%) and remains fixed in the heart. MIBI clears rapidly from the blood and localizes in skeletal muscle, liver, and kidneys (Fig. 9-13). Hepatic uptake is initially high with radiotracer then clearing into the biliary system and bowel. Subdiaphragmatic tumor detection is more difficult due to intestinal and urinary clearance.

Mechanism of Tumor Uptake

The cellular uptake of Tc-99m MIBI is related to its lipophilic properties and appears to lead to passive diffusion into the cell. A strong electrostatic attraction

Box 9-6	**Factors Determining Tumor Cell Uptake of Thallium-201 and Technetium-99m Sestamibi**
THALLIUM-201	**TC-99M SESTAMIBI**
Blood flow	Blood flow
Tumor viability	Tumor viability
Tumor type	Tumor type
Sodium-potassium ATPase system	Lipophilic cation
Co-transport system	Large negative transmembrane potential
Calcium ion channel system	

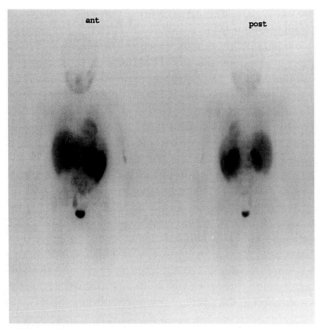

Figure 9-13   Normal resting technetium-99m sestamibi distribution. Imaging at 60 minutes after injection reveals prominent uptake by heart and liver. Hepatobiliary clearance and gallbladder filling are seen, as is intestinal and urinary clearance.

occurs between the positive charge of the lipophilic Tc-99m MIBI molecule and the negatively-charged mitochondria. Approximately 90% of Tc-99m MIBI is concentrated within the mitochondria. Tumors are detected as abnormal areas of uptake.

A cellular membrane glycoprotein, P-glycoprotein (Pgp), is responsible for pumping cationic and lipophilic substances out of the cell, including Tc-99m MIBI and chemotherapy agents. Malignant cells have increased expression of the multidrug resistance gene (MDR-1), which encodes for Pgp. Thus, increased amounts of the chemotherapeutic drugs are transported out of the tumor cells and may play an important role in drug resistance. With high levels of Pgp, more MIBI is transported out of the tumor cells. It has been postulated that Tc-99m sestamibi clearance might be used as an MDR-1 indicator and thus predictive of chemotherapy efficacy.

Technetium-99m Tetrofosmin

Chemistry and Physics

Tc-99m tetrofosmin (Myoview) is a lipophilic cationic diphosphine (trans-dioxo-bis) complex. When Tc-99m pertechnetate is added to tetrofosmin in the presence of the reducing agent stannous ion, a lipophilic, cationic Tc-99m tetrofosmin complex is formed.

Pharmacokinetics and Normal Distribution

Myocardial uptake of Tc-99m tetrofosmin is rapid. Like Tc-99m MIBI, it is not cleared from the myocardium. Tc-99m tetrofosmin is cleared more rapidly from the lung, blood, and liver than Tc-99m MIBI, which may be

advantageous for detection of tumors in the inferior quadrant of the right breast.

Mechanism of Tumor Uptake

The mechanisms of tetrofosmin uptake and sestamibi uptake are probably similar. Both are lipophilic cationic complexes and the uptake of both correlates with perfusion, high intracellular levels of mitochondria, and cell viability. Accumulation and retention in the mitochondria are mediated by the negative potential of the mitochondrial membrane. Tetrofosmin is also a substrate for Pgp. The Na^+/K^+ ATPase pump is only partially involved in the cellular uptake of tetrofosmin.

Dosimetry

Tl-201 results in a somewhat higher radiation dose to the patient than that of the Tc-99m-labeled agents (Table 9-2). The kidney is the critical organ for Tl-201, receiving 1.2 rads per 3 mCi (0.03 cGy/37 MBq). With a 30-mCi (1110 MBq) administered dose of the technetium agents (Tc-99m sestamibi and Tc-99m tetrofosmin), the organs receiving the largest radiation dose are the large bowel. The gallbladder receives the next highest dose.

Methodology

The imaging protocol should be modified for the particular clinical indication. Whole-body planar views, regional "spot views," and SPECT imaging are all possible. The optimal time to begin tumor imaging with these agents is approximately 5–30 minutes after injection. Specific protocols are discussed in the next section.

The technetium radiolabeled agents have better imaging characteristics than Tl-201. Thallium is suboptimal because of its low-energy (69- to 83-keV) mercury x-ray emission and low allowable administered dose (3 mCi or 111 MBq), which limits photon yield. Because of the better dosimetry of the Tc-99m-labeled agents, higher doses (25–30 mCi) are administered. Thus imaging time can be shorter and the images better.

Clinical Applications

Breast Cancer

Mammography detects breast cancer with a high degree of sensitivity (85–90%). However, its positive predictive value for malignancy is low (20–30%) and thus many women undergo unnecessary surgical biopsies. Mammography also has a poor negative predictive value in women who have dense breasts, implants, or those who have undergone breast surgery or radiotherapy. The false-negative rate in this group of patients approaches 30%.

Ultrasonography can differentiate cyst from solid tumor, but it is often otherwise nonspecific. MRI is very sensitive for tumor detection and can add diagnostic information in some cases, but its specificity is not high.

A noninvasive imaging test with high positive and negative predictive values could obviate the need for surgical biopsy in many women.

Tl-201 is taken up by adenocarcinomas of the breast. In a study of 45 patients with breast lesions greater than 1.5 cm, Tl-201 had a sensitivity of 97% for detecting breast cancer. In that study, fibrocystic disease showed no Tl-201 uptake. The smallest detectable primary lesion was approximately 1 cm in diameter. Most of these patients had palpable lesions.

Because of the better imaging characteristics of Tc-99m MIBI, studies of its utility for breast imaging were undertaken. Over 20 studies have been reported. In 1997, Tc-99m MIBI became the first radiopharmaceutical to be approved by the U.S. Food and Drug Administration (FDA) for breast imaging.

In a large multicenter trial of 673 patients from 30 institutions, an overall sensitivity of 85% and specificity of 81% were reported for diagnosis of breast cancer in patients who had a palpable breast mass or a mammographically detected lesion. Sensitivity was better for palpable masses (sensitivity 95%, specificity 74%) than for nonpalpable lesions (sensitivity 72%, specificity 86%). Sensitivity was also lower for lesions less than 1 cm in diameter. Another large, multicenter study of 530 patients with a palpable breast mass reported a sensitivity of 90% and specificity of 87.5%. In this study, the negative predictive value was nearly 99%, whereas the positive predictive value was only 50.8%.

Fibroadenomas are the most common cause for false-positive studies. The positive and negative predictive values for axillary node metastatic involvement are approximately 83% and 82%, respectively.

Methodology

A typical imaging protocol is described in Box 9-7. Tc-99m MIBI scintimammography is best performed with the patient lying on a specially designed imaging table with cutouts that allow one breast to hang dependent with the patient in the prone position. This setup allows lateral images of each breast without background activity from the chest wall and heart. Supine images are obtained for two-dimensional tumor localization. A narrow window of 10% rather than the typical 20% window around the 140-keV photopeak is recommended to minimize table scatter. SPECT has not proven advantageous.

Image Interpretation

Breast tumor scintigraphy should be interpreted in conjunction with the physical examination, mammography, and ultrasound if available. An abnormal study consistent with malignancy will show focal increased uptake in the region of the palpable or mammographically detected mass (Fig. 9-14). Diffuse uptake is nonspecific and usually does not indicate malignancy.

Clinical Role

Although Tc-99m MIBI breast imaging has a limited clinical role currently, the technique is clearly useful

---

Box 9-7   Scintimammography: Protocol Summary

PATIENT PREPARATION

None

DOSE

Tc-99m sestamibi 25 mCi (925 MBq)

INSTRUMENTATION

Camera: Large field of view with low-energy all-purpose collimator; 10% photopeak over 140 keV.

IMAGING PROTOCOL

Position patient prone on table with cutouts so that breasts hang dependent.
Inject Tc-99m sestamibi intravenously.
Begin imaging 5 min after injection. Ten minutes per image. Marker images may be shorter.
Prone: Lateral of breast with palpable nodule or mammographically detected mass. Repeat lateral image with radioactive marker over palpable nodule. Lateral of opposite breast.
Supine: Chest, including axilla

---

for certain subsets of patients. For example, patients with nondiagnostic mammograms, those with dense breasts or architectural distortion (e.g., from surgery and breast implants), and those with fibrocystic disease who are at increased risk for malignancy may benefit.

The current false-negative rate of 15% means an unacceptably high number of patients with tumor are not detected. Continued developments, such as new dedicated breast imaging devices with better camera sensitivity and image resolution, may increase the role of Tc-99m MIBI in breast imaging.

Bone and Soft Tissue Tumors

Tl-201 can successfully differentiate malignant from benign bone lesions. A high degree of correlation has been found between Tl-201 uptake and response to chemotherapy (Fig. 9-15). The lack of Tl-201 uptake in a mass indicates tumor necrosis, and tumor response results in decreasing Tl-201 uptake. Tl-201 is superior to both Tc-99m MDP and Ga-67 for imaging of bone and soft tissue tumors. This is not surprising because uptake of the latter two radiopharmaceuticals is determined by factors other than tumor response to therapy, such as bone repair. Frequently, extensive edema is associated with the tumor on MRI and may obscure tumor margins. Better definition of tumor may be possible with Tl-201. Tc-99m sestamibi has performed similarly to Tl-201 in evaluating bone primary sarcomas.

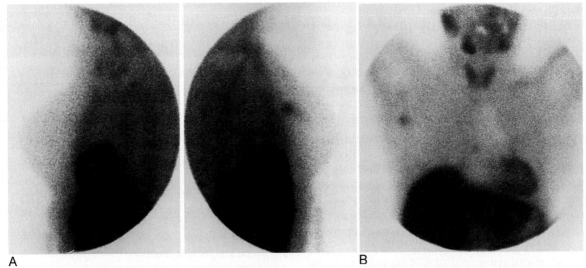

Figure 9-14 Scintimammography. Large palpable breast mass imaged with technetium-99m sestamibi. **A,** Laterals of right and left breast show intense focal uptake in right breast near the axilla consistent with malignancy. **B,** Anterior view helps localize the uptake to the upper outer quadrant.

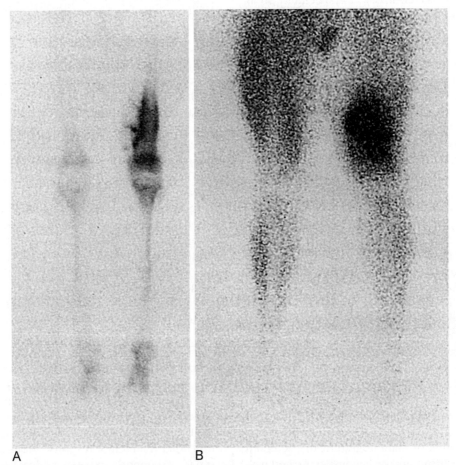

Figure 9-15 Thallium-201 uptake in osteosarcoma. **A,** Tc-99m HDP bone scan shows uptake in the distal left femur extending into soft tissue medially in a young patient with an osteosarcoma. **B,** Tl-201 study shows a pattern of uptake similar to that with Tc-99m HDP, but Tl-201 more clearly shows soft tissue involvement superomedially. Thallium study demonstrates viable tumor.

Thyroid Cancer

Although iodine-131 (I-131) is the primary agent for imaging and therapy of differentiated thyroid cancer, it does not accumulate in poorly differentiated tumors, anaplastic tumors, and medullary thyroid cancer. Tl-201 has been used for tumor localization when the I-131 whole body scan is negative but the patient's serum thyroglobulin level is elevated. Some of these Tl-201 positive patients will still show a response to I-131 therapy as evidenced by decreased thyroglobulin after therapy. F-18 FDG is now approved for this same indication.

Medullary thyroid cancer (MTC) arises from the parafollicular C-cells and does not accumulate I-131. MTC is a component of the familial multiple endocrine neoplasia type 2 (MEN-2) syndrome (Box 9-8). Tl-201 and Tc-99m MIBI accumulate in the primary tumor and can be used to detect recurrence. However, Tc-99m(V)-dimercaptosuccinic acid [Tc-99m(V)-DMSA] has been shown the most sensitive of these agents. The reported sensitivity of Tc-99m(V)-DMSA has ranged from 50% to 95%. The variability in sensitivity may be the result of various isomeric forms of the DMSA depending on the preparation. It is not available in the United States. F-18 FDG PET is useful in the evaluation of MTC and the use of In-111 pentreotide (OctreoScan) is discussed later.

Kaposi's Sarcoma

Tl-201 can be used in the diagnosis of pulmonary disease in AIDS patients. Kaposi's sarcoma is Ga-67 negative but Tl-201 positive. Most other infectious pulmonary diseases are gallium avid (e.g., *Pneumocystis*, atypical and typical *Mycobacterium*). Tl-201 scintigraphy is usually negative in infectious and inflammatory disease.

Other Tumors

A variety of other tumors, such as lung cancer, lymphoma, and head and neck tumors, have been imaged with the thallium and technetium radiopharmaceuticals. However, the clinical role of these agents is limited.

PEPTIDE RECEPTOR IMAGING

Numerous endogenous peptides that modulate tumor cell growth and metabolism have been identified. These peptides include several hormones and growth factors that interact with receptors on the tumor cell membrane. Among these are somatostatin, vasoactive intestinal peptide (VIP), tumor necrosis factor, and angiogenesis factor. This section discusses somatostatin derivatives which are available for therapy and clinical imaging.

Neuroendocrine Tumors

Neuroendocrine cells derive from embryonic neural crest cells. They share the ability to synthesize amines and produce peptide hormones and neurotransmitters. Neuroendocrine tumors have long been associated with the inheritable multiple endocrine neoplasia syndromes (MEN syndromes) along with other tumors (*see* Box 9-8).

Tumors arising from these cells fall into one of three categories: (1) neuroendocrine tumors or amine precursor uptake decarboxylation tumors (APUDomas), including pituitary adenomas, gastric endocrine tumors (carcinoid, gastrinoma, insulinoma), pheochromocytomas, medullary thyroid carcinoma, and small cell lung cancer; (2) central nervous system tumors (astrocytomas, meningiomas, and neuroblastoma); and (3) other tumors including lymphoma, breast, lung, and renal cell cancer.

Somatostatin receptors have been identified on many different cells and tumors of neuroendocrine origin (Fig. 9-16). Somatostatin is a 14–amino-acid long peptide produced in the hypothalamus, pituitary gland, brainstem, gastrointestinal tract, and pancreas. Somatostatin acts as a neurotransmitter in the central nervous system. Outside of the brain, it functions as a hormone that inhibits release of growth hormone, insulin, glucagon,

Box 9-8	Multiple Endocrine Neoplasia (MEN) Syndromes		
LESION	**MEN-I**	**MEN-IIA**	**MEN-IIB**
Pituitary adenoma	+		
Pancreatic islet cell tumor	+		
Parathyroid adenoma	+	+	
Pheochromocytoma		+	+
Medullary thyroid cancer		+	+
Ganglioneuroma			+

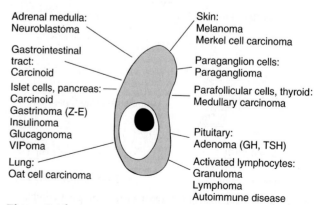

Figure 9-16 Neuroendocrine cells and the tumors originating from each type.

gastrin, serotonin, and calcitonin. Somatostatin has an antiproliferative effect on tumors. It appears to play a role in angiogenesis inhibition and is involved in the immune function of white blood cells.

Several agents have been developed which readily bind to somatostatin receptors (Fig. 9-17). Octreotide is an 8–amino-acid segment of somatostatin that maintains active binding properties of the native peptide hormone. Unlike the native molecule, it is resistant to enzymatic degradation in the body. This is reflected in the half-life of 2–3 hours rather than 2–3 minutes, as seen with endogenous somatostatin. Nonradiolabeled Octreotide (Sandostatin) has been approved by the FDA as a therapeutic agent suppressing growth in acromegaly and controlling symptoms in metastatic carcinoid and vasoactive intestinal peptide.

Indium-111 Pentreotide (In-111 OctreoScan)

Octreotide was initially radiolabeled with iodine-123. However, this is a technically demanding process and images obtained with this radiotracer are limited by a significant amount of bowel activity. Improved images are seen with indium-111 (In-111) labeled octreotide. The In-111 label allows delayed imaging not possible with a technetium label. Also, In-111 labeled octreotide has a low level of bowel activity. This agent, In-111 pentetreotide or In-111 OctreoScan (OctreoScan, Mallinckrodt), has been approved by the FDA for imaging of neuroendocrine tumors.

Chemistry and Pharmacokinetics
The In-111 pentreotide radiolabeling process involves complexing octreotide with diethylenetriamine pentaacetic acid (DTPA) to bind In-111. In-111 OctreoScan is rapidly cleared by the kidneys. There is also a low level (only 2%) of hepatobiliary excretion. At 4 hours after injection, 10% of the dose is still in circulation; at 24 hours, less than 1% is in circulation. This rapid clearance enhances the target-to-background ratio.

Five different subtypes of human somatostatin receptors (SSTR) have been identified (SSTR1 to SSTR5). These receptors are expressed to varying degrees on different tumors. This explains the differing sensitivities of somatostatin receptor imaging radiopharmaceuticals. The commercially available radiopharmaceutical In-111 pentetreotide binds with high affinity to the SSTR2 and SSTR5 subtypes, to a lesser extent with SSTR3, and not at all with SSTR1 or SSTR4. Identifying the specific receptor subtypes on tumors is also important as future therapeutic agents are developed to target tumors.

Accuracy
The accuracy of In-111 pentetreotide for diagnosis of various neuroendocrine tumors is noted in Table 9-6. Many of these tumors are small and can easily be missed on conventional imaging. However, sensitivity for small lesions (less than 1 cm) is limited. The ability to perform SPECT in addition to whole-body imaging increases detectability.

For most neuroendocrine tumors, such as gastrinoma and carcinoid, the sensitivity is very high. Two exceptions are insulinoma and medullary carcinoma of the thyroid, with only 50% sensitivity. The sensitivity for pheochromocytoma and neuroblastoma is high (approximately 90%), similar to that obtained with I-131 MIBG imaging (see Chapter 5). For adults, MIBG scanning is generally preferred, even though the image quality is poorer and the radiation dose is higher than with OctreoScan. The advantage of I-131 MIBG is the higher

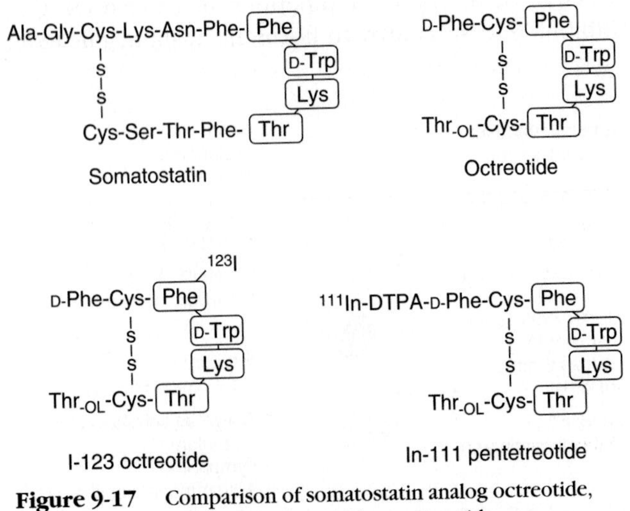

Figure 9-17 Comparison of somatostatin analog octreotide, iodine-123 octreotide, and indium-111 pentetreotide (OctreoScan).

Table 9-6 Accuracy of Indium-111 OctreoScan in Multicenter Trial

Tumor type	Consistent/total patients (n)*	Percent
Carcinoid	190/237	80
Insulinoma	8/11	31
Gastrinoma	40/42	95
Glucagonoma	8/11	73
Small cell carcinoma of lung	2/2	100
Pheochromocytoma	9/9	100
Paraganglioma	6/7	86
Medullary thyroid carcinoma	12/22	54
Vipoma	6/7	86
Pituitary adenoma	24/30	80

*Other methods included biopsy, computed tomography, ultrasonography, magnetic resonance imaging, and angiography.

target-to-background ratio and better specificity. An important disadvantage of In-111 pentreotide is its persistent high kidney activity, which makes interpretation of the adjacent adrenal gland more difficult. The reported sensitivity for other tumors, such as lymphoma and lung and breast cancer, is about 70% each; however, clinical utility has not been established.

Methodology

Box 9-9 describes a typical imaging protocol for In-111 OctreoScan. Because Sandostatin competes with In-111 OctreoScan for uptake, the therapeutic agent Sandostatin is usually discontinued 3–7 days before the study. However, there are case reports of better visualization of metastases while patients were taking the drug. Imaging is normally done at 4 and 24 hours. Early imaging at 4 hours is a dvantageous because bowel activity is absent at this early time, although the background activity is still high. The tumor detectability improves on 24-hour images due to background clearance. Additional images can be done at 48 hours after bowel cleansing if needed.

Dosimetry

The estimated radiation-absorbed dose to the patient from OctreoScan is shown in Table 9-7. The spleen is the target organ, receiving the highest absorbed dose followed by the kidneys.

Table 9-7   Radiation Dosimetry of In-111 Pentetreotide (OctreoScan)

Organ	rads/mCi (cGy/37 MBq)
Large intestine	0.27
Kidney	1.8
Urinary bladder	1.02
Liver	0.4
Adrenal glands	0.25
Spleen	2.5
Thyroid	0.25
Testes	0.1
Red marrow	0.12
Total body	0.44

Target organ (highest radiation absorbed dose) appears in boldface type.

Image Interpretation

Normal uptake occurs in the thyroid gland, liver, gallbladder, spleen, kidneys, and bladder. The kidneys retain considerable radiotracer and appear quite intense even on delayed imaging (Fig. 9-18). Bowel uptake should be absent or insignificant on the 4-hour images. By 24 hours, significant bowel activity is often seen normally.

Approximately 80–90% of tumors are visible by 4 hours. Due to decreasing background, more lesions will be visible on 24-hour images. Many tumors can be diagnosed with planar imaging (Figs. 9-19 and 9-20). However, SPECT is essential in the abdomen. The region between the kidneys can be difficult to scan because of the high renal uptake.

Tc-99m NeoTect

NeoTect (Tc-99m Depreotide, Diatide) is a synthetic peptide with high-affinity binding to somatostatin receptors. Originally developed to diagnose neuroectodermal tumors, it proved inferior to octreotide, due in part, to a high level of abdominal background activity. Delayed imaging at 24 hours was not realistic because of the Tc-99m radiolabel. NeoTect binding has been demonstrated in somatostatin receptor-positive pulmonary malignancies, and it has been approved by the FDA for evaluating lung masses seen on x-ray or CT.

The clinical indications are similar to that of F-18 FDG (i.e., to evaluate a solitary pulmonary nodule for malignancy). In one study, NeoTect differentiated malignancy from benign processes with an overall sensitivity of 70% and specificity of 86%. It was able to improve the predictive value of malignancy from 85% with CT to 97% with NeoTect. NeoTect appears to have a similar accuracy to F-18 FDG PET.

Box 9-9   Indium-111 OctreoScan: Protocol Summary

RADIOPHARMACEUTICAL

Dose: 6 mCi (222 MBq) In-111 OctreoScan intravenously

PREPARATION

Bowel preparation with laxative and enema; hydration
Discontinue octreotide therapy 3–7 days before
  injection

INSTRUMENTATION

Camera: Large-field-of-view SPECT gamma camera
  Dual-headed camera preferable
Collimator: Low-energy high-resolution collimator
Photopeaks: 20% window around 173 and 245 keV
Computer: 128 × 128 word mode matrix size

IMAGING PROCEDURE

4 hr: Planar images of abdomen and pelvis, 500,000
  counts or 15 min; SPECT of abdomen
24 hr: Planar whole body imaging, 300,000 counts or 15
  min; SPECT of abdomen and other regions as clinically
  indicated

4 Hours Imaging

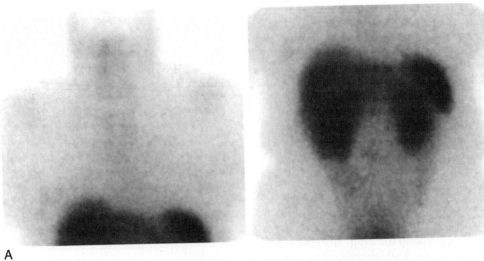

A

24 Hours Imaging

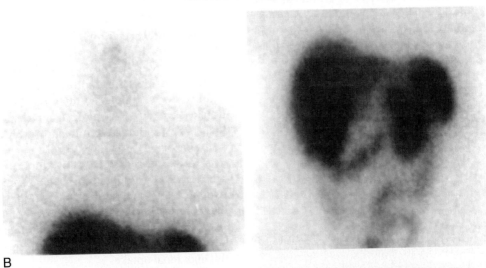

B

Figure 9-18   Normal distribution of In-111 OctreoScan. **A,** Planar images at 4 hours show intense uptake in the kidneys and spleen with liver activity nearly as intense. **B,** Delayed images at 24 hours reveal diffuse bowel activity which is frequently seen and may obscure disease.

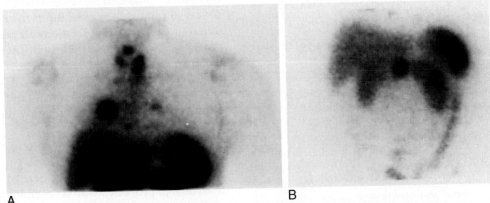

A   B

Figure 9-19   Metastatic carcinoid tumor on In-111 OctreoScan. Anterior planar views of chest **(A)** and abdomen **(B).** Multiple sites of thoracic, mediastinal, and paratracheal uptake, as well as uptake in the midabdomen, representing paraaortic adenopathy. The patient also had multiple other sites not shown here, including many soft tissue metastases.

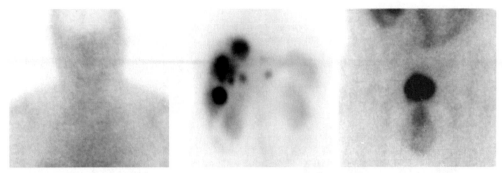

Figure 9-20   Anterior In-111 OctreoScan images reveal diffuse hepatic metastasis in a patient with gastrinoma.

Method

A dose of 15–20 mCi (555–740 MBq) is administered containing approximately 47 μg of Tc-99m radiolabeled depreotide peptide. No patient preparation is necessary, although patients should be well hydrated. Planar and SPECT images of the chest are obtained between 2–4 hours after injection.

Dosimetry

Because NeoTect is a Tc-99m radiolabeled radiopharmaceutical, the radiation absorbed dose is low. The kidneys are the critical organs with 0.33 rad/mCi (cGy/37 MBq). The spleen receives 0.16 rad/mCi (cGy/37 MBq), and the marrow receives 0.078 rad/mCi (cGy/37 MBq).

Tumor Therapy

In recent years, significant advances have occurred in the use of targeted antibodies as a means to deliver radiation therapy. Although preliminary results are promising, targeted peptide radiotherapy is still investigational. It has been shown that high doses of In-111 OctreoScan will inhibit tumor growth in patients with somatostatin receptor-positive tumors. In-111 emits an Auger electron that travels only short distances but has been noted to cause damage in the nucleus. This Auger electron damage can be used for therapeutic purposes if higher doses than the normal scan dose are given. High-energy beta-emitting radioisotopes including Yttrium-90 (Y-90) and Lutetium-177 (Lu-177) bound to octreotide have been used effectively in early therapeutic trials against neuroendocrine tumors.

MONOCLONAL ANTIBODIES

Monoclonal antibody imaging has the potential for targeting specific tumor types. In recent years, important clinical advances have been made in the development of antibodies for diagnosis and therapy. Four radiolabeled monoclonal antibodies have been approved by the FDA

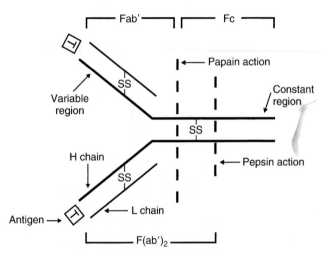

Figure 9-21   IgG antibody. The molecule can be digested enzymatically by papain, resulting in three parts, two Fab′ fragments and one Fc fragment, or by pepsin to produce $F(ab')_2$ fragments and subfragments of Fc. Fab′ may be produced by splitting the disulfide bond of $F(ab')_2$.

for imaging cancer of the colon, ovary, prostate, and lung. Two radiolabeled antibodies have been approved for therapy in B-cell lymphoma. Other antibodies are under investigation and await the results of further clinical trials and approval.

Background

Antibodies are proteins produced by lymphocyte plasma cells in response to exposure to foreign antigens. An IgG antibody consists of two identical heavy (H) and two light (L) chains linked by a disulfide bridge (Fig. 9-21). Each chain is made up of two regions. The *variable* region (Fab′) is responsible specifically binding to a cell surface antigen. The *constant* region (Fc) is involved with cell destruction through complement fixation and antibody-dependent cell cytotoxicity.

Each plasma cell produces one specific antibody against a single antigenic determinant. However, animals immunized with an antigen produce and secrete into

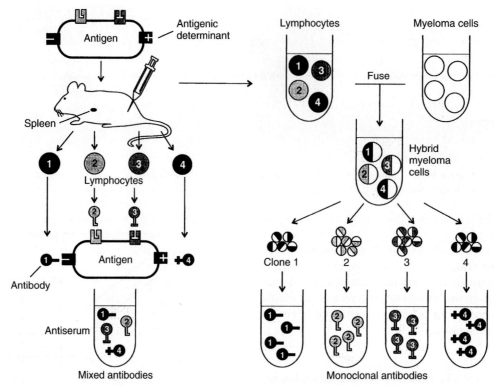

Figure 9-22   Monoclonal hybridoma antibody production. The process starts with injection of an antigen into a mouse, causing proliferation of B-lymphocytes that can make antibody to the antigen. The mouse spleen is removed and the B-cells are harvested. Many of the B-cells are capable of making antibody to the specific antigen. If they were cultured at this point (*left*), they would make a mix of antibodies and would soon die off. If instead the B-cells are mixed with mouse myeloma cells in polyethylene glycol, some of the normal B-cells will fuse with the myeloma cells, producing a population of hybridomas that can be cultured indefinitely. When this population is selectively cloned for those that make the desired antibody, a pure culture of target antibody-producing cells can be grown in great quantities. Its product is the desired monoclonal antibody.

their blood a mixture of antibodies from many plasma cells, each against different antigenic determinants. Some medically useful antibodies (e.g., gamma globulin) have been produced in rabbits or other animals for human use, but these polyclonal antibodies bind to multiple different antigenic sites and are thus nonspecific. Early antibody imaging studies used polyclonal antibodies, often labeled with I-131. Although they showed promising results in a variety of tumors, I-131 had imaging and dosimetric disadvantages for diagnostic studies.

Kohler and Milstein won the Nobel Prize in 1975 for describing a method for unlimited production of a single monoclonal antibody (MoAb). Myeloma cancer cells from a mouse are fused with lymphocytes from the spleen of mice immunized with a particular antigen (Fig. 9-22). These "hybridoma" cells retain both the specific antibody production capacity of the lymphocytes and the immortality of the myeloma cancer cells. Immunoassays screen the hybrid cells to identify the specific cell line that produces the murine (or mouse) MoAb clone desired. A MoAb with high affinity and

specificity for the antigen of interest is harvested. The individual hybridoma cells can be maintained in culture to produce large quantities of the monoclonal antibody for future use.

MoAbs that are produced by the immunization of mice are mouse proteins, and as such are recognized by the human immune system as foreign. The human immune system mounts an immunological response against the MoAb. This human antimouse antibody (HAMA) response ranges from mild with fever and hives to severe with shortness of breath and hypotension. The reaction may even be fatal as a result of anaphylaxis.

The HAMA response is related to the amount of antibody the patient is exposed to as well as the size of the antibody. Rather than delivering a whole intact antibody, a fragment can be used which will be less immunogenic. The active regions are kept and the large constant portions of the antibody that contribute the most to the HAMA response are deleted.

Proteolytic enzymes such as pepsin and papain will cleave off the Fc portion of the antibody. Pepsin produces a larger F(ab')$_2$ fragment and papain a smaller F(ab') fragment (Fig. 9-21). These fragment antibodies not only have fewer immunogenic side effects but are also better suited for imaging. These fragments are cleared from the background much more rapidly, thus improving tumor detection.

Despite the development of MoAb fragments, the potential for serious reactions remains a serious clinical concern. In an attempt to overcome the problems with using foreign mouse proteins, new production methods have been developed. One first step was the creation of chimera MoAbs by replacing the murine Fc portion of the antibody with a human component. Further steps have lead to fully human MoAbs through phage display and recombinant DNA technology. Although not yet available with the FDA-approved MoAb imaging agents described here, these new antibody production techniques will likely play an important clinical role in the near future.

The MoAb imaging agents currently available for clinical use are derived from both whole murine antibodies and fragments. They are selected based on a high level of tumor-specific binding. Many tumors express specific antigens on their surfaces, which can be targeted. An example of this is carcinoembryonic antigen (CEA) on colon cancer cells. Other tumors express increased numbers of normal antigens or receptors on their surfaces, such as the CD20 receptor on certain lymphomas.

Radiolabeling

Chemists have attached various radionuclides (such as I-131, I-123, In-111, and Tc-99m) to MoAbs. Each has distinct advantages and disadvantages (Table 9-8). Radiolabeling must be done without changing the antibody's immunoreactivity or biological properties so that the resulting radiopharmaceutical can be used successfully for immunoscintigraphy.

Although I-131 can be easily bound to other molecules, it creates very limited images because of its physical prop-

erties. I-123 has very good imaging characteristics but has been difficult and expensive to obtain in the past, and it is only recently that production methods became available that create a product with lower dosimetry by eliminating I-124 and I-125 radiocontaminants.

In-111 was frequently used for MoAb radiolabeling because it has better imaging characteristics than I-131. The 2.8-day half-life of In-111 allows time for the slow radiopharmaceutical accumulation and background clearance of whole antibodies. The best target-to-background ratio for imaging occurred 48–72 hours after injection.

With the development of antibody fragments and their more rapid background clearance, high target-to-background ratios can be obtained on the day of injection. Thus, imaging with Tc-99m–labeled MoAbs became a possibility. The optimal imaging characteristics of a technetium label may lead to significant improvements in lesion detection.

Clinical Imaging Applications

The FDA has approved four radiolabeled monoclonal antibodies for oncological diagnostic imaging: OncoScint for colorectal and ovarian cancer, CEA-Scan for colorectal cancer, ProstaScint for prostate cancer, and Verluma for small cell carcinoma of the lung.

Colorectal Cancer

Colorectal cancer is the second most common malignancy in the United States. Prognosis is strongly dependent on tumor staging (Box 9-10). Five-year survival is 85% with localized disease, 50% with regional spread, and less than 7% with distant metastases. The first recurrence occurs at a single site in 75% of cases. These sites include the liver (33%), local or regional sites (21%), intra-abdominal sites (18%), and retroperitoneal lymph nodes (10%).

CEA arises from ectodermally-derived epithelial cells of the digestive system. It is normally only expressed during embryological development but is also found in

Radionuclide	Energy (keV)	Half-Life	Advantages	Disadvantages
Technetium-99m	140	6 hr	Pure gamma, inexpensive, high-photon flux	Complex chemistry, short half-life, high counts in kidney and bladder
Indium-111	173, 247	2.8 days	Gamma emitter	Affinity for liver and RES, delayed imaging possible
Iodine-123	159	2.8 days	Gamma emitter, ease of labeling	Dehalogenates, cyclotron produced, expensive due to short half-life
Iodine-131	364	8 days	Ease of labeling	Dehalogenates, low count rate, poor image quality, high radiation dose

Table 9-8 Radionuclides Used for Immunoscintigraphy: Advantages and Disadvantages

Box 9-10	Dukes' Classification for Colorectal Cancer Staging
DUKES A	Involvement into bowel wall but not beyond muscularis
DUKES B	Spread beyond pericolonic tissue; No lymph nodes involved
DUKES C	Locoregional lymph node involvement
DUKES D	Distant metastasis

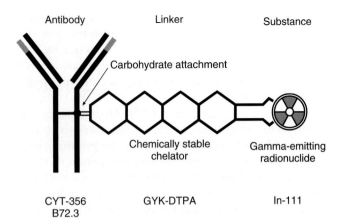

Figure 9-23   Indium-111 OncoScint CR/OV and In-111 ProstaScint formulation. The site of attachment of the linker does not interfere with the effector or binding functions of the antibody. (Courtesy of Cytogen, Princeton, NJ.)

colorectal cancer and other solid tumors. Over 95% of colorectal cancers express membrane surface CEA. It is shed into the bloodstream and is detectable in 65% of patients with colorectal carcinoma. Although serum CEA levels are used as a marker of residual and recurrent tumor, nearly one-third of patients with recurrence do not have elevated serum CEA levels.

Most recurrences and metastases occur in the abdomen and pelvis. Colonoscopy and barium studies produce a low yield in determining sites other than local recurrence because they detect only intraluminal disease. CT is a sensitive method for detecting metastatic colon cancer. However, CT often misses lymph node involvement, especially as lymph nodes must be enlarged (>1 cm) before they are usually considered abnormal. In addition, postoperative and radiation changes may obscure tumor. F-18 FDG-PET has proven highly effective in detecting distant colorectal metastasis. However, it has limitations. Local lymph node involvement is frequently missed, due in part to adjacent bowel activity. Also, the sensitivity of F-18 FDG PET is lower in certain tumors types (e.g., mucinous rectal tumors).

Radiopharmaceuticals

OncoScint CR/OV   OncoScint (satumomab) was the first monoclonal antibody approved as a tumor-imaging agent by the FDA (1994). It is a B72.3 murine IgG monoclonal antibody directed against a high molecular-weight tumor-associated glycoprotein (TAG-72), which is expressed by the majority of colorectal and ovarian cancers. Although not currently available commercially in the United States, OncoScint detects several types of tumor, most commonly ovarian and colorectal cancer. In ovarian carcinoma, sensitivity and specificity were 95% and 56%, respectively. In colorectal carcinoma, it showed sensitivities ranging from 70–89% and a specificity of 76%.

The antibody is linked to In-111 by conjugation to the Fc portion, which avoids the area of active antigen binding and preserves the immunoreactivity of the antibody (Fig. 9-23). OncoScint is approved for localization and determination of the extent of extrahepatic metastatic tumor in patients with known colorectal or ovarian can-

cer (Fig. 9-24). Although the urinary clearance is lower than fragment antibodies, leading to low levels of kidney uptake, there is significant liver background which interferes with the detection of liver metastasis.

Tc-99m CEA-Scan   CEA SCAN was approved in 1996 for imaging of colorectal cancer. It is a Tc-99m-labeled Fab′ fragment of the CEA antibody IMMU-4. Removal of the Fc group of IgG, the most immunogenic part of the molecule, eliminates much of the immunogenicity ordinarily observed with mouse-derived antibody products.

Pharmacokinetics   The pharmacokinetics of Onco-Scint and Tc-99m CEA-Scan are very different, largely because the former radiopharmaceutical is a whole antibody and the latter is an antibody fragment. Table 9-9 compares the pharmacokinetics of OncoScint and CEA-SCAN. Liver metabolism is low but renal activity is high compared with that for the whole antibody (Fig. 9-25).

An advantage of the Tc-99m-labeled Fab′ fragment is its rapid renal clearance from the blood, allowing for same day high tumor-to-background ratio imaging. At 1, 5, and 24 hours after infusion, 63%, 23%, and 7%, respectively, of the injected dose is present in the circulation. Over 24 hours, 28% of the dose is excreted in the urine.

Indications   The FDA approved CEA-Scan for detection and localization of recurrent, metastatic, and occult colorectal carcinoma in patients with histologically confirmed colorectal carcinoma (Fig. 9-26). Its major role to date has been in the evaluation of recurrent disease. The two clinical indications are a patient with a rising serum CEA level but negative conventional imaging, and a patient with known potentially resectable disease who requires preoperative evaluation to exclude the presence of unresectable disease. The CEA-Scan can assure the surgeon that the patient has no other metastatic disease that would contraindicate surgical treatment. Due to the increasing clinical role of PET,

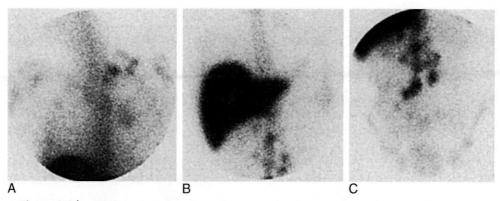

Figure 9-24   Distant recurrent colorectal cancer with indium-111 OncoScint. Tumor uptake is seen in the left supraclavicular nodes and left hilum (**A**), in the periaortic nodes, and more diffusely throughout the abdomen (**B** and **C**). Retrosternal uptake was detected with SPECT.

Table 9-9 Comparison of OncoScint CR/OV and CEA-SCAN		
	OncoScint CR/OV	**CEA-SCAN**
Radionuclide	In-111	Tc-99m
Monoclonal antibody type	B72.3, whole antibody	IMMU-4 reactive with CEA, Fab′ fragment
HAMA	40%	<1%
Liver metabolism and uptake	High	Low
Renal metabolism and uptake	Low	High
Plasma half-life	Slow (50 hr)	Rapid (initial T ½ 1 hr, final T ½ 13 hr)
Urinary excretion	10% at 72 hr	28% at 24 hr

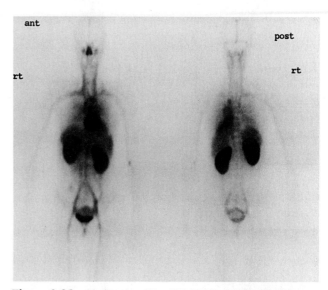

Figure 9-25   Technetium-99m CEA-SCAN normal distribution. The kidneys have the greatest uptake of the radiopharmaceutical. Renal clearance into the bladder is seen. Cardiac and vascular blood pool is prominent. Lesser distribution is seen in the liver and spleen. The focal uptake above the bladder is the uterine blood pool.

CEA-Scan is often reserved for F-18 FDG PET negative tumors (e.g., mucinous cellularity) or for cases where PET is unavailable.

The role of Tc-99m CEA in primary disease is not well established. Possible applications might be the detection of synchronous lesions, preoperative determination of the extent of regional disease, or search for occult metastases.

Accuracy   In a multicenter trial, 192 patients with colorectal carcinoma were imaged with OncoScint CR/OV and CT. The overall sensitivity was 69%, specificity was 76%, positive predictive value was 97%, and negative predictive value was 19%. Scans detected occult disease in 10% and changed patient management in 25%. Although CT was more sensitive than antibody imaging of the liver, OncoScint was superior for the pelvis and extrahepatic abdomen (Table 9-10). The combined sensitivity of CT and OncoScint immuno-scintigraphy (88%) was higher than the sensitivity of either study alone.

In a multicenter trial of 210 patients with advanced recurrent or metastatic colorectal carcinomas, the sensitivity of Tc-99m CEA for detection of metastatic colon cancer in the abdomen, liver, and pelvis was superior to CT (Table 9-10). Tc-99m CEA was superior to CT in the extrahepatic abdomen and pelvis. The accuracy of CT and CEA-Scan was similar in the liver. The combination of Tc-99m CEA and CT increased the overall sensitivity from 66% to 78% while only slightly decreasing specificity (from 89% to 83%).

Tc-99m CEA is superior to OncoScint in several respects. First, it has better imaging characteristics

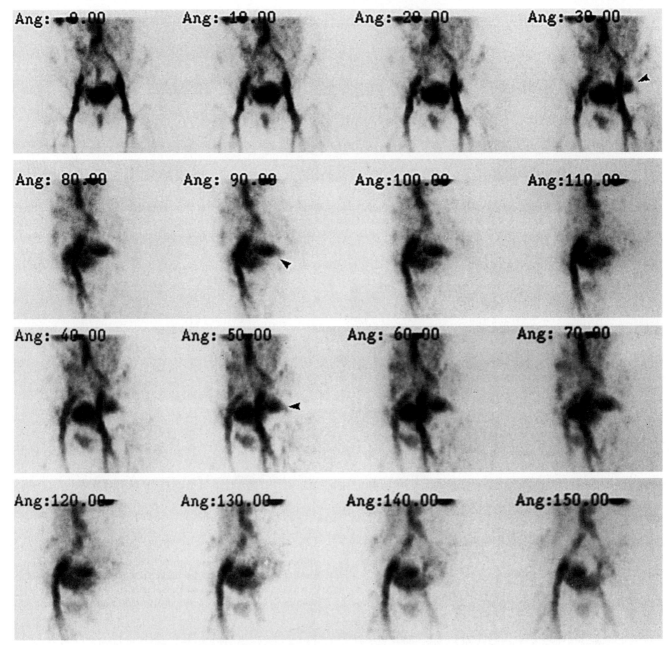

Figure 9-26 Technetium-99m CEA, local recurrence of colorectal cancer. Patient had rising serum CEA level several months after primary resection of tumor in the rectosigmoid area. This reconstructed volume display of sequential projection angles (Ang = degrees) shows tumor recurrence in the rectal area (*arrowheads*).

because of the Tc-99m radiolabel. Second, the antibody fragments of Tc-99m CEA clear more rapidly. This results in a higher target-to-background ratio at an earlier imaging time (day 1 versus day 2 or 3). Because of the absence of high liver uptake with Tc-99m CEA-Scan, it is also superior to In-111 OncoScint in detecting liver metastases. Although liver metastases are often photopenic with OncoScint, they are usually hot or target lesions with Tc-99m CEA. Finally, CEA-Scan has a much lower incidence of HAMA response, less than 1% versus 40% for OncoScint.

One disadvantage of the CEA F(ab′) fragment is the high level of renal uptake, which can obscure disease.

Methodology Imaging protocol for Tc-99m CEA Scan is described in Box 9-11.

Dosimetry The estimated radiation absorbed patient doses for OncoScint CR/OV and CEA-Scan are detailed in Table 9-11. The highest radiation dose from In-111 OncoScint occurs in the spleen and red marrow. For Tc-99m CEA the highest dose is in the kidney, followed by the urinary bladder and spleen.

Table 9-10   Imaging Sensitivity of OncoScint and CEA-SCAN versus Computed Tomography by Anatomical Site

	Sensitivity for colorectal tumor localization (%)			
Anatomical site	In-111 OncoScint	CT	Tc-99m CEA-Scan	CT
Pelvis	74	57	69	39
Abdomen (extrahepatic)	66	34	55	32
Liver	41	84	63	64

Box 9-11   Tc-99m CEA-Scan Sample Protocol

PREPARATION

None

RADIOPHARMACEUTICAL

Dose: 30 mCi (1110 MBq) intravenously

INSTRUMENTATION

Camera: Large-field-of-view gamma camera, Dual-headed camera preferable
Collimator: Low-energy, high-resolution
Photopeaks: 15% symmetric window around 140 keV
Computer: 128 × 128 word matrix size

IMAGING PROCEDURE

Image: imaging 2 hr after injection
Planar images: 10 min/view spot images chest to pelvis
SPECT: Abdomen and pelvis, with tow-headed camera: 60 stops/head, 40 sec each
Optional 24-hr planar imaging (20 min/view) or SPECT (50% increased acquisition time)

Adverse Effects   The incidence of side effects with OncoScint is less than 4%. Most are not serious and are readily reversible, generally without intervention. Adverse effects with Tc-99m CEA have also been uncommon and self-limiting.

The incidence of elevated HAMA with CEA-Scan is less than 1%, compared with a 40% incidence with OncoScint. Generally HAMA levels decrease with time and half of cases become seronegative. This has implications for using OncoScint in a serial manner to evaluate the effectiveness of therapy or as a prelude to therapy with a MoAb. At present, only a single administration has been approved. HAMA can interfere with murine-based immunoassays of CEA and CA-125, producing falsely high values. Alternative assay methods that are not adversely affected are available. HAMA can alter the biodistribution and pharmacokinetics of MoAbs and may interfere with the quality or sensitivity of the imaging study.

Ovarian Cancer

Ovarian cancer is the fourth most frequent cause of cancer deaths in women. The overall 5-year survival rate is 39%. Ovarian cancer is difficult to diagnose and stage with current imaging methods because it frequently metastasizes as small (<2 cm) miliary peritoneal implants not detectable on CT. Nor can CT detect tumor in normal-sized lymph nodes or distinguish adhesions or scar from tumor. Although F-18 FDG PET has added sensitivity when used with the CT, the pattern of uptake may be misleading due to nonspecific normal bowel activity. Serum CA-125 assay, a tumor marker, has a high false-negative rate and does not predict the location or extent of disease. Exploratory laparotomy is the best approach to surgical staging. However, it does not detect extraabdominal tumors, is expensive, has a 20% complication rate, and gives false-negative results in 20–50% of patients based on the results of second-look surgery.

In a multicenter trial of patients with primary or recurrent disease, OncoScint had a sensitivity of 60–70% and a specificity of 55–60% for ovarian cancer. It was superior to CT for patients with recurrent disease and carcinomatosis (60% versus 30%). Tc-99m CEA-Scan has not been used clinically or approved for ovarian cancer. F-18 FDG PET has proven useful in ovarian carcinoma, although it may miss very small tumors which often stud the peritoneum.

Prostate Cancer

Cancer of the prostate is the most frequently diagnosed malignant tumor in men in the United States and the second leading cause of cancer death. Its incidence is increasing. The 5-year survival is approximately 50%. Although many patients have symptoms for which they seek medical evaluation, the diagnosis is often suspected on the basis of screening prostate-specific antigen (PSA) levels drawn on men older than 50 years. Ultrasound-guided needle biopsy is used to obtain tissue from suspect nodules.

Staging of prostate cancer is based on the combination of physical examination, histopathological Gleason's score, and serum PSA. Bone scans are indicated for patients with serum PSA greater than 10–20 ng/ml or with a high Gleason's score. In patients who have undergone prostatectomy, any increase in PSA is suspicious. Lymph node involvement is the most common pattern of metastatic spread, usually occurring in a stepwise fashion from periprostatic or obturator nodes, to internal and external iliac nodes, and then to common iliac and periaortic nodes (Fig. 9-27). Frequent sites of distant metastases are the skeleton, liver, and lungs.

Table 9-11   Dosimetry of Approved Monoclonal Imaging Agents

Organ	In-111 Satumomab Pendetide OncoScint rads/5 mCi cGy/185 MBq	Tc-99m Arcitumomab CEA-Scan rads/30 mCi cGy/1110 MBq	In-111 Capromab Pendetide ProstaScint rads/5 mCi cGy/185 MBq
Gallbladder wall			7.3
Large intestine	3.1		7.6
Kidney	9.7	**11.1**	12.4
Urinary bladder	2.8	1.8	2.2
Liver	15.0	1.1	**18.5**
Lungs	4.9		5.6
Adrenal glands	4.5		5.32
Ovaries	2.9	0.5	
Heart wall	3.2		7.8
Spleen	**16.0**	1.8	16.3
Thyroid	1.5		1.4
Testes	1.4	0.5	5.6
Red marrow	12.0		4.3
Total body	2.7	0.5	2.7

Target organ (highest radiation absorbed dose) appears in boldface type.

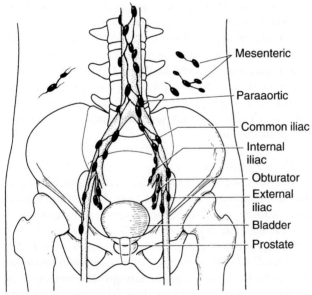

Figure 9-27   Pelvic and abdominal lymph node anatomy. Knowledge of this anatomy is critical for proper interpretation of indium-111 ProstaScint studies.

Initial therapy involves either surgery or radiation therapy. Radical prostatectomy, the best chance for cure, is not undertaken when there is evidence of nodal involvement or distant spread. Thus, assessing the status of pelvic lymph nodes draining the prostate gland is critical to staging and management. CT and MRI have limited value owing to their low sensitivity for detecting nodal involvement. F-18 FDG PET has low sensitivity for prostate cancer. Even when inactions are favorable that the tumor is contained intracapsularly before surgery, patients are frequently found to have extracapsular dis-

ease at surgery. The rate of local recurrence after surgery is 15–20%.

Lymphadenectomy, the most accurate technique for detecting nodal involvement, may fail and lead to surgery for patients with occult disseminated disease. Patients with high PSA levels and a high Gleason's score are usually treated with local radiation therapy because they are at risk for local recurrence. Radiation therapy can be performed as the initial treatment or following radical prostatectomy.

If after initial treatment the PSA fails to fall to undetectable levels or subsequently rises, residual or recurrent cancer is likely. Radiation therapy of the prostate fossa or the pelvis is often given, even in the absence of positive biopsy or positive imaging results. If disease is localized to the prostate fossa or pelvis, radiation therapy offers the potential for effective treatment. However, if recurrence involves periaortic lymph nodes or other distant sites, radiation therapy exposes the patient to significant morbidity with no potential for cure, owing to the presence of tumor outside the radiation therapy field. In this situation, In-111 ProstaScint can play an important role.

Indium-111 ProstaScint

In-111 ProstaScint (Capromab Pendetide, Cytogen, Princeton, NJ) is a conjugate of the monoclonal antibody 7E11-C5.3 (CYT-356), a linker-chelator (GYK-DTA), and In 111 (Fig. 9-28). This is an intact murine immunoglobulin reactive with prostate-specific membrane antigen (PMSA), a glycoprotein expressed by more than 95% of prostate adenocarcinomas. ProstaScint was approved in 1996 as an imaging agent for the detection of soft tissue metastases for patients with prostate cancer who were at high risk for metastatic disease.

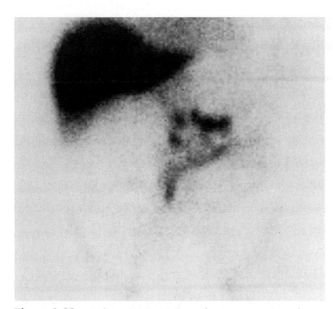

Figure 9-28   Indium-111 ProstaScint shows paraaortic and mesenteric lymph nodes. This planar abdominal image showed no change in distribution between days 3 and 6, excluding bowel activity as the cause for this activity.

	ProstaScint scan positive	ProstaScint scan negative	
Biopsy positive	40	24	Sensitivity 62%
Biopsy negative	24	63	Specificity 72%

Table 9-12   Comparison of ProstaScint with Pelvic Lymph Node Dissection

Pharmacokinetics and Normal Distribution   In-111 ProstaScint follows a monoexponential clearance pattern with a biological half-life of 72 hours. Ten percent is excreted in the urine within 72 hours, and a smaller amount is excreted through the bowel. Normal distribution includes the liver, spleen, bone marrow, and blood pool structures. Clearance occurs into the bowel and bladder.

Accuracy   In a multicenter trial, 152 patients with a tissue diagnosis of prostate cancer scheduled for pelvic lymphadenectomy had ProstaScint scans. Other standard noninvasive imaging including bone scans, CT, and MRI were negative or equivocal. The patients were considered at high risk for the presence of lymph node metastases based on PSA or Gleason's score. The imaging results were correlated with histological analysis of pelvic lymph nodes. ProstaScint correctly identified lymph node metastases in 40 of 64 patients (sensitivity 62%), compared with a sensitivity of 4% for CT and 15% for MRI. Of 88 patients without pelvic nodal metastases, 63 were correctly identified as normal (specificity 72%) (Table 9-12). The specificity of ProstaScint may actually be higher than these results suggest because 15 patients with a false-positive study had biochemical evidence of disease after radical prostatectomy, suggesting that disease was missed.

Results were similar in a multicenter series of 183 patients in whom residual or recurrent prostate cancer after radical prostatectomy was strongly suspected based on rising PSA levels, but bone scans and standard imaging methods gave negative results. Although the accuracy of ProstaScint scanning is only fair, it far surpasses all other available imaging modalities.

Minor adverse events have been reported in 4% of patients. Most common have been liver enzyme elevations, hypotension, and hypertension, each occurring in 1% of patients or less. Elevated HAMA titers have been observed in 8%. A similar incidence (4%) of adverse events was seen in patients undergoing repeated injections.

Indications   In-111 ProstaScint is indicated for the assessment of nodal metastases in two different situations. First, it can be used to stage patients at high risk for pelvic lymph node metastases but with apparently localized disease after standard diagnostic evaluation tests. Most commonly, In-111 ProstaScint is used in postprostatectomy patients when occult metastatic disease is suspected because of a rising PSA level but the standard workup is negative or equivocal. Radiation therapy is indicated if disease is localized to the prostate bed and pelvic lymph nodes, but not if the scan shows activity in periaortic lymph nodes or other distant sites. In the latter case hormonal manipulations, systemic chemotherapy, or orchiectomy would be more appropriate treatment options.

Methodology   An imaging protocol for In-111 ProstaScint is described in Box 9-12. SPECT of the abdomen and pelvis is mandatory. Blood pool images are necessary for correct interpretation. They may be acquired either by imaging on day 1 at 30 minutes after In-111 ProstaScint injection or, preferably, by radiolabeling the patient's red blood cells and acquiring dual-isotope Tc-99m RBC and In-111 ProstaScint planar and SPECT images at 96 hours (3–5 days). The day 3 images often have problematic bowel activity, and the day 5 images are occasionally limited by a low count rate. Review of the two study days together gives us the most confidence in interpretation. In addition, software fusion packages are available which can combine the ProstaScint images with a CT to optimize lesion localization or characterization. If available, SPECT-CT can be very helpful.

Dosimetry   The highest In-111 ProstaScint radiation dose is received by the liver, followed by the spleen

---

Box 9-12 Indium-111 Capromab Pendetide ProstaScint Imaging: Dual Isotope Protocol Summary

RADIOPHARMACEUTICAL CAPROMAB PENDETIDE

Dose: 5 mCi (185 MBq) In-111 ProstaScint intravenously over 5 minutes. Observe patient 30 minutes

PATIENT PREPARATION

Well hydrated, bowel cleansing preparation 2 days before imaging

PLANAR IN-111 PROSTASCINT IMAGING

96 Hours after injection: patient voids
Whole body images performed by either multiple overlapping spot views (10 min/view, 256 × 256 matrix) OR whole body scan mid femur to head (4-6 cm/min)
Collimator: Medium-energy collimator
Photopeaks: 20% window around 173, 247 keV
Computer: 256 × 256 matrix size for spots, 512 × 1024 for whole body scan
Draw and label red blood cells

SPECT IMAGING PROCEDURE

96 hours (3-5 days) Image after planar images:
    patient voids
Re-administer 2-3 mCi (74-111MBq) Tc-99m tagged RBCs
Positioning: SPECT pelvis make sure symphysis included

ACQUISITION

128 × 128 matrix, 64 stops/head; 50-60 sec/stop
140 keV peak window at 5%; 173 keV window at 15%; 247 keV window at 20%

PROCESSING

Fusion software for overlie and localization with CT
Occasionally, repeat delayed imaging required to permit time for blood pool, bladder, or bowel clearance

---

and kidneys. Table 9-11 lists dosimetry estimates for the body.

Interpretation There is a steep learning curve for interpretation of In-111 ProstaScint SPECT studies. The FDA approved this radiopharmaceutical for clinical use and interpretation only by physicians who have undergone specific training in the acquisition and interpretation of these studies. There are several reasons for the concern about interpretive difficulty. In the pelvic SPECT, there is a paucity of normal anatomical landmarks. The individual cross-sectional images have low counts and poor resolution. Bowel and bladder clearance can complicate interpretation. Increased uptake may be seen in the prostate bed following radiation therapy.

The dual-isotope acquisition method allows single-day imaging and perfect image registration of the two studies. For correct interpretation, the physician must be familiar with pelvic lymph node anatomy and common patterns of tumor spread (Fig. 9-28). The lymph nodes lie along the blood vessels. Therefore, the In-111 ProstaScint images must be carefully correlated with the blood pool images, because right-to-left vascular asymmetries may otherwise be misinterpreted as nodal disease

on the In-111 ProstaScint images. An abnormal scan shows increased uptake in the prostate fossa, at pelvic, abdominal, or chest lymph node sites, or less commonly in bony structures. Pelvic lymph node metastases are best seen on the SPECT studies and rarely seen on planar studies (Fig. 9-29). However, both planar and SPECT images may show periaortic lymph or thoracic lymph node metastases. ProstaScint is considerably less sensitive (50%) than bone scan for detecting bone metastases.

SPECT images software fused with CT or SPECT-CT improves anatomical certainty in interpretation.

Lung Carcinoma

Lung cancer can be divided into two distinct diseases based on tumor biology and chemotherapy responsiveness: small-cell carcinoma of the lung (SCLC) and nonsmall-cell lung cancer (NSCLC). SCLC accounts for 25% of all new lung cancers in the United States. Survival is poor, 18% at 5 years with limited disease and only 2% with distant metastases. Two thirds of patients with SCLC have metastatic spread at the time of diagnosis, thus only one third would be expected to respond to local therapy. Staging determines the extent of disease at the time of

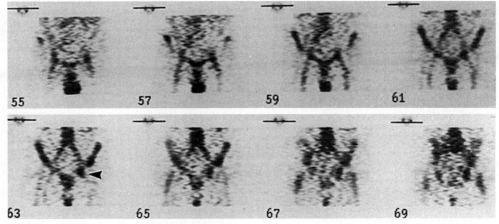

Figure 9-29   Indium-111 ProstaScint detects metastases to regional nodes. Sequential coronal images show prominent uptake in external iliac nodes (*arrowhead*).

presentation and guides therapy. Patients with limited disease are treated with local radiation therapy and systemic chemotherapy, whereas patients with extensive disease receive palliative treatment with chemotherapy alone.

NSCLC is primarily a surgical disease; resection is the treatment of choice for localized disease. Accurate staging is essential to determine whether the patient is potentially curable. The standard diagnostic imaging staging method is CT. Mediastinoscopy with lymph-node biopsy is indicated to evaluate enlarged or equivocal lymph nodes. The patient is considered a candidate for primary tumor resection if no evidence of tumor spread to extrathoracic sites, the contralateral chest, or the mediastinum is found. CT relies on lymph-node size to detect metastatic disease. However, normal-sized nodes may contain microscopic tumor. Because of this, CT lacks sensitivity and may underestimate the extent of lung cancer. Thus patients may undergo unnecessary surgery. In addition, enlarged nodes may be due to reactive hyperplasia or infection, resulting in false-positive findings. Although mediastinoscopy may improve accuracy, it is invasive and expensive.

Tc-99m Verluma

Verluma (Tc-99m Nofetumomab, DuPont Pharmaceuticals) is a Tc-99m-labeled Fab′ fragment of a murine IgG2b monoclonal antibody NR-LU-10 directed against a 40-kilodalton glycoprotein expressed on a variety of carcinomas, including SCLC, NSCLC, and cancers of the breast, ovary, prostate, colon, and rectum. Tc-99m Verluma was approved by the FDA in 1996 as a diagnostic imaging agent for staging of patients with newly diagnosed SCLC.

Pharmacokinetics   Renal clearance is the main route of excretion, with 64% of the injected dose excreted within the first 22 hours. The secondary route of elimination is hepatobiliary, with clearance into the gallbladder and intestines. HAMA develops in only 6% of patients.

Accuracy   Tc-99m Verluma was compared with conventional diagnostic methods in a multicenter trial of 96 patients with SCLC, of whom 42% had limited and 58% had extensive disease as evaluated with standard imaging modalities. Tc-99m Verluma correctly staged 82% of patients. The positive predictive value for demonstrating extensive disease was 94%. Sensitivity for tumor detection was 77%, compared with 88% for a battery of standard diagnostic tests. Tc-99m Verluma had the highest accuracy for clinical staging of any single diagnostic test.

Although approved for SCLC, Tc-99m Verluma is taken up by other tumors. In addition to NSCLC, uptake has been reported in gastrointestinal, breast, ovarian, pancreatic, renal, and cervical cancers. The ultimate role of Tc-99m Verluma in these cancers is uncertain and will require further investigation. However, Tc-99m Veraluma is not commercially available.

Methodology   Imaging is performed about 18 hours after injection of the radiopharmaceutical (30 mCi or 1110 MBq). SPECT of the chest is routine.

Monoclonal Antibody Therapy of Lymphoma

Non-Hodgkin's lymphoma (NHL) is the most common hematologic cancer and the sixth most common cause of death. The most common forms of NHL are follicular cell and diffuse large B-cell lymphoma. Although large B-cell NHL can be cured, low-grade follicular NHL is considered incurable. Initial response rates are high but patients ultimately relapse and die. The mean survival is 8–10 years with conventional chemotherapy and radiation therapy. Response rates of recurrent episodes become progressively less, and these patients frequently transform into a higher-grade lymphoma.

There are several immunologic targets on the B-cell surface that MoAbs can specifically bind. The CD20 antigen is present on 90% of the B-cell lymphomas on mature

Table 9-13	Comparison of Low-Grade NHL Monoclonal Antibody Therapies: Y-90 Zevalin and I-131 Bexxar	
	Y-90 Zevalin	**I-131 Bexxar**
Radiolabel half-life	64 hrs	8 days
Beta particle	2.293 MeV	0.606 MeV
	5 mm path	8 mm path
Gamma emission	No	Yes; 364 keV
Pretreatment dosimetry	No	Yes
Pretreatment unlabeled antibody	Rituximab chimeric	Tositumomab murine
HAMA	1-2%	60%
Outpatient therapy	+	+/−

B-lymphocytes. CD20 is not expressed on the membranes of normal hematopoietic cells, antibody-producing mature plasma cells, early B-cell precursors, or other lymphoid tissues.

This CD20 antigen is the target for the currently approved immunologic therapies Yttrium-90 ibritumomab (Y-90 Zevalin) and I-131 tositumomab (I-131 Bexxar) (Table 9-13). Radiolabeled MoAb therapies show better tumor response than treatment with nonradiolabeled MoAb. They each recruit immune system response to aid in tumor cell killing, but they also irradiate the cell they are bound to and cause "crossfire" killing of tumor cells. Crossfire is the result of beta-radiation traveling a short distance from the site of antibody binding and killing adjacent tumor cells not bound to the MoAb.

Y-90 Ibritumomab tiuxetan (Y-90 Zevalin)

Y-90 Ibritumomab tiuxetan (Zevalin, IDEC-Y2B8) was the first FDA-approved radiolabeled antibody therapy agent (Fig. 9-30). It is a murine IgG1 kappa monoclonal antibody that targets the CD20 receptor on lymphocytes. The short half life of the radiotracer is ideal for effective clearance. Tiuxetan is a chelator that binds either In-111 or Y-90 and provides a stable link between the radioisotope and the antibody.

Yttrium-90 has a physical half-life of 64 hours and is a high energy (2.29 MeV) pure beta-emitter. The beta-particle travels only a short distance of 5 mm. An effective dose of radiation will be deposited very close to the site of radiolabeled antibody binding. No imaging can be done with this agent because no significant radiation leaves the patient (e.g., no gamma ray emission). However, this also means the dose requires no special shielding and the therapy can be done as an outpatient. In fact, few special radiation safety precautions are needed. This situation contrasts with I-131 Bexxar therapy, which is stored and administered through heavily shielded equipment.

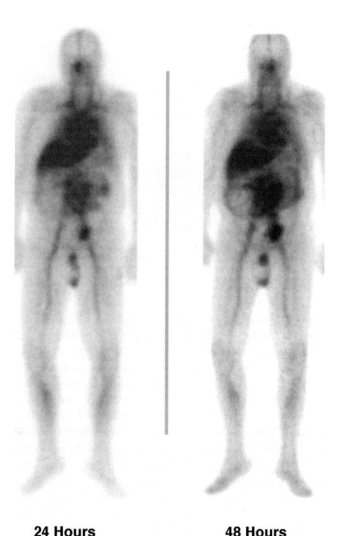

24 Hours   **48 Hours**
A   B

Figure 9-30   Biodistribution scan for Y-90 zevalin lymphoma therapy. Prior to therapeutic infusion of the pure beta-emitter, Y-90 zevalin, a biodistribution scan is performed with In-111 ibritumomab tiuxetan (zevalin) planar images. In-111 Zevalin images at 24 hours (**A**) and 48 hours (**B**) show an expected biodistribution. Normal activity is seen in the kidneys, liver and blood pool. Expected uptake is present in the lymph nodes involved with tumor in the midabdomen, left groin and left pelvis. This patient may go on to receive the therapeutic Y-90 zevalin dose.

Indications

Y-90 Zevalin is used for the treatment of relapsed, refractory, or transformed CD20+ non-Hodgkin's lymphoma. It is absolutely contraindicated in patients with a known hypersensitivity reaction to murine proteins (HAMA), greater than 25% tumor involvement of marrow, and those with impaired marrow reserves. Patients should not have had myelotoxic therapies with autologous bone marrow transplant or stem cell rescue. External beam radiation should not have involved over 25% of the marrow. The neutrophil count must be over 1500 cells/mm³ and platelet count must be over 100,000.

Dosimetry

Y-90 Zevalin has a biologic half-life of 46–48 hours with a typical dose to the tumor of 15–17 Gy. Elimination is primarily through the urine, although most of the agent remains in the body. The radiation dose to various organs is listed in Table 9-14.

Methods

The protocol consists of three parts (Table 9-15). Rituximab (Rituxan) is given to block CD20 antigens on cells circulating in the blood and spleen. The patient must be closely monitored during this infusion as serious, potentially fatal reactions can occur. Then, within 4 hours of receiving the rituximab, 5.0 mCi (185 MBq) of In-111 labeled zevalin is administered over 10 minutes. Then whole body planar images are done within 2–24 hours and between 48–72 hours later to assess distribution of the radiopharmaceutical. An optional third image can be obtained over the next 90–120 hours. Normally, low urinary tract uptake and low bowel activity is seen, but fairly high liver and spleen uptake are present. The blood pool activity should markedly decrease over the studies. Altered blood pool distribution would include activity increasing rather than decreasing over time in lung, liver,

heart, urinary tract, or bowel uptake. Any of these changes could lead to unacceptable radiation to the organ in question, such as the kidneys.

Toxicity

Significant side effects may occur from this therapy. Usually within 7–9 weeks, blood counts reach a nadir (median neutrophil count 800, platelet count 40,000, hemoglobulin 10.3). The cytopenia may last from 7 to 35 days. In particular, roughly 7% of neutropenic patients are prone to febrile neutropenia and infections. Thrombocytopenia may result in hemorrhage. Up to one third of patients will subsequently transform to a more aggressive lymphoma. It is uncertain if this is a side effect of therapy or the natural course of the disease. A small number (1.4%) of patients will develop myelodysplasia or acute myelogenous leukemia.

Results

This is a very effective therapy. Overall, 67–83% of patients experience some response, with 15–37% of patients showing complete remission. These values are significantly better than the results of nonlabeled rituxan MoAb therapy alone. The duration of response ranges from 0.5 to 24.9 months.

I-131 Tositumomab (I-131 Bexxar)

I-131 Tositumomab (I-131 Bexxar) is a murine IgG2a monoclonal antibody developed to target CD20 which is the same target for Y-90 zevalin. There are several similarities and differences between Y-90 zevalin and I-131 Bexxar.

Indication

I-131 Bexxar is not a first line therapy. It is recommended for CD20+ follicular NHL (with or without transformation), which is refractory to rituximab.

Method

A protocol outline is provided in Table 9-16. Unlike Y-90 zevalin, the I-131 Bexxar therapy dose can be imaged using the 364-keV gamma emissions. Whereas a therapy patient receiving zevalin will first receive In-111 zevalin for biodistribution imaging then Y-90 zevalin for therapy, I-131 Bexxar is used for both the image and

Table 9-14   Radiation Dosimetry of Y-90 Ibritumomab Tiuxetan (Zevalin) and I-131 Tositumomab (Bexxar)

Organ	Y-90 Zevalin (mGy/MBq)	In-111 Zevalin	T-131 Bexxar (mGy/MBq)
Spleen	9.4	0.9	1.14
Testes	9.1	0.6	0.83
Liver	4.8	0.7	0.82
Colon	4.8	0.4	1.34
Heart	2.8	0.4	1.25
Thyroid	0.3	0.1	2.71
Lungs	2.0	0.2	0.79
Bladder	0.9	0.2	0.64
Kidney	0.1	0.2	1.96
Total body	0.5	0.1	0.24

Table 9-15   Therapy Protocol for Y-90 Ibritumomab (Zevalin)

I. Day 1	II. Biodistribution scans	III. Therapy (Day 7-9)
Pretreatment: Rituximab 250 mg/m² < 4 hrs: 5 mCi (185 MBq) In-111 Zevalin Over 10 min	First scan 2–24 hours Second scan 48–72 hours Optional: Third scan 90–120 hours	Pretreatment Rituximab 250 mg/m² < 4 hours: Y-90 Zevalin 0.4 mCi/kg platelet >150k 0.3 mCi/kg platelet 100–150k

Table 9-16	Therapy Protocol for I-131 Tositumomab (Bexxar)			

Day 0	Day 1	Day 2, 3, or 4	Day 6 or 7	Day 7 (up to day 14)
Thyroid block	1. Premedicate: acetaminophen, diphenhydramine	Whole-body dosimetry scan	Whole-body dosimetry scan	Therapy administration
SSKI: 4 drops **TID OR** potassium iodide: 130 mg QD	2. Pretreatment Tositumomab (450 mg) over 60 min		Calculate patient specific dose:	1. Pretreat Tositumomab (450 mg) over 60 min
			Plate >150k 75 cGy	
Note: begin day before and continue for 2 weeks	3. I-131 Bexxar (5 mCi or 185 MBq) over 20 min			2. Therapy dose I-131 Tositumomab over 20 min
			Plate 100-150k 65 cGy	
	4. Dosimetric whole-body scan prevoid			

therapy. The Bexxar regimen also uses the same tositumomab monoclonal antibody for pretreatment (in the nonradiolabeled form) as for dosimetry and therapy (in the I-131 labeled form). The I-131 label means that, unlike a pure beta-emitter, the dose requires shielding. Also, it must be determined before discharging the patient that the exposure to others will not be greater than 500 mrem from the patient.

One potential problem with I-131 Bexxar is the need to perform additional scans after dosing to determine dosimetry. This is less convenient than Y-90 zevalin, where two scans rather than three or four are done to examine biodistribution and not for dose calculations.

Because the I-131 radiolabel can disassociate from the MoAb and result in unwanted thyroid exposure, the patient must receive thyroid blocking medication at least one day before beginning the studies. This usually involves supersaturated potassium iodide (SSKI) four drops three times a day or potassium iodide 130 mg tablets once a day. This should be continued for 2 weeks.

The patient is first treated with nonlabeled tositumomab to block excess CD20 sites. This helps decrease nonspecific antibody targeting. Following this, the patient receives a low dosimetry dose of I-131 tositumomab. The first scan is done after infusion but before the patient voids to determine the maximal initial activity in the patient. Dosimetry scans are then done serially to calculate how fast activity clears from the body (or residence time) before dosing can be calculated. Then a patient-specific dose is calculated based on this information as well as the desired dose based on platelet levels.

Toxicity

Like Y-90 zevalin, similar significant hematologic side effects can occur. Up to 15% of patients may require supportive care such as transfusions and colony-stimulating

factor. Long-term side effects are possible, such as the myelodysplastic syndrome and secondary leukemia. Hypothyroidism may occur if proper premedication is not given to block the thyroid from taking up I-131.

The other concern with any murine MoAb is the HAMA response. HAMA is common initially with an incidence that ranges widely in clinical use. The patients who had extensive previous chemotherapy became seropositive roughly 10% of the time, whereas those patients who received I-131 Bexxar as a first-line therapy had initially elevated titers up to 70% of the time.

Results

Overall, 63% of patients refractory to rituximab showed response. Of these, 29% of the patients experienced complete response. The median duration of response was 26 months. This is significantly longer than with Y-90 zevalin.

PALLIATION OF BONE PAIN

Metastatic disease to the bone is a common problem causing significant pain and disability to patients with cancer. Although this can occur with almost any cancer, it most commonly involves tumors originating from prostate, breast, and lung. Red marrow involvement is most common, although cortical lesions are also frequently seen. Numerous methods are available for the treatment of bone pain. These include analgesics, chemotherapy drugs, hormonal therapy, bisphosphonates, external beam radiation, and even surgery. Radiopharmaceuticals are an important addition to this list of treatments. Radiopharmaceuticals available for treatment of bone pain are listed in Table 9-17.

Bone-seeking radiopharmaceuticals have been used to treat bone pain from cancer for decades. These agents

Table 9-17 Radiopharmaceuticals for Bone Pain Palliation

Radionuclide	Pharmaceutical	Physical half-life (days)	β Max (MeV)	β Mean (MeV)	Maximal tissue distance (mm)	γ Photon (keV)
P-32	Orthophosphate	14.3	1.71	0.695	8	–
Sr-89	Chloride	50.5	1.46	0.583	6.7	–
Sm-153	EDTMP	1.95	0.8	0.224	3.4	103
Re-186	HEDP	3.8	1.07	0.349	4.7	137

all localize to bone, in areas of bone repair and turnover. Therefore, they deposit in areas of metastasis. The therapeutic effects depend on the emission of beta particles. Beta particles are high energy but only travel millimeters from the site of deposition. This ensures the effects are limited to the abnormal bone and normal tissue is spared. These agents are extremely useful as they can be given in addition to other therapies such as external beam radiation, or even after external beam therapy has reached maximal limits.

Phosphorus-32 (P-32)

P-32 is one of the earliest known bone-seeking radioisotopes. It has been used via intraperitoneal infusion for the treatment of tumors such as ovarian cancer and in the treatment of polycythemia vera. It is available for intravenous administration for bone pain palliation. A range of skeletal absorbed doses have been calculated (25–63 rad/mCi or 0.68–1.733 cGy/MBq). However, it appears that the normal marrow receives a high dose relative to the tumor due to the distribution of P-32 in the inorganic matrix as well as the cellular regions. Also, the lack of a gamma emission means no external imaging can be done to assess distribution.

Strontium-89 (Sr-89)

Sr-89 (Metastron, Amersham) is also a pure beta-emitter which has been approved by the FDA for the management of metastatic bone pain under the trade name Metastron (Amersham). It selectively localizes in areas of boney turnover, predominantly in blastic lesions. It is retained longer in regions of metastasis than normal bone. The pathway of excretion is predominantly through the urine with about one third bowel excretion. Dosimetry is outlined in Table 9-18.

A 4-mCi (148 MBq) dose is administered intravenously slowly over 1–2 minutes. An alternative dose of 55 uCi/kg (2.04 MBq/kg) may be used. Repeat dosing is possible, but factors such as initial response, hematologic status, and current status must be considered in each case. In general, a repeat administration is not recommended before 90 days have elapsed.

Table 9-18 Dosimetry of Bone Pain Therapeutic Agents Strontium-89 (Sr-89) and Samarium-153 (Sm-153)

Organ	Sr-89 rad/mCi (cGy/37 MBq)	Sm-153 rad/mCi (cGy/37 MBq)
Bone surface	63.0	25.0
Red marrow	40.7	5.7
Colon	4.7	0.037
Bladder	4.8	3.6
Testes	2.9	0.02
Ovaries	2.9	0.032
Whole body	2.9	0.04

Toxicity

Because toxicity occurs to marrow components platelets and white blood cells, the hematologic status of each patient must be evaluated before therapy. After obtaining a baseline platelet count, platelets should be measured at least every other week. Typically, platelets will decrease 30% from baseline and reach the nadir between 12–16 weeks after therapy. Toxicity is generally mild; however, Sr-89 must be used with caution in those with white cell counts less than 2400 and platelets less than 60,000. A small number of patients experience transient worsening of symptoms.

Approximately 20% of patients will become pain free. Roughly 75% of patients will experience some significant decrease in pain, although some series have reported up to 90% of patients experience some symptom relief. Pain relief begins about 7–20 days after injection and generally lasts 3–6 months.

Samarium-153 (Sm-153)

Sm-153 (Quadramet, DuPont) is a beta-emitting radiopharmaceutical that has the added advantage of a gamma emission that can be detected for external imaging. It has been approved for use in patients with osteoblastic

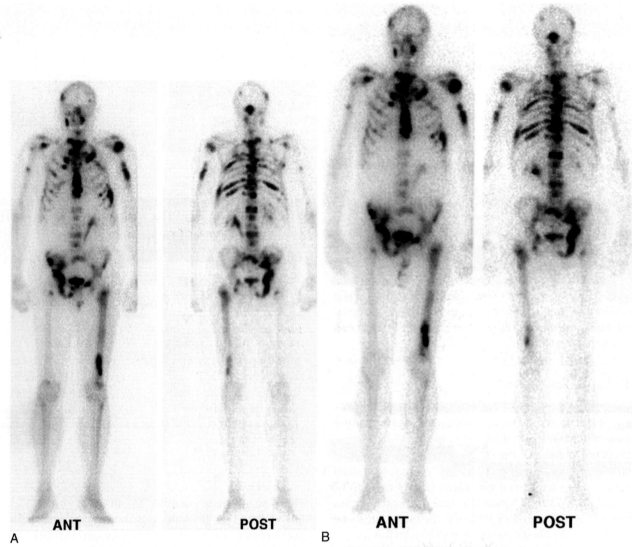

ANT **POST** A **ANT** **POST** B

Figure 9-31   Samarium-153 (Sm-153) palliation of metastatic disease bone pain. **A,** The whole body Tc-99m MDP bone scan prior to therapy confirms the presence of osseous metastasis that will accumulate the therapy agent. **B,** The whole body scan done with the Sm-153 therapy dose shows close correlation with the lesions seen on bone scan.

metastases that can be visualized on a nuclear medicine bone scan (Fig. 9-31).

It is administered in a 1.0-mCi/kg (37 MBq/kg) dose intravenously over the course of 1 minute. Approximately 50% of the dose is localized to normal and abnormal bone. It accumulates in metastatic lesion in a 5:1 ratio compared with normal bone. Patients should be well hydrated and void frequently as the primary route of clearance is through the urine. Approximately 35% of the dose is excreted in the first 6 hours.

As in Sr-89, the bone marrow toxicity is a limiting factor. Toxicity is usually mild, although serious side effects and even fatalities have been reported. Platelets decreased on the order of 25% from baseline and white blood cells by 20%.

The short range of the Sm-153 beta particle should be advantageous when considering the dose to normal marrow. A response rate on the order of 83% has been reported. Pain relief is generally noted within 2 weeks, with a duration of 4–40 weeks.

Re-186 HEDP

Re-186 HEDP or rhenium-186 hydroxylidene diphosphonate (Rh-186 HEDP) is formed by combining a diphosphonate useful for bone pain therapy, etidronate, with a beta emitter. Re-186 HEDP is another agent that may be useful for the palliation of bone pain. It emits a gamma ray useful for imaging and lesion identification. It rapidly localizes to bone with approximately 14% retained in bone. The remainder is rapidly cleared with roughly 70% of the dose excreted in the urine 6 hours after injection.

LYMPHOSCINTIGRAPHY

Melanoma

Malignant melanoma can be cured by surgery if the disease is localized, but advanced disease is invariably fatal. The main prognostic factors are thickness of the primary lesion and metastatic lymph node involvement. Patients with regional lymph node metastases have a 10% 10-year survival rate; those with distant metastases have a less than 1% 10-year survival.

Patients with a primary cutaneous melanoma thickness of less than 1 mm have a greater than 90% 10-year survival. Those with a primary lesion thickness greater than 4 mm have a poor prognosis with a 4-year survival of 40%, and the benefit of lymph node dissection is questionable. It is the patient with an intermediate thickness lesion (greater than 1 mm but less than 4 mm) that can benefit from lymph node dissection.

Lymph node metastases are found in approximately 20% of patients undergoing draining nodal bed resection. Complications of this surgery include chronic lymphedema and nerve injury. Histopathologic evaluation of the first lymph node draining the tumor, the sentinel lymph node, predicts the presence or absence of lymphatic spread and nodal involvement.

Lymphoscintigraphy can localize the sentinel lymph node (Fig. 9-32) and determine the need for nodal basin resection. Absence of tumor in the sentinel lymph node has a very high negative predictive value because skip metastases are rare (<2%). Sentinel lymph node biopsy is associated with a very low incidence of late lymphedema (<2%).

The pattern of lymphatic drainage is usually predictable when the lesion is located in the extremities. Activity generally drains into axillary and groin lymph node basins, although popliteal and epitrochlear nodes are more common than previously thought. The pattern of lymphatic drainage from lesions of the head, neck, and trunk is much less predictable, sometimes crossing midline, having multiple drainage patterns, and unusual pathways (e.g., the triangular intermuscular back space and paravertebral and retroperitoneal nodal beds).

Vital blue dye has been used to detect the sentinel node intraoperatively but this has limitations because of its rapid transit. If surgery is not prompt, the dye may move beyond the sentinel node to other nodes. Although some surgeons still use this technique, many combine both dye and radionuclide techniques. An intraoperative gamma probe detector is often used to provide accurate localization of the node at the time of surgery.

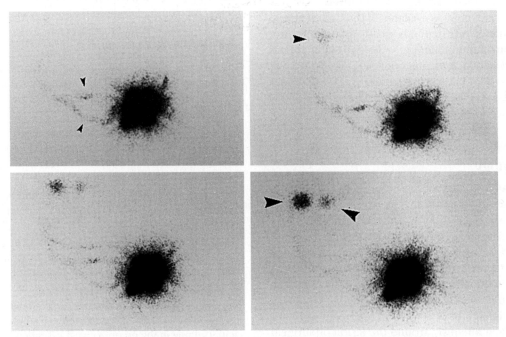

Figure 9-32   Melanoma lymphoscintigraphy. Filtered Tc-99m sulfur colloid injected intracutaneously around the melanoma lesion. Note the early lymphatic drainage (*small arrowheads, upper left*) at 10 minutes, first appearance of sentinel node (*medium arrowhead, upper right*) at 20 minutes, and visualization of two nodes at 40 minutes (*lower left*) and 1 hour (*large arrowheads, lower right*).

Breast Cancer

The surgical management of breast cancer has evolved over recent years from radical surgical procedures toward lesser surgical procedures. With the success of sentinel node identification for melanoma, surgeons became interested in this approach to determine whether a patient with newly diagnosed breast cancer has regional tumor spread to axillary nodes. Involvement of the regional nodal basin is the single most important independent variable in predicting prognosis. However, axillary lymph node dissection is associated with considerable morbidity including wound infection, seroma, paresthesia, and chronic limb edema.

Increasingly, the sentinel lymph node approach has gained favor with surgeons. Sentinel node lymphoscintigraphy using an intraoperative gamma probe has greater than 90% accuracy for detecting sentinel lymph nodes. A histopathologically negative node has a very high negative predictive value for metastatic axillary involvement.

Radiopharmaceuticals

Over the years, a number of radiopharmaceuticals have been used for lymphoscintigraphy, including Tc-99m sulfur colloid (Tc-99m SC), Tc-99m human serum albumin (HSA), Tc-99m nanocolloid, and Tc-99m antimony sulfur colloid. Only Tc-99m SC is available in the United States. Colloidal clearance rate depends greatly on particle size. A large portion of unmodified larger Tc-99m sulfur colloid particles are retained at the injection site. Therefore, the Tc-99m sulfur colloid is first filtered using a 0.22-μm filter to ensure a more uniform, smaller colloidal particle that is more conducive to lymphatic drainage.

Methodology

Melanoma

The methodology of scanning in cases of melanoma varies. Some surgeons order lymphoscintigraphy before surgery and mark the location of the sentinel node on the patient's skin. Others do not request imaging but use a radiation detector probe at surgery to find the sentinel node, on which they then perform biopsy. The combination of the two methods is common.

Four to six injections of 100 μCi in tuberculin syringes are made intracutaneously around the lesion or surgical site. Sequential imaging is performed every 5 minutes for 60–90 minutes until the sentinel node is detected. The location of the node can then be marked on the skin with an indelible marker pen.

Breast Cancer

Various injection methods have been investigated and used on a clinical basis. One method uses an injection around the tumor or biopsy site itself. This may require ultrasound guidance for deep tumors. The lymphatic channels are more limited in the deep subcutaneous tissues compared with the dermal regions of the breast. In addition, the lymphatics may be disrupted by the tumor or surgery. Therefore, a dose injected in the peritumoral location may not migrate. Some physicians use an intradermal or subdermal injection overlying the tumor. Another approach utilizes a periareolar injection that takes advantage of rich lymphatic drainage. Although this location may be distant from the tumor, lymphatic drainage follows this pathway. The migration failure rate using this periareolar method is extremely low. Finally, a subareolar injection just proximal to the tumor or biopsy site can be used. Care must be taken that activity in the injection site will not obscure adjacent axillary lymph nodes. The use of two methods together produces the best results.

On the day of surgery or even the day before surgery, several injections of the radiopharmaceutical (around 100 μCi each) are made in a peritumoral location, proximal to the biopsy site, or periareolar region. Imaging may or may not be performed, although it is recommended to visualize unusual routes of migration. Vigorous injection site massage for 5 minutes improves the chance migration will occur. An intraoperative gamma probe is used to detect the sentinel node so that biopsy can be performed.

SUGGESTED READING

Alazraki NP, Eshima D, Eshima LA, et al: Lymphoscintigraphy, the sentinel node concept, and the intraoperative gamma probe in melanoma, breast cancer, and other potential cancers. Semin Nucl Med 27:55-67, 1997.

Isreal O, Mor M, Epelbaum R, et al: Clinical pretreatment risk factors and Ga-67 scintigraphy early during treatment for prediction of outcome of patients with aggressive non-Hodgkin's lymphoma. Cancer 94:873-878, 2002.

Krag D, Weaver D, Ashikaga T, et al: The sentinel node in breast cancer: a multicenter validation study. N Engl J Med 339:941-946, 1998.

Krenning EP, Kwekkeboom DJ, Bakker WH, et al: Somatostatin receptor scintigraphy with [111 In-DTPA-Dphe-1] and [123I-Tyr-3]-octreotide: The Rotterdam experience with more than 1000 patients. Eur J Nucl Med 20:716-731, 1993.

Kurtaran A, Scheuba C, Kaserer K, et al: Comparison of In-111 DTPA-D-Phe[1]-octreotide and Tc-99m-(V)-dimercapto-succinic acid scanning in the preoperative localization of medullary thyroid carcinoma. J Nucl Med 39:1907-1909, 1998.

Mariani G, Gipponi M, Moresco L, et al: Radioguided sentinel lymph node biopsy in malignant cutaneous melanoma. J Nucl Med 43:811-827, 2002.

Moffat FL, Pinsky CM, Hammershaimb L, et al: Clinical utility of external immunoscintigraphy with IMMU-4 technetium-99m Fab' antibody (Tc-99m CEA-SCAN) fragment in patients undergoing surgery for carcinoma of the colon and rectum: results of a pivotal, phase III trial, J Clin Oncol 14:2295-2305, 1996.

Newman LA: Lymphoscintigraphy and sentinel lymph node biopsy in breast cancer: a comprehensive review of variations in performance and technique. J Am Coll Surg 199:804-816, 2004.

Raj GV, Partin AW, Polascik TJ: Clinical utility of Indium-111-Capromab pentreotide immunoscintigraphy in the detection of early, recurrent prostate carcinoma after radical prostatectomy. Cancer 94: 987-996, 2002.

Serafini AN: Current status of bone palliation with systemic radioisotopes. Nucl Med Ann: 253-274, 2002.

Taillefer R: The role of 99mTc-sestamibi and other conventional radiopharmaceuticals in breast cancer diagnosis. Semin Nucl Med 29:16-40, 1999.

Weiner RE, Thakur ML: Radiolabeled peptides in diagnosis and therapy. Semin Nucl Med 31:296-311, 2001.

Willkomm P, Bender H, Bangard M, et al: FDG PET and immunoscintigraphy with 99mTc-labeled antibody fragments for the detection of colorectal carcinoma. J Nucl Med 41:1657-1663, 2000.

Witzig TE, Gordon LI, Cabanillas F, et al: Randomized controlled trial of yttrium-90-labeled ibritumomab tiuxetan radioimmunotherapy versus Rituximab immunotherapy for patients with relapsed or refractory low-grade, follicular, or transformed B-cell non-Hodgkin's lymphoma. J Clin Oncol 20:2453-2463, 2002.

Oncology: Positron Emission Tomography

INTRODUCTION AND BACKGROUND

For decades, positron emission tomography (PET) has been used for many research applications. In recent years, changes in reimbursement and availability have led to the rapid expansion of PET for clinical patient care. The majority of these PET scans are performed to evaluate cancer. Uses include cancer diagnosis, staging, restaging and monitoring response to therapy (Table 10-1).

In most cases, cancer cells are more metabolically active and divide more rapidly than normal tissues. By using radiopharmaceuticals that target physiological parameters such as glucose metabolism, PET enables imaging and quantification of cellular function and tumor detection. This approach has several potential advantages over anatomic modalities like computed tomography (CT).

CT imaging relies on size and architectural changes to diagnose malignancy, which limits sensitivity and specificity. For example, when lymph nodes are identified in patients with cancer, enlarged nodes are assumed to harbor malignancy, whereas normal-sized nodes are characterized as benign. Therefore, nodes seen on CT are often inaccurately characterized as benign because they are not pathologically enlarged.

Often, it is not possible to determine if a residual mass seen on CT after therapy contains tumor, and a change in the size of a mass does not accurately predict tumor response to therapy. Another limitation of CT is that tumor evaluation after therapy is difficult, and scarring from surgery and radiation may obscure malignant disease. PET, on the other hand, permits monitoring of

Table 10-1 Historical Perspective on Medicare-approved Indications of F-18 FDG PET in Oncology

Clinical condition	Effective date	Coverage
Solitary pulmonary nodule	January 1998	Characterization
Lung cancer (non-small cell)	January 1998	Initial staging
Lung cancer (non-small cell)	July 2001	Diagnosis, staging, restaging
Esophageal cancer	July 2001	Diagnosis, staging, restaging
Colorectal cancer	July 1999	Locating tumors if rising CEA suggests recurrence
Colorectal cancer	July 2001	Diagnosis, staging, restaging
Lymphoma	July 1999	Staging and restaging (only when used as an alternative to Gallium scan)
Lymphoma	July 2001	Diagnosis, staging, restaging
Melanoma	July 1999	Evaluate recurrence prior to surgery instead of Gallium scan
Melanoma	July 2001	Diagnosis, staging, restaging (evaluating regional nodes not covered)
Breast cancer	October 2002	Staging when distant metastasis, restaging locoregional recurrence or metastasis, monitoring treatment response for locally advanced and metastatic cancer when change in therapy is anticipated
Head and neck cancers (excluding central nervous system and thyroid)	July 2001	Diagnosis, staging, restaging
Thyroid cancer	October 2003	Restaging recurrent or residual cancers of follicular cell origin that were previously treated by thyroidectomy and radioiodine ablation with serum thyroglobulin >10 ng/ml and negative I-131 whole body scan
Cervical cancer	Under CMS consideration for coverage	Possible detection of residual or recurrent tumor after therapy
Ovarian cancer	Under CMS consideration for coverage	Initial staging, detecting recurrence, detecting recurrence when CA-125 titre is rising but computed tomography is negative
Pancreatic cancer	Under CMS consideration for coverage	Possibly differentiating benign from malignant, detect metastases
Small cell lung cancer	Under CMS consideration for coverage	Initial staging, restaging, diagnosis of occult tumor in paraneoplastic syndrome
Testicular cancer (pure seminoma or nonseminomatous germ cell)	Under CMS consideration for coverage	Initial staging, evaluate residual mass, recurrence when computed tomography is normal but serum factors rising

CEA, Carcinogen embryonic antigen; CMS, Centers for Medicare and Medicaid.

activity levels on serial studies. Changes in metabolic activity better characterize a mass and better predict therapy outcome than anatomic measurements of size.

However, PET is limited by a lack of anatomic detail. Normal uptake in structures like bowel, muscles, and ureters can be mistaken for tumor. Therefore, correlation with CT or magnetic resonance imaging (MRI) is critical for image interpretation. If the CT is performed separately from the PET, comparison of the two data sets can be done side-by-side or after processing with image fusion software. Increasingly, PET is acquired sequentially with the CT on a PET-CT scanner. This allows the most precise image fusion as differences in position are minimal. The combination of anatomic information with metabolic data is the most accurate method for evaluating malignancy.

Radiopharmaceuticals

Many commonly used positron-emitting radioisotopes are based on atoms found in organic substances: oxygen-15, nitrogen-13, carbon-11, and the hydroxyl analog, fluorine-18 (Table 10-2). Short half-lives limit the clinical usefulness of many positron emitters, requiring a cyclotron to be in close proximity. However, F-18 has a 110-minute half-life and can be delivered from regional, commercial cyclotrons.

The various positron emitters can be attached to various biological carrier molecules. Carrier molecules such as nucleosides, amino acids, fatty acid components, and glucose analogs are chosen to form radiopharmaceuticals that target components of cellular metabolism and

Table 10-2	Physical Characteristics of Important Positron-emitting Isotopes in Oncology					
Radio-isotope	Half-life (min)	Decay mode (%)	γ (keV)	β^+E_{max} (MeV)	Range (mm)	
O-15	2.07	β^+ (99.9) EC (0.1)	511	1.72	8.0	
N-13	9.96	β^+ (100)	511	1.19	5.4	
C-11	20.4	β^+ (99.8) EC (0.2)	511	0.96	4.1	
F-18	109.7	β^+ (97) EC (3)	511	0.635	2.4	

β^+, positron emission; EC, electron capture.

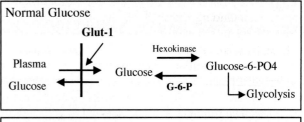

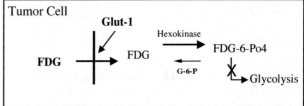

*G-6-P: Glucose-6-Phosphatase

Figure 10-1   Glucose and F-18 FDG intracellular kinetics.

division. Targets include DNA synthesis, membrane synthesis, and glucose metabolism (Table 10-3). The chemistry of labeling carrier molecules with positron emitters is usually much simpler than labeling with gamma emitters such as technetium-99m. Currently, the only PET radiopharmaceutical approved by the Food and Drug Administration for clinical use in oncologic imaging is F-18 fluorodeoxyglucose (F-18 FDG).

F-18 Fluorodeoxyglucose

Cancer cells generally have a higher level of metabolic activity than normal tissues and use more glucose. In malignant cells, higher levels of glucose membrane transporters increase intracellular glucose uptake. Within the cancer cell, hexokinase (hexokinase II) activity levels are increased, and the phosphorylated glucose then moves through the glycolysis pathway.

F-18 FDG is a glucose analog that is taken into the cell and phosphorylated by the same mechanism as glucose. Increased F-18 FDG activity is seen in tumors for several reasons. First of all, increased glucose transporter activity is present. In addition, glucose-6-phosphatase levels are low in cancer cells, and the phosphorylated FDG cannot diffuse out of the cell. Unlike glucose, F-18 FDG is not metabolized further and remains trapped (Fig. 10-1).

Table 10-3	Carrier Molecules for PET Imaging in Oncology	
Agent	Target	Label
Deoxyglucose	Glucose metabolism	F-18
Thymidine	DNA synthesis	F-18, C-11
Acetate	Lipid synthesis	F-18, C-11
Choline	Lipid synthesis, membrane synthesis	C-11
Tyrosine	Protein synthesis	F-18, C-11
Methionine	Protein synthesis	C-11

After intravenous injection, F-18 FDG rapidly distributes throughout the body. Cellular uptake and phosphorylation occur as background activity clears. The primary route of radiotracer excretion occurs by the kidneys, although F-18 FDG excretion also takes place through the bowel. Optimal imaging time is between 40 to 60 minutes, based on maximum uptake, background clearance, and physical half-life.

Many factors affect F-18 FDG uptake, distribution, and clearance. Serum glucose actively competes with F-18 FDG uptake. Insulin occurring endogenously after eating or administration to diabetics will increase uptake to the liver and soft tissues, thereby decreasing uptake in tumors. Also, inflammation and infection may result in uptake that rivals or exceeds that of a malignancy.

Investigational PET Imaging Agents

F-18 FDG uptake in tumor is not specific for malignancy. Clinically, it is often critical to differentiate cancer from inflammation. Many radiotracers that are more specific for malignancy by imaging the increased cellular division seen with cancer are under investigation. Other agents may be superior to F-18 FDG because of better tumor uptake or reduced background activity.

The radiolabeled nucleoside F-18 fluorothymidine (F-18 FLT) is a marker of cellular proliferation. It has shown a promising ability to predict tumor grade in lung cancer evaluation, better evaluates many brain tumors, and may be an earlier predictor of tumor response. C-11 methionine, an amino acid, has accurately evaluated various cancers including brain tumors. C-11 choline and C-11 acetate have shown promise in prostate cancer that may be due, in part, to the lack of urine activity in bladder adjacent to the prostate bed as well as differences in uptake activity. F-18 misonidazole is a marker of tumor hypoxia and may play a role in therapeutic decision-making. Additional PET radiopharmaceuticals are being developed that bind to receptors, including estrogen receptors in breast carcinoma. These agents are not available for clinical use.

In addition to these newer agents, F-18 sodium fluoride (F-18 fluoride) is gaining renewed interest. F-18 fluoride was originally used as a bone-scan agent, and it may be superior to Tc-99m MDP or F-18 FDG in the evaluation of several skeletal tumors. This includes highly lytic tumors such as multiple myeloma.

F-18 FDG PET Dosimetry

Radiation dosimetry values for F-18 FDG are listed in Table 10-4. The whole body effective dose from a standard 400-MBq scan is 1.6 mSv (160 mrem). The effective radiation dose of a low-dose whole-body CT performed for PET-CT varies, but may be 2 mSv (200 mrem). This compares to a typical diagnostic chest CT, in which the effective dose frequently reaches 8 mSv due to increased radiation used to visualize structures optimally.

Protocol

An example of a protocol for F-18 FDG PET in oncology patients is included in Box 10-1. Because glucose competes with F-18 FDG, protocols include measures to limit the impact of serum glucose of the scan. Patient preparation generally includes fasting overnight or for at least 4-6 hours before injection and avoiding carbohydrates in the meal before injection. The serum glucose level of patients should be checked before injection. The upper-limit cutoff varies among institutions, but a value under 200 mg/dl is generally considered acceptable. Diabetics are asked to follow the same preparation routine and take their insulin. However, insulin should not be given within 2 hours of radiotracer injection. Non–insulin-dependent diabetics are treated in a similar fashion.

Claustrophobic patients may require sedation, particularly when a PET-CT is performed because the machine has a deep bore. Sedatives and beta-adrenergic blockers are

sometimes used to decrease uptake in the supraclavicular fat (so-called "brown fat"), although this is often with limited effectiveness. Patients should be kept warm, quiet, and relaxed during the injection and uptake phases to decrease muscle and brown-fat uptake. Patients should be instructed to avoid strenuous exercise for a couple of days before the study.

The standard F-18 FDG dose is 10-15 mCi (370-555 MBq) intravenously. An absorption and clearance period necessitates a delay of 40-60 minutes before scanning. Immediately before being placed on the scanner, patients must void.

Patients are usually imaged in a supine position. Because attenuation correction with CT causes beam-hardening

Box 10-1 Protocol for F-18 FDG Imaging in Oncology

PATIENT PREPARATION

Avoid strenuous exercise for several days
Diabetics well controlled, take medication on day of scan but no insulin within 2 hours of FDG injection
NPO 4-6 hours or overnight, avoid carbohydrates
Check serum glucose (<180-200)
Patient kept warm and relaxed
Consider sedation for: claustrophobia, anxiety/tense muscles, cancer in head and neck, prior brown fat uptake

DOSE

Adults: 10-15 mCi (0.21 mCi/kg) intravenously
Children: 150 uCi/kg
Wait 45-60 minutes, patient to avoid movement and speech
Void

ACQUISITION AND PROCESSING
Field of view

Varies by patient size (50 cm)

Transmission scan
Stand-alone PET

External rod source
Minute/bed position

PET-CT

Low-dose CT (70-80 mA, 140 kvP)

Emission scan

5-10 minutes/bed position
Repeat imaging each section or bed position until area covered

Processing

Filtered backprojection or iterative reconstruction

Table 10-4 F-18 FDG Dosimetry

Organ	rad/mCi (cGy/37 MBq)
Bladder wall	**0.32**
Myocardium	0.22
Brain	0.07
Liver	0.058
Kidneys	0.074
Red marrow	0.047
Testes	0.041
Ovaries	0.053
Colon	0.046

Critical organ in bold.
From package insert for MetaTrace, PETNET Pharmaceuticals, Knoxville, TN.

artifact when the arms are in the field of view, arm position must always be taken into consideration. Arms are placed above the head when the pathology is in the chest, abdomen, and pelvis. In cases where the tumor is in the head and neck, patients are imaged with arms at their sides. Scanning usually begins at the head but will begin at the thighs when tumor is in the pelvis to minimize the impact of urine activity accumulating in the bladder.

The imaging is done in two stages. First, a transmission scan using an external positron or x-ray source is performed for attenuation correction. The positron emission scan is then acquired, which detects the photons from the F-18 FDG. As the administered dose is known and can be time-decay corrected, the number of photons striking the detector will reflect the metabolic activity of a lesion once a correction for differences in tissue attenuation is applied. Therefore, attenuation correction allows the levels of activity in the patient to be accurately quantified. An attenuation correction factor is calculated by comparing the counts striking the detector from the transmission scan through the patient to a blank scan where no patient is present: attenuation correction factor = (counts blank scan) / (counts transmission scan).

External rods (germanium-68 or cesium-137) rotating around the patient can be used for this attenuation correction transmission scan. The process requires 4–6 minutes per image level (or bed position) with a typical whole-body scan requiring 5–7 bed positions. A PET-CT scanner uses the CT transmission data for attenuation correction, as well as for image fusion for anatomic localization. The CT takes only seconds to complete.

The emission scan data are then acquired from the F-18 FDG activity emitted from the patient. Depending on patient size and radiopharmaceutical dose, the emission scan takes 5–10 minutes per bed position. A whole-body scan has traditionally been considered a scan from skull base to mid-thigh. Such a whole-body scan will require approximately 35–40 minutes. If the entire brain or the lower extremities are included, more bed positions are added.

Currently, most scans done on a PET-CT are performed without intravenous or oral contrast. Contrast administration requires additional time, support personnel, equipment, and patient supervision. Also, CT contrast agents cause increased attenuation on the transmission scan, which can lead to areas of artifactually increased activity on attenuation-corrected PET images. Using dilute oral contrast or water minimizes the impact of this artifact. Performing the attenuation-correction CT scan after the arterial phase of the intravenous contrast bolus will reduce the artifact from intravenous contrast. In practice, examining the nonattenuation-contrast images should allow an experienced reader to avoid confusion caused by contrast artifact. Newer software may decrease the artifacts from contrast.

Following the scan, reconstruction is performed. Although ititerative reconstruction is becoming the norm, some scanners will use filtered backprojection, including for nonattenuation-corrected images. Data is displayed as a maximal intensity projection (MIP) rotating image and/or as transaxial, coronal and sagittal slices. Both attenuation-corrected images and nonattenuation-correction images should be reviewed as artifacts and lesions may be more obvious in one or the other. PET-CT scanners will automatically provide images fused to the CT in each orthogonal plane. If the CT is done in a separate imaging session, post-image fusion software may require manual alignment or may offer semiautomatic capabilities. A current correlative CT is needed for optimal interpretation.

IMAGE INTERPRETATION

Normal Distribution and Variants of F-18 FDG

The normal distribution of F-18 FDG reflects glucose metabolism (Fig. 10-2). The brain is an obligate glucose user, so uptake is high. The kidneys, ureters, and bladder also show intense activity due to urinary clearance of F-18 FDG. Moderate and sometimes heterogeneous activity is seen in the liver. Variable activity occurs in the heart, gastrointestinal tract, salivary glands, and testes. The uterus may show endometrial uptake depending on the menstrual cycle stage. Low-level activity is normal in the bone marrow.

The urinary activity can lead to interpretation difficulties. Although the ureters usually appear as long tubular structures, they may be seen as very focal areas of activity that may be confused with pathology. CT correlation or PET-CT can help localize the activity to a visible ureter or show that no mass or lymph node is present. F-18 FDG in the bladder and kidneys can prevent visualization of tumors in those structures. The bladder may also limit evaluation of other tumors in the pelvis.

When imaging tumors located near the heart, minimizing cardiac activity is desirable. The myocardium uses glucose as an optional fuel. In a fasting state, fatty acid metabolism dominates over glucose use, leading to decreased FDG uptake. However, fasting yields inconsistent results. In fact, significant cardiac uptake is seen in up to 50% of fasting patients. Myocardial uptake is usually not seen in the right ventricle and may be heterogeneous in the left ventricle.

Normal excretion of F-18 FDG is highly variable throughout the gastrointestinal tract. Low-level activity can be seen focally or diffusely in the esophagus. In general, this normal uptake is less than that seen with esophagitis or cancer. Intense activity in the stomach sometimes limits the use of F-18 FDG PET in the evaluation of gastric adenocarcinoma and gastric lymphoma. Activity

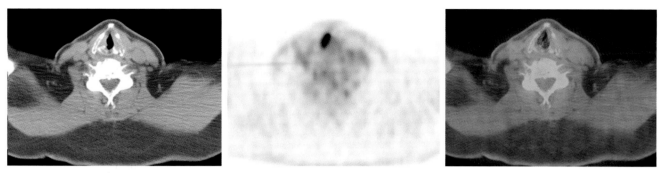

Figure 10-A   Paralyzed vocal cord artifact on positron emission tomography (PET). Axial computed tomography (CT), PET, and fused PET-CT images reveal unilateral uptake in the neck localizing to the right vocal cord. The left vocal cord was found to be paralyzed on physical exam after radiation therapy for lung cancer affected the left recurrent laryngeal nerve. This uptake could be confused with a lymph node metastasis on PET if CT correlation is not used.

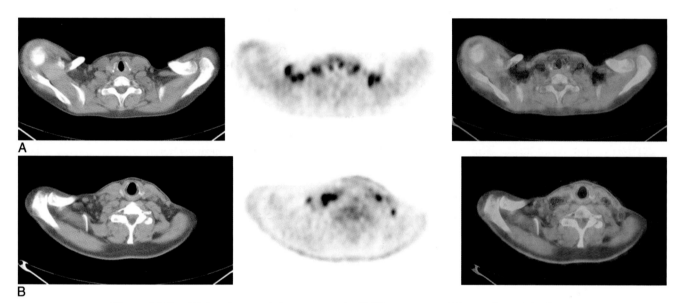

Figure 10-B   FDG positron emission tomography (PET) appearance of "brown fat" activity. **A,** Abnormal supraclavicular uptake localizes to the fat on fused PET-CT images. The fused images help to differentiate this common benign variant from muscle activity or malignant adenopathy. **B,** Lymphoma involvement in the supraclavicular region can appear similar to brown fat uptake on PET images, but fused images localize the activity to involved lymph nodes.

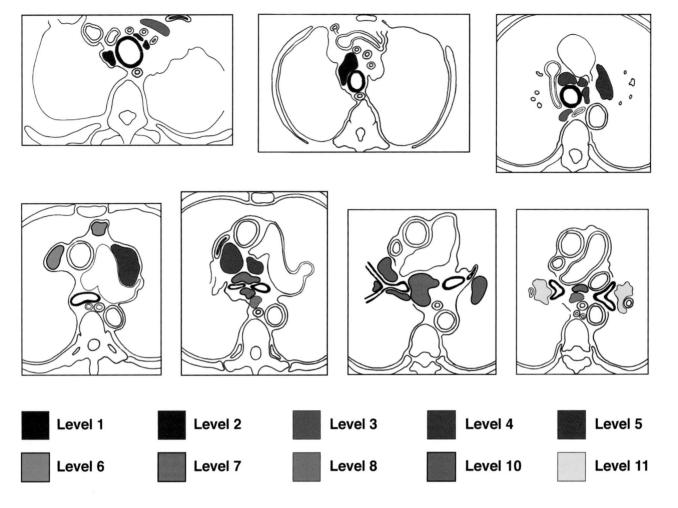

Figure 10-C   Lymph node stations or levels of the mediastinum.

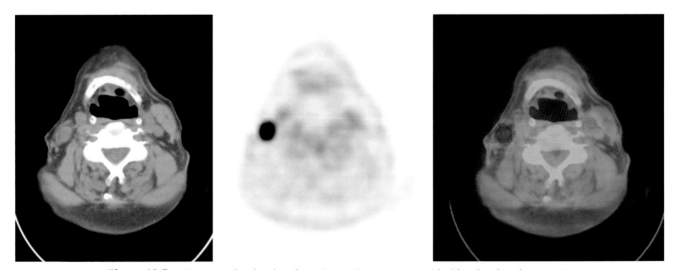

Figure 10-D   Recurrent head and neck carcinoma. Recurrent or residual head and neck cancer is often difficult to diagnose by computed tomography (CT) or magnetic resonance imaging due to the distorted anatomy from surgery and radiation. Positron emission tomography (PET) better demonstrates tumor even in cases of marked anatomical asymmetry. PET-CT makes localization easier such as in this patient following removal of the sternocleidomastoid muscle and other structures.

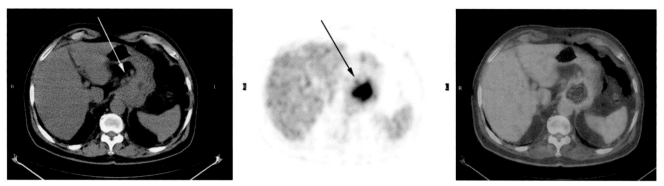

Figure 10-E   Tumor involvement in regional lymph nodes. Small lymph nodes are seen in the lesser curvature of the stomach on computed tomography. Positron emission tomography images show only mild activity in one of the lymph nodes (*arrow*) near the tumor in the gastroesophageal junction and fundus. This is better localized on the fused image (*right*). Endoscopic biopsy later showed tumor involvement in the regional nodes during staging.

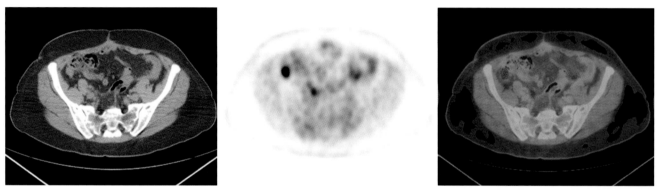

Figure 10-F   Metastatic ovarian cancer along the right colon. Ovarian cancer spread often presents as focal activity studding the peritoneal organs on positron emission tomography (PET). Fused PET-CT images improve accuracy over PET alone or PET and CT read side-by-side. Uptake is often subtle and can be confused with normal structures such as benign activity in bowel lumen.

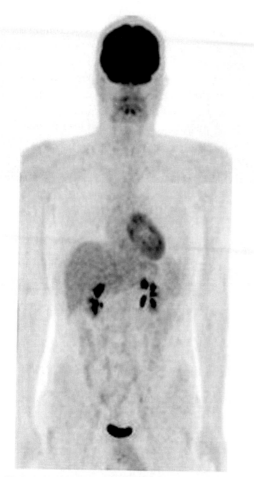

Figure 10-2   Normal distribution of F-18 fluorodeoxyglucose: F-18 FDG uptake is normally intense in the brain and urinary tract, moderately intense in the liver, and variable in muscles (especially of the oropharynx), heart, and bowel.

in both large and small bowel is especially problematic as it may obscure tumor in the bowel and mesentery (Fig. 10-3A). Fusion of the PET and CT often helps localize focal uptake to bowel wall or mesentery. Focal accumulation of F-18 FDG may be caused by malignant and villous adenomas, but it is frequently a normal, transient finding.

Activity in the oropharyngeal cavity is highly variable. Low-level activity is normally seen in the salivary glands. Nonspecific diffuse uptake is occasionally seen in the parotid glands bilaterally in patients undergoing therapy. Focal, intense uptake is often seen in oropharyngeal lymphoid tissue, including palatine and lingual tonsils (Fig. 10-3B). Although it is most often symmetric, asymmetry can occur normally or due to therapy. This may make it difficult to evaluate tumor.

Benign Variants

Many processes alter F-18 FDG distribution (Box 10-2) and may affect the scheduling of a PET scan (Box 10-3).

In addition, there are many reasons for the radiotracer distribution to be altered in clinical use.

Activity is frequently seen in muscles that can sometimes pose interpretative problems. The muscles of the oropharynx will show variable activity, and patients should avoid speaking after injection to decrease artifact. The skeletal muscles may show prominent uptake due to recent exertion and tension. Insulin administered to diabetics or increased endogenous insulin occurring after eating may also cause intense levels of muscle activity necessitating a repeat exam (Fig. 10-4). Unilateral uptake may occur in a normal vocal cord in a patient with contralateral vocal cord paralysis (Fig. 10-5 and 10-A [see color insert]) or when surgery, such as for head and neck cancer, causes contralateral muscles to be unbalanced.

One interesting and common variant is supraclavicular F-18 FDG accumulation in so-called "brown fat" (Figs. 10-6 and 10-B [see color insert]). This activity was originally thought to occur in the muscles of the neck, but fused PET-CT images showed the uptake actually localized to areas of fat on the CT scan. This variant occurs more commonly in cold weather and cold patients, which relates to the origin of the tissue as a primitive, nonshivering warming mechanism. Brown fat contains adrenergic receptors that contribute to uptake in anxious patients. Although the pattern is simple to recognize, it may decrease sensitivity for tumor detection in the region. Variable degrees of improvement have been obtained with sedation and adrenergic blocking agents in anxious patients or those with a previously abnormal scan. Warming the patient before injection and keeping them warm is most effective in diminishing this uptake.

Focal F-18 FDG accumulation may localize to vessels, particularly in the aortic arch. This may be associated with calcifications from atherosclerotic disease. In general, this activity is nonspecific, although intense uptake could indicate arteritis.

The thyroid gland may show different uptake patterns (Fig. 10-7). Diffusely increased activity may be seen in thyroiditis, goiter, and Graves' disease. The significance of low-level diffuse uptake in patients without identifiable thyroid disease is uncertain; it may be normal or the result of subclinical thyroiditis. Focal uptake can be seen in benign nodules. However, focal activity can be the result of malignancy in up to 50% of cases and evaluation is warranted.

Benign adenomas and tumors outside the thyroid gland may also accumulate F-18 FDG. This includes adenomas in colon, parotid gland, and benign ovarian tumors.

Effects of Inflammation and Therapy

F-18 FDG uptake is not specific for tumor. Increased activity can be seen in inflammation and infection, and the cause has been attributed to glycolytic activity in

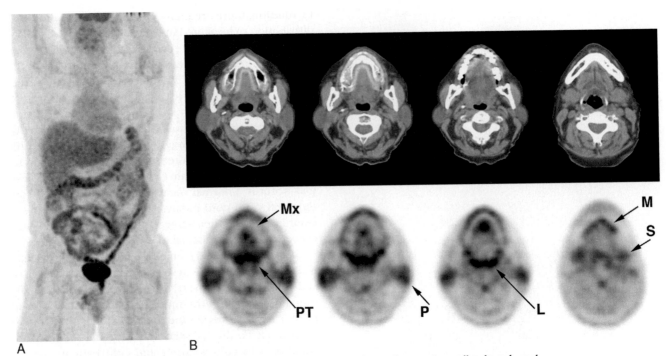

Figure 10-3   Normal variants. **A,** Normal intense uptake can be seen in small or large bowel. **B,** Axial PET and corresponding CT images show normal uptake in the oropharynx. Normal uptake is often symmetric and may be very intense when patients swallow excessively or talk. *L,* Lingual tonsils; *M,* mandible; *Mx,* maxilla; *P,* parotid gland; *PT,* palatine tonsils; *S,* submandibular gland.

Box 10-2   Factors Affecting F-18 FDG Uptake

INCREASE UPTAKE

Higher tumor grade
Large number of viable cells
Increased tumor blood flow
Inflammation
Tumor hypoxia
Acute radiation
Acute chemotherapy
Recent surgery

DECREASE UPTAKE

Benign lesion
Necrosis
Low-grade or low-cellularity tumor, mucinous tumors, bronchoalveolar carcinoma
Hyperglycemia
High insulin
Chronic radiation
Prior chemotherapy
Scar

Box 10-3   Clinical Factors Altering Patient Scheduling

History	Course of Action
Prior surgery	Delay scan 4-6 weeks
Chemotherapy	Delay scan several weeks or schedule scan just before next cycle
Radiation therapy	Delay scan at least 3 months
Colony stimulating factor (G-CSF)	Delay scan 1 week for short acting agents or several weeks for long acting
Serum glucose >200	Reschedule scan to control glucose
Insulin administration	Wait at least 2 hours
Breastfeeding	Discontinue feeding at least 6 hours

leukocytes. Infections such as pneumonia will have intense radiotracer accumulation. Inflammatory uptake in a lymph node or mass cannot be differentiated from malignancy. Such uptake may be problematic in sarcoidosis and granulomatous disease in the chest (e.g., histoplasmosis and tuberculosis). Other inflammatory processes in the lungs, such as occupational lung diseases and active interstitial fibrosis and pneumonitis, may also cause markedly abnormal uptake (Fig. 10-8).

Increased activity around a joint in the soft tissues or joint capsule may be confused with a metastatic lesion. This pattern is most common in the hip and shoulder. Fused PET-CT images can help localize the uptake. Activity involving the joint surface or both side of the joint may be present with degenerative disease. Acute and healing fractures normally accumulate F-18 FDG (Fig. 10-9). Correlation with the CT can usually help differentiate this from a metastatic lesion, as the fracture will be seen radiographically.

Therapy often results in an inflammatory response causing increased activity (Figs. 10-10 and 10-11). There are no hard and fast rules on how long to wait following therapy to perform a PET scan. At times, repeat or even serial imaging may be needed to confirm that increased activity is iatrogenic. Radiation therapy causes intense F-18 FDG uptake acutely. Because this uptake may persist for many months, delaying the PET scan for 3 months is recommended. Chemotherapy may cause a lesion to show a transient apparent worsening. A delay in scanning of several weeks or until just before beginning the next chemotherapy cycle is currently recommended. However, increasing data indicates that imaging early can predict therapeutic response. The postoperative inflammatory

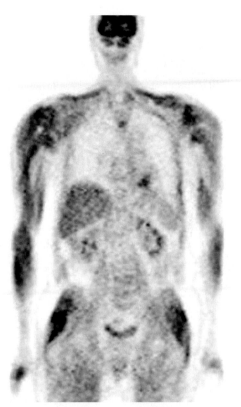

Figure 10-4 Muscle activity from increased insulin levels. Intense, diffuse uptake in the muscles caused by eating prior to radiotracer injection might obscure malignancy and require a repeat exam.

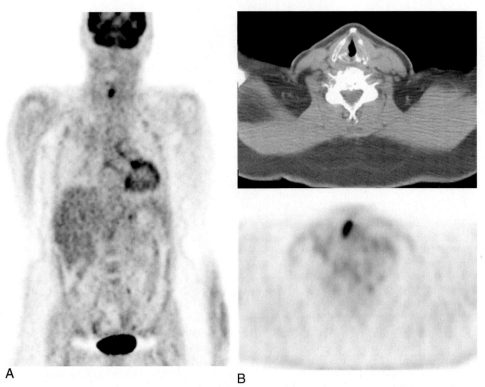

A   B

Figure 10-5 Vocal cord paralysis. **A,** Maximum-intensity projection whole-body image for restaging lung carcinoma reveals suspicious focal right neck. Faint posttherapy change is seen in the right upper lobe from radiation. **B,** Axial CT and PET images localize the neck uptake to the right vocal cord, ruling out malignant adenopathy. Although therapy was to the right chest, mediastinal radiation affected the recurrent laryngeal nerve on the left. The paralyzed left vocal cord has no uptake.

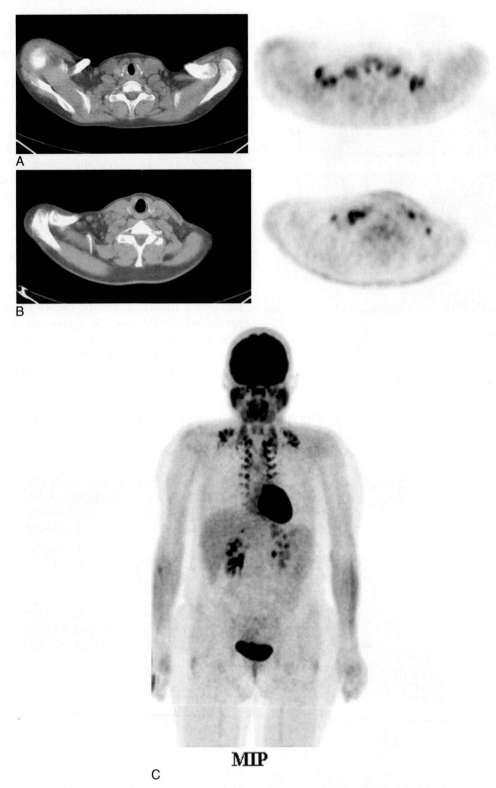

Figure 10-6 Brown fat uptake. **A,** CT and axial PET images show intense supraclavicular activity in the fat. **B,** Supraclavicular activity can also be caused by malignant adenopathy as in this patient with lymphoma or benign muscular activity. Fusion images can help clarify the etiology. **C,** Commonly, whole-body PET may show benign intense costovertebral uptake in these same patients, as well as the supraclavicular brown-fat activity.

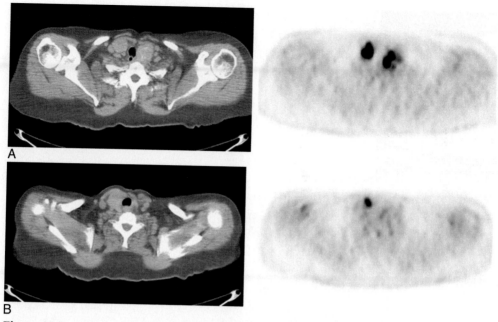

Figure 10-7   Patterns of thyroid activity. **A,** Diffuse thyroid uptake suggests a benign process as in this patient with Hashimoto's thyroiditis, although the etiology of uptake is not always known. **B,** Focal uptake due to a benign right adenoma in this patient will have a similar appearance to a malignant nodule so follow-up is needed.

response in the wound healing process results in F-18 FDG uptake that is usually mild to moderate (Fig. 10-12) and a delay of at least 2–4 weeks to minimize the effects of inflammation on uptake is recommended.

Evaluation of the bone marrow may be limited by the effects of therapy. When marrow-stimulating drugs are used on patients with anemia or undergoing chemotherapy, a diffuse increase in radiotracer uptake may result. Usually this pattern is easily differentiated from metastatic disease (Fig. 10-13). However, increased marrow background can mask actual lesions from tumor involvement. If at all possible, scans should be delayed until the effects of marrow-stimulating therapy has resolved. In short-acting agents, this typically takes 5–7 days but it is prolonged with newer, long-acting drugs.

Low-level activity may be seen in the thymus in young patients. Activity in the anterior chest may have a characteristic shield shape of the thymus (Fig. 10-14). In cases where activity appears following therapy, careful correlation with the CT can help determine if normal-appearing thymic tissue is present in the anterior mediastinum. Increased uptake following therapy is known as "thymic rebound" and can be seen on gallium scanning as well. It may be difficult to differentiate from tumor involvement and response.

Artifacts

When metal or dense-iodinated contrast is present, the attenuation-correction images may mistakenly show increased radiotracer activity around the area (Fig. 10-15). Examining the nonattenuation-corrected images, which

will show no increased activity, can lead to the correct interpretation. Correlation with a current CT should be done to help identify sources of such artifact.

Areas of intense F-18 FDG activity, such as in the bladder and infiltration at the injection site, can cause a reconstruction artifact manifested by a band of artifactually decreased activity across the patient. This was more common with older systems that relied on filtered backprojection and is less of a problem with iterative reconstruction. Again, the nonattenuation-corrected images show less effect.

Although combined PET-CT scanners have been a major advance, these hybrid systems can generate certain artifacts. A common artifact is caused by misregistration of PET and CT data due to respiration. A CT acquired with breath-holding will greatly alter the position of organs compared with the PET, which must be done in quiet respiration. If the CT is done in quiet respiration, structures more closely match the PET, but motion and low lung volumes may obscure lesions. Respiratory motion artifact can also cause abnormal uptake from a lesion to appear in an incorrect location on the CT, particularly for pathology near the diaphragm. This most frequently involves a liver lesion projecting over the lung or rib on the CT (Fig. 10-16). If the patient is large or imaged with arms at their sides, truncation artifact may lead to thin linear bands of activity running the length of the patient on the maximum-intensity projection image. CT beam-hardening artifact is a common problem that affects the quality of the CT and fused PET-CT images (Fig. 10-17). This can be minimized by

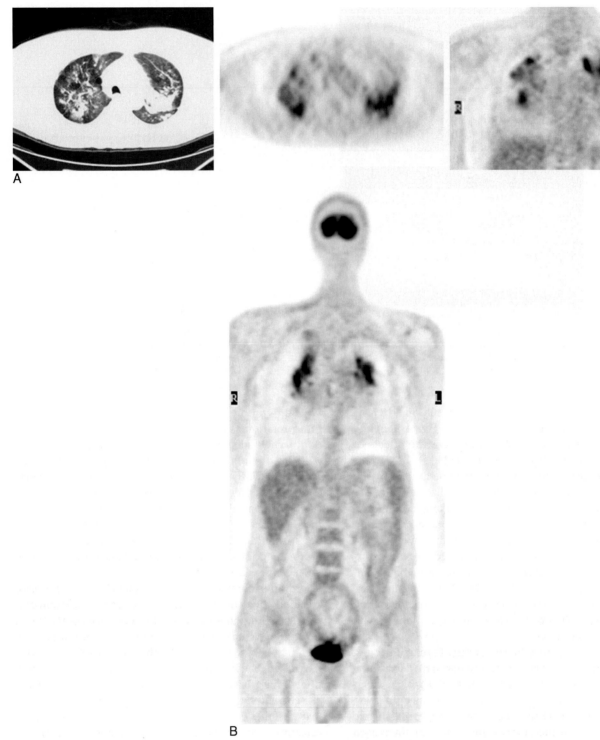

Figure 10-8   Abnormal activity with inflammatory processes on PET. **A,** CT (*left*) reveals severe changes from occupational lung disease. Uptake is seen in areas of active inflammation on axial (*middle*) and coronal (*right*) PET images. FDG PET does not differentiate tumor from benign inflammatory change. **B,** Bilateral hilar uptake is seen on the coronal PET image of a patient with marked adenopathy worrisome for lymphoma. Biopsy later proved this to be secondary to sarcoidosis.

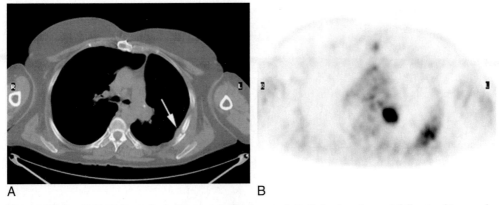

Figure 10-9   F-18 FDG uptake in fracture. **A,** CT shows a left rib fracture (*arrow*) following biopsy of a lung cancer. **B,** PET shows uptake in the fracture as well as the left suprahilar mass, which is not well seen on the single noncontrast CT slice.

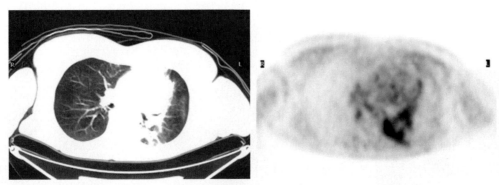

Figure 10-10   FDG posttherapy uptake. CT and PET images show acute radiation changes in the posterior medial left lung. The uptake may decrease on follow-up scans.

moving the arms out of the field of view. Another common, subtle artifact is a thin horizontal band or seam perpendicular to the patient's axis from adjoining bed positions.

Patterns of Malignancy

Usually, there is a greater degree of uptake in more aggressive tumors due to higher levels of metabolic activity. This pattern must be differentiated from the intense activity often seen in infection or following radiation therapy. Low-level activity may be seen in low-grade tumors and tumors with lower relative numbers of cells such as bronchoalveolar carcinoma and mucinous adenocarcinoma. Malignant pleural effusions most often have low-level F-18 FDG activity and some are even negative, which may be due to the dispersion of tumor cells in the fluid so uptake is not detected.

Areas of tumor necrosis will have diminished F-18 FDG accumulation. This is often seen as absent activity centrally in very large masses. By determining areas of necrosis and intense activity, PET scans can help direct biopsy for more sensitive accurate sampling. It may not be possible to differentiate a cavitary infectious process from a necrotic tumor on PET, as both will have a cold center and a peripheral rim of increased activity (Fig. 10-18).

Levels of background activity play a role in the detection of malignant lesions. For example, the high background activity of the brain limits sensitivity for metastatic disease, with perhaps only a third of lesions being visualized. Also, if background uptake is heterogeneous, as may happen in the liver, it can make lesion detection more difficult. It is helpful to describe or grade the severity of abnormal activity in terms of lesion to background differential. For example, lymph node activity in the hila and mediastinum are compared to the background mediastinal activity. The uptake can be graded as mild, moderate, or severe depending on the level above normal adjacent tissue.

Lesion activity can be quantified with a lesion-to-background ratio, lesion-to-liver ratio, or with a standard uptake value (SUV). Quantification can help confirm the visual impression and help follow abnormalities. The SUV is a measure of the relative uptake in a region of interest. It is corrected for body mass or body surface area. F-18 FDG distribution is very low in fat that leads to higher values in tumor and normal tissues in heavier patients than thin patients.

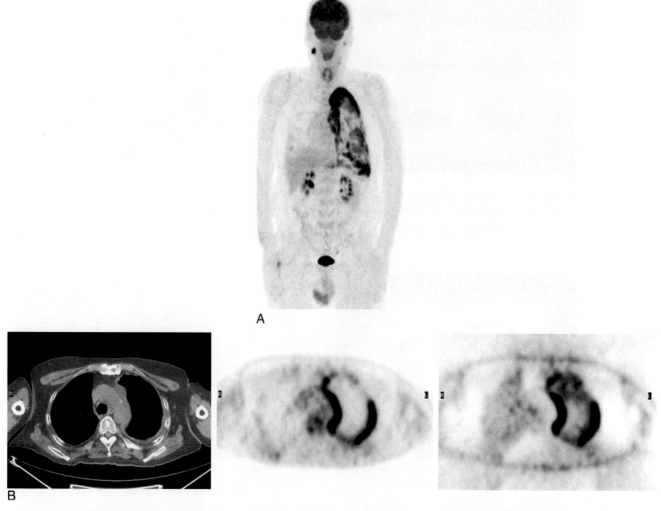

Figure 10-11   Positive PET scan caused by pleurodesis. Maximal-intensity projection **(A)** images and PET and CT images **(B)** show thickened left pleura on the CT (*left*) and intense FDG uptake on attenuation corrected images (*middle*). This uptake may be difficult to differentiate from tumor. Note the typical differences on the nonattenuation-corrected image (*right*) where the lungs appear "hotter," as does the skin.

$$SUV = \frac{tissue\ activity\ (mCi/ml)}{injected\ dose\ (mCi)\ /\ body\ surface\ area}$$

In general, an SUV >2.5 is considered suspicious for malignancy. Most tumors have an even higher SUV. There is a great deal of overlap with inflammatory processes. Numerous factors affect SUV levels (Box 10-4). For example, when comparing serial exams, different imaging at different times after injection may alter SUV values. Lesion size is also an important consideration. Volume averaging can artifactually lower SUV values, as regions of interest may include pixels from normal surrounding tissue in small tumors or from motion.

CLINICAL USES OF PET IN ONCOLOGY

The use of PET scanning in primary tumors of the brain is discussed in Chapter 13. Evaluation of lung cancer in solitary pulmonary nodules was the first approved clinical indication for F-18 FDG PET scanning in the U.S by the Centers for Medicare and Medicaid (CMS). Since that time, the number of applications for PET has increased. Although the list continually changes, indications for F-18 FDG PET approved by the CMS are listed in Table 10-1. New indications are continually being evaluated and added to the list, and private insurers may cover other indications. Box 10-5 lists tumors that show a low degree of F-18 FDG uptake, causing a lower sensitivity.

Lung Carcinoma

Lung carcinoma is the most common malignancy and has the highest cancer-related death rate. The histologic classification of lung cancer is outlined in Box 10-6. Non–small-cell lung carcinoma (NSCLC) accounts for roughly 80% of cases and small-cell lung carcinoma

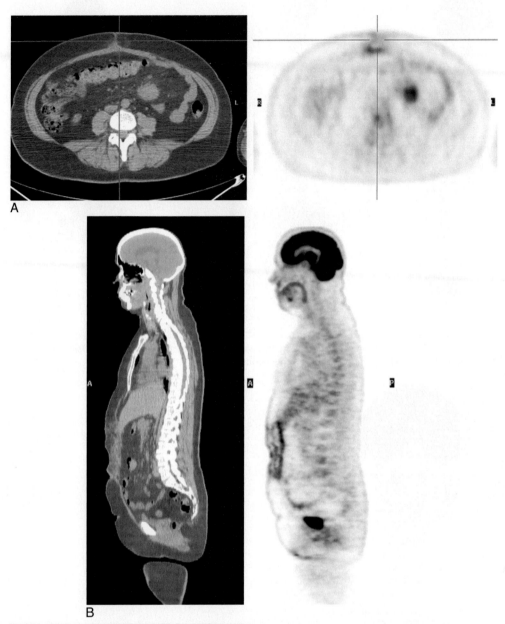

Figure 10-12   Postoperative change. **A,** Two months after laparotomy, the CT shows secondary changes in the midline anterior abdominal wall and stranding of the left lower quadrant peritoneal fat. The corresponding PET image has mild anterior soft tissue uptake as well as normal uptake in bowel and marrow. **B,** More intense uptake can be seen in the sagittal image from 6 months earlier.

(SCLC) accounts for the remaining 20%. Approximately 75% of SCLC cases present with disseminated disease. Therefore, surgery is rarely indicated and chemotherapy and radiation therapy are used. NSCLC, on the other hand, is often resectable. Early diagnosis and proper staging are critical to therapeutic planning in NSCLC.

Presenting clinical and radiographic findings are variable in lung cancer. Patients may be asymptomatic or experience hemoptysis, cough, weight loss, and symptoms of metastatic disease. Radiographic findings are also nonspecific. A mass with an irregular, spiculated border is malignant in up to 85% of cases, but lesions with smooth margins may be cancerous over a third of the time. Workup for patients with these abnormal radiographs might include sputum cytology, bronchoscopy, transthoracic needle biopsy, and mediastinoscopy. Each of these procedures has limitations. For example, although bronchoscopy has a sensitivity of 85% for central tumors, it is much lower for small and peripheral lesions. The false-negative rate for transthoracic

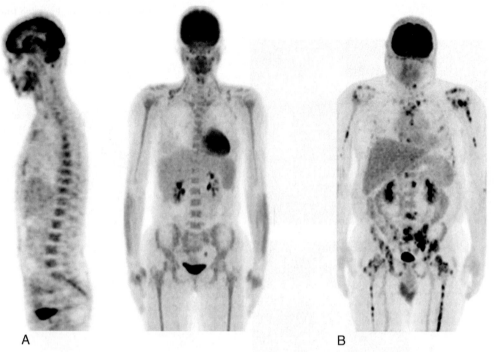

A   B

Figure 10-13   Patterns of bone marrow FDG uptake. **A,** Diffuse uptake in the marrow is frequently seen in cancer patients following colony stimulating factor therapy. **B,** Osseous metastases usually present with a heterogeneous pattern.

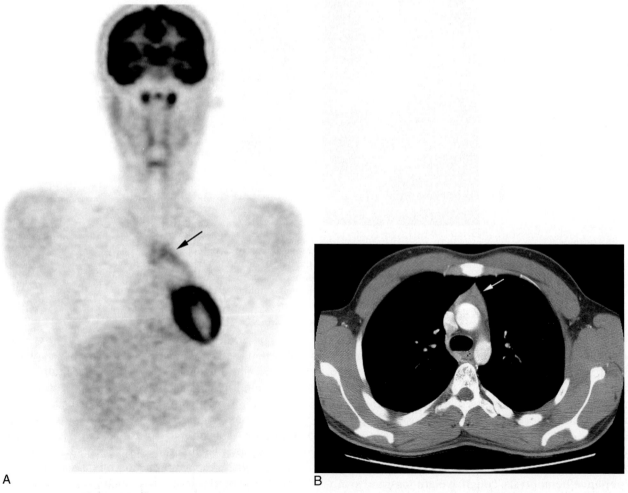

A   B

Figure 10-14   FDG uptake in the thymus. Area of uptake above the heart (*arrow*) in the typical configuration of the thymus (**A**) corresponds to a normal thymus (**B**) on CT. After chemotherapy, this uptake may be even more intense, the so-called thymic "rebound."

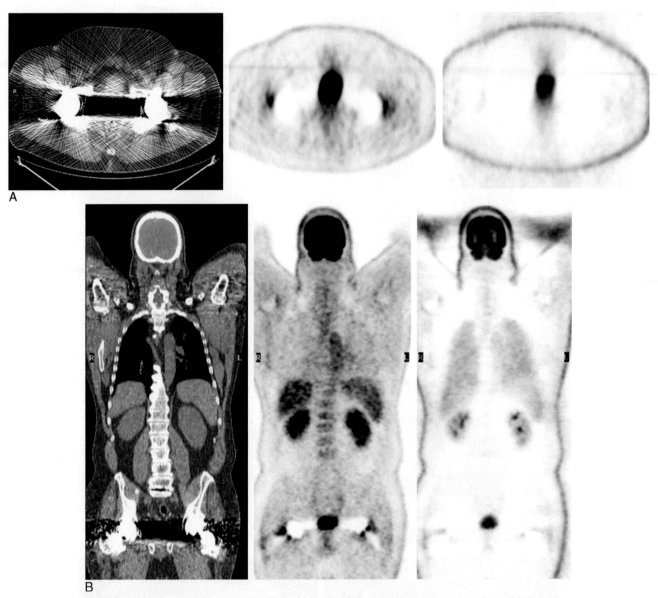

Figure 10-15   Metal artifact. Axial (**A**) and coronal (**B**) CT and PET images show beam hardening artifact on the CT (*left*) from bilateral hip prostheses. The attenuation corrected PET images (*middle*) show artifactually increased uptake along the lateral margins of the prostheses, which is significantly decreased on nonattenuation-corrected images (*right*).

needle biopsy is approximately 25%. Transthoracic needle biopsy also carries a 10–25% risk of a pneumothorax requiring a chest tube. Patients may require thoracotomy and surgical biopsy for definitive diagnosis.

Diagnosis of Solitary Pulmonary Nodule

The use of F-18 FDG PET for pulmonary nodule evaluation was one of the first indications in which PET was proven to be clinically useful. A pulmonary nodule is defined as a well-circumscribed lesion measuring <4 cm in size. With the increased use of CT, the incidental detection of these nodules has risen tremendously; about one half will prove to be malignant.

The presence of central calcifications in some nodules indicates they are benign granulomas. However, most pulmonary nodules are indeterminate based on radiographic appearance. The conventional workup of an indeterminate nodule is biopsy or serial radiographic follow-up for 2 years. If a nodule is stable in size over a 2-year period, it is presumed benign. Suspicious-appearing nodules and those that seem to increase in size are sent to biopsy. This method results in biopsy of many benign lesions and delayed diagnosis of some malignant cases. F-18 FDG PET has proven to be an accurate method to differentiate benign from malignant nodules and decrease biopsy of benign lesions (Fig. 10-19A).

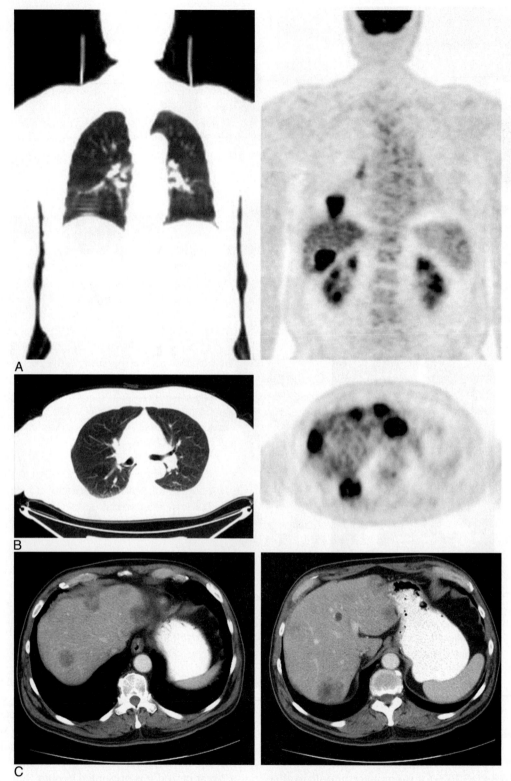

Figure 10-16   Respiratory motion artifact. Coronal (**A**) and axial (**B**) CT scans in lung windows and corresponding PET scans show intense FDG activity in liver metastases as well as in the right lung base. However, no lung mass is seen on CT. **C,** Two axial enhanced CT images show liver metastases. Differences in respiration have caused misregistration and a posterior liver lesion projects over the lung on PET.

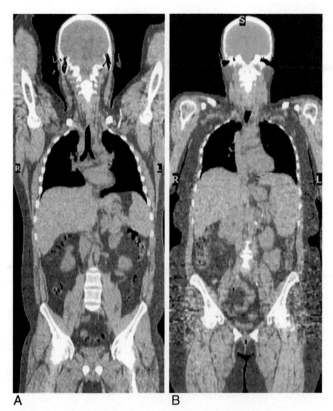

Figure 10-17   Effects of arm position and beam hardening on CT images. Soft tissue window CT image with the patient's arms up **(A)** compared with arms down **(B)** demonstrates the effect of beam hardening with artifact throughout the abdomen on **B**.

Malignant nodules generally have increased F-18 FDG uptake with an SUV >2.5, although most cancers have considerably higher SUVs (Fig. 10-19B). The sensitivity of PET is reported to be about 95% and the specificity approximately 81%. The high negative predictive value of PET means that biopsy can usually be avoided when the PET scan is normal. Because there is still a chance that malignancy is present, these patients should be followed with CT. The incidence of malignancy in patients with a negative PET scan depends on the prevalence of disease; it may be as low as 1% for patients at low risk for cancer, but can be 10% in high-risk cases.

PET scans can change the surgical approach for nodules demonstrating increased uptake. This includes identification of mediastinal lymph nodes with abnormal uptake and distant metastases (Figs. 10-20 and 10-21). In these patients, thoracotomy and surgical biopsy may be changed to mediastinoscopy.

However, PET has some limitations. False-negative results can be seen in small lesions <1 cm. The resolution of PET is on the order of 7–8 mm, and volume averaging of small tumors with surrounding normal tissue may result in low- or normal-appearing uptake. The greater motion occurring with tachypnea or in the more mobile lung bases may accentuate volume averaging. False-negative PET results can also occur in certain tumors. In the lungs, the most common of these are bronchoalveolar cell carcinoma and carcinoid.

The positive predictive value of PET is not as high as the negative predictive value, and a positive result cannot be assumed to represent malignancy. An inflammatory process such as granuloma commonly causes false positive findings. In some areas of the country where granulomatous disease is highly prevalent, this is a very significant problem.

A malignant solitary nodule is most commonly caused by primary bronchogenic carcinoma, although a single metastatic lesion is also a possibility. Close examination of the PET scan and correlative CT are essential to detect any unexpected primary tumor outside of the lungs.

Staging NSCLC

Staging of NSCLC lung carcinoma is critical in assessing prognoses and deciding the appropriate course of therapy.

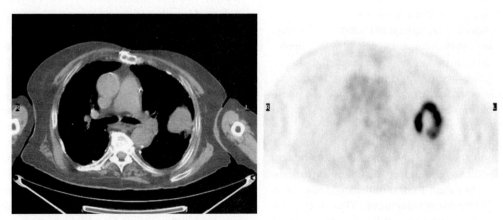

Figure 10-18   Central tumor necrosis on PET. A left upper lung carcinoma seen as a solid mass on CT actually contains significant central necrosis that is revealed as absent uptake on PET. Visualization of regional differences in tumor metabolic activity with PET can help direct a biopsy.

Box 10-4 Factors Affecting Standard Uptake Value (SUV) Levels

Factor	Change in SUV
↑ Serum glucose	↓
↑ Body mass	↑
↓ Dose delivery: extravasated dose	↓
↑ Uptake period	↑
↓ Region-of-interest size	↑
↓ Pixel size	↑

Box 10-5 Tumors with Low F-18 FDG PET Uptake

Prostate cancer
Renal cell carcinoma
Bronchoalveolar cell lung cancer
Mucinous adenocarcinomas
Carcinoid
Low-grade sarcomas
Low-grade lymphoma
    MALT mucosa-associated lymphoma
    Small cell lymphocytic non-Hodgkin lymphoma
Differentiated thyroid cancer (iodine-avid)
Hepatocellular carcinoma
Metastasis to brain

Box 10-6 World Health Organization Histologic Classification of Lung Carcinoma

SMALL CELL

Pure small cell (oat cell)
Mixed (small cell and large cell)
Combined (small cell and squamous cell or adenocarcinoma)

NON-SMALL CELL
Large cell

Undifferentiated large cell
Giant cell
Clear cell

Squamous cell carcinoma

Epidermoid
Spindle cell

Adenocarcinoma

Acinar
Papillary
Bronchoalveolar
Solid carcinoma with mucus production

Adenosquamous carcinoma

Bronchial gland carcinoma
Adenoid cystic carcinoma
Mucoepidermoid tumor

Carcinoid

Lung cancer staging is based on the tumor-node-metastasis (TNM) classification (Boxes 10-7 and 10-8). Generally, stage I and stage II patients are considered resectable, although a subset of stage III patients might benefit from surgery. Only about 25% of patients present with stage I or stage II disease. However, improved methods of staging are needed, as up to 50% of patients with NSCLC who undergo curative surgery suffer a recurrence.

CT and PET often have complementary roles in the staging, restaging, and surveillance of NSCLC. CT better assesses tumor size, invasion of the pleura and mediastinum, and the distance of the tumor from the carina. Also, abnormalities such as atelectasis and aspiration pneumonia can cause abnormal F-18 FDG uptake that may be confused with the primary tumor.

However, radiographic staging has its limitations. For example, CT examination of the lymph nodes depends on size criteria to determine if tumor involvement is present. Any lymph node larger than 1 cm is considered abnormal and suspicious for tumor involvement. This frequently leads to understaging patients. PET can often detect abnormal activity from tumor in normal-sized lymph nodes. In addition, a whole-body PET scan may detect lesions not seen on a chest and abdomen CT examination (Fig. 10-22). The sensitivity of PET for tumor involvement in any one lymph node is 75%, but it averages 91% for overall mediastinal involvement. This compares well to reported sensitivities of CT at 63–76%.

Both CT and PET can have false-positive results in the lymph nodes. Inflammatory conditions can cause enlarged lymph nodes on CT, with false positive interpretations occurring in up to 40% of patients. Inflammatory processes and the effects of therapy also cause increased uptake of radiotracer. However, lymph nodes may remain enlarged after disease has resolved and PET has normalized. Following therapy, PET provides information on response that CT cannot. Patients who respond to therapy will show PET changes more quickly than on CT.

The results of PET can help direct the method and location of biopsy. Patients with no mediastinal involvement or distant metastases can go to thoracotomy for curative resection at the time of biopsy. C, However, PET may not be able to differentiate N1 disease from N2 disease. This is a critical difference, as N1 involvement is operable but N2 is not. Mediastinoscopy may be needed to differentiate N1 from N2 disease or to further evaluate the mediastinum

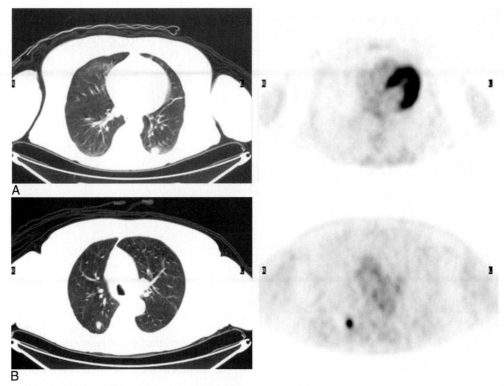

Figure 10-19   Characterization of solitary pulmonary nodules. **A,** A left lung nodule on CT had no FDG uptake on PET consistent with a benign process. This lesion remained stable on CT follow-up confirming this impression. **B,** A small, well-circumscribed right lower-lobe nodule with increased FDG accumulation on PET was later found to be an adenocarcinoma.

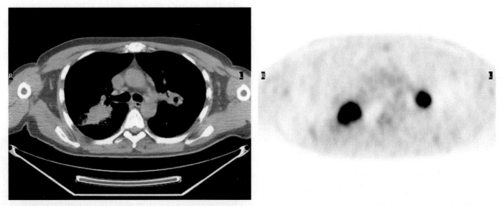

Figure 10-20   Detection of distant disease with PET. A large right-lung nodule showed markedly increased FDG uptake consistent with tumor. Contralateral hilar lymph nodes were also abnormal, which meant this patient was not a candidate for surgical resection.

when PET is positive. It is important to describe lymph node involvement in uniform terms. The commonly used classification system is outlined in Box 10-9 and Figures 10-23, 10-24, and 10-C [see color insert].

PET is superior to conventional imaging modalities for the detection of distant metastases. Bone involvement is detected with a somewhat higher sensitivity than the bone scan, and a considerably higher specificity. Tumor involvement that might be overlooked on CT may be seen with PET. This includes retroperitoneal and supra-clavicular lymph nodes, soft tissue lesions, and small adrenal metastases. Assessment of the adrenal glands is important, as they are a frequent site of lung cancer metastasis (Fig. 10-25). CT reveals adrenal lesions in roughly 20% of cases, but the majority are later proven to be benign adenomas. PET can help differentiate benign

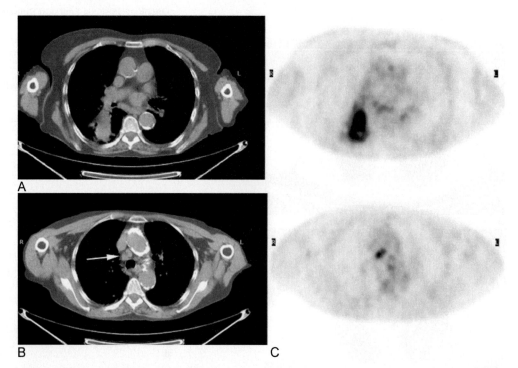

Figure 10-21 PET improves lung cancer staging. **A,** The right upper lobe bilobed pulmonary nodule appears malignant on PET. **B,** Small lymph nodes on CT would not be read as positive based on size criteria alone. **C,** However, PET revealed these small lower paratracheal lymph nodes to be abnormal. Biopsy confirmed malignancy in both regions.

<table>
<tr><td colspan="2">Box 10-7   Tumor-Node-Metastasis (TNM) Staging of Lung Carcinoma</td></tr>
</table>

PRIMARY TUMOR (T)

Tx: Malignant cells; primary not seen

T0: No evidence of primary tumor

T1: <3 cm; surrounded lung or visceral pleura; not in mainstem bronchus

T2: Any of the following:
>3 cm
Involves mainstem bronchus >2 cm from carina
Invades visceral pleura
Associated atelectasis or obstructive pneumonia extends to hilar region but does not involve whole lung

T3: Any size invades chest wall, pericardium, mediastinal pleura, diaphragm
<2 cm carina
Atelectasis entire lung

REGIONAL LYMPH NODES (N)

N0: No involvement

N1: Nodes within lung, ipsilateral bronchopulmonary or hilar

N2: Ipsilateral mediastinal, mid-line prevascular, and/or subcarinal

N3: Contralateral mediastinal, contralateral hilar, contralateral scalene, supraclavicular

DISTANT METASTASIS (M)

M0: No distant metastasis

M1: Distant metastasis

---

and malignant adrenal gland lesions with a high degree of accuracy based on the level of uptake.

Overall, PET has a significant effect on patient staging and management. Unsuspected metastases are detected 10–14% of the time. A significant change in management has been reported in 19–41% of cases based on PET findings.

Restaging NSCLC and Assessing Response to Therapy

When surgery and therapy distort anatomy, PET can detect residual and recurrent tumor not found on CT.

Box 10-8   Staging of Lung Carcinoma Based on Tumor-Node-Metastasis (TNM) Classification Scheme

Stage	TNM
Ia	T1 N0 M0
Ib	T2 N0 M0
IIa	T1 N1 M0
IIb	T2 N1 M0
	T3 N0 M0
IIIa	T3 N1 M0
	T1–3 N2 M0
IIIb	T4 N0–2 M0
	T1–4 N3 M0
IV	Any T, any N, M1

Based on the AJCC staging system, 1997.

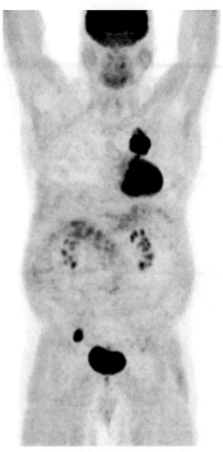

Figure 10-22 Added value of whole-body scanning. The MIP image of a patient with a left upper lobe non-small carcinoma (above the heart) demonstrates a metastasis to an external iliac node in the right pelvis, not detected previously as CT scans were only done through the adrenal glands.

Caution must be used as increased F-18 FDG accumulation may occur following therapy. The most significant problem occurs after radiation. The accuracy of PET can be improved by delaying imaging until at least 3 months after therapy. Even given these limitations, PET can provide valuable information by identifying residual disease or relapse. For example, distant recurrence after complete resection of tumor occurs over 20% of the time. PET restaging frequently leads to changes in management.

The use of PET to measure a response to treatment is more limited. Although a decrease in the size of a mass on CT has been used to assess response, this does not always provide the best indicator of the efficacy of therapy. A response to therapy with PET has been defined as a decrease in uptake on the SUV by at least 50%. Limited data suggests a decrease in F-18 FDG activity may provide a better measure of response and normalization of uptake may be associated with a favorable prognosis.

Box 10-9 Classification of Lymph Node Stations in the Chest

Station	Designation
SUPERIOR MEDIASTINAL NODES	
1 Highest mediastinal	Above top of left brachio-cephalic vein crossing trachea
2 Upper paratracheal	Below station 1 to top aortic arch
3 Prevascular	Anterior to great vessels above top aortic arch
Retrotracheal	Behind trachea, thoracic inlet to bottom azygous vein
4 Lower paratracheal	Below top of aortic arch
	Above top right upper lobe bronchus
	Azygous arch divides superior from inferior
AORTIC NODES	
5 Subaortic or AP window	Medial first branch pulmonary artery, lateral ligamentum arteriosum
6 Para-aortic	Anterior and lateral to aortic arch
INFERIOR MEDIASTINAL NODES	
7 Inferior mediastinal	Subcarinal
8 Paraesophageal	Lateral to esophagus or anterior if below subcarinal nodes
9 Pulmonary ligament	In pulmonary ligament
N1 NODES—DISTAL TO MEDIASTINAL PLEURAL REFLECTION	
10 Hilar	
11* Interlobar	Between lobar bronchi and adjacent to lobar bronchi
12* Lobar	
13* Segmental	
14* Subsegmental	

*Intrapulmonary.

Small Cell Lung Carcinoma

SCLC staging usually involves categorizing the disease as limited or extensive. If disease that is confined to one hemithorax, it can be treated more successfully by adding radiation to the chemotherapy. Small cell lung carcinoma shows intense F-18 FDG accumulation. In general, data on the use of PET in SCLC is more limited than for NSCLC. PET may help detect additional metastasis and lead to upstaging of some patients. The cost effectiveness of F-18 FDG PET in SCLC has not been proven.

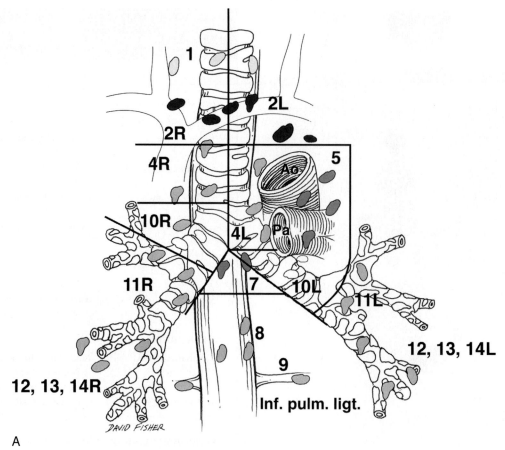

Figure 10-23   **A–B,** Lymph node classification of the chest. Coronal images of the chest outline the location of lymph node stations described in Box 10-9.

Continued

Head and Neck Carcinoma

The prognosis of head and neck cancer depends on the disease stage. As distant metastases at initial diagnosis occur only 5% of the time, local lymph node status is most critical in determining which patients are candidates for surgical resection. At diagnosis, roughly 40% of patients have localized disease and 60% have advanced cases (Figs. 10-26 and 10-27). F-18 FDG PET has been found to be useful in staging, monitoring therapy response, and detecting recurrence of head and neck cancers (Box 10-10). PET reportedly changes patient management in 20–30% of patients with head and neck cancer.

Although FDG PET is sensitive, it plays a more limited role in head and neck tumor diagnosis than lung cancer. Conventional modalities adequately visualize most tumors and are generally better able to assess tumor size. However, head and neck cancer often presents with palpable adenopathy. These lymph node metastases may be much larger than the primary tumor in head and neck

cancer. In 5% of cases, the primary cannot be identified by endoscopy, CT, or MRI, which means that a patient might have to undergo large-field radiation therapy. Although small primary tumors may not be detected, PET can identify the unknown primary tumor in 20–50% of patients.

In the staging of head and neck cancer, PET has been found equivalent if not superior to CT and MRI in the detection of nodal metastases. When lymph nodes are normal in size, this is particularly helpful. For restaging, PET appears superior to conventional imaging modalities. When the anatomy is distorted from surgery and radiation, restaging and detection of recurrent tumor by PET is superior to CT. The reported sensitivity of PET for recurrence ranges from 79–96%, with a negative predictive value >90%. CT, on the other hand, has a sensitivity of 54–61%.

PET-CT is particularly useful in evaluating the postoperative neck (Figs. 10-28 and 10-D [see color insert]). With a loss of symmetry, evaluation is difficult; fusion images allow better identification of increased uptake in

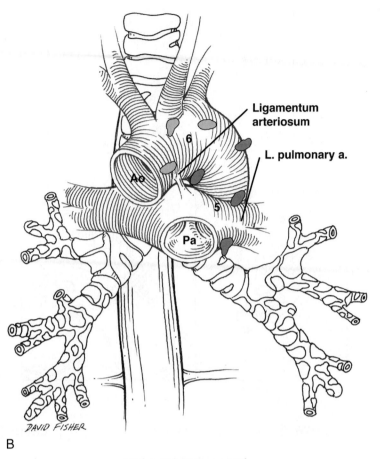

B

Figure 10-23 B, cont'd.

normal structures, such as discriminating muscles, from sites of tumor recurrence or metastases. Recent studies suggest additional imaging after a further delay of an hour or so may increase specificity.

Consistent terms must be used to describe the location of head and neck cancer. Different methods of describing the location of cervical lymph nodes have been utilized over the years. Currently, an imaging-based method of lymph node classification proposed by Som optimizes recent updates by the AJCC (Box 10-11; Figs. 10-29 and 10-30).

Thyroid Carcinoma

Thyroid cancer must be considered separately from other cancers occurring in the head and neck. In most cases, thyroid cancer derives from the follicular cells of the gland giving rise to papillary, follicular, or mixed cellularity variants. These differentiated tumors accumulate iodine-131 (I-131) and are best evaluated and treated with radioactive iodine. The sensitivity of F-18 FDG in these patients is low.

Clinical utility of FDG PET scanning is limited to thyroid malignancies that do not accumulate I-131. These include poorly differentiated, aggressive tumors. This may occur in metastatic and recurrent tumors that degenerate from a previously well-differentiated, iodine-avid tumor. In cases where the I-131 scan is negative but serum thyroglobulin levels remain elevated, the sensitivity of PET is >90%. PET may help direct surgical resection or external beam radiation therapy. Unlike I-131 scanning, patients do not need to undergo thyroid hormone replacement therapy withdrawal or stimulation with recombinant TSH. PET may also be of some benefit in the more aggressive Hürthle cell variant of follicular carcinoma and in some anaplastic tumors.

PET scanning may also be useful in medullary thyroid carcinoma. This tumor arises from the parafollicular cells of the thyroid and does not accumulate I-131. These tumors have been evaluated with somatostatin receptor analogs, pentavalent DMSA, and thalium-201 and Tc-99m sestamibi. However, FDG PET may be superior to these agents and can be helpful in difficult

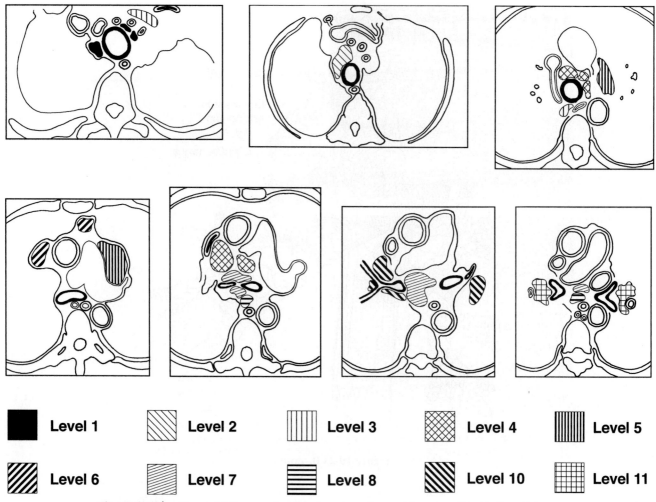

Figure 10-24   Transaxial diagram chest lymph node station positions as outlined in Box 10-9 (pulmonary ligament [level 9] not included) and Figure 10-23.

cases. The sensitivity of PET has been reported to be 78% with a specificity of 79%.

It must be noted that F-18 FDG may accumulate with equal intensity in benign adenomas, thyroiditis, and malignant lesions. Although an incidentally detected F-18 FDG avid nodule should be pursued to exclude malignancy, PET has no role in the diagnosis of thyroid cancer.

Esophageal Carcinoma

Esophageal carcinoma is most commonly due to squamous cell cancer in the upper two-thirds of the esophagus, whereas adenocarcinoma typically occurs in the lower third. It frequently presents as dysphagia or is detected by endoscopic biopsy in patients with Barrett's esophagus, a known precursor of many cases of esophageal cancer. Because whole-body scanners have limited sensitivity and specificity for detecting tumor in patients with Barrett's, PET has not proven useful in screening these patients.

Diagnosis

Overall, the sensitivity of PET is 95% in esophageal cancer. The diagnosis of the primary esophageal tumors by PET may be limited by a small tumor volume. In adenocarcinoma, 10–15% of patients may be falsely negative by PET due to low uptake in mucinous and signet cell varieties. PET is not able to determine the extent of the primary tumor and may not offer any substantial advantage over the standard diagnostic modalities such as endoscopic ultrasonography.

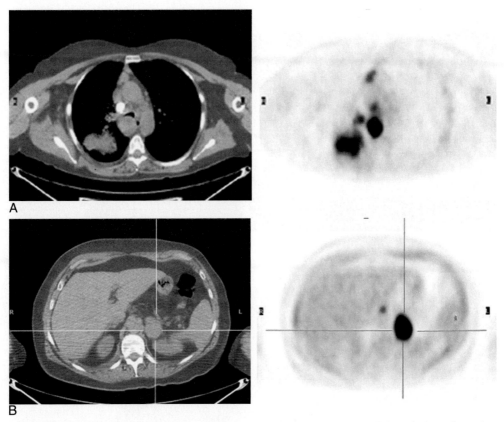

Figure 10-25   Adrenal metastases on PET. **A,** A non-small cell carcinoma of the right lung showed mediastinal involvement on PET. **B,** The enlarged adrenal gland seen on CT also appeared malignant by PET. Adrenal metastases can also be detected with PET in normal appearing glands by CT.

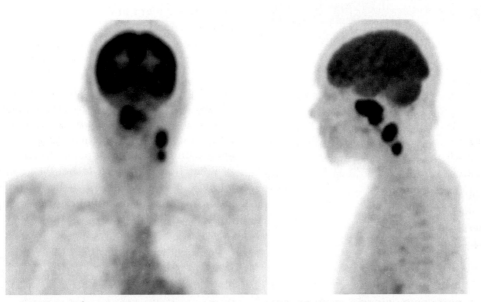

Figure 10-26   Recurrent squamous cell carcinoma of the head and neck. Coronal and sagittal PET images demonstrate tumor activity in enlarged palpable left cervical lymph nodes, as well as the primary tumor posteriorly along the oropharynx extending up to the skull base.

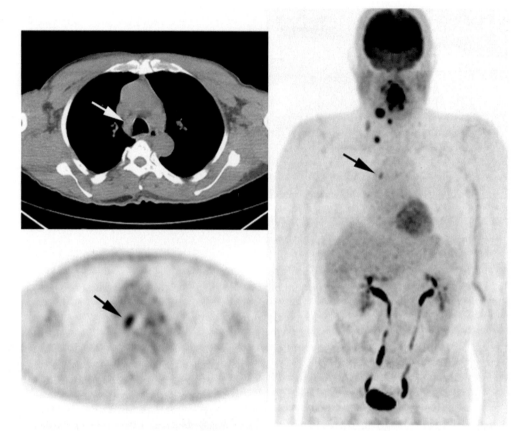

Figure 10-27   Head and neck carcinoma staging. PET images reveal several abnormal lymph nodes in the right cervical and supraclavicular region, as well as an unexpected mediastinal metastasis to a normal-sized lower paratracheal (*arrow*).

Box 10-10	F-18 FDG Imaging in Head and Neck Carcinoma

Indication	Utility of FDG PET
Surveillance	Very useful
Restaging recurrence	Very useful, especially postoperative neck but limited by radiation change
Response to therapy	May be useful
Diagnosis in unknown primary	Useful; positive only 25–30%
Staging	
Clinical N1–N3 neck	Useful, detect distant metastasis
Clinical N0 neck	Low yield

Staging

Esophageal cancer most commonly spreads to regional lymph nodes. The location of these nodes depends to a certain extent on the level of the primary tumor. For example, cervical metastases are more common in proximal tumors and abdominal lymph node involvement may be more frequent in distal masses. However, spread is unpredictable.

Although the sensitivity of PET for lymph node involvement is not high (>70%), the specificity is >90% (Figs. 10-31 and 10-E [see color insert]). Identification of paraesophageal nodes is limited by PET as they may be inseparable from the primary mass and very small lesions may be below the resolution of the PET detection systems. However, the detection of distant metastases with F-18 FDG is superior to CT. The accuracy of PET has been reported to be 83%, compared to 68% with CT. PET may result in a change in patient management in a significant number of cases, approximately 20% of the time.

Restaging and Monitoring Response to Therapy

PET has proven value in assessing patients during therapy and following therapy for recurrence. A scan following neoadjuvant chemotherapy may better predict patient survival after subsequent therapy than standard imaging methods (Fig. 10-32). The ability to detect

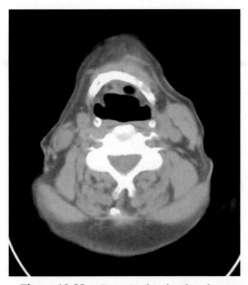
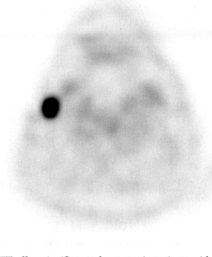

Figure 10-28   Restaging head and neck cancer. PET offers significant advantages in patients with postoperative change where landmarks are gone or distorted. Following modified radical neck dissection, this patient shows considerable asymmetry, but recurrent disease is obvious on the PET scan.

Box 10-11   Comparison of Nodal Classification Systems for Head and Neck Cancer

Rouviere System	AJCC System	Imaging-Based System	
Submental	I	**IA:** medial to medial edge anterior belly digastrics	Below mylohyoid muscle, above hyoid bone
Submandibular	I	**IB:** lateral to IA and anterior to back of submandibular gland	
Internal jugular	**II:** skull base to hyoid, anterior to back edge sternocleidomastoid	**II:** skull base to bottom of hyoid, anterior to back edge sternocleidomastoid	**IIA:** anterior, lateral, or inseparable from internal jugular vein
			IIB: posterior to internal jugular vein with fat plane between
Retropharyngeal	**III:** hyoid to cricothyroid membrane, anterior to back edge sternocleido-mastoid	**III:** bottom of hyoid to bottom of cricoid arch, anterior to back edge sternocleidomastoid	Lateral to carotid, level VI nodes are medial to carotids
Midjugular	**IV:** cricothyroid membrane to clavicle, anterior to back edge of sternocleido-mastoid	**IV:** bottom of cricoid arch to top of manubrium, anterior to back edge sternocleidomastoid	Lateral to carotids, level VI nodes are medial to carotids
Spinal accessory	**V:** posterior to sternocleido-mastoid, anterior to trapezius, above clavicle	**V:** posterior to sternocleido-mastoid, anterior to trapezius, above clavicle	**VA:** skull base to bottom of cricoid arch
			VB: bottom cricoid arch to level clavicle Visceral nodes
Anterior compartment	**VI:** below hyoid, above suprasternal notch, between carotid sheaths	**VI:** below bottom of hyoid, above top of manubrium, medial to carotid arteries	
Upper mediastinal	**VII:** below suprasternal notch	**VII:** below top manubrium and above innominate,	Overlaps highest mediastinal nodes of chest classification between carotids
Supraclavicular		Clavicles in field of view, above and medial to ribs	

All systems use facial, parotid, retropharyngeal, and occipital groups.

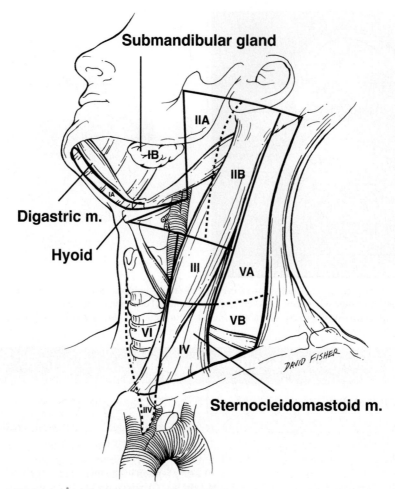

Figure 10-29   Cervical lymph node levels according to the imaging based classification system described in Box 10-11.

residual and recurrent disease is also significant. However, caution must be taken when evaluating patients immediately after therapy as an artifactual increase in activity may be seen (Fig. 10-33).

Normal physiologic activity in the esophagus may confound interpretation. Similarly, intense F-18 FDG uptake in normal stomach limits the usefulness of PET in evaluating tumors of the stomach and gastroesophageal junction. However, when a gastric tumor is F-18 FDG avid, PET scanning may be useful in monitoring therapy.

Colorectal Carcinoma

Colon cancer is known to develop in colon polyps. Dysplastic elements are found in approximately one third of adenomatous polyps. A progression to invasive

cancer occurs slowly. The diagnosis of colorectal carcinoma depends on direct visualization by colonoscopy as well as imaging with CT and barium enema. Staging with CT often identifies regional adenopathy and distant metastases. The staging of colorectal carcinoma is important in determining therapy and prognosis (Boxes 10-12 and 10-13).

The ability of PET to diagnose primary colorectal tumors may be limited as small tumors and cancerous polyps are frequently not detected, and the high levels of F-18 FDG activity normally occurring in the bowel can decrease sensitivity and specificity. However, even given these limitations, PET detects primary colon carcinomas >90% of the time. In comparison, CT has a sensitivity of about 60%.

Although contrast-enhanced CT is the primary modality for the staging of colorectal carcinoma, it often

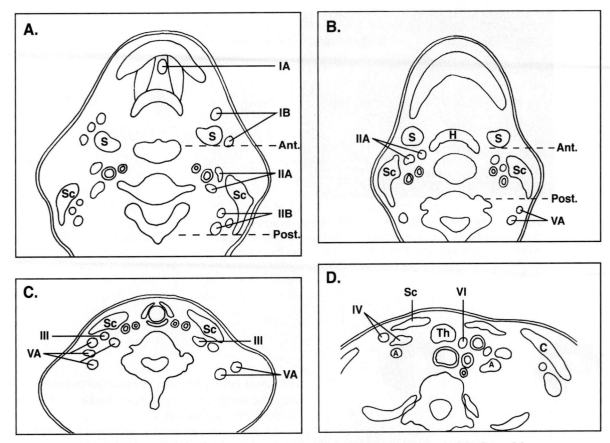

Figure 10-30   Transaxial diagram of cervical lymph node stations at the level of the floor of the mouth and submandibular gland (*S*) **(A)**, the hyoid bone (*H*) **(B)**, thyroid cartilage and cricoid cartilage **(C)**, and just above the clavicles (*C*) **(D)** with a portion of the thyroid gland (*Tb*) in view. Note the appearance of the sternocleidomastoid muscle (*SC*), which is a key landmark.

fails to identify nodal disease. F-18 FDG PET is superior to CT for initial staging and the detection of recurrent colon cancer. Local recurrence can be difficult to detect on CT due to scarrin following therapy, but may be easily visible on PET images. The obturator and iliac nodal regions of the pelvis are often particularly difficult to evaluate on CT, and PET is very helpful in evaluating these regions. However, PET is also superior to CT in the retroperitoneal nodes. The detection of hepatic metastases is good with CT, but PET often compliments this information or detects new lesions (Fig. 10-34). Sensitivity of PET has been reported at 85–99%, with specificity of 71–87%. PET may directly alter patient management in 29–36% of staging and restaging cases. Data are limited concerning the use of PET in monitoring therapy effects.

Other Tumors of the Gastrointestinal Tract

The use of PET in other tumors of the gastrointestinal tract is more limited, and CT remains critical in the analysis of these tumors. However, PET may be helpful in tumors of pancreatic, biliary, and hepatic origin. PET is often used in patients with CT scans that are difficult to evaluate or in patients with elevated serum tumor markers. These include alpha-feto protein in hepatocellular carcinoma and Ca 19-9 in pancreatic cancer.

PET is highly sensitive for the detection of pancreatic cancer (Fig. 10-35). However, CT is essential in defining tumor extent and determining resectability. Some masses seen on CT are actually benign, and PET can often differentiate benign and malignant processes (with accuracies ranging from 85–93%). This can support a negative fine-needle biopsy finding. PET may also detect occult cancers not seen on CT in symptomatic patients. The detection of nodal disease is comparable between PET and CT. However, PET may identify lymph nodes difficult to visualize on CT, such as in the upper portal regions. Also, PET can identify undiagnosed distant metastases in 14% of cases. These factors can lead to alterations in surgical

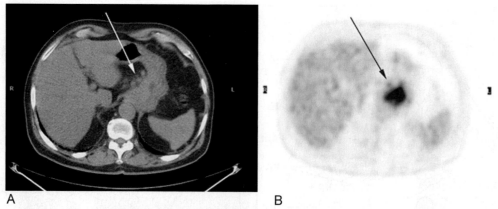

A   B

Figure 10-31   Identification of regional lymph nodes in head and neck cancer. **A,** Small lymph nodes along the lesser curvature of the stomach (*arrow*) are seen on CT. **B,** Only low-level FDG activity was present despite the presence of metastases on endoscopic biopsy. The difficulty in identifying regional nodes may relate to activity in adjacent tumor or microscopic amounts of tumor present.

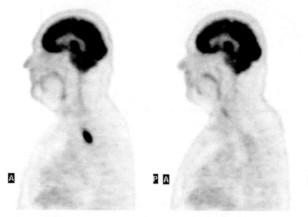

Figure 10-32   Monitoring esophageal tumor response to therapy. Sagittal PET scans (*left*) before and (*right*) after chemotherapy show rapid resolution of the abnormal activity within an esophageal tumor. This type of response has been linked to a better prognosis in recent studies.

management in up to 41% of cases. PET is often limited by poor sensitivity in small tumors and in acute pancreatitis. The uptake in acute pancreatitis can be as intense as in malignancy and can mask underlying tumor. Acute pancreatitis often accompanies therapy or obstruction by tumor, and PET in these cases is often nondiagnostic.

Primary tumors of the liver are much less common and are most often evaluated by CT. The two most common primary liver tumors are hepatocellular carcinoma and cholangiocarcinoma. Although F-18 FDG PET is highly accurate for detecting metastases to the liver, it is considerably less sensitive for primary hepatic tumors.

PET may detect 50–70% of hepatocellular carcinomas, but the sensitivity is reportedly higher (90%) for other hepatic primary tumors.

Cholangiocarcinoma is a rare cancer of the bile ducts that may not be detected on CT. It may occur in an extrahepatic or an intrahepatic location. Tumors arising peripherally have a better prognosis as they may be resected, whereas those near the hilum are infrequently resectable. Tumors can be infiltrating, exophytic, or a polypoid intraluminal mass. The sensitivity of PET is lower for the infiltrating type. Gallbladder cancer is a rare tumor that is generally diagnosed late in the course of disease and may present with distant metastases. PET may identify nodal metastases difficult to detect with CT, including distant nodes and those high along the common biliary duct.

One tumor where PET has proven useful is the gastrointestinal stromal tumor (GIST). These tumors usually show high levels of F-18 FDG accumulation. Rapid response to Gleevac therapy seen with PET can predict improved patient survival (Fig. 10-36).

Lymphoma

Malignant lymphoma is classified as either Hodgkin disease (HD) (15%) or the more common non-Hodgkin lymphoma (NHL) (85%). For Hodgkin disease, 10-year survival rates are 80–85% for the early stages and ~40% for very advanced (Stage IV) disease. Survival rates are much lower for NHL, with a 60% 5-year survival for the potentially curable tumors, which are the high-grade, more aggressive forms of the disease.

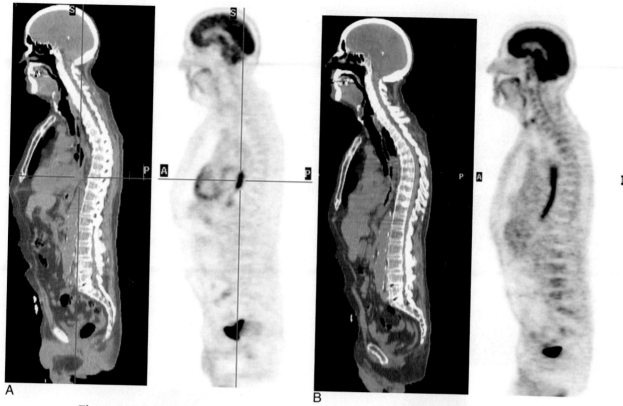

Figure 10-33   Effects of radiation therapy on PET interpretation. **A,** Initial sagittal CT and PET images reveal abnormal uptake in the esophagus from tumor. **B,** Two months following radiation therapy, diffusely increased activity is seen in an extensive region of thickened esophagus. Although this was presumed secondary to therapy, underlying tumor could go undetected and further follow-up was needed.

Box 10-12	Tumor-node-metastasis (TNM) Classification of Colon and Rectal Carcinoma	
Primary Tumor	**Regional Lymph Nodes**	**Distant Metastases**
Tx: cannot be assessed	Nx: cannot be assessed	Mx: cannot be assessed
T0: no evidence of tumor	N0: none	M0: none
TIS: carcinoma in situ	N1: 1–3 positive nodes	M1: distant metastases
T1: invades submucosal	N2: ≥4	
T2: invades muscularis propria	N3: central nodes	
T3: through propria		
T4: invades other organs		

HD tends to spread in an orderly fashion in contiguous lymph node chains. Staging of HD is important in treatment planning and assessing prognosis, but surgical staging has largely been replaced by imaging (Box 10-14). Prognosis is good for stage I and stage II disease, which can be treated with local radiation therapy. More advanced disease requires the addition of chemotherapy.

NHL is often widely disseminated at the time of diagnosis and is more frequently fatal. Prognosis is closely related to histopathological classification and tumor grade. High-grade and intermediate-grade tumors are treated with chemotherapy and radiation therapy with the goal of a cure. Patients with low-grade tumors typically have an

Box 10-13	Dukes Staging of Colorectal Carcinoma
A	T1,T2; N0; M0
B	T3,T4; N0; M0
C	T1–4; N1; M0
D	Any T; Any N; M1

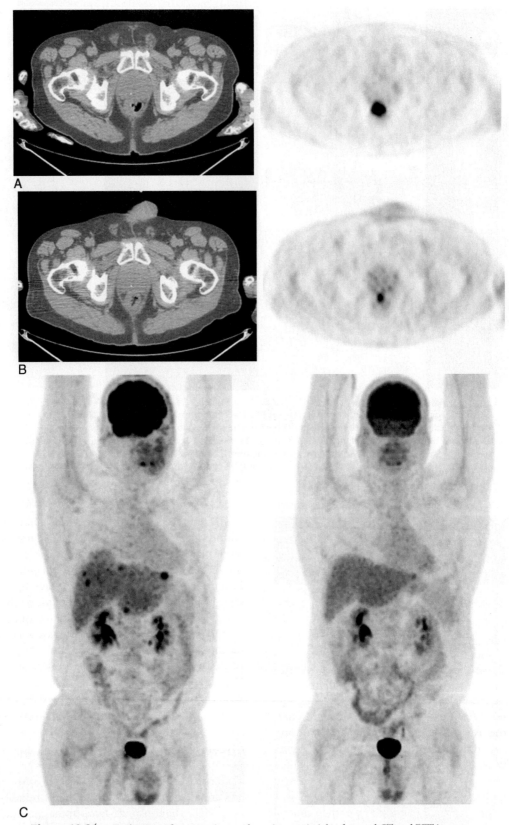

Figure 10-34 Evaluation of metastatic rectal carcinoma. Axial-enhanced CT and PET images before (**A**) and after (**B**) chemotherapy show a decrease in activity in a malignant rectal mass. **C,** Coronal images before (*left*) and after (*right*) therapy in this patient show a decrease in hepatic lesions, only one of which was ever detected by CT.

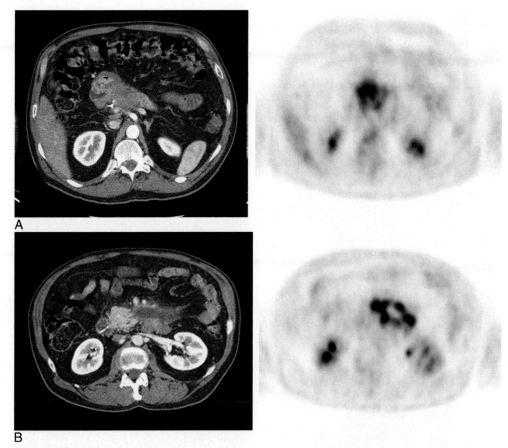

Figure 10-35 PET imaging of the pancreas. **A,** A malignant pancreatic head mass seen on contrast-enhanced CT had a high level of F-18 FDG uptake consistent with malignancy. However, the inflammation that accompanies pancreatitis can also cause intense uptake. **B,** CT following biopsy of a pancreatic mass showed inflammatory changes around the pancreatic tail. These were positive with PET. Note the central "cold" area corresponding to a pancreatic duct dilated due to proximal obstruction from the mass.

indolent course initially. However, although therapy may prolong survival, low-grade tumors relapse and eventually transform to aggressive and fatal tumors.

Imaging

Developments in imaging and therapy have led to significant improvements in the treatment of lymphoma. CT remains a critical component of diagnosis and staging. Gallium-67 (Ga-67) has long been used to stage, restage, and evaluate the response of lymphoma to therapy. However, there are drawbacks to this radiotracer. Spatial resolution is limited, even when imaging is performed with SPECT. The exam often requires multiple sessions over the course of several days. The sensitivity of Ga-67 is limited below the diaphragm and in low-grade tumors. Ga-67 imaging is discussed further in Chapter 9.

Recently, F-18 FDG PET imaging was proven to be useful in the assessment of lymphoma. PET offers several significant advantages over Ga-67, including improved

sensitivity (Fig. 10-37). Imaging is usually completed within hours and not days. Resolution is much higher, radiation dose is lower, and quantification is possible with PET. Specificity may be improved with image fusion to the CT.

Detection

PET is highly sensitive in the detection of HD and high-grade NHL and usually shows high levels of radiotracer uptake. Some low-grade NHL cases caused by follicular NHL are also accurately evaluated. Other low-grade NHL tumors such as small cell lymphocytic lymphoma and mucosa-associated lymphoma tissue (MALT) have much less uptake and are not visualized reliably with F-18 FDG PET. Diagnosis of lymphoma generally relies on histopathologic characterization of tissue samples, and PET has not played a significant role in diagnosis of lymphoma. PET might be useful in directing biopsy to the most accessible site.

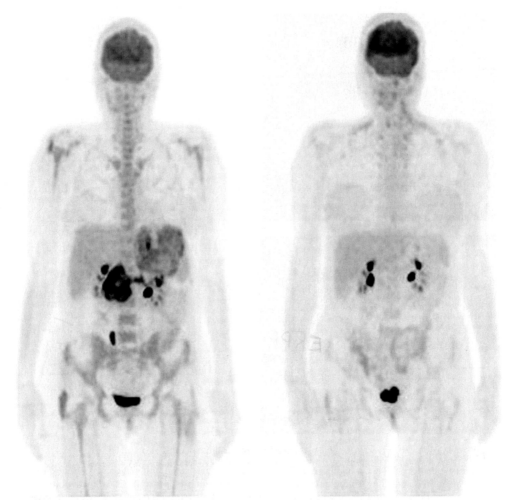

Figure 10-36   FDG PET in gastrointestinal stromal tumor (GIST). PET has proven useful in monitoring the remarkable effects of Gleevac therapy on GIST tumors. A baseline study (*left*) is needed to confirm the tumor is FDG avid. Rapid improvement is often seen within days of therapy (*right*).

Staging, Monitoring Therapy, and Restaging

Although CT remains the primary modality for staging lymphoma, the accuracy of PET is 96% compared to 56% with CT. With sensitivity >91%, PET scans are 10% more sensitive than CT. The stage of the patient may be altered based on the PET in anywhere from 10–40% of cases. PET is more accurate in assessing extranodal disease, including bone marrow and spleen. Focal lesions are generally caused by tumor, whereas diffuse uptake may be the result of therapy. As bone marrow biopsy can miss disease, a combination of PET and biopsy may provide the most accurate evaluation of the marrow.

FDG PET can accurately evaluate the effectiveness of therapy. Decreased radiotracer uptake is seen in patients responding to therapy (Figs. 10-38 and 10-39). This can be evaluated after as little as one cycle of chemotherapy or even after a few days of therapy. Responders identified by PET had longer disease-free remission periods or were cured, whereas patients with residual disease (or nonresponders) all relapsed or progressed. This indicates PET may help optimize therapy in patients with lymphoma.

Like Ga-67, PET can assess for tumor viability in a residual mass found on CT following therapy. PET is

Box 10-14	Ann Arbor Classification of Lymphoma
I	Single lymph node or lymphoid structure
IE	I+: growth into adjacent tissue or extralymphatic involvement (not liver)
II	Involving ≥2 regions on the same side of the diaphragm
IIE	II+: extralymphatic involvement
III	Disease on both sides of the diaphragm (IIIS: splenic involvement)
IIIE	III+: involvement extranodal tissue localized
IV	Nonlocalized or disseminated disease

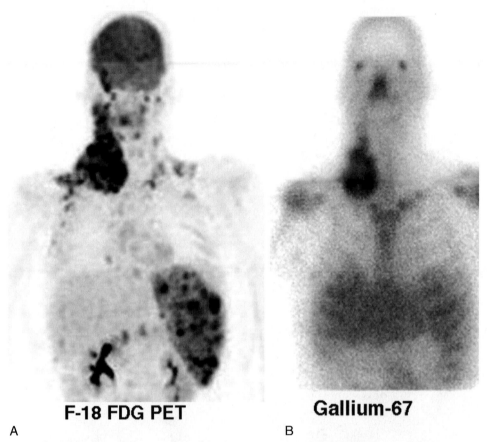

F-18 FDG PET

A

Gallium-67

B

Figure 10-37   Improved sensitivity of FDG PET over gallium-67. PET shows a large right neck mass as involvement in the left neck, spleen and abdomen from lymphoma **(A)** whereas a 10-mCi Ga-67 scan at 96 hours fails to detect lesion outside of the right neck **(B)**.

much more specific than CT (86% compared with 31%) in these cases (Fig. 10-40). PET is often used in the restaging of patients as information compliments that gained by CT scanning.

Melanoma

The incidence of malignant melanoma is increasing dramatically. Survival depends on the stage at the time of diagnosis. The thickness of the primary lesion is the most important prognostic factor, and this is graded according to the Breslow classification. Prognosis is extremely poor with nodal or distant metastases. Even after potentially curative surgery is performed, patients frequently present with metastatic disease because of early hematogenous spread. Some patients would benefit from further surgery or directed therapy if they were accurately restaged.

Diagnosis of these metastases is difficult by conventional modalities alone, such as CT. Metastatic disease may occur in unusual locations such as other cutaneous and subcutaneous sites, spleen, distant nodes, liver, and gallbladder. Metastases are frequently found on PET in an extensive pattern or widespread from the primary tumor

location (Fig. 10-41). Thus, many sites perform head-to-toe imaging on patients with melanoma. Lesions that are not detected are likely microscopic. PET is generally more sensitive than conventional imaging methods. However, CT is more sensitive than PET in detecting small parenchymal lung lesions and MRI best identifies brain metastases. The sensitivity of PET is reported to be over 90% with a specificity of 87%. PET frequently alters therapy in 20–26% of patients. PET is useful in staging patients at high risk for metastases and in those who relapse.

PET does not replace sentinel lymph node scintigraphy in patients with melanoma. Lymphoscintigraphy involves Tc-99m sulfur colloid injection around the primary lesion to identify the first draining sentinel lymph node. Evaluating the resected sentinel lymph node with histochemical staining is the most sensitive method to determine patients at risk for metastatic disease. This allows detection of microscopic disease not detected with PET.

Breast Carcinoma

Breast cancer is classified as being a noninvasive or invasive tumor of ductal or lobular type. Of invasive carcinomas,

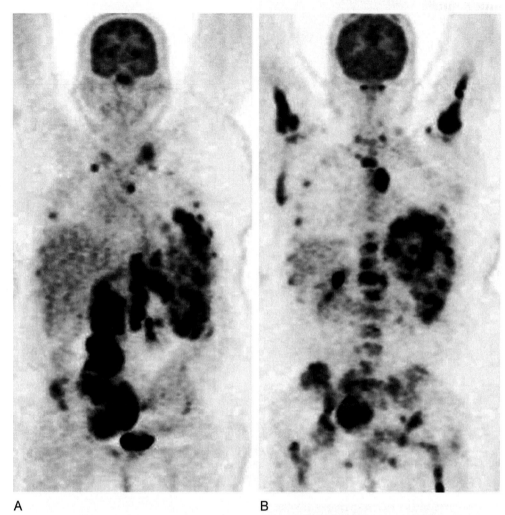

A   B

Figure 10-38   Restaging lymphoma. **A,** The initial PET image in a patient with non-Hodgkin's lymphoma shows extensive abdominal adenopathy, involvement of the spleen, chest and supraclavicular nodes. **B,** Following two cycles of chemotherapy, much of the adenopathy has resolved in the abdomen, but worsening disease is seen in spleen, bone marrow, and mediastinum, requiring a change in therapy protocol.

ductal carcinoma accounts for 80% of cases, lobular 10%, and medullary 5%. Noninvasive carcinoma, or carcinoma in situ, may be detected by mammography when microcalcifications are present (i.e., ductal carcinoma in situ [DCIS]), but may be difficult to detect when it presents as architectural distortion found in lobular carcinoma in situ (LCIS).

Diagnosis

Mammography is a sensitive screening tool for detecting breast carcinoma (81–90%). However, the specificity of mammography is low and biopsy performed after an abnormal mammogram results in a histopathological diagnosis of malignancy only 10–50% of the time. MRI continues to be investigated due to its high sensitivity

(up to 90–95%) for the detection of breast cancer, although its specificity is also low. MRI is recommended for patients with dense breasts, where the diagnostic ability of mammography is limited. It can also better visualize multifocal disease, recurrence, and disease in patients with implants. Ultrasound has also added considerably to the evaluation of the breast in cases of palpable masses and discrete masses found on the mammogram. Recently, F-18 FDG PET imaging has proven to be useful in breast carcinoma staging and restaging.

Primary Breast Cancer

The ability of F-18 FDG PET to detect primary breast cancer is related to tumor size. One meta-analysis of

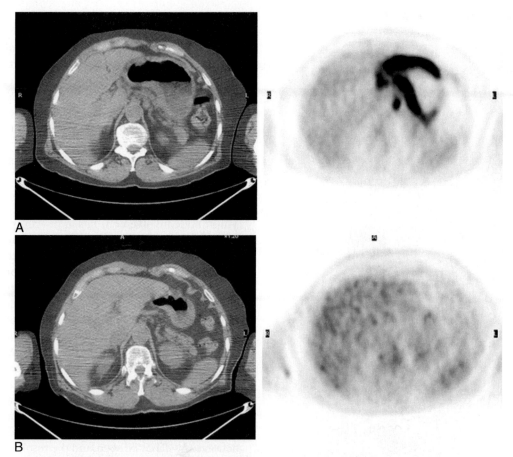

Figure 10-39   Monitoring therapy of lymphoma. **A,** PET-CT images show intense uptake in a gastric lymphoma as well as an adjacent lymph node. Gastric involvement may not be detected, but when seen, PET may be useful for follow-up. **B,** After one cycle of chemotherapy, no tumor could be identified. This suggests a better prognosis than for a late or nonresponder.

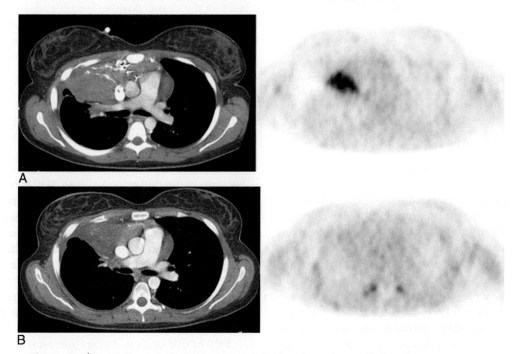

Figure 10-40   Evaluation of a residual mass. **A,** During chemotherapy for lymphoma, a large partially enhancing anterior mediastinal mass on CT showed markedly abnormal FDG accumulation. **B,** When the follow-up CT showed residual mass, a follow-up PET was done. No FDG uptake was seen consistent with fibrosis and scar.

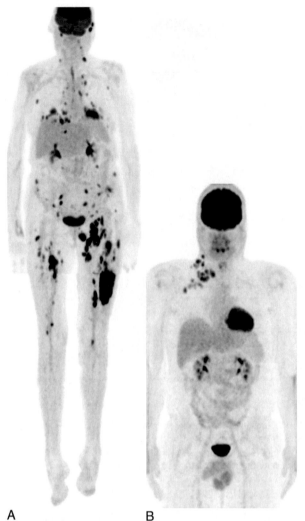

A   **B**

Figure 10-41   FDG PET in melanoma. **A,** Diffuse tumor involvement including uptake near the primary tumor in the left thigh, multiple lymph nodes, organs, and soft tissue metastases in this patient with melanoma. This result led to changing planned radiation therapy to systemic chemotherapy. PET can identify subtle disease not found on CT. **B,** Regional involvement is seen in metastases involving numerous right cervical lymph nodes in a patient with a recently resected melanoma of the right ear.

well. PET scanning may help detect multicentric disease. Also, PET may occasionally detect breast carcinoma during evaluation of other malignancies.

One factor limiting the sensitivity of FDG PET is the inherent resolution of whole-body PET scanners with lesion detectability on the order of 6–8 mm. Dedicated PET breast imaging systems are being developed, which may significantly improve detection rates compared to whole-body scanners.

Lymph Node Evaluation

Lymph node involvement has important prognostic and therapeutic implications in breast carcinoma. Axillary lymph node dissection fully evaluates the draining lymph nodes. However, this is a highly invasive procedure with side effects (e.g., lymphedema). In patients with nonpalpable lymph nodes, sentinel lymph node localization with Tc-99m sulfur colloid, with or without blue dye, is still the best method to select which patients should undergo this highly invasive procedure. A negative PET scan does not exclude the need for further workup.

F-18 FDG PET imaging is able to visualize lymph node metastases by detecting changes in metabolism, often before any anatomical change occurs on CT. Not all lymph nodes will be visualized because microscopic metastases will not be seen, and the resolution of PET prevents evaluating the number of nodes involved. Reported sensitivities of PET range from 79–100% and specificities range from 66–100%. The accuracy depends on the size of the primary tumor and the approach to reading the exam. Positive lymph nodes are found more often in larger tumors >2 cm with a sensitivity of 94%, whereas metastases in small tumors may only be detected one third of the time. If scans are interpreted in a highly sensitive mode, a sensitivity of 95% is seen, resulting in a high negative predictive value of 95%. However, this method of reading lowers specificity to 66% because inflammatory conditions frequently affect the axillary lymph nodes and cause increased FDG accumulation.

Clinical Use of PET

Because of the limitations of F-18 FDG PET, it is not generally recommended in the initial diagnosis or screening of most patients. However, it was proven to be useful for staging patients with advanced disease, monitoring response to therapy, restaging, and detecting recurrent disease. Although PET cannot detect every metastatic deposit, it frequently adds significant information to that obtained with conventional imaging such as CT, MRI, and bone scan. One study reported that PET added information in 29% of cases (Fig. 10-42).

PET better detects distant metastases than conventional modalities in chest, liver, and bone. In the bone, PET is best able to identify more aggressive or lytic

the literature suggests the sensitivity of PET is 88% and the specificity 79% for detecting primary tumors. Reported sensitivity of PET is 92% for tumors measuring 2–5 cm but is only 68% for tumors <2 cm. The false-negative rate of F-18 FDG PET is not sufficient for a screening test.

There may be a role for PET in the differentiation of benign and malignant lesions. However, false negatives may occur with well-differentiated and slow-growing tumors, including lobular carcinoma, tubular carcinoma, and DCIS. Lobular carcinoma is more difficult to detect than invasive ductal carcinoma by mammography as

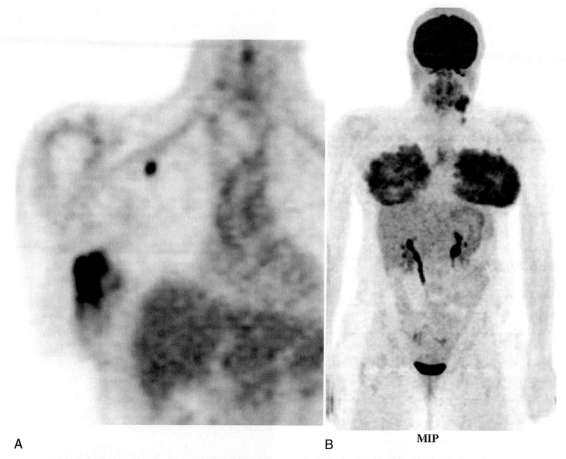

A   B   **MIP**

Figure 10-42   Breast cancer staging. **A,** PET often identifies malignant adenopathy in advanced and recurrent breast cancer. In this case, the large right breast tumor shows markedly increased uptake, as does an axillary lymph node. **B,** Abnormal breast uptake may not be due to primary tumor. Increased uptake can be caused by therapy and hormonal stimulation. This postpartum patient presented with lymphoma in the left cervical region and intense benign breast uptake.

lesions while the technetium bone scan visualizes sclerotic disease. Therefore, PET should not replace bone scan in patients at highest risk for metastases. When abnormalities are detected by CT, PET is often able to differentiate benign from malignant processes.

More accurate assessment of tumor response to therapy is possible with PET. Although CT can be used to monitor therapy, it can only examine changes in size. PET reveals changes in metabolic activity, which is a more accurate indication of response. Limited data suggests a 55% decrease in activity was able to accurately differentiate responders from nonresponders after only one cycle of chemotherapy. This allows rapid protocol modifications to optimize therapy.

The detection of local recurrence is often difficult due to distortion of the anatomy from surgery and radiation. Yet detection is critical as recurrence occurs in up to 30% of patients. PET has a sensitivity of 90% for the detection of recurrence (Fig. 10-43). Caution must be

exercised because false-positive results can occur from therapy, particularly radiation.

Ovarian Carcinoma

Tumors may arise from any of the cellular elements of the ovary (Box 10-15). Ovarian carcinoma diagnosis is challenging because physical examination may not reveal disease and symptoms do not present until late in the course of disease. Tumor staging is outlined in Box 10-16. Hematogenous spread is rare, but direct spread and seeding of the omentum and organ surfaces is common (Figs. 10-44 and 10-F [see color insert]). Lymphatic spread can lead to malignant pleural effusions. Although patients with localized disease have more than a 90% survival chance, most patients present with stage III and IV disease. The prognosis of ovarian carcinoma is poor, with overall survival of only 46% at 5 years.

Preoperative evaluation of patients often includes imaging with sonography, CT, and MRI. Staging with CT has 70–90% accuracy. However, small peritoneal lesions found with surgical exploration are frequently overlooked or undetectable by CT. PET often highlights abnormal activity in lesions that were overlooked on CT and this may be easiest to identify when the PET and CT are fused.

F-18 FDG PET has been used for staging and restaging but is most widely used to detect recurrent disease. Often, this involves patients with elevated serum markers (Ca-125, Ca 19-9, alpha fetoprotien [AFP], and human chorionic gonadotropin [HCG]) and negative or inconclusive CT findings. The reported sensitivity of PET varies from 50–90% and the specificity from 60–80%. The accuracy of PET depends on tumor size and cell type. Small peritoneal nodules seen during laparoscopy and small primary tumors confined to the ovary may be missed. Well-differentiated and mucinous tumors may not be seen, causing false negative results (Box 10-17). Also, PET scanning may not be useful for initial tumor diagnosis because several benign conditions may accumulate F-18 FDG (Box 10-18). Despite these limitations, PET alters management in approximately 15% of cases.

Cervical Carcinoma

Cervical carcinoma is the most common gynecological cancer. It may be treated effectively by surgery when localized, but radiation and chemoradiation may be required for locally advanced disease. The spread of cervical carcinoma can occur by local extension or by lymphatic spread to pelvic, para-aortic, retroperitoneal, and even supraclavicular lymph nodes. Detection of nodal involvement is important in therapy planning but may be difficult by CT. In patients who have had prior

---

Box 10-15   Histopathologic Classification of Ovarian Carcinoma

EPITHELIAL TUMORS

Serous
Mucinous
Endometrioid
Brenner
Transitional cell
Mixed epithelial
Small cell
Clear cell

SEX CORD STROMAL TUMORS

Granulosa cell
Serotoli-Leydig cell

GERM CELL

Dysgerminoma
Yolk sac
Embryonal
Teratomas

Box 10-16   Outline of Ovarian Carcinoma Staging

Stage I: Growth limited to ovaries with an intact capsule
Stage II: Extension onto pelvic organs or into ascites
Stage III: Peritoneal implants outside of the pelvis; retroperitoneal or inguinal lymph node involvement
Stage IV: Distant metastasis

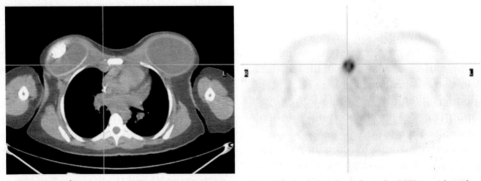

Figure 10-43   Recurrent breast carcinoma in an internal mammary lymph node. PET can identify metastases to regional lymph nodes as well as distant disease. Internal mammary node involvement is frequent in cancers of the inner or medial breast.

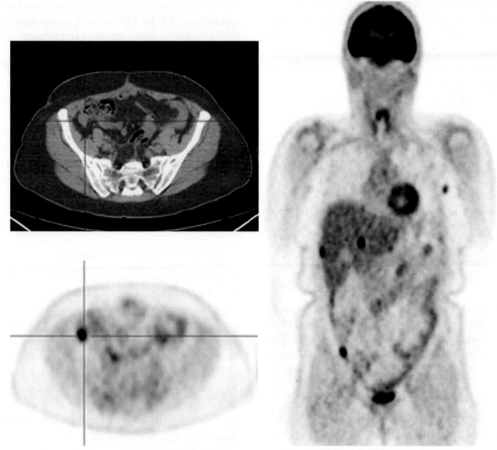

Figure 10-44   Recurrent ovarian carcinoma. A patient with a rising CA-125 had numerous metastases on the coronal PET including a left axillary lymph node, metastases studding the surface of the liver, and a right lower quadrant peritoneal lesion studding the right colon on axial images.

resection, scar may make detection of recurrent disease by CT difficult.

PET has shown >90% sensitivity for detection of cervical cancer. Markedly abnormal F-18 FDG uptake is seen in recurrent cancers and lymph node metastases (Fig. 10-45). The use of PET requires careful correlation with CT. Evaluation may be complicated by normal uptake in bowel and urinary tract, as well as increased uptake in tissues affected by radiation therapy.

Testicular Carcinoma

Testicular cancer can be divided into seminoma and nonseminoma germ-cell tumors. The spread of testicular tumor is most commonly to retroperitoneal lymph nodes. Although the overall prognosis for these tumors is good, accurate staging and surveillance are necessary, but patients are frequently incorrectly staged by CT. Patients initially classified as stage I are commonly then found to have nodal involvement at surgery. Other patients placed

---

Box 10-17   Processes Causing False-Negative Results in Ovarian Cancer

Well-differentiated serous cystadenocarcinoma
Mucinous cystadenocarcinoma
Disseminated peritoneal carcinomatosis
Borderline tumors
Stage I tumors confined to the ovary

---

incorrectly in high-risk groups may undergo unnecessary therapy. For example, it has been common practice to treat all patients with seminoma with radiation.

Standard imaging of testicular carcinoma consists of ultrasound for diagnosis and CT for staging. PET is accurate for tumor staging and detecting recurrence. PET has a high negative predictive value of 94% and a sensitivity of 85%. Detection of small tumors and well-differentiated teratomas is limited with PET. Relapse of testicular carcinoma is a frequent occurrence and PET is useful for surveillance.

Prostate Carcinoma

F-18 FDG PET has very limited sensitivity for prostate carcinoma. Uptake in primary tumor is low and similar as for benign prostatic hypertrophy. In terms of staging, F-18 FDG PET detected less than two thirds of osseous metastases found on bone scintigraphy and approximately one half of nodal metastases. CT is superior to PET for the detection of pulmonary metastases.

Renal and Bladder Carcinomas

CT is the most common imaging modality for the diagnosis and staging of renal cell carcinoma and bladder carcinoma. PET is not useful in the diagnosis of primary tumors. Although some have suggested that the urinary excretion of F-18 FDG might obscure adjacent tumors, these masses often show no radiotracer uptake (Fig. 10-46). The cause for this finding, such as variations in glucose transporter expression, is being investigated. However, F-18 FDG PET may play a role in diagnosing distant metastases and detecting recurrent disease.

There are limited data concerning the use of F-18 FDG PET in bladder and renal tumors. Recent studies detected only two thirds of primary bladder carcinomas, but PET showed a high sensitivity for distant metastases. In renal cell carcinoma, anywhere from 50–75% of primary tumors were identified by PET, although metastatic lesions may be identified that are not seen on CT.

Musculoskeletal Tumors

Malignant primary bone tumors are usually F-18 FDG avid, as are many benign conditions. Benign tumors such as giant cell tumor, fibrous dysplasia, and eosinophilic granulomas have been shown to accumulate F-18 FDG. PET may be useful both in the evaluation of patients who cannot undergo MRI imaging and in monitoring the effects of therapy. If a nonresponder is identified early by showing little change in SUV values on PET, the course of therapy can be altered. F-18 FDG may be impact therapy by identifying other sites of disease, such as in patients with plasmacytoma.

For the evaluation of soft tissue sarcomas, the accuracy of F-18 FDG PET appears related to tumor grade. The increased uptake in high-grade tumors such as malignant fibrous histiocytoma allows detection with a high degree of sensitivity. Low-grade tumors, on the other hand, show minimal or nonexistent uptake, leading to poor sensitivity. Although MRI remains the main imaging modality of the primary tumor, the ability of MRI to detect recurrence is limited in the postoperative patient. PET may help detect recurrent tumors, although the effects of surgery and radiation therapy lower sensitivity.

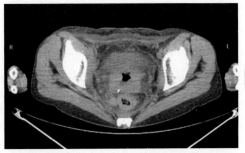 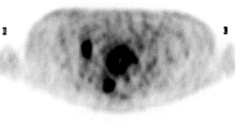

Figure 10-45   Cervical carcinoma. Residual tumor uptake is seen around air in the vaginal cuff and increased metabolic activity is seen in a metastasis to the right pelvic sidewall.

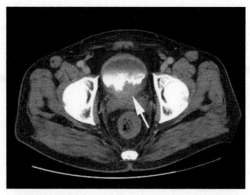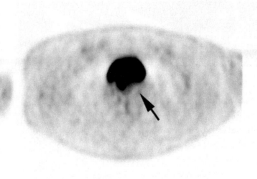

Figure 10-46   Bladder carcinoma. Renal cell carcinoma and bladder tumors are often negative on FDG PET. A mass along the posterior bladder (*arrow*) on CT (*left*) shows no FDG uptake on the PET portion of the exam (*right*).

SUGGESTED READING

Been LB, Suurmeijer AJ, Cobben DC, et al: F-18 FLT-PET in oncology: current status and opportunities. Eur J Nucl Med 31:1659-1672, 2004.

Beyer T, Antoch G, Muller S, et al: Acquisition protocol considerations for combined PET/CT imaging. J Nucl Med 45:25S-35S, 2004.

Delbeke D, Martin WH: PET and PET-CT for the evaluation of colorectal carcinoma. Semin Nucl Med 34:209-223, 2004.

Eubank WB, Mankoff DA: Evolving role of positron emission tomography in breast cancer imaging. Semin Nucl Med 35:84-95, 2005.

Gupta NC, Maloof J, Gunel E: Probability of malignancy in solitary pulmonary nodules using fluorine-18-FDG and PET. J Nucl Med 37:943-947, 1996.

Ko JP, Drucker EA, Shepard JO, et al: CT depiction of regional node stations for lung cancer staging. AJR 174:775-782, 2000.

Kresnik E, Mikosch P, Gallowitsch HJ, et al: Evaluation of head and neck cancer with F-18 FDG PET: a comparison with conventional methods. Eur J Nucl Med 28:816-821, 2001.

Kubota K, Yokoyama J, Yamaguchi K, et al: FDG-PET delayed imaging for the detection of head and neck cancer recurrence after radio-chemotherapy: comparison with MRI/CT. Eur J Nucl Med 31:590-595, 2004.

Kumar R, Alavi A: PET imaging in gynecologic malignancies. Radiol Clin North Am 42:1155-1167, 2004.

Macapinlac HA: FDG PET and PET/CT imaging in lymphoma and melanoma. Cancer J 10:262-270, 2004.

Mountain CF, Dresler CM: Regional lymph node classification for lung cancer staging. Chest 111:1718-1723, 1997.

Som PM, Curtin HD, Mancuso AA: Imaging-based nodal classification for evaluation of neck metastatic adenopathy. AJR 174:837-844, 2000.

Vesselle H, Pugsley JM, Vallieres E, et al: The impact of fluorodeoxyglucose F-18 positron-emission tomography on the surgical staging of non-small cell lung cancer. J Thorac Cardiovasc Surg 124:511-519, 2002.

Wahl RL: Principles and Practice of Positron Emission Tomography. Baltimore, Lippincott Williams & Wilkins, 2002.

Wong RJ, Lin DT, Schöder H, et al: Diagnostic and prognostic value of F-18 fluorodeoxyglucose positron emission tomography for recurrent head and neck squamous cell carcinoma. J Clin Oncol 20:4199-4208, 2002.

Zanzonico P: Positron emission tomography: a review of basic principles, scanner design, and performance, and current systems. Semin Nucl Med:87-111, 2004.

Gastrointestinal System

Radionuclide studies of the gastrointestinal tract provide noninvasive functional imaging and quantification of gastrointestinal function not available from other methodologies.

The gastric emptying study is the standard clinical test for quantification solid and liquid motility. Gastroesophageal reflux scintigraphy is an extremely sensitive and noninvasive method for diagnosis and quantification of reflux, used most commonly for pediatric patients. Gastrointestinal bleeding scintigraphy has long been used to localize the site of active bleeding prior to angiography. Tc-99m pertechnetate can localize a Meckel's diverticulum responsible for small-bowel bleeding or other heterotopic gastric mucosa.

Nonimaging radionuclide studies of gastrointestinal function date back to the earliest days of nuclear medicine. The Schilling test has long been the standard method for the diagnosis of vitamin B_{12} malabsorption and pernicious anemia. Our new understanding of the infectious origin of gastritis and ulcer disease has led to a simple diagnostic radionuclide C-14 breath test for detection of the bacteria responsible, *Helicobacter pylori*.

ESOPHAGEAL MOTILITY

The esophagus has multiple functions, including the transport of food from the mouth to the stomach, clearance of regurgitated substances, and prevention of tracheobronchial aspiration and acid reflux (Fig. 11-1). The most common clinical complaint of patients with abnormal esophageal motility is pain with swallowing (dysphagia).

Esophageal Motor Disorders

Esophageal motor disorders have been classified as primary (e.g., achalasia) and secondary (e.g., scleroderma) or by the type of dysfunction (amotility, hypomotility, hypermotility) (Box 11-1).

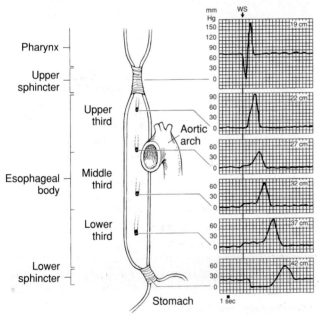

Figure 11-1 Esophageal anatomy and function. Swallowing initiates a coordinated peristaltic contraction that propagates down the esophagus. The esophagus has three distinct regions: the upper esophageal sphincter (UES), which allows food to pass from the mouth to the esophagus and prevents tracheobronchial aspiration; the esophageal body, with striated muscle proximally and smooth muscle distally; and the lower esophageal sphincter (LES), a high-pressure smooth muscle region that prevents gastric reflux but relaxes during swallowing to allow passage of food into the stomach. Manometric pressure changes with a water swallow (*WS*) of an 8-ml bolus. Following swallowing, the UES pressure falls transiently. Then the LES pressure falls and remains low until peristaltic contraction passes aborally through the UES and esophageal body, which closes the LES.

The diagnosis of esophageal motility disorders is most often made by contrast radiography and esophageal manometry. Although a barium-swallow study can demonstrate anatomical lesions and mucosal changes, it provides only a qualitative assessment of motility. Esophageal manometry is the accepted reference standard for the diagnosis of motility disorders. It can quantify peristaltic contraction, sphincter pressure, and upper and lower esophageal sphincter (LES) relaxation, but it is invasive and technically demanding. Although scintigraphy has been used as a diagnostic technique, it has been found most valuable in evaluating response to therapy.

Achalasia

This primary esophageal motor disorder manifests as partial or absent relaxation of the lower esophageal sphincter and loss of esophageal body peristalsis, resulting in esophageal retention of food and dilation, producing symptoms of dysphagia, weight loss, nocturnal regurgitation, cough, and aspiration. Etiology is unknown.

Upper gastrointestinal radiographic studies show retention of contrast in a distended column, narrowed sphincter, and delayed clearance. Esophageal manometry reveals an absence of peristalsis in the distal two thirds of the esophagus, increased lower esophageal sphincter pressure, and incomplete sphincter relaxation with swallowing.

Scleroderma

Smooth muscle involvement of the esophagus is a common manifestation of this connective tissue disorder.

Box 11-1 Classification of Esophageal Motility Disorders

PRIMARY/SECONDARY
Primary

Achalasia
Esophageal spasm
Nutcracker esophagus

Secondary

Scleroderma
Diabetic enteropathy

DEGREE OF MOTILITY
Amotility

Achalasia
Scleroderma

Hypomotility

Presbyesophagus

Hypermotility

Diffuse spasm
Nutcracker esophagus

Contrast radiography demonstrates a dilated aperistaltic esophagus with barium retention and gastroesophageal reflux. Manometry confirms decreased or absent lower esophageal sphincter pressure and reduced contraction amplitude.

Diffuse Esophageal Spasm

Symptoms include intermittent chest pain and dysphagia. Barium swallow and manometry detect abnormal nonperistaltic contractions of the esophageal body. No organic lesion is demonstrable.

Nutcracker Esophagus

Patients present with noncardiac chest pain. Radiographic studies are normal. The diagnosis is made with esophageal manometric findings of high-amplitude, prolonged peristaltic contractions.

Other Esophageal Disorders

Smooth muscle disease of the esophagus also occurs with systemic lupus erythematosus and polymyositis. Esophageal striated muscle abnormalities are problems for patients with muscular dystrophy, myasthenia gravis, and myotonia dystrophica. Diabetes and alcoholism are associated with abnormalities of esophageal motor function. Severe esophagitis may also cause disordered motility.

Scintigraphy

Esophageal transit scintigraphy provides noninvasive functional diagnostic information about esophageal motility. The procedure is relatively simple to perform and quantitative. It can be used to screen symptomatic patients and evaluate the effectiveness of therapy for patients with diagnosed esophageal motility disorders.

Radiopharmaceuticals

Esophageal transit scintigraphy is performed with technetium (Tc)-99m sulfur colloid (SC) or Tc-99m diethylene-triamine-pentaacetic acid (DTPA), 200–300 μCi (7.4–11.1 MBq), dispersed in a liquid bolus (usually water). Reports suggest that semisolid food boluses are more sensitive than liquid boluses for detecting dysmotility. Transit is faster for less viscous materials, for small versus larger volumes, and in the upright versus the supine position.

Dosimetry

Table 11-1 provides the radiation absorbed dose (rad) for gastroesophageal scintigraphy (esophageal transit, gastroesophageal reflux, and gastric emptying) for children of different ages. Table 11-2 reports the dosimetry based on the radiopharmaceutical and particular meal used. The large intestine receives the highest radiation absorbed dose.

Table 11-1 Dosimetry for Tc-99m SC Gastroesophageal Scintigraphy for Children

Organ	Rad/100 μCi by age*			
	Newborn	1 year	5 years	10 years
Stomach	0.383	0.093	0.050	0.031
Large intestine	0.927	0.380	0.194	0.120
Ovaries	0.099	0.042	0.033	0.072
Testes	0.018	0.007	0.003	0.011
Whole body	0.020	0.011	0.006	0.004

*Usual dose, 200–300 μCi (7.4–11.1 MBq).
Modified from Castronovo FP: Gastroesophageal scintiscanning in a pediatric population: dosimetry. J Nucl Med 27:1212-1214, 1986.

Table 11-2 Adult Dosimetry for Esophageal and Gastric Scintigraphy

	Millirads/study meal, by organ					
	Stomach	Small intestine	Large intestine	Ovaries	Testes	Total body
LIQUID						
300 μCi Tc-99m SC	28	83	160	29	2	5
1 mCi Tc-99m DTPA	93	280	520	98	5	20
250 μCi In-111 DTPA	110	490	2000	420	27	60
SOLID						
500 μCi Tc-99m SC ovalbumin	120	120	230	42	2	9
500 μCi Tc-99m chicken liver	120	120	230	42	2	9

Modified from Siegel JA, Wu RK, Knight C, et al: Radiation dose estimates for oral agents used in the upper gastrointestinal diseases. J Nucl Med 24:835-837, 1983.

Box 11-2 Esophageal Transit Scintigraphy: Protocol Summary

PATIENT PREPARATION

Order an overnight fast.
Place radioactive marker on cricoid cartilage.
Position the patient supine.
Practice swallows with nonradioactive bolus.

RADIOPHARMACEUTICAL

Tc-99m SC or DTPA, 11 mBq (300 µCi) in 10 ml of water.

INSTRUMENTATION

Camera setup: Tc-99m photopeak with 20% window
Computer setup: 0.8-sec frame × 240; byte mode,
64 × 64

SWALLOWING PROCEDURE

Swallow Tc-99m SC or DTPA as a bolus.
Dry swallow at 30 sec, then radiolabeled bolus
every 30 sec × 4.
No swallowing between boluses.

PROCESSING

Time–activity curves, condensed dynamic images

QUANTIFICATION

Time to 90% emptying
Transit time

Box 11-3 Esophageal Transit Scintigraphy (Semisolid Meal): Protocol Summary

PATIENT PREPARATION

Overnight fast.
Patient position: seated
Posterior camera acquisition

RADIOPHARMACEUTICAL

Tc-99m SC or DTPA , 37 MBq (1.0 mCi), mixed with
120 ml milk, 19 g of cornflakes and 1 g sugar

COMPUTER SETUP

Feeding phase: 10 sec frames × 12 (64 × 64 matrix)
Spontaneous emptying phase: 10 sec frames × 120
Water ingestion phase: 10 sec × 6
Carbonated beverage phase (150 ml): 10 sec × 6

PROCESSING

Draw a region of interest around the esophagus.
Display the time–activity curve
Display a condensed image

QUANTIFICATION

Calculate the percent retention = esophageal
counts/total counts × 100
Normal percent retention, <5% at 20 minutes

Methodology

Box 11-2 describes a standard liquid esophageal motility protocol and Box 11-3 describes a semisolid transit protocol.

Although both anterior and posterior views can be acquired, posterior acquisition allows for easier administration of the bolus and closer observation of the patient. The supine position is preferable because it eliminates the effect of gravity on esophageal emptying. Because gravity is the only mechanism of emptying in achalasia, upright positioning is preferable for serial studies in this disease. Emptying occurs in both the supine and the upright position in systemic sclerosis.

Multiple swallows are often necessary for complete emptying even in normal subjects because of a 25% incidence of "aberrant" swallows, or extra swallows, which occur between the two prescribed swallows. Aberrant swallows inhibit subsequent swallows and delay transit. Any normal residual remaining after an initial swallow will clear when followed by a dry swallow.

Analysis and Quantification

Image analysis and computer cinematic movie display is often adequate for diagnosis of severe motility abnormalities (Figs. 11-2 and 11-3). However, quantitative analysis is helpful for diagnosing less severe abnormalities, comparing serial studies, and evaluating the effectiveness of therapy. Time–activity curves can be derived for the entire esophagus or for the proximal, middle, and distal thirds (Figs. 11-3C and 11-4).

Esophageal transit can be quantified by calculating either the transit time or the residual activity in the esophagus. *Transit time* is the time from the initial entry of the bolus into the esophagus until all but 10% of peak activity clears. Abnormal for liquid bolus is >15 seconds (*see* Box 11-2).

$$\text{Residual esophageal activity (\%)} = [(E_{max} - E_t)/E_{max}] \times 100$$

where E_{max} is the maximum counting rate in the esophagus (15-second intervals) and E_t is the counting rate after dry swallow number t (abnormal, >20%). For a semisolid meal, the abnormal retention at 20 minutes is >5% (*see* Box 11-3).

Functional images can be helpful for assimilating and interpreting the many images acquired in a single transit study. Because craniocaudal transit, not lateral motion, is needed, the dynamic data can be condensed into a single image with one spatial (vertical) and one temporal dimension (Figs. 11-5 and 11-6).

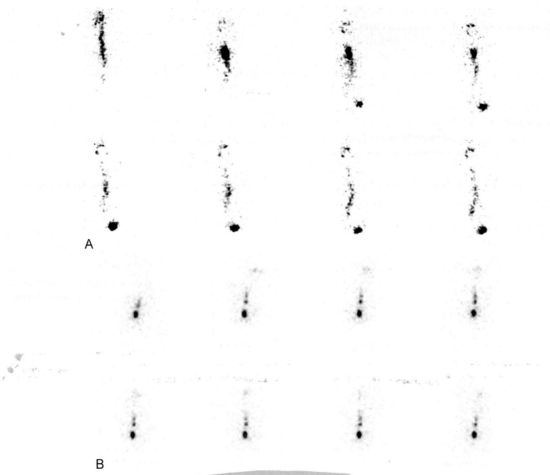

Figure 11-2 Normal esophageal clear liquid transit. **A,** Images were obtained supine at 2-second intervals. The swallowed bolus travels rapidly through the esophagus. Transit time is 11 seconds (normal, 15 seconds). **B,** Scleroderma. Dysmotility with poor propagation of bolus and retention of activity in the distal esophagus.

Accuracy

Esophageal transit studies have a high sensitivity for the diagnosis of achalasia but a generally lower detection rate for other conditions, thus limiting their routine use as screening tests. The specificity of scintigraphic findings (e.g., for differentiating achalasia from scleroderma) is also not high. Thus, in current practice, esophageal transit studies are most commonly done to evaluate response to pharmacological, medical, or surgical therapy.

GASTROESOPHAGEAL REFLUX

Symptomatic reflux of gastric contents into the esophagus is a common medical problem. Serious complications of gastroesophageal reflux include esophagitis, bleeding, perforation, Barrett's esophagus, cancer, and stricture. The clinical presentation of infants and children differs considerably from that of adults. In adults, heartburn is the usual complaint. Common pediatric symptoms include respiratory symptoms, iron deficiency anemia, and failure to thrive.

Gastroesophageal reflux occurs in infants as a normal physiological event that resolves spontaneously by 7–8 months of age. Clinically important reflux becomes evident by 2 months of age. Most children have a benign course and are symptom free by 18 months of age. However, approximately one-third have persistent symptoms until age 4 years and 5–10% percent may have serious sequelae of strictures, recurrent pneumonia, and inanition.

The adequacy of esophageal clearance is an important factor in determining whether reflux becomes clinically evident. Delayed clearance increases the duration of mucosal exposure to refluxate. Other factors include the efficacy of the antireflux mechanism, the volume of gastric contents, the potency of refluxed material (acid, pepsin), mucosal resistance to injury, and mucosal reparative ability. Most adult patients with moderate to severe esophagitis have a sliding hiatal hernia; however, the majority of individuals with a hiatal hernia do not have reflux disease.

Although lower esophageal sphincter pressure is reduced in many patients with reflux, overlap exists between healthy and ill subjects. Reflux events result from either a transient sphincter relaxation not associated with swallowing, transient increases in intra-abdominal pressure, or free reflux across an atonic sphincter.

Diagnosis

Various tests have been used to diagnose gastroesophageal reflux. *Barium esophagography* can detect mucosal damage, stricture, and tumor, but has a low sensi-tivity for detecting reflux and results in considerable radiation from fluoroscopy. *Esophageal endoscopy* provides a direct view of the esophageal mucosa and allows biopsy of ulcerations and areas suspicious for malignancy; however, histological evidence of esophagitis is not sensitive for diagnosing reflux disease. Hydrochloric acid (0.1 N) infused into the distal esophagus (*Bernstein acid infusion test*) can reproduce symptoms of reflux and confirm their esophageal origin.

The *Tuttle acid reflux test* is considered the reference standard but is technically demanding. Reflux events are detected by positioning a pH electrode in the distal esophagus and monitoring over 24 hours. An abrupt drop in pH (<4) is diagnostic of a reflux event. However, a second reflux event cannot be detected until acid has cleared the pH probe. Although reflux volume clears within seconds, acid clearance takes several minutes because neutralization by swallowed saliva is necessary. This limits its temporal sensitivity for detection of reflux.

Scintigraphy

The radionuclide method is the most sensitive noninvasive method for detecting gastroesophageal reflux and

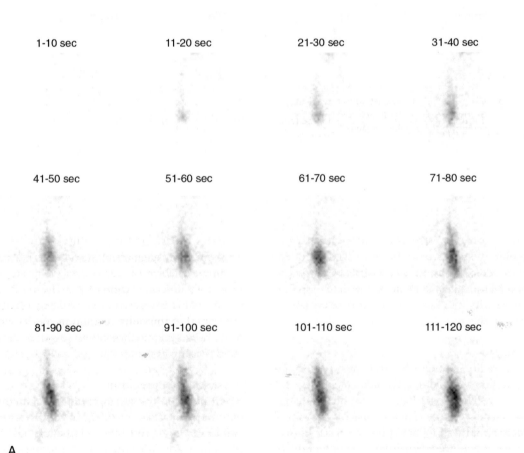

1-10 sec	11-20 sec	21-30 sec	31-40 sec
41-50 sec	51-60 sec	61-70 sec	71-80 sec
81-90 sec	91-100 sec	101-110 sec	111-120 sec

A

Figure 11-3 Achalasia: semisolid meal. **A,** Ten second frames × 12. Retention of activity in the esophagus, most prominently in the distal portion.

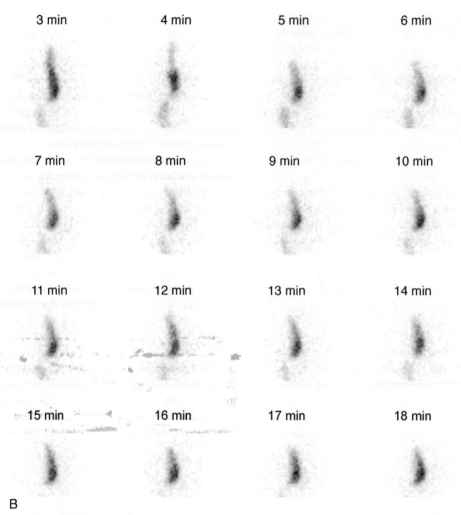

3 min   4 min   5 min   6 min

7 min   8 min   9 min   10 min

11 min   12 min   13 min   14 min

15 min   16 min   17 min   18 min

B

Figure 11-3, cont'd **B,** Two minute frames × 22. Persistent retention in distal esophagus with minimal evidence of clearance into the stomach.

Continued

has a low radiation exposure compared with barium studies. It is physiological, easy to perform, well-tolerated, and quantitative. Scintigraphic results are most affected by the volume of the ingested meal and the rate of gastric emptying. Sensitivity for detection of reflux decreases as the stomach empties.

Methodology

In the past, the radionuclide reflux study was performed differently in adults and children. The adult technique was done in a manner similar to barium contrast methodology, using Valsalva maneuvers and an abdominal binder to progressively increase intra-abdominal pressure. Static 30-second images were acquired. Sensitivity for detection of reflux was not particularly high and the methodology was not physiologic. This method is no longer recommended.

The standard pediatric reflux study is acquired with a rapid framing rate of 5–10 seconds during ingestion of the infant's usual formula or milk meal ("Milk study"). A typical protocol is described in Box 11-4. The high temporal acquisition rate increases sensitivity for detection of reflux events compared to the older method of 30–60 second acquisitions. The same methodology is recommended for adults as well as children, although with orange juice.

Image Interpretation

All frames should be reviewed individually or in cinematic display. Gastroesophageal reflux is seen as distinct spikes of activity into the esophagus (Fig. 11-7). A simple semiquantitative method of interpretation is to grade each reflux event as high-level or low-level (greater or less than midesophagus), by its duration (e.g., lasting less

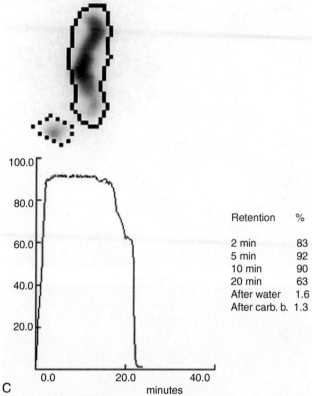

Retention	%
2 min	83
5 min	92
10 min	90
20 min	63
After water	1.6
After carb. b.	1.3

Figure 11-3, cont'd   C, Quantification. 63% retention after 20 minutes (<5% is normal). After ingestion of water and carbonated beverage, rapid emptying ensues.

or greater than 10 seconds), and by the temporal relationship to meal ingestion (events at low gastric volume carry greater significance). The study is usually performed for 60 minutes. Delayed imaging at 2 hours can be used for calculation of gastric emptying. The total number of reflux events can be summed in four categories: low-level, <10 seconds; low-level, ≥10 seconds; high-level, <10 seconds; high-level, ≥10 seconds.

Alternatively, time–activity curves can be generated and regions-of-interest drawn for the oropharynx, esophagus, and stomach. Various quantitative indices have been used (Box 11-5). Peaks greater than 5% generally correspond to reflux.

Normal values for neonates have never been established. The greater the number of high events and the longer the reflux events, the more severe is the disease. Reflux events that occur with small gastric volumes have more clinical significance because reflux is occurring without the effect of the increased pressure of a full meal volume and acid buffering.

Gastric emptying can be quantified by drawing a stomach region-of-interest on computer for the initial time 0, 1-hour, and 2-hour images and is usually expressed as the percent emptying. Between 40% and 50% emptying of milk at 1 hour and 60–75% at 2 hours is generally considered to be normal. The 2-hour emptying is considered more reliable than the 1-hour emptying. Pulmonary

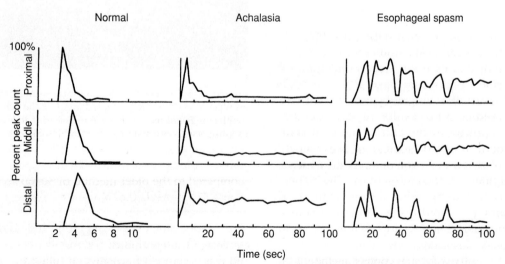

Figure 11-4   Esophageal time–activity profiles: normal, achalasia, and esophageal spasm. Regions of interest are drawn on computer for the proximal, middle, and distal esophagus and time activity curves generated. *Left:* Normal subject. Bolus proceeds promptly sequentially from proximal to distal esophagus. *Middle:* Achalasia. Retention predominantly in the lower esophagus. *Right:* Spasm, uncoordinated contraction. Bolus shows poor progression through the esophagus.

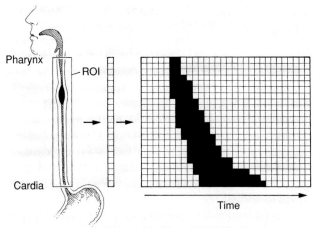

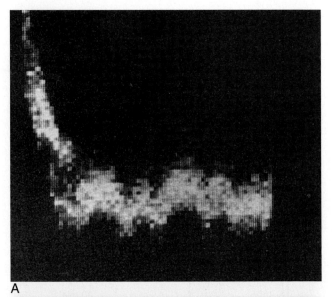

Figure 11-5 Generation of condensed dynamic images. In each consecutive frame, the data in an esophageal region of interest are compressed into a single column, displaying the distribution of the tracer from the pharynx to the proximal stomach for each 0.8-second interval. The columns are arranged consecutively, generating a space and time matrix, with vertical and horizontal dimensions representing spatial and temporal activity changes.

aspiration should be looked for with the aid of computer enhancement.

Salivagram is a more sensitive method of detecting aspiration than the reflux study. It is essentially a variation of an esophageal transit study (Box 11-2). A small volume labeled bolus of radiotracer is placed in the infant's posterior pharynx and the study is acquired with a rapid framing rate followed by static imaging (Fig. 11-8).

Accuracy

The early reported poor sensitivity (60–70%) for radionuclide esophageal reflux studies was the result of the long framing rates used. More rapid framing methods described previously have reported high sensitivities of 75–100%. Scintigraphy is more sensitive than barium studies and results in considerably less radiation exposure to the child. The gold standard is considered to be pH monitoring; however, its limitations were discussed previously (e.g., 24-hour monitoring and poor temporal resolution). The highest sensitivity is achieved by using a combination of scintigraphy and pH monitoring. However, scintigraphy is noninvasive and more commonly used clinically.

The reported sensitivity for detection of aspiration on gastroesophageal reflux studies is quite low, from 0–25%. However, the salivagram study can often demonstrate aspiration when it is clinically suspected but the gastroesophageal reflux study is negative.

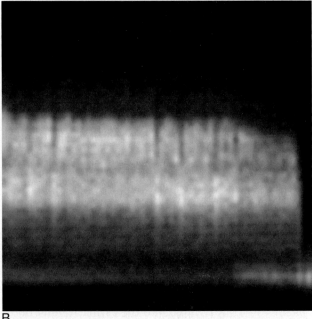

Figure 11-6 Condensed dynamic images. **A,** Normal esophageal swallow. Uninterrupted transit of the bolus down the esophagus. **B,** Achalasia. Persistent retention of activity in the esophagus with minimal clearance towards end of study.

GASTRIC MOTILITY

The radionuclide gastric emptying study is the standard method for evaluating gastric motility because the technique is noninvasive, sensitive, accurate, quantitative, and simple to perform in the nuclear medicine clinic. Nonradionuclide techniques have serious limitations. Gastric intubation methods require serial aspiration. Marker-dilution techniques with duodenal recovery are

Box 11-4 Gastroesophageal Reflux (Milk Study): Protocol Summary

PATIENT PREPARATION

Overnight fast.

COMPUTER SETUP

Framing rate of 5 to 10 sec/frame for 60 min.

RADIONUCLIDE

Tc-99m sulfur colloid, 0.2 to 1 mCi (5 µCi/ml)

FEEDING MEAL

Infants: Normal feeding meal (formula or milk). The radionuclide is mixed with half of the meal and fed to the child. The second "cold" half of the meal is then fed to the child. Orange juice for older children and adults.

IMAGING PROCEDURE

After burping infant, place supine with gamma camera positioned posteriorly and the chest and upper abdomen in the field of view. Place radioactive marker at the mouth for several frames.

Acquire delayed image of chest. Review for aspiration with computer enhancement.

Quantify reflux and gastric emptying

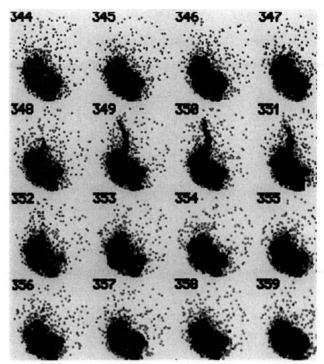

Figure 11-7   Gastroesophageal reflux. Sequential 5-second frames show episode of long-lasting (greater than 15 seconds) high-grade (higher than mid-esophagus) gastroesophageal reflux.

Box 11-5 Methods Used for Quantifying Gastroesophageal Reflux in Children

Mean value of the esophageal time–activity curve (TAC) as a percentage of the initial gastric activity.

Reflux index, derived by integrating esophageal TAC over 60 min and dividing by initial gastric activity.

Percent activity relative to gastric activity in a specified episode multiplied by duration of the episode.

Number of episodes of high-level and low-level reflux and their duration, <10 seconds or >10 seconds.

cumbersome, disliked by patients, and the tubing may alter the rate of emptying. Radiographic contrast studies detect gross mechanical obstruction, but are insensitive to motility disorders of the stomach and are not quantitative.

Physiology

Anatomically, the stomach is a smooth-muscle hollow viscus, anatomically divided into the cardia, fundus, body, antrum, and pylorus (Fig. 11-9). The mucosa contains glands that produce hydrochloric acid and digestive enzymes. Gastric motility is produced by an interaction of muscular and neural activity with feedback regulation from the small bowel. The proximal and distal portions of the stomach have distinct functions.

The proximal stomach, or *fundus,* acts as a reservoir, accepting large ingested solid and liquid volumes with only minimal increase in pressure (receptive relaxation and accommodation). The muscular contractions of the fundus are not rhythmic but rather tonic in character, producing a constant pressure gradient between the stomach and duodenum, which moves the stomach contents distally. Liquid emptying is the result of this fundal-produced pressure gradient. Emptying is volume dependent; the larger the volume, the more rapid the emptying, thus the emptying pattern is exponential

(Fig. 11-10). There is no delay before emptying begins. Nutrients, salts, and acidity in the liquid all slow the rate of emptying.

The distal stomach, or *antrum,* has a neural pacemaker initiating rhythmic phasic contractions, which are responsible for solid emptying. After ingestion of solid food, muscular contractions sweep down the antrum in a ringlike pattern, squeezing the food toward the pylorus. Large food particles are not allowed to pass and are retropelled back toward the antrum. The food particles become progressively ground up, eventually becoming small enough (1–2 mm) to pass through the pyloric sphincter. The pylorus, at the junction of the antrum and

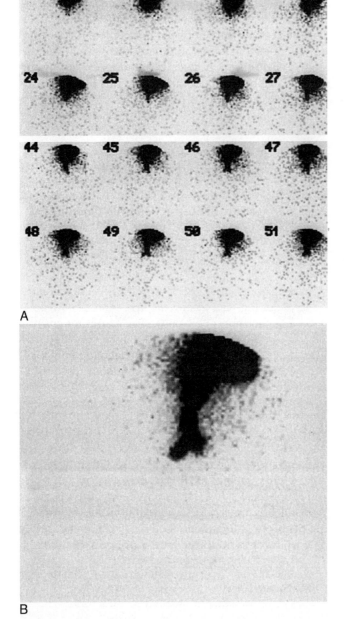

A

B

Figure 11-8   Salivagram: aspiration. Neonate with neurological problems and swallowing difficulties. Prior gastroesophageal reflux (milk) study (not shown) revealed numerous reflux events, but no aspiration. **A,** After radiotracer was placed in the posterior pharynx, sequential 5-second frames showed transit into the tracheal bifurcation. **B,** High-count image at the end of 60 minutes. Radiotracer remains at the tracheal bifurcation. No esophageal transit to stomach.

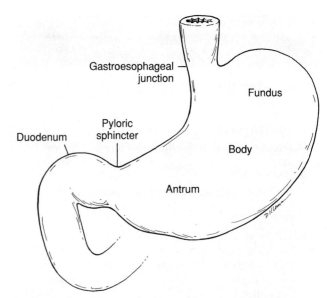

Figure 11-9   Gastric anatomy and function. The proximal stomach (fundus) accommodates and stores food and is responsible for liquid emptying. The distal stomach (antrum) is responsible for solid emptying. The antrum mixes and grinds food into small enough particles that they can pass through the pylorus.

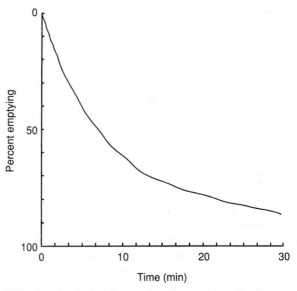

Figure 11-10   Normal clear liquid emptying. Ingestion of 300 ml of water with Tc-99m sulfur colloid. One-minute frames for 30 minutes. Time–activity curve generated by drawing a whole stomach region of interest on computer. Emptying began immediately. The clearance curve pattern is exponential with a half-emptying time of 9 minutes (normal <20 minutes).

duodenal bulb, acts as a sieve, regulating outflow of gastric contents.

The time required for grinding food into small particles before solid emptying begins is called the *lag phase*. During this phase there is no emptying. The solid material is converted into chyme through contact with acid and peptic enzymes and mechanical grinding. Once solid emptying begins, clearance into the duodenum occurs at a constant rate, usually in a linear manner (Fig. 11-11). The rate of emptying depends on the size and contents of the meal.

Fat, acid, protein, and carbohydrates all act to slow emptying (Box 11-6). An increasing volume of liquids slows the rate of solid emptying; however, the liquids empty faster than the solid meal component (Fig. 11-12).

In the fasting state between meals there are forceful contractions that empty nondigestible debris from the stomach. *Motilin,* a peptide hormone secreted by the upper small bowel mucosa, initiates this interdigestive event. Gastric motility is further modulated by sympathetic and parasympathetic neural innervation and a variety of hormones with complex interactions.

Gastric Stasis Syndromes

The radionuclide gastric emptying study cannot differentiate an anatomical obstruction from functional gastroparesis. Mechanical causes of gastric stasis, such as obstruction by tumor or pyloric channel ulcer, have to be excluded by endoscopy or contrast barium radiography.

Acute gastroparesis is seen in a variety of clinical situations, including viral gastroenteritis, trauma, and metabolic derangements (Box 11-7). The causes for *chronic gastric stasis* are diverse and have been classified into various categories (e.g., electrical, metabolic, neurologic, and systemic) (Box 11-8). Various commonly used therapeutic drugs may cause delayed gastric emptying, such as anticholinergics, antidepressants, oral contraceptives, and beta adrenergic agonists (Box 11-9). Furthermore,

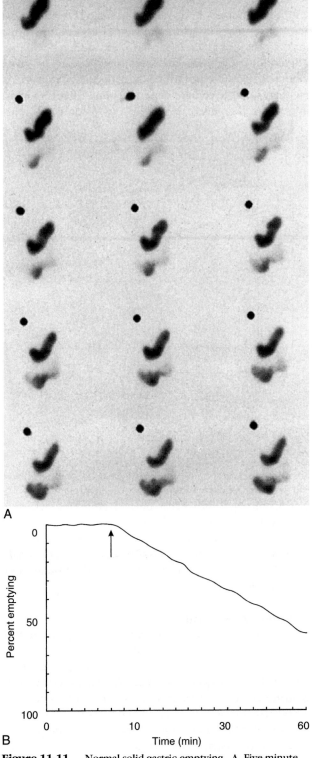

A

B

Figure 11-11   Normal solid gastric emptying. **A,** Five-minute sequential images acquired for 60 minutes. The egg-sandwich meal moves from the gastric fundus to the antrum in a normal manner. Radioactive marker placed at the right upper chest to check for motion. **B,** Computer-generated time-activity curve with delay (lag phase) of 9 minutes (*arrow*) before emptying begins (normal 5–25 minutes). A linear pattern of emptying follows. Greater than 50% emptying occurred by 90 minutes (normal, >35%).

Box 11-6   Factors that Affect the Rate of Gastric Emptying

PHYSIOLOGICAL

Meal content
Fat, protein, acid, osmolality
Volume
Weight
Caloric density
Particle size
Time of day
Patient position (standing, sitting, supine)
Gender
Metabolic state
Stress
Drugs

TECHNICAL

Radioisotope decay
Attenuation correction method
Scatter and septal penetration
Single-head versus dual-head camera
Frequent versus infrequent image acquisition
Method of quantification

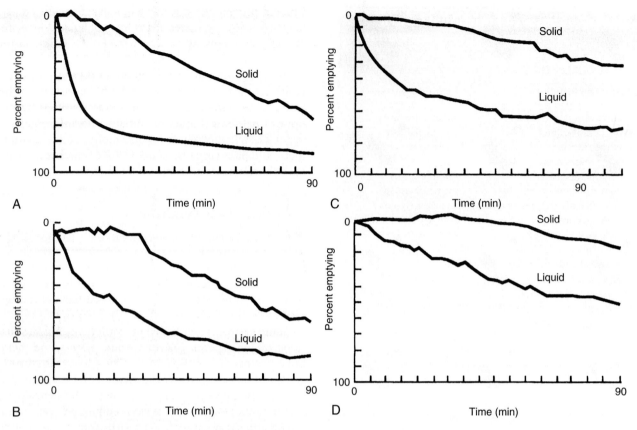

Figure 11-12   Diabetic gastroparesis: dual-phase solid-liquid emptying. **A,** Normal nondiabetic subject: Linear solid emptying after a short lag phase and prompt exponential liquid emptying. **B,** Diabetic with normal solid and liquid emptying. **C,** Diabetic with delayed solid but normal liquid emptying. **D,** Diabetic with delay in solid and liquid emptying.

nicotine, opiates, and alcohol all inhibit gastric emptying. Rapid gastric emptying is seen in patients who have had prior surgery (e.g., pyloroplasty and gastrectomy) or diseases such as gastrinoma and hyperthyroidism (Box 11-10).

Gastroparesis is clinically manifested by symptoms that include early postprandial satiety, bloating, nausea, and vomiting. Mild-to-moderate disease may be asymptomatic. As the disease progresses, symptoms become clinically manifest. Rapid gastric emptying can also produce symptoms (at times severe) including palpitations, diaphoresis, weakness, and diarrhea (*dumping syndrome*).

Diabetic Gastroparesis

Long-standing insulin-dependent diabetes mellitus is one of the more common causes for chronic gastroparesis. Pathophysiologically, it is the result of vagal nerve damage as part of a generalized autonomic neuropathy. In addition to producing disagreeable postprandial symptoms, abnormal emptying may exacerbate the problem of diabetic glucose control because timing of the insulin dose with food ingestion and absorption is critical. Rapid gastric emptying, rather than delayed emptying, occurs in some diabetics.

Delayed gastric emptying may also be caused acutely by hyperglycemia per se. Gastric motility studies thus should ideally be performed with the patient under optimal diabetic control.

Nonulcer Dyspepsia

A common clinical syndrome evaluated by gastroenterologists is the entity of nonulcer dyspepsia. It is characterized by upper abdominal symptoms, ulcerlike in some patients but dyspeptic in others. To make the diagnosis of nonulcer dyspepsia, organic conditions must have been excluded by radiologic and endoscopic studies. It is considered a functional disease and some of the patients have delayed gastric emptying.

Pharmacological Therapy

Various drug therapies are used to treat gastroparesis. Their prokinetic properties are mediated by different mechanisms. *Metoclopramide* (Reglan) has both central and peripheral antidopaminergic properties.

Box 11-7 Causes of Functional Gastric Stasis Syndromes—Acute and Chronic

Acute Dysfunction	Chronic Diseases
Trauma	Diabetes mellitus
Postoperative ileus	Hypothyroidism
Gastroenteritis	Progressive systemic
Hyperalimentation	sclerosis
Metabolic disorders:	Systemic lupus
hyperglycemia, acidosis,	erythematosus
hypokalemia, hypercalcemia,	Dermatomyositis
hepatic coma, myxedema	Familial dysautonomia
Physiological effects:	Pernicious anemia
labyrinth stimulation,	Bulbar poliomyelitis
physical and mental stress,	Amyloidosis
gastric distention, increased	Gastric ulcer
intragastric pressure	Postvagotomy
Hormones: gastrin,	Tumor-associated
secretin, glucagon,	gastroparesis
cholecystokinin,	Fabry disease
somatostatin,	Myotonic dystrophy
estrogen, progesterone	

Box 11-8 Common Causes of Delayed Gastric Emptying

ANATOMIC	NEUROMUSCULAR DISORDERS
Peptic ulceration	Diabetic gastroparesis
Surgery/Vagotomy	Smooth muscle disorders
Pyloric hypertrophy	Ileus
Postradiotherapy	Systemic diseases
Tumors	Scleroderma
METABOLIC DISORDERS	**AMYLOIDOSIS**
Electrolyte disturbances	Anorexia nervosa
Diabetic acidosis	Acute viral infections
Uremia	

Box 11-9 Drugs that Delay Gastric Emptying

Drug Type	Specific Drugs
Cardiovascular	Nifedipine, beta adrenergic agonists
Respiratory	Isoproterenol, theophylline
Gastrointestinal	Sucralfate, anticholinergics
Neuropsychiatric	Levodopa, diazepam, tricyclic antidepressants, phenothiazine
Reproductive	Progesterone, oral contraceptives
Drug abuse	Alcohol, nicotine, opiates

Neurological side effects (e.g., drowsiness, lassitude) are not uncommon. *Cisapride* (Propulsid) works by releasing acetylcholine from the myenteric plexus. *Domperidone,* not available in the United States, is a peripheral dopamine antagonist that penetrates the blood–brain barrier poorly, rarely producing neurological side effects. *Erythromycin* is a motilin agonist with prokinetic properties. Nausea as a side effect is common. All improve emptying by increasing the amplitude of antral contractions. Anticholinergics can be effective in slowing rapid emptying and ameliorating the symptoms (e.g., in patients with pylorospasm).

The side effects of therapeutic drugs discussed previously are reasons to confirm the diagnosis of abnormal gastric motility before treating.

Scintigraphy

The radionuclide gastric emptying study is the accepted standard for evaluation of gastric transit. Various other methods have been investigated, but none provide this physiological information so accurately, reproducibly, and are so relatively simple to perform.

Box 11-10 Causes of Rapid Gastric Emptying

POSTOPERATIVE

Pyloroplasty
Hemigastrectomy (Billroth I, II)

DISEASES

Duodenal ulcer
Gastrinoma (Zollinger-Ellison syndrome)
Hyperthyroidism

HORMONES

Thyroxine
Motilin
Enterogastrone

Clinical Indications

Recommendations have been published regarding generally agreed-upon indications for a radionuclide gastric emptying study (Box 11-11). They include diabetic patients with symptoms of gastroparesis (particularly those with poor glucose control, nonulcer dyspepsia, severe reflux esophagitis, unexplained nausea, and vomiting) and to assess response to a motility drug.

Radiopharmaceuticals

For accurate quantification of solid gastric emptying, the radioactive tracer must be tightly bound to the ingested food. Elution of the radiolabel will result in a part-solid, part-liquid labeled mixture resulting in an erroneously shortened solid emptying time because liquids empty faster than solids.

A physiologically superb in vivo method of radiolabeling chicken liver was described and used by early investigators. Tc-99m SC was injected into the wing vein of a chicken. After extraction by Kupffer cells of the liver where it is fixed intracellularly, the chicken was sacrificed and the liver was removed and cooked. The liver was mixed with beef or chicken stew for palatability and volume. This radiolabel was highly stable and did not dissociate after ingestion. Although of proven utility, this method is not generally used for obvious reasons.

Alternative in vitro methods of labeling liver have proven acceptable. Good radiolabeling results by cooking (fry, grill, microwave, etc.) Tc-99m SC in liver pâté, injecting it into liver cubes, or even surface-labeling it; the radionuclide is bound within the meat.

However, in current practice, most nuclear medicine clinics radiolabel eggs with Tc-99m SC. Frying or scrambling the eggs with Tc-99m SC produces good binding to the egg albumin. Egg substitutes can be used. Often administered as an egg sandwich, this semisolid meal is easy to prepare and palatable to most patients. Liquid meal markers should equilibrate rapidly and be nonabsorbable. Tc-99m SC or Tc-99m DTPA in water meet these criteria.

Two-phase markers, one for the solid meal and another for the liquid phase, have been used. In these dual-isotope, solid-liquid studies, In-111 DTPA is often used as the liquid marker (171 and 247 keV) in combination with the Tc-99m SC (140 keV) solid meal (see Fig. 11-12).

Methodology

The radionuclide gastric emptying study is straightforward. After the patient ingests a radiolabeled meal, intermittent or dynamic imaging is performed for the duration of the study. On computer, regions of interest are drawn around the stomach and gastric emptying is quantified.

Numerous protocols have been used for radionuclide gastric emptying. Meal composition, patient positioning, instrumentation, frequency of data acquisition, study length, and quantitative methods have varied (Table 11-3). Because many of these factors affect the rate of emptying, no general normal values can be used. In each clinic, the test must be standardized (i.e., performed the same way for all studies, at the same time of day, with the same meal, instrumentation, and computer processing). Normal values must be determined for the protocol used or one must closely follow a protocol in the medical literature and use its normal values. Some of the factors that affect the rate of gastric emptying and normal values are listed in Box 11-6.

Meal

The food content of the ingested meal is the major factor affecting the rate of gastric emptying. Clear liquids empty faster than liquids containing nutrients. Liquids empty faster than semisolids, which empty faster than solids. Large meals empty faster than small meals. Increases in volume, weight, caloric density, and particle size all slow the rate of gastric emptying. Normal emptying values are meal-specific. Normal values apply to a meal of a specific type with a specific volume and calorie content.

Routine Solid versus Liquid Meal

The solid or semisolid meal is more sensitive than liquid emptying for detection of abnormal gastric emptying. Liquid emptying is always normal when solid emptying is normal. When solid emptying is delayed, liquid emptying may be normal or delayed, depending on the severity of the gastroparesis (see Fig. 11-12). A liquid-only study should be reserved for patients who cannot tolerate solids (Fig. 11-13).

Single versus Dual Isotope

A dual-isotope study allows for simultaneous evaluation of liquid and solid gastric emptying. Although dual-phase may be important for the investigation of gastric physiology and pharmacology, it adds complexity, cost, and increased radiation exposure to the patient. Furthermore,

---

Box 11-11   Clinical Indications for Radionuclide Gastric Emptying Study

Insulin dependent diabetics with persistent
   postprandial symptoms
Diabetics with poor blood glucose control
Nonulcer dyspepsia
Severe reflux esophagitis.
Unexplained nausea and vomiting
Assess response to a motility drug

Table 11-3   Gastric Emptying Protocols

	Single-headed camera (LAO method)*	Dual-headed camera (geometric mean)†
Preparation	Overnight fast	Overnight fast
Meal	Tc-99m sulfur colloid egg white sandwich, 200 ml water	Tc-99m sulfur colloid egg white sandwich, 200 ml water
Dose	Tc-99m sulfur colloid, 1 mCi (37 MBq)	Tc-99m sulfur colloid, 1 mCi (37 MBq)
Window	15% 140 keV	15% 140 keV
Patient position	Semi-upright (60°)	Supine
Projections	LAO	Anterior and posterior simultaneously
Framing rate	90 sec/frame for 90 min	60 sec/frame for 90 min
Decay correct	Yes	Yes
Attenuation correction	LAO nonmathematical method	Geometric mean
Computer processing	ROI around summed gastric image	ROI around summed gastric image
Data presentation	TAC of counts versus time	TAC of anterior, posterior, and geometric mean counts versus time
Quantification	Percent emptying at 90 min	Percent emptying at 90 min
Abnormal	Less than 35%	Less than 34%

LAO, Left anterior oblique; ROI, region of interest; TAC, time–activity curve.

*From Ziessman HA, Fahey FH, Collen MD: Biphasic solid and liquid gastric emptying in normal controls and diabetics using continuous acquisition in the LAO view. Dig Dis Sci 37:744-750, 1992.

†From Ziessman HA, Fahey FH, Atkins FB, Tall J: Standardization and quantification of radionuclide solid gastric emptying studies. J Nucl Med 45:760-764, 2004.

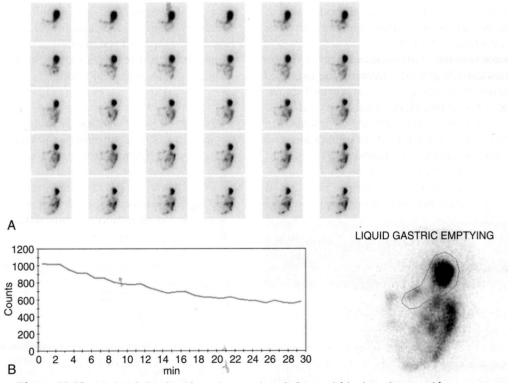

LIQUID GASTRIC EMPTYING

Figure 11-13   Delayed clear liquid gastric emptying. **A,** Sequential 1-minute images with delayed emptying of water from the stomach. **B,** A region-of-interest drawn around stomach and a time–activity curve generated. $T_{1/2}$ of 38 minutes (normal 10–20).

the dual-isotope study has no added clinical benefit over a single-isotope solid emptying study.

Study Length

Protocol length varies from clinic to clinic, ranging from 60 minutes to 4 hours, although 90–120 minutes is the most common. To some extent, this decision depends on the meal ingested. Large, difficult-to-digest meals (stew) empty slowly and may require 2.5–3 hours for acquisition, whereas smaller, more easily digestible semi-solid meals (eggs) require a shorter study length, about 1.5 hours.

Recent publications have recommended that gastric emptying studies can be simplified in methodology while maximizing sensitivity by acquiring images at time 0, 2 hours, and 4 hours, and utilizing a large published database for normal values. Further confirmation is needed.

Decay Correction

Correction for radioactive decay is mandatory for Tc-99m labeled meals because of the short half-life of the radionuclide (6 hours) and the relatively long duration of the study.

Attenuation Correction

The ingested radiolabeled meal moves from the gastric fundus to the gastric antrum, which is more anteriorly located. The posterior-to-anterior movement of the radiolabeled gastric contents results in variable attenuation. A radiolabeled meal is detected with increasing efficiency as it moves towards the gamma camera because of the decreasing amount of attenuating soft tissue between the camera and stomach contents.

In a gastric emptying study acquired with a single-headed gamma camera placed anteriorly, the detected radioactive counts often rise as the meal moves from the fundus to the antrum, although the amount of food in the stomach is unchanged. This artifact of attenuation adversely affects the accuracy of quantification and results in an underestimation of emptying. The amount of error varies from patient to patient, depending on size and anatomy. This artifact is a particular problem in obese patients, but often occurs in nonobese patients as well. The average error resulting from attenuation is 10–15%, but can be as high as 30–50% in some individuals. The percent error is unpredictable prior to the study; thus, routine correction for attenuation should be routinely performed to ensure accurate gastric emptying quantification.

Geometric Mean Method   Conjugate views are used to reduce the variability in sensitivity for radiotracer detection as a function of location in the body. The geometric mean (GM) method for attenuation correction is the accepted gold standard. Opposed images are routinely acquired in the anterior and posterior projections. Ideally, both images are obtained simultaneously with a dual-headed gamma camera. With a single-headed camera, the two opposing views can be obtained sequentially. The GM method is a mathematical correction performed at each data point (Fig. 11-14).

$$\text{Geometric mean (GM)} = \sqrt{(\text{counts}_{\text{anterior}} \times \text{counts}_{\text{posterior}})}$$

Left Anterior Oblique Method   An alternative to the GM method for attenuation correction is the left anterior oblique (LAO) method. This technique compensates for attenuation using a single-headed gamma camera and allows for frequent image acquisition. It requires no mathematical correction.

The rationale is that in the LAO oblique projection, the stomach contents move roughly parallel to the head of the gamma camera, thus minimizing the effect of attenuation (Fig. 11-15). The LAO method results correlate well with the GM method (Fig. 11-16). The GM method is still the standard and in general superior to the LAO method; however, the LAO method is adequate for most clinical purposes and definitely superior to the anterior view-only acquisition.

Frequency of Image Acquisition

Frequent image acquisition (e.g., a 1–5 minute framing rate) permits dynamic temporal visualization of emptying. With infrequent image acquisition (e.g., 30–60 minute framing rate) considerable information is lost. Potential sources of error may not be appreciated with infrequent imaging (e.g., gastroesophageal reflux, motion, overlap of stomach, and small bowel activity). Fewer data points are available for determining the rate of emptying. Thus, there is the potential for quantitative errors. Despite these potential problems, for many clinical

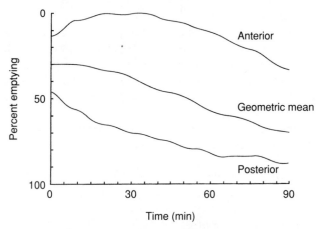

Figure 11-14   Geometric mean (GM) attenuation correction. The time–activity curves of both anterior and posterior projections show the effect of varying attenuation. Anterior data has a rising time–activity curve before it begins to empty. Posterior data shows decreasing counts from time zero. The GM curve is a normal two-phase solid emptying pattern.

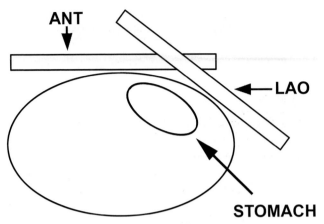

Figure 11-15   Left anterior oblique method. If the camera is placed in the LAO projection, the radiolabeled stomach contents move roughly parallel to the head of the gamma camera, compensating for the effect of varying attenuation. No mathematical correction is needed.

purposes, infrequent image acquisition provides generally reliable results.

Scatter Correction
With dual-isotope meals (e.g., In-111 and Tc-99m), correction for downscatter (In-111 into the Tc-99m window) and correction for upscatter (Tc-99m into the In-111 171 keV window) may be necessary. If and how much correction is needed can be determined from a simulated phantom study. However, the error is inconsequential when the dose ratio of Tc-99m to In-111 is at least 4:1 to 5:1.

Quantitative Analysis
The best method for processing a gastric emptying study depends to some extent on how the study is acquired (e.g., frequency of image acquisition, static versus dynamic acquisition, anterior and posterior views acquired sequentially or simultaneously). Generally, a gastric region of interest is drawn on the computer for individual or summed images. After correction for decay and attenuation, a time–activity curve is generated and a parameter of gastric emptying calculated, usually a half-time of emptying or a percent emptying at the end of the study.

The specific protocol used is to some extent determined by factors unique to each clinic. Table 11-3 describes two typical and validated protocols with normal values.

Liquid Emptying   Clear liquids have no lag phase. Emptying begins immediately after ingestion. The clearance time–activity curve is monoexponential, with a normal half-time of emptying of 10–20 minutes (Figs. 11-10 and 11-13). Liquids with nutrients empty slower than clear liquids. Liquids in a dual-phase meal also empty slower than a liquid-only meal (Fig. 11-12).

Solid Emptying   After an initial delay before emptying begins (lag phase), solid meals usually empty in a linear manner. The length of the lag phase is affected by many of the same factors that affect the rate of emptying.

Various different methods for quantifying solid emptying have been used. From a physiological standpoint, one might wish to calculate the length of the lag phase and then a rate of emptying. However, the clinical importance of the lag phase is uncertain. A few investigators have reported that a prolonged lag phase is the cause of delayed emptying in certain diseases and others have reported that the prokinetic effect of certain drugs improves emptying by shortening the lag phase. However, data are limited and conflicting. Differences in methodologies likely account for the discrepant results. Further investigations with frequent image acquisition are required to answer this question.

The rate of emptying is best calculated after the lag phase using a curve fitting method to determine either a linear (%/min) or exponential rate of emptying ($t_{1/2}$). A linear rate of emptying would be more physiologically correct in most cases, although the difference between a linear and exponential fit may not be great in many cases.

Thus, one of two methods of quantification has been generally used for clinical purposes, either a *half-time of emptying* beginning from time 0 (start of the study) or a *percent emptying* (at the end of the study) calculated at the end of the study. These approaches incorporate both phases of solid emptying into the overall result.

Evaluation of Therapeutic Effectiveness

The radionuclide gastric emptying study is uniquely able to evaluate the effectiveness of therapy. A patient with gastroparesis should have a repeat study after initiation of prokinetic therapy to judge whether in fact emptying has improved (Fig. 11-17). In some cases, prokinetic drugs improve the patient's symptoms without discernable improvement in emptying. This knowledge would be particularly important in insulin-dependent diabetic patients. The success of various surgical interventions (e.g., gastroplasty, surgical relief of obstruction) can also be effectively judged (Fig. 11-18).

HELICOBACTER PYLORI INFECTION

A major medical advance was the discovery that ulcer disease was caused by a bacteria, which led to antibiotic cure of the disease rather than the prior chronic medical treatment of symptoms and, in many cases, surgery.

Helicobacter pylori, a gram-negative bacterium, is the causative organism which infects the gastric mucosa of patients with duodenal ulcer disease, gastric ulcer disease, and antral gastritis. Bacterial eradication greatly decreases ulcer recurrence rates, reverses histological changes, and promotes healing of active ulcers.

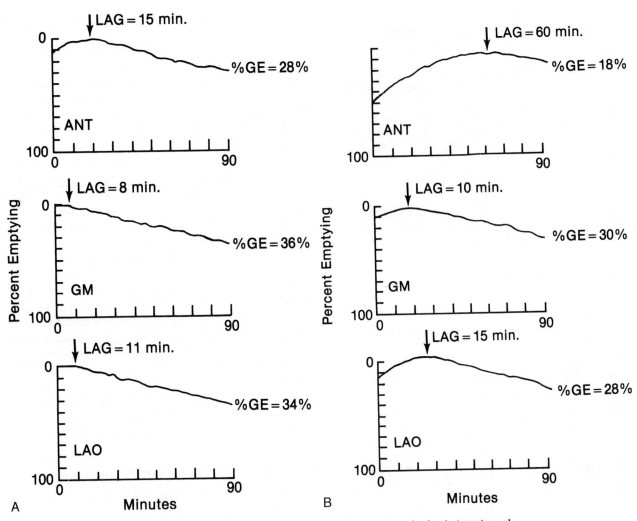

Figure 11-16   Attenuation correction using both GM and LAO methods. **A,** Anterior-only acquisition shows moderate rise in counts over 15 minutes (*top*). GM correction (*middle*). Lag phase shortened to 8 minutes and gastric emptying quantification is increased. LAO method (*bottom*). Results very similar to GM method. **B,** Anterior-only acquisition shows very long lag phase of 50 minutes (*top*). GM correction shortens the lag phase considerably, although there is still some initial rise suggesting incomplete correction (*middle*). Percent gastric emptying is much improved. LAO method shows similar results (*bottom*).

Urea Breath Test

In the presence of the bacterial enzyme urease, orally administered urea is hydrolyzed to carbon dioxide (CO_2) and ammonia. If the urea carbon is labeled with either the stable isotope carbon-13 or radioactive beta-emitter C-14, it can be detected in the breath as labeled CO_2. *H. pylori* is the most common urease-containing gastric pathogen; therefore, a positive urea breath test can be equated with *H. pylori* infection. The radioactive method is the most cost-effective.

The urea breath test is now widely available. This test is simple to perform, noninvasive, accurate, and inexpensive. An onsite analyzer is not needed because an expired air-filled balloon can be mailed for breath gas analysis. The overall accuracy is high. However, false-negative results may occur because of the recent use of antibiotics or bismuth-containing medications. False-positive results occur in patients with achlorhydria, contamination with oral urease-containing bacteria, and colonization with another *Helicobacter,* such as *H. felis.*

The initial diagnosis is usually made by gastric biopsy. The urea breath test is most commonly used to determine the effectiveness of therapy against *H. pylori.* Serological tests cannot determine the effectiveness of therapy because the antibody titer falls too slowly to be diagnostically useful.

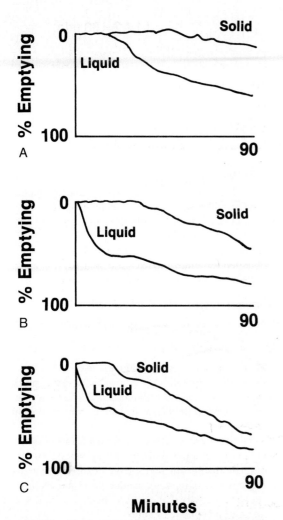

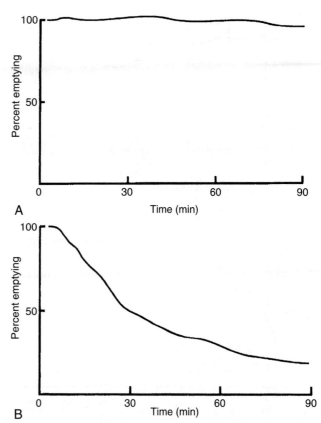

Figure 11-18 Pyloric obstruction. **A,** Referred for postprandial symptoms. Solid gastric emptying shows no emptying. Pyloric obstruction secondary to peptic ulcer disease was subsequently diagnosed and partial gastrectomy performed. **B,** Postoperative study shows a short lag phase and relatively rapid emptying.

Figure 11-17 Monitoring response to therapy. **A,** Baseline delayed solid and liquid gastric emptying. **B,** With metoclopramide treatment, both solid and liquid emptying improved. **C,** Because the patient had persistent symptoms, cisapride therapy was given. Both liquid and solid emptying improved further.

GASTROINTESTINAL BLEEDING

Effective and prompt therapy for acute gastrointestinal bleeding depends on accurate localization of the site of hemorrhage. The history and clinical examination can often distinguish upper from lower tract bleeding (e.g., melena versus bright red rectal bleeding). Upper-tract hemorrhage can be confirmed with gastric intubation and localized with a flexible fiberoptic endoscopy. Lower-tract bleeding is more problematic. During active hemorrhage, colonoscopy and barium radiography are of limited value.

Contrast Angiography

Angiography is diagnostic when positive, but it is invasive and will demonstrate the bleeding site only if the contrast agent is injected at the time of active hemorrhage. Gastrointestinal bleeding is typically intermittent and the clinical evaluation of whether the patient is actively bleeding at any one time is unreliable. Clinical signs of active hemorrhage often develop after bleeding has ceased.

Because repeated angiographic studies are not practical, it is often the angiographer who requests that a radionuclide gastrointestinal bleeding study be performed prior to the contrast study. The radionuclide study ensures that the patient is indeed actively bleeding and helps localize the bleeding site to the likely vascular origin of the bleed (e.g., celiac, superior, or inferior mesenteric) so that the angiographer can inject contrast promptly into the appropriate artery, limiting the duration of the study and the amount of contrast media required.

Radionuclide Scintigraphy

Tc-99m Sulfur Colloid

In 1977 at the University of Pennsylvania, Alavi et al. first described using Tc-99m SC for scintigraphic detection of

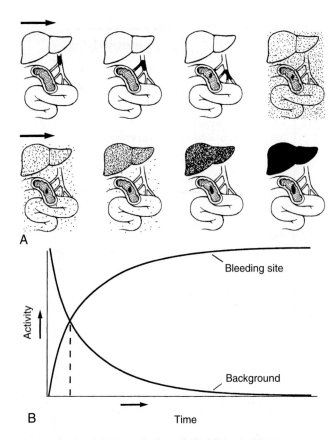

Figure 11-19   Tc-99m sulfur colloid gastrointestinal bleeding study. **A,** After injection, Tc-99m SC is cleared rapidly by the reticuloendothelial system, with a serum half-life of 3 minutes. Tc-99m SC will extravasate at the site of bleeding with each recirculation. Because of rapid background clearance, a high-contrast image results. **B,** Time–activity curves demonstrate rapid clearance of background and increasing activity at the bleeding site.

gastrointestinal bleeding. The rationale for this method is that after intravenous injection, Tc-99m SC is rapidly extracted from the serum (half-life of 3 minutes) by the reticuloendothelial cells of the liver, spleen, and bone marrow. By 15 minutes after injection, it is cleared from the vascular system. During active bleeding, the radiopharmaceutical extravasates at the bleeding site into the bowel lumen, increasing with each recirculation of blood. Continued extravasation with simultaneous background clearance results in a high target-to-background ratio, permitting visualization of the intra-abdominal active bleeding site (Fig. 11-19).

Methodology
Ten mCi (370 MBq) of Tc-99m SC are administered. Flow images (1–2 seconds/frame) are followed by serial 500k–750k count images of the abdomen and pelvis acquired every 1–2 minutes for 20–30 minutes (Box 11-12).

Image Interpretation
Rapid bleeding may be detected on the initial blood flow images. Vascular blushes of tumors, angiodysplasia, and

---

Box 11-12   Tc-99m SC Scintigraphy for Gastrointestinal Bleeding: Protocol Summary

PATIENT PREPARATION
None

RADIOPHARMACEUTICAL
Tc-99m sulfur colloid, 10 mCi (370 MBq)

INSTRUMENTATION
Camera: Large-field-of-view gamma camera. Collimator: high resolution, low energy, parallel hole. Interface with nuclear medicine computer; intensity set so that bone marrow can be seen
Computer setup: 1-sec/frame anterior flow images obtained for 1 min, then acquire 500k to 750k images of the abdomen every 1 to 2 min for 20 min

PATIENT POSITION
Supine; entire abdomen and pelvis in field of view

IMAGING PROCEDURE
Inject radiopharmaceutical intravenously.
Acquire on computer.
Acquire anterior views. Oblique, lateral, and posterior views may be obtained as needed to confirm the site of bleeding.
If no bleeding site is detected, obtain a 1000k count image of the upper abdomen with oblique views to evaluate the hepatic and splenic flexures. If negative, repeat views of the lower abdomen 15 min later to check for activity that may have been obscured in the hepatic and splenic flexures.
If the scan is negative and recurrent active bleeding is suspected, a repeat dose of Tc-99m sulfur colloid is given and the protocol repeated.

---

arteriovenous malformations may be seen in the absence of active bleeding. Active hemorrhage is most often detected in the first 5–10 minutes of imaging on the static high-count images (Fig. 11-20).

Active bleeding will move in an intestinal tract pattern, usually antegrade, but retrograde movement is not uncommon. A fixed region of radiotracer accumulation is not diagnostic of bleeding and likely is due to fixed uptake of the Tc-99m SC (e.g., ectopic spleen, renal transplants, and bone marrow) rather than intraluminal hemorrhage. Asymmetrical bone marrow uptake may be due to marrow replacement by tumor, infarction, or fibrosis, making the adjacent marrow appear as focal accumulation and perhaps suggesting a bleeding site.

Detection of bleeding in the region of the splenic flexure or transverse colon is complicated by intense normal liver and spleen uptake. Oblique views may help. A major

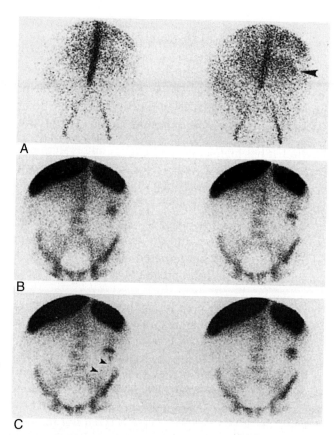

Figure 11-20 Tc-99m sulfur colloid study: descending colon bleed. **A,** Two 3-second flow images; the second image indicates extravasation at the site of bleeding (*large arrowhead*). **B** and **C,** Four sequential 5-minute images confirm the site of bleeding. Images in **C** show movement to the more distal left colon (*small arrowheads*).

disadvantage of the Tc-99m SC method is that bleeding must be active at the time of injection, similar to angiography. However, if the initial study is negative, a repeat injection can be administered and imaging repeated.

Tc-99m Red Blood Cells

In 1979 at Massachusetts General Hospital, Winzelberg et al. described the Tc-99m-labeled red blood cells (RBCs) method that is now in general use. The advantage of this method over Tc-99 SC is that imaging can be performed for a longer length of time, increasing the likelihood for detection of intermittent bleeding. The study length is limited only by the physical half-life of Tc-99m and the stability of the radiolabel.

A high-labeling efficiency ensures a high target-to-background ratio and optimal image quality, which can affect scan interpretation. Free (unbound) Tc-99m pertechnetate is taken up by the salivary glands and gastric mucosa and then secreted into the gastrointestinal tract, potentially complicating interpretation. Various labeling techniques (e.g., in vivo, modified in vivo [in-vivtro], and in vitro) with different labeling efficiencies have been used (Box 11-13).

Box 11-13 Methods of Tc-99m Red Blood Cell Labeling

IN VIVO METHOD (LABELING EFFICIENCY, 75–80%)
1. Inject stannous pyrophosphate.
2. Wait 10–20 min.
3. Inject Tc-99m sodium pertechnetate.

MODIFIED IN VIVO (IN VIVTRO) METHOD (LABELING EFFICIENCY, 85–90%)
1. Inject stannous pyrophosphate.
2. Wait 10–20 min.
3. Withdraw 5 to 8 ml of blood into shielded syringe with technetium-99m.
4. Gently mix syringe contents for 10 min at room temperature.

IN VITRO (BROOKHAVEN) METHOD (LABELING EFFICIENCY, 98%)
1. Add 4 ml of heparinized blood to reagent vial of 2 mg Sn^{+2}, 3.67 mg Na citrate, 5.5 mg dextrose, and 0.11 mg NaCl.
2. Incubate at room temperature for 5 min.
3. Add 2 ml of 4.4% EDTA.
4. Centrifuge tube for 5 min at 1300 g.
5. Withdraw 1.25 ml of packed red blood cells and transfer to sterile vial containing Tc-99m.
6. Incubate at room temperature for 10 min.

IN VITRO COMMERCIAL KIT (ULTRATAG) (LABELING EFFICIENCY, >97%)
1. Add 1-3 ml of blood (heparin or acid citrate dextrose as anticoagulant) to reagent vial (50–100 μg stannous chloride, 3.67 mg Na citrate) and mix. Allow 5 min to react.
2. Add syringe 1 contents (0.6 mg sodium hypochlorite) and mix by inverting four or five times.
3. Add contents of syringe 2 (8.7 mg citric acid, 32.5 mg Na citrate, dextrose) and mix.
4. Add 370-3700 MBq (10–100 mCi) of Tc-99m to reaction vial.
5. Mix and allow to react for 20 min, with occasional mixing.

The in vitro method is preferable because of its superior labeling efficiency (>97%).

Radiolabeling Red Blood Cells

Tc-99m RBC labeling requires that the technetium-99m be reduced intracellularly so that it will bind with the intracellular protein of the beta chain of the hemoglobin molecule. The stannous ion in the form of stannous pyrophosphate (tin) is used for this purpose. The dose is optimized to maximize the percentage of technetium bound inside the erythrocyte and minimize extravascular and circulating free technetium.

ble kit technique for labeling red blood cells
commercially available (UltraTag, Mallinckrodt,
Louis, MO) (Fig. 11-21). This method uses whole
blood and does not require centrifugation or transfer of
erythrocytes. The in vivo and modified in vivo methods
depend on biological clearance of undesirable extracellular reduced stannous ion. The original in vitro method
removed it by centrifugation. The in vitro commercial
kit method prevents extracellular reduction of stannous
ion by adding an oxidizing agent (sodium hypochlorite),
which cannot enter the red blood cells.

Drugs, intravenous solutions, and various clinical conditions may interfere with red blood cell labeling.
Heparin is the most common cause. It oxidizes the stannous ion and complexes with pertechnetate, thus reducing labeling efficiency. Direct injection of tin or pertechnetate into intravenous lines containing heparin should
be avoided. Dextrose, mannitol, and sorbitol and the
presence of antibodies to erythrocytes reduce labeling
efficiency.

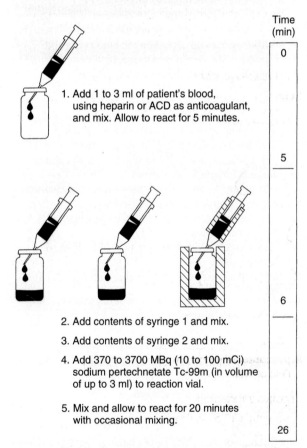

Time (min)

0

5

6

26

1. Add 1 to 3 ml of patient's blood, using heparin or ACD as anticoagulant, and mix. Allow to react for 5 minutes.

2. Add contents of syringe 1 and mix.

3. Add contents of syringe 2 and mix.

4. Add 370 to 3700 MBq (10 to 100 mCi) sodium pertechnetate Tc-99m (in volume of up to 3 ml) to reaction vial.

5. Mix and allow to react for 20 minutes with occasional mixing.

Figure 11-21 In vitro erythrocyte labeling with Tc-99m (UltraTag RBC). Each kit consists of three nonradioactive components: a 10-ml vial containing stannous chloride, syringe 1 containing sodium hypochlorite, and syringe 2 containing citric acid, sodium citrate, and dextrose (*ACD*). Typical labeling efficiency is >97%.

Various different methodologies have been used over
the years for labeling of red blood cells with Tc-99m (Box
11-13). The in vivo method was the original methodology. It was simple to perform but had suboptimal labeling
efficiency. A modified in vivo method was subsequently
developed and widely used because of its improved
labeling efficiency. However, today most nuclear medicine clinics use an in vitro commercially available
method. It has high labeling efficiency and is simple to
prepare.

In Vivo Nonradioactive stannous pyrophosphate
(15 µg/kg body weight) is reconstituted with saline and
injected intravenously. After 15–30 minutes, Tc-99m
pertechnetate is injected intravenously. The pertechnetate diffuses across the erythrocyte membrane,
where it is reduced by the stannous ions administered
previously. The Tc-99m label binds to the beta chain of
hemoglobin.

Although the in vivo technique is simple, the labeling
yield is less than ideal, on the order of 80% but frequently
as low as 60–65%. Tc-99m activity not labeled to red
blood cells can contribute to background activity and also
reduces the number of counts available from the cardiac
blood pool. In some cases, the labeling fails dramatically
because of drug–drug interactions or other causes of poor
labeling (Box 11-14). Special care is taken not to inject
through heparinized intravenous tubing. For these reasons, most laboratories have adopted either the modified
in vivo approach or preferably the in vitro approach.
Excessive gastric, thyroid, and soft tissue background activity suggests poor labeling with free Tc-99m pertechnetate.

Box 11-14 Causes of Poor Tc-99m Red Blood Cell Labeling

Drug	Mechanism or Comment
Stannous ion	Too little or too much will result in poor labeling
Heparin	A Tc-99m labeled heparin complex may form when Tc-99m is injected through a heparinized catheter
Methyldopa; hydralazine	Oxidation of stannous ion, diminution of reduction capacity
Doxorubicin	Decreased labeling efficiency; effect related to drug concentration
Quinidine	May increase production of antibodies to red blood cells
Iodinated contrast	Multiple mechanisms: lowering of stannous reduction capacity, altering stannous distribution, competition for erythrocyte binding sites between Tc-99m and iodide media, alterations in Tc-99m binding sites

Modified In Vivo (In Vivtro) First, cold stannous pyrophosphate is administered intravenously. After the 15- to 30-minute wait for equilibration of stannous ion in RBCs, 3–5 ml of blood is withdrawn through an intravenous line into a shielded syringe containing Tc-99m pertechnetate and a small amount of either acid-citrate-dextrose (ACD) solution or heparin. The blood is incubated at room temperature for at least 10 minutes. The syringe is agitated periodically and its contents are reinjected into the patient. The syringe is left attached to the intravenous line during the procedure so that the entire system is closed with respect to the patient's circulation. The labeling efficiency in the modified in vivo approach is approximately 90%.

In Vitro Blood is first withdrawn from the patient and added to a reaction vial containing cold stannous chloride. The stannous ion diffuses across the RBC membrane and binds to the hemoglobin. Sodium hypochlorite is added to oxidize excess extracellular stannous ion to prevent reduction of Tc-99m pertechnetate. A sequestering agent is added to remove extracellular stannous ion. Radioactive labeling is then accomplished by adding Tc-99m pertechnetate, which crosses the RBC membrane and is reduced by stannous ion in the cell. The mixture is incubated for 20 minutes before reinjection. Labeling efficiency is greater than 95%. This approach is less subject to drug–drug labeling interference and to problems of excessive or deficient stannous ion. A simple in vitro kit (UltraTag RBC, Mallinckrodt) is commercially available.

Dosimetry
The radiation absorbed dose to the patient both using the Tc-99m SC technique and the Tc-99m-labeled red blood cell method is relatively low, particularly when compared with contrast angiography. The target organ for Tc-99m SC is the liver; for Tc-99m erythrocytes, the liver and the myocardial wall. The whole-body dose for labeled erythrocytes is 0.15 cG/925 MBq (0.4 rad/25 mCi) (Table 11-4).

Methodology
A detailed imaging protocol is described in Box 11-15. An initial flow study is acquired at a 1–2 second framing rate (Fig. 11-22). The patient is supine and the camera placed anteriorly. Then, 1-minute images are acquired for 90 minutes (Figs. 11-23 to 11-26). A left lateral view of the pelvis can help differentiate activity in the bladder from that in the rectum, and even occasionally, from penile activity (Fig. 11-27). If the study is not diagnostic, delayed imaging can be obtained for up to 24 hours. Delayed images should always be acquired at the same framing rate, usually for 30 minutes.

Image Interpretation
Rapid hemorrhage may be seen on the flow phase of the study which can occasionally be helpful at a bleeding site difficult to see on later dynamic imaging (e.g., adja-

Table 11-4 Dosimetry for Gastrointestinal Bleeding: Tc-99m Red Blood Cells (RBCs) and Tc-99m Sulfur Colloid

	Tc-99m RBCs (UltraTag) cGy/740 MBq (rads/20 mCi)	Tc-99m Sulfur colloid cGy/370 MBq (rads/10 mCi)
Heart wall	2.0	
Bladder wall	0.48	
Spleen	2.2	2.10
Blood	0.80	
Liver	0.58	3.40
Red marrow	0.30	0.27
Ovaries	0.32	0.06
Testes	0.22	0.01
Whole body	0.3	0.19

From package inserts: Mallinckrodt, St. Louis, MO.

Box 11-15 Tc-99m Red Blood Cell Scintigraphy for Gastrointestinal Bleeding: Protocol Summary

PATIENT PREPARATION
None

RADIOPHARMACEUTICAL
Tc-99m labeled red blood cells

INSTRUMENTATION
Camera: Large-field-of-view gamma.
Collimator: high resolution, parallel hole.
Computer setup: 1-sec frames for 60 sec; 1-min frames for 60 to 90 min.
If needed: 2-4-hr delayed image sequence as 1-min frames for 20 to 30 min.
Static images: 2- to 3-sec flow images and 1000k count images every 2 to 5 min.
Set intensity so that aorta, inferior vena cava, and iliac vessels are well visualized.

PATIENT POSITION
Supine; anterior imaging, with abdomen and pelvis in field of view.

IMAGING PROCEDURE
Inject patient's Tc-99m-labeled erythrocytes intravenously.
Acquire flow images, followed by static images for 60 to 90 min.
If study is negative or bleeding is recurrent, repeat 30-min acquisition.

cent to the bladder). The flow phase can help localize the site of bleeding even if bleeding is not active (e.g., detection of a vascular blush due to angiodysplasia or tumor) (Fig. 11-22). Furthermore, vascular structures can be defined (e.g., kidneys, ectatic vessels, or uterus) to help with image interpretation on delayed images.

Active bleeding is most often diagnosed by review of the sequential 1-minute images obtained during the first 90 minutes of the study (Figs. 11-23 to 11-26). Over 80% of bleeding sites are detected during this initial imaging time. Cinematic display on a computer can be very helpful for determining the pattern of flow (e.g., whether small or large bowel). Because bleeding is intermittent, delayed imaging beyond 90 minutes can sometimes be helpful. The timing will depend on the patient's condition and the logistics of the clinic.

Diagnostic Criteria

The purpose of the gastrointestinal bleeding study is to diagnose active bleeding and to localize the site of bleeding. Specific criteria must be used to avoid incorrect interpretations (Box 11-16). The radiotracer activity must appear where there was none before, increase over time, and conform to intestinal anatomy. The intraluminal activity may move antegrade and/or retrograde. Activity that is not moving should not be diagnosed as an active bleeding site and is likely due to a fixed vascular structure (e.g., hemangioma, accessory spleen, or ectopic kidney).

Frequent image acquisition is important for localizing the site of bleeding because hemorrhage can be rapid and may move both antegrade and retrograde. Review of 1-minute dynamic frames displayed on a computer in cinematic mode is very helpful for confirming and better defining the site of bleeding.

Carefully noting the pattern of intestinal transit of the radioactivity is critical for determining the anatomical bleeding site. An appreciation of gastrointestinal vascular anatomy and its embryological development is helpful in pinpointing the vascular bed for the angiographer (Fig. 11-28).

Bleeding in the large intestines typically appears as activity moving along the periphery of the abdomen in elongated loops of bowel (Figs. 11-23 and 11-24). The small bowel is more centrally located and blood progresses rapidly through its curvilinear segments. Localization of the site of bleeding to the small intestine may be difficult (Fig. 11-25). Slow small intestinal bleeds may be hard to localize. They may first be detected by pooling of radiotracer in the cecum. Intravenous glucagon may be useful for inhibiting bowel peristalsis and allow pooling of activity at the site of active bleeding in the small bowel.

Because of scintigraphic limitations in exact anatomical localization of the bleeding site, it is often described as in the general region of the small bowel, cecum, ascending colon, hepatic flexure, transverse colon, splenic flexure, descending colon, or rectosigmoid colon. This is usually sufficient for the angiographer to determine which vessel (celiac, superior mesenteric, or inferior mesenteric artery) to inject with contrast.

Although the radionuclide gastrointestinal bleeding study is not generally ordered to diagnose upper gastrointestinal bleeding, the first indication of an upper gastrointestinal source is sometimes revealed on the bleeding scan (Fig. 11-29). It is important to differentiate upper gastrointestinal bleeding from free Tc-99m pertechnetate. Free Tc-99m pertechnetate may simulate gastric bleeding due to uptake by the gastric

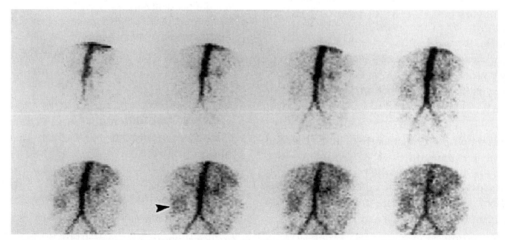

Figure 11-22   Positive blood flow: no active bleeding. Increased focal blood flow to the region of the ascending colon (*arrowhead*). Ninety-minute Tc-99m red blood cell study was negative, as well as a second acquisition for 30 minutes at 3 hours. Colonoscopy with biopsy diagnosed colon cancer in the region of increased abnormal flow.

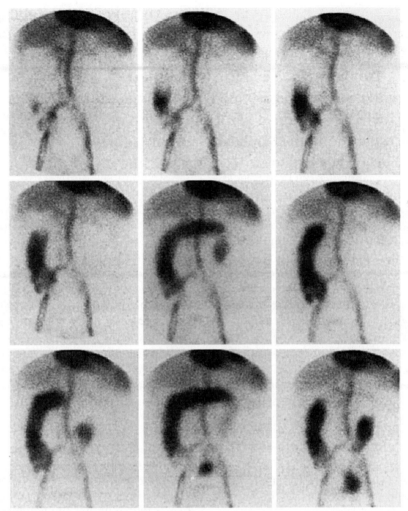

Figure 11-23   Tc-99m RBC: ascending colon bleed. Active hemorrhage originates in the proximal ascending colon, then transits the transverse colon and enters the left colon by the end of the 60-minute study. Etiology was colon cancer.

mucosa (Fig. 11-29). Over time, activity may be seen to move distal to the stomach in the small bowel and even the large bowel on delayed images. Images of the thyroid and salivary glands should be obtained to confirm or exclude free Tc-99m pertechnetate as a source of gastric activity.

Pitfalls

Pitfalls are defined as normal, technical, or pathological findings that may be misinterpreted active hemorrhage (Box 11-17). The presence of free Tc-99m pertechnetate caused by poor radiolabeling or dissociation of the label in vivo would be considered a technical pitfall. A common anatomical pitfall as a cause for misinterpretation is focal activity in the genitourinary tract. This could be due to pelvic or focal ureteral retention either free pertechnetate or another Tc-99m labeled reduced compound. This activity will usually move with time, possibly making interpretation even more problematic. Upright positioning, oblique, or posterior views may be helpful to clarify the etiology. Renal transplants and ectopic kidneys may also be causes for concern.

Activity seen in the region of the pelvis can be misinterpreted. The differential diagnosis should include bleeding in the rectum, bladder activity, uterine activity during menses, and normal penile blood pool. A left lateral view is essential for making the correct interpretation (Figs. 11-26 and 11-29).

Intraluminal radioactivity first detected on delayed images can pose a diagnostic dilemma. Blood first seen in the sigmoid colon or rectum on a single delayed image obtained between 8 to 24 hours may have originated from anywhere in the gastrointestinal tract. Misinterpretation of this isolated finding can be avoided

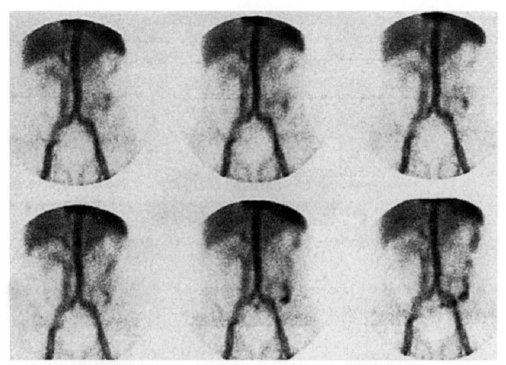

Figure 11-24 Tc-99m RBC: left colonic bleed. Dynamic images acquired over 60 minutes show increasing activity in the region of the descending colon which moves distally to the sigmoid colon.

by acquiring dynamic 1-minute images whenever delayed imaging is performed. An active bleeding site should be diagnosed only by using the criteria already described (Box 11-16).

A pathological pitfall might include abdominal varices, hemangioma, accessory spleen, arterial grafts, and aneurysms (Fig. 11-30). Activity clearing through the hepatobiliary system and gallbladder may be related to hemobilia; however, patients with renal failure have gallbladder visualization because of radiolabeled fragmented heme breakdown products (e.g., porphyrins).

Accuracy
Only 2–3 ml of extravasated blood is necessary for detection. In experimental studies, bleeding rates as low as 0.05–0.1 ml/min could be detected. This compares favorably with the ability of contrast angiography to detect bleeding rates of 1 ml/min or greater, at least a 10-fold difference.

Many investigations over the years have reported generally high accuracy for radionuclide gastrointestinal bleeding scintigraphy; however, there are reports that have found lower accuracy and have not found the study helpful (Table 11-5). Thus, controversy exists regarding its clinical utility.

The reasons for the discrepancy in reported accuracy of localization are several. Misinterpretation may be from infrequent image acquisition, pitfalls described previously, and incorrect localization based on single delayed images. However, other factors are likely. Patient referral bias is one. Whether the patients had the radionuclide bleeding study early in the course of their workup or only after hospitalization with extensive negative radiologic and endoscopy evaluation is a critical factor in biasing the investigation. The scintigraphic study will have the highest yield when performed soon after arrival in the emergency room or on admission.

The gold standard is often a problem with these investigations. The majority of patients do not get angiography, and when they do, it may be a false-negative because the patient is no longer actively bleeding. Colonoscopy is not usually possible during active bleeding. Detection of pathological abnormalities on radiographic studies or colonoscopy after bleeding has ceased does not necessarily indicate that they were the source of bleeding.

Overall, the majority of investigations have found the gastrointestinal bleeding study is accurate in bleeding site localization and therefore is clinically useful. A telling point is that angiographers are the ones at many institutions that aggressively demand scintigraphy prior to their invasive procedure. Being available when needed and having good communication with referring physicians is critical for success.

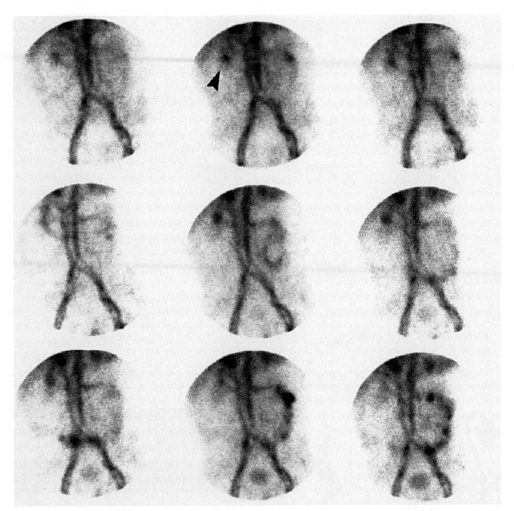

Figure 11-25 Tc-99m RBC: duodenal bleed. Active bleeding is initially seen in the region of the duodenum (*arrowhead*) and sequential images show transit through the small intestines.

Tc-99m Red Blood Cells versus Tc-99m Sulfur Colloid

The general consensus is that Tc-99m-labeled red blood cell studies are superior to Tc-99m SC for diagnosing acute gastrointestinal scintigraphy (Table 11-6). A large multicenter prospective study by Bunker et al. compared these two approaches in 100 patients referred with clinical evidence of acute bleeding. The Tc-99m SC study was performed first, followed by labeled Tc-99m red blood cells. Tc-99m SC localized only five sites of hemorrhage, compared to 38 localized with Tc-99m RBC imaging. The sensitivity and specificity of the Tc-99m red blood cell study were 93% and 95%, respectively. Continuous imaging for 90 minutes revealed 83% of all active hemorrhages. Smaller studies have reported similar results.

The advantage of Tc-99m RBC scintigraphy is the ability to image over a longer time period. Tc-99m SC may still have a limited role (e.g., in patients with active bleeding who are clinically unstable). The quick preparation time and 20-minute total imaging time may provide valuable information to the angiographer.

HETEROTOPIC GASTRIC MUCOSA

Meckel's diverticulum is the most common and clinically important form of heterotopic gastric mucosa. The terminology often used is "ectopic" gastric mucosa; however, it is not truly correct. Ectopic refers to an organ that has migrated (e.g., ectopic kidney). Heterotopic refers to a tissue at its site of origin. For example, other manifestations of heterotopic gastric mucosa are in gastrointestinal duplications, postoperative retained gastric antrums, and Barrett's esophagus.

Radiopharmaceutical

Tc-99m pertechnetate has been used since 1970 to diagnose heterotopic gastric mucosa. The most common

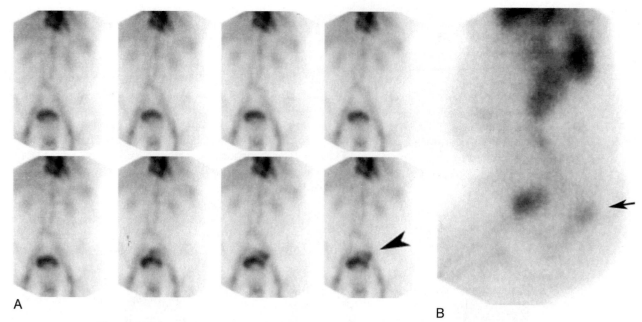

Figure 11-26   Tc-99m RBC: rectal bleed.   **A,** The last three of the 1-minute images show increasing activity just superior and to the left of the bladder (*arrowhead*) very suggestive of rectosigmoid colon bleed. **B,** Left lateral view. Blood is seen in the region of the rectum (*arrow*).

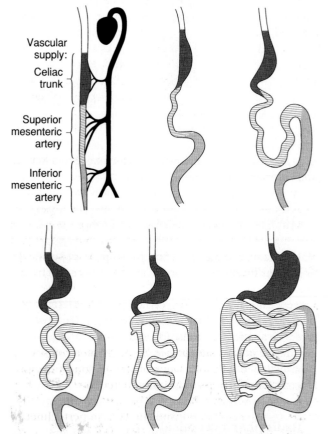

Figure 11-27   Vascular supply of gastrointestinal tract.   The embryological development of the gastrointestinal tract explains its anatomical configuration and its vascular distribution.   This schematic diagram also relates the gastrointestinal anatomy to its arterial supply (celiac, superior mesenteric, and inferior mesenteric arteries).

Box 11-16   Criteria for Diagnosis of Localization of Bleeding Site with Tc-99m Red Blood Cell Scintigraphy

Focal activity appears
Activity increases over time
Activity movement conforms to intestinal anatomy
Movement may be antegrade or retrograde

---

clinical indication has been to detect a Meckel's diverticulum as the cause of gastrointestinal bleeding in a child. However, it can be used to diagnose and localize other types of heterotopic gastric mucosa listed previously.

Mechanism of Uptake

The mucosa of the gastric fundus contains parietal cells, which secrete hydrochloric acid and intrinsic factor, and chief cells, which secrete pepsinogen.   The antrum and pylorus contain G cells, which secrete the hormone gastrin. Columnar mucin-secreting epithelial cells are found throughout the stomach; they excrete an alkaline juice that protects the mucosa from the highly acidic gastric fluid.

Parietal cells were originally thought to be responsible for Tc-99m pertechnetate gastric mucosal uptake and secretion. Some experimental evidence supports this hypothesis; however, most evidence points to

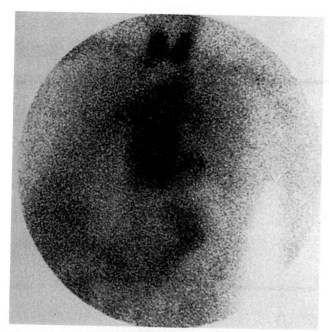

Figure 11-28 Free Tc-99m pertechnetate. A gastrointestinal bleeding study showed increasing gastric activity (not shown). This subsequent image confirmed thyroid uptake, consistent with free Tc-99m pertechnetate rather than active bleeding. The poor target-to-background ratio is also due to considerable free pertechnetate.

the mucin-secreting cells. Tc-99m pertechnetate uptake has been found in gastric tissue with no parietal cells and autoradiographic studies localize Tc-99m pertechnetate uptake to the mucin cell rather than the parietal cell.

A hypothesis explaining the conflicting data suggests that the predominant mechanism is specific mucin cell uptake and secretion, which is suppressible by potassium or sodium perchlorate in a manner similar to iodide, whereas parietal cell uptake is a minor factor, nonspecific, secondary, and (as in chloride uptake) not suppressed by perchlorate.

Dosimetry

The target organ for Tc-99m pertechnetate is the stomach, followed by the thyroid gland (Table 11-7).

Clinical Indications

Meckel's Diverticulum

The most common congenital anomaly of the gastrointestinal tract is Meckel's diverticulum, occurring in 1–3% of the population. The diverticulum results from failure of closure of the omphalomesenteric duct in the embryo. The duct connects the yolk sac to the primitive foregut through the umbilical cord. This true diverticulum arises on the antimesenteric side of the small bowel, usually 80–90 cm proximal to the ileocecal valve. It is typically 2–3 cm in size but may be considerably larger.

Heterotopic gastric mucosa is present in 10–30% of patients with Meckel's diverticulum, in approximately 60% of symptomatic patients, and in 98% of those that manifest bleeding (Box 11-18).

Clinical Manifestations

Gastric mucosal secretions can cause peptic ulceration of the diverticulum or adjacent ileum, producing pain, perforation, or most commonly, bleeding. Sixty percent of patients with complications of Meckel's diverticulum are under age 2 years. Adults present with intussusceptions, obstruction, infection, and abnormal fixation of the diverticulum. Bleeding from Meckel's diverticulum after age 40 is unusual.

Diagnosis

Meckel's diverticulum is often missed on small bowel radiography because it often has a narrow or stenotic ostium, fills poorly, and has rapid emptying. Small bowel enteroclysis is superior because the higher pressure of the barium column more reliably fills the diverticulum. Angiography is useful only with brisk active bleeding and rarely used. The Tc-99m pertechnetate scan is considered the standard method for preoperative diagnosis of a Meckel's diverticulum.

Methodology

A typical protocol is described in Box 11-19. Patient preparation is important. Because a full stomach or urinary bladder may obscure an adjacent Meckel's diverticulum, fasting for 3–4 hours prior to the study or continuous nasogastric aspiration to decrease the size of the stomach is recommended and the patient should void before, during, and after the study. Potassium perchlorate should *not* be used to block thyroid uptake because it will also block uptake of Tc-99m pertechnetate by the gastric mucosa. It may be administered after the study to wash out the radiotracer from the thyroid and thus to minimize radiation exposure.

Barium studies should not be performed for several days before scintigraphy because attenuation by the contrast material may prevent lesion detection. Procedures (e.g., colonoscopy or laxatives that irritate the intestinal mucosa) can result in nonspecific Tc-99m pertechnetate uptake and should be avoided. Certain drugs (e.g., ethosuximide [Zarontin]) may also cause unpredictable uptake.

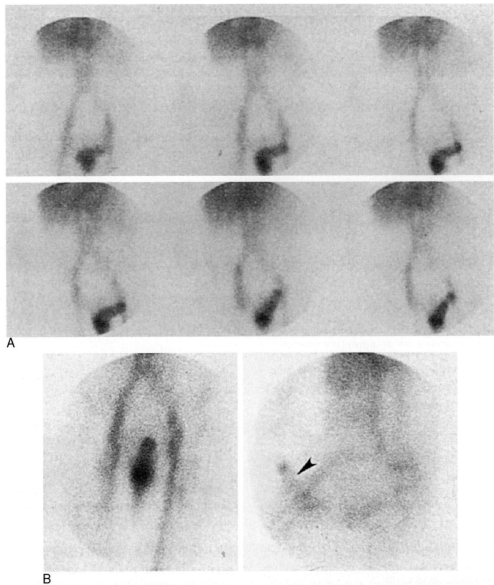

Figure 11-29 Potential false-positive for gastrointestinal bleeding. **A,** Images acquired every 10 minutes × 6 show changing, increasing activity in the lower left and middle pelvic region. **B,** Anterior (*left*) and left lateral (*right*) images acquired 90 minutes after tracer injection show the activity to be the penile blood pool (*arrowhead*). Left lateral views should be obtained whenever pelvic activity is seen in order to separate rectal, bladder, and penile activity.

Pharmacological Augmentation

Various pharmacological maneuvers have been reported to improve the detection of Meckel's diverticulum, including pentagastrin, glucagon, and cimetidine.

Cimetidine The histamine H_2-receptor antagonist cimetidine increases uptake of Tc-99m pertechnetate by inhibiting its release from the gastric mucosa. No large or controlled studies have been done to evaluate its diagnostic utility; however, some recommend its routine use because of its possible effectiveness and its lack of

significant risks or side effects. Others reserve its use for a patient with a suspected false-negative Tc-99m pertechnetate scan for Meckel's diverticulum. The usual dose is 20 mg/kg orally for 2 days prior to the study.

Pentagastrin and Glucagon Pretreatment with pentagastrin has been used because it increases the rapidity, duration, and intensity of Tc-99m pertechnetate uptake. The mechanism may be the result of increased acid production, leading to increased activity of the mucin-producing cells and thus increased Tc-99m pertechnetate

Box 11-17 **Pitfalls in Interpretation of Tc-99m Red Blood Cell Scintigraphy**

PHYSIOLOGICAL
Common

Gastrointestinal (free Tc-99m pertechnetate)—stomach, small and large intestine
Genitourinary
Pelvic kidney
Ectopic kidney
Renal pelvic activity
Ureter
Bladder
Uterine blush
Penis

Uncommon

Accessory spleen
Hepatic hemangioma
Varices, esophageal and gastric

RARE

Vascular
Abdominal aortic aneurysm
Gastroduodenal artery aneurysm
Abdominal varices
Caput medusae and dilated mesenteric veins
Gallbladder varices
Pseudoaneurysm
Arterial grafts
Cutaneous hemangioma
Duodenal telangiectasia
Angiodysplasia

MISCELLANEOUS

Gallbladder (heme products in uremia)
Factitious gastrointestinal bleeding

posterior location of renal or ureteral activity. Upright views may distinguish fixed activity (e.g., duodenum) from ectopic gastric mucosa, which moves inferiorly, and this also serves to empty renal pelvic activity. The intensity of activity may fluctuate because of intestinal secretions, hemorrhage, or increased motility washing out radiotracer. Postvoid images can empty the renal collecting system and aid in visualization of areas adjacent to the bladder.

Accuracy

False-negative studies can result from poor technique, washout of the secreted Tc-99m pertechnetate, or lack of sufficient gastric mucosa. Diverticula smaller than 2 cm^2 may not be detectable by scintigraphy. An impaired blood supply to a diverticulum from intussusception, volvulus, or infarction can give false-negative studies.

The reported accuracy of scintigraphy in the detection of Meckel's diverticulum has varied, depending on the referral population studied (children or adults), the presenting symptom (rectal bleeding or abdominal pain), and the technology used (old rectilinear scanners or modern gamma cameras). However, one large report summarized the results in 954 patients (mostly children) who had undergone scintigraphy for suspected Meckel's diverticulum using modern imaging methods, and found an overall sensitivity of 85% and a specificity of 95%.

Scintigraphy for Meckel's diverticulum in adults appears to have a poorer sensitivity than in children. One series reported a sensitivity of only 63%. There were 10 false-positive studies, although 7/10 of the subjects had surgically treatable disease. False negatives are probably related to the lack of gastric mucosa in the many adult diverticula.

Causes for false-positive studies are listed in Box 11-20. Normal structures may be confused with ectopic gastric mucosa if careful technique is not followed. Activity in the genitourinary tract may cause false interpretation. False positives may also result from inflammatory or obstructive lesions of the intestines.

Gastrointestinal Duplications

Duplications are cystic or tubular congenital abnormalities that have a mucosa, smooth muscle, and an alimentary epithelial lining attached to any part of the gastrointestinal tract, but often the ileum. Most are symptomatic by age 2 years. Twenty percent are found in the mediastinum. Presenting symptoms are often those of Meckel's diverticulum because 30–50% have heterotopic gastric mucosa.

The diagnosis is usually made at surgery. Occasionally a preoperative diagnosis is made by barium radiography or ultrasonography. Scintigraphy occasionally may be helpful; for example, mediastinal gastrointestinal cysts have been diagnosed with Tc-99m pertechnetate.

uptake. However, pentagastrin also increases intestinal motility, leading to rapid movement into the small bowel. Glucagon, because of its antiperistaltic effect, has been used with pentagastric to decrease bowel peristalsis and prevent tracer washout from a diverticulum. However, pentagastrin is associated with significant side effects and is no longer commercially available in the United States.

Image Interpretation

Scintigraphically, Meckel's diverticulum appears as a focal area of increased intraperitoneal activity, most frequently in the right lower quadrant (Fig. 11-31). Uptake is usually first seen 5-10 minutes after tracer injection, increasing over time at a rate similar to normal gastric uptake.

Lateral or oblique views can be helpful in confirming the anterior position of the diverticulum versus the

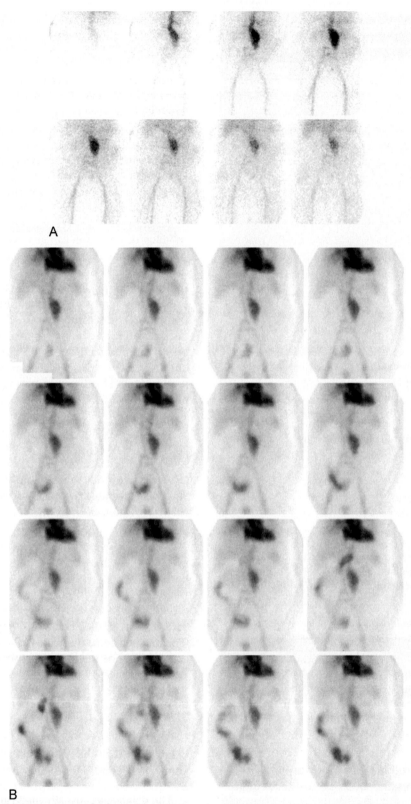

Figure 11-30   Aortic aneurysm and acute bleed. **A,** Flow study demonstrates a distal aortic aneurysm. **B,** On dynamic imaging over 60 minutes, an acute bleed is seen to originate in the mid lower pelvis, moving with time to the ascending and transverse colon, most consistent with a cecal bleed. The midabdominal aortic aneurysm showed persistent activity from the beginning to the end of the study. The fixed activity suggests that this is not active bleeding but anatomical.

Table 11-5 Correct Localization of Gastrointestinal Bleeding with Tc-99m Red Blood Cells

First author	Year	No. scans	% Positive	% Correct
Suzman	1996	224	51	96
Orechhia	1985	76	34	94
O'Neill	2000	26	96	88
Emslie	1996	75	28	88
Leitman	1989	28	43	86
Bearn	1992	23	78	82
Dusold	1984	74	59	75
Rantis	1995	80	47	73
Van Geelen	1994	42	57	69
Nicholson	1989	43	72	67
Hunter	1990	203	26	58
Bentley	1991	182	60	52
Garofalo	1997	161	49	19
Voeller	1991	111	22	0

Table 11-6 Comparison of Tc-99m Sulfur Colloids (SC) and Tc-99m Red Blood Cells (RBCs) for Gastrointestinal Bleeding

	Tc-99m SC	Tc-99m RBCs
Dose	10 mCi (370 MBq) (may be repeated)	25 mCi
Dosimetry		
Whole body	0.2 rad	0.4 rad
Target organ	3.6 rads (liver)	1.2 rads (heart)
Minimal bleeding detectable	0.1 ml/min	0.05–0.4 ml/min
Labeling	Commercial kit	Commercial kit
Imaging duration	20–30 min (repeat once)	60–90 min (repeat as needed for 24 hr)
Advantages	Short imaging time High target-to-background ratio	Repeat imaging up to 24 hr
Disadvantages	Difficulty detecting hepatic and splenic flexure bleeding Detects bleeding only over short time	False positive studies due to excretion of free Tc-99m pertechnetate

Table 11-7 Radiation Absorbed Dose for Tc-99m Pertechnetate (Meckel's Scan)

Target organ	rad/mCi	cGy/185 MBq (rad/5 mCi)
Bladder wall	0.053	0.265
Stomach wall	0.250	1.250
Large intestine wall	0.068	0.340
Ovaries	0.022	0.110
Red marrow	0.019	0.095
Testes	0.009	0.045
Thyroid	0.130	0.650
Total body	0.014	0.070

From MIRD Primer, Society of Nuclear Medicine, Reston, VA, 1988.

Box 11-18 Epidemiology of Meckel's Diverticulum

1–3% incidence in the general population.

50% occur by age 2 years.

10–30% have ectopic gastric mucosa.

25–40% are symptomatic; 50–67% of these have ectopic gastric mucosa.

95–98% of patients with bleeding have ectopic gastric mucosa.

through the gastrojejunostomy. The high acid production leads to marginal ulcers.

Endoscopy or barium radiography may demonstrate the retained gastric antrum. Tc-99m pertechnetate scintigraphy can be confirmatory. The protocol used is similar to that used for imaging a suspected Meckel's diverticulum. Uptake in the gastric remnant occurs simultaneously with gastric uptake and is seen as a collar of radioactivity in the duodenal stump of the afferent loop. The retained antrum usually lies to the right of the gastric remnant. In one series, Tc-99m pertechnetate uptake was demonstrated in 16 of 22 patients with a retained antrum.

Barrett's Esophagus

Chronic gastroesophageal reflux can cause the distal esophagus to become lined by gastric columnar epithelium rather than the usual esophageal squamous epithelium. This condition is known as Barrett's esophagus and is associated with complications of ulcers, strictures, and an 8.5% incidence of esophageal adenocarcinoma.

Tc-99m pertechnetate scans first demonstrated Barrett's esophagus in 1973; however, today the diagnosis is typically made with endoscopy and mucosal biopsy. Positive scintigraphy shows intrathoracic uptake contiguous with the stomach but conforming to the shape

Duplications often appear as large, sometimes multilobulated areas of increased activity. They are a cause for a false-positive interpretation of Meckel's diverticulum.

Retained Gastric Antrum

The gastric antrum may be left behind in the afferent loop after a Billroth II gastrojejunostomy. The antrum continues to produce gastrin, which is no longer inhibited by acid in the stomach because it has been diverted

Box 11-19   Meckel's Diverticulum: Protocol Summary

PATIENT PREPARATION

4-6 hr fasting before study to reduce size of stomach.

No pretreatment with sodium perchlorate; may be given after completion of study.

No barium studies should be performed within 3 to 4 days of scintigraphy.

Void before, during if possible, and after study.

PREMEDICATION

Optional: Cimetidine, 20 mg/kg orally for 24 hours prior to the study and 1 hour prior to the study.

RADIOPHARMACEUTICAL

Tc-99m pertechnetate

Children: 30-100 μCi/kg (minimal dose 200 uCi) (7.4 MBq)

Adults: 5-10 mCi intravenously

INSTRUMENTATION

Camera: large-field-of-view gamma.

Collimator: low energy, all purpose or high resolution.

PATIENT POSITION

Supine under camera with xiphoid to symphysis pubis in field of view

IMAGING PROCEDURE

Obtain flow images: 60 1-sec frames.

Obtain static images: 500k counts for first image, others for same time every 5-10 min for 1 hr.

Erect, right lateral, posterior, or oblique views may be helpful at 30-60 min.

Obtain postvoid image.

and posterior location of the esophagus. Scintigraphy should be performed with the patient erect to minimize reflux. To avoid misinterpreting accumulation in a hiatal hernia as Barrett's, the scan should be interpreted in conjunction with an upper gastrointestinal contrast series. False-negative results have been reported.

INTESTINAL FUNCTION AND TRANSIT

Schilling Test

Although most often ordered to diagnose pernicious anemia, the Schilling test is really a test of vitamin B_{12} (methylcobalamin) absorption. Vitamin B_{12} can be absorbed from the ileum only if it is complexed with intrinsic factor, which is produced by gastric parietal cells in the stomach. After absorption, vitamin B_{12} is

bound to storage sites in various tissues and slowly metabolized.

Vitamin B_{12} deficiency manifests clinically as a megaloblastic anemia and neurological disease. The most common cause is an intrinsic factor (IF) deficiency in patients with pernicious anemia and associated gastric atrophy. Intestinal causes of vitamin B_{12} malabsorption include Crohn's disease, ileal resection, gluten enteropathy, tropical sprue, bacterial overgrowth syndromes, and fish tapeworm (*Diphyllobothrium latum*) infestation. Pancreatic insufficiency can also cause vitamin B_{12} malabsorption.

Vitamin B_{12} is usually labeled with cobalt-57 (Co-57). Co-57 has a physical half-life of 272 days and a 122-keV photopeak. An intramuscular flushing dose of unlabeled vitamin B_{12} is administered to saturate tissue and plasma binding sites, maximizing the renal excretion of absorbed cobalt-labeled vitamin B_{12}. Thus, the healthy person will absorb the labeled vitamin and excrete it in the urine through glomerular filtration. A urine collection is made for 24 hours and sometimes 48 hours.

Renal excretion of cobalt is not continuous and one or two missed samples in the collection could erroneously result in an abnormal result. The urine volume should be examined to ensure adequate function and collection. The 48-hour sample may be used in cases of poor renal function. A small sample is taken from the total collection and counted in a scintillation counter. The Schilling test measures the fraction of the administered dose that is excreted in the urine (normal, >9% in 24 hours).

The traditional approach first measures Co-57–labeled vitamin B_{12} excretion (stage I). If it is abnormal, the study is repeated (stage II) with the addition of IF. If excretion is abnormal without IF but increases significantly with IF, the diagnosis of pernicious anemia is confirmed. If both are abnormal, pernicious anemia is ruled out and the cause is small bowel malabsorption or pancreatic insufficiency. An alternative second or third stage can be performed (e.g., after antibiotic therapy for assumed bacterial overgrowth or with pancreatic enzyme replacement).

The second approach to the Schilling test administers vitamin B_{12} and IF simultaneously, with Co-58–labeled vitamin B_{12} and Co-57–labeled vitamin B_{12} bound to IF. The advantage of this method is convenience. The disadvantage of the dual method is scatter, making calculations more complex.

Intestinal Transit Scintigraphy

Small and large intestinal transit scintigraphy is not routine in most laboratories and optimal methods are still under investigation. This section is meant to provide a limited overview of the subject. A detailed review of methodologies for intestinal transit studies is listed under *Suggested Reading* (Maurer and Kevsky). Because a clinician may inquire regarding such a study, clinical indications,

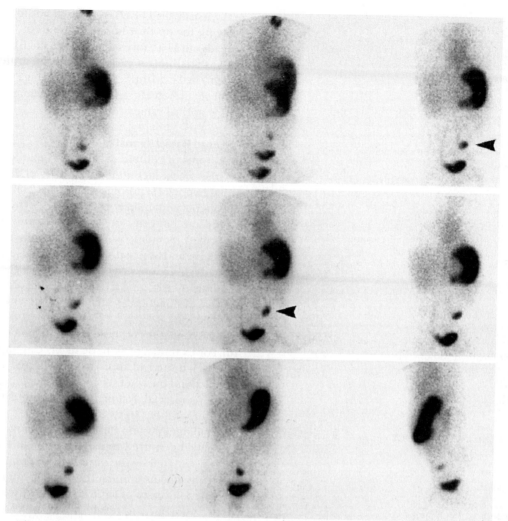

Figure 11-31   Meckel's diverticulum. A 7-year-old boy with rectal bleeding. Sequential images show focal uptake in left lower quadrant confirmed at surgery to be a Meckel's diverticulum (*arrowheads*). Note simultaneous rate of uptake of the Meckel's diverticulum and stomach. Motion artifact can be seen in second image.

nonscintigraphic methodologies, and scintigraphic methodologies are briefly reviewed.

Technical problems exist for accurately measuring intestinal transit. The radiolabeled meal must withstand the acidic environment of the stomach and the alkaline milieu of the small bowel. Quantification is more complex than for gastric emptying, where all the radiolabeled meal resides in the stomach at the start of the study and quantification depends only on the clearance rate. With intestinal transit, there is a protracted infusion from the stomach and no single time zero.

Small Bowel Transit

Chronic intestinal pseudo-obstruction, a disease of the enteric nervous system, has delayed gastric and small bowel motility. Small bowel transit may sometimes be altered in irritable bowel syndrome, although primarily a large bowel disease. Transit is typically faster through the small and large bowel in patients with irritable bowel syndrome with diarrhea and slower in patients with constipation.

Nonscintigraphic Methods

The *hydrogen breath test* measures hydrogen produced when a carbohydrate (C-14 lactose) is fermented by colonic bacteria. The test measures the transit time of the meal's leading edge from mouth to cecum, but is not an index of the transit of the meal's bulk. The transit rate is affected by the rate of gastric emptying. Fermentative bacteria in the colon are required but absent in one fourth of the population. The test is not widely available. A *small bowel barium follow-through study* is not quantitative, although mixing barium with food and plotting

Box 11-20   Causes for False-Positive Meckel's Scan

URINARY TRACT

Ectopic kidney
Extrarenal pelvis
Hydronephrosis
Vesicoureteral reflux
Horseshoe kidney
Bladder diverticulum

VASCULAR

Arteriovenous malformation
Hemangioma
Aneurysm of intraabdominal vessel
Angiodysplasia

OTHER AREAS OF ECTOPIC GASTRIC MUCOSA

Gastrogenic cyst
Enteric duplication
Duplication cysts
Barrett's esophagus
Retained gastric antrum
Pancreas
Duodenum
Colon

HYPEREMIA AND INFLAMMATORY

Peptic ulcer
Crohn's disease
Ulcerative colitis
Abscess
Appendicitis
Colitis

NEOPLASM

Carcinoma of sigmoid colon
Carcinoid
Lymphoma
Leiomyosarcoma

SMALL BOWEL OBSTRUCTION

Intussusception
Volvulus

its movement provides an index of the transit rate. The radiation dosimetry is relatively high compared to scintigraphic methods and the meal is nonphysiological.

Radionuclide Small Intestinal Transit

Small bowel transit can be measured most rapidly and accurately by direct placement of the radiotracer via intubation at the site of the proximal small bowel. However, this is invasive and not usually practical. Alternatively, transit can be measured using a liquid marker taken orally, usually In-111 DTPA, with or without a solid meal. Imaging for up to 4 hours is required. The radiolabel spreads out as it moves through the small bowel. That, as well as anatomical variation (e.g., identification of the cecum) make quantification challenging. Normal variability in small bowel transit variation makes it difficult to define normal values.

Large Bowel Transit

Symptoms of colonic dysmotility include constipation, diarrhea, fecal incontinence and lower abdominal pain. Irritable bowel syndrome is the most common diagnosis in patients with mild constipation.

Several patterns of abnormal motility have been described, including isolated anal sphincter dysfunction (adult onset Hirschsprung's disease), isolated rectosigmoid dysfunction, slow transit through the entire colon (colonic inertia), and a generalized disorder of gastrointestinal dysfunction as seen in chronic intestinal pseudo-obstruction.

Differentiation of these patterns can be clinically useful. For example, prokinetic drugs can improve colonic inertia. If a surgical approach is indicated, the procedure will depend on whether the entire colon, rectosigmoid, or only anorectal dysfunction is the problem.

Radiographic Methods

Cineradiography and fluoroscopy with radiopaque markers have been used to estimate transit times. Interpretation is limited by the infrequent abdominal images and difficulty in determining the exact location of the markers due to overlap of large and small bowel. The study is not physiologic and results in a relatively large radiation dose to the patient.

Large Bowel Transit Scintigraphy

The various different patterns of colonic transit described previously have been differentiated with scintigraphy. The study requires 72–96 hours, giving the radiotracer orally. In-111 DTPA has been most commonly used. Gallium-67 citrate has also been used as a measure of small and large intestinal transit. Given orally, Ga-67 is not absorbed from the bowel and 98% of the ingested dose is excreted in the feces.

Various other creative radiopharmaceuticals have been investigated that will not breakdown before reaching the large bowel (e.g., radiolabeled cellulose fiber). In-111 polystyrene cation exchange resin pellets have been placed in a gelatin capsule coated with a pH-sensitive polymer that resists disruption at pH levels of the stomach and proximal small bowel but breaks down at the ileocecal valve because of the increasing pH.

Various quantitative methods have been used (e.g., orocecal transit times or initial arrival times). Cecal arrival time has been defined as the time for accumulation of 10% of total abdominal counts in the cecum and

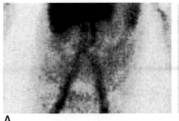
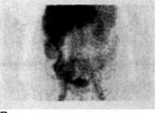
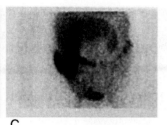

A   B   C

Figure 11-32 Protein-losing enteropathy. Patient received Tc-99m human serum albumin. Immediate **(A)**, 1-hour **(B)**, and 2-hour **(C)** images. Increasing activity is seen in the small bowel initially **(B)**, with subsequent transit to the colon **(C)**, consistent with protein-losing enteropathy.

ascending colon. More complicated methods of quantification have generally been used (e.g., determining the geometric center, which is a weighted average of the counts in each region of the bowel).

Protein-Losing Enteropathy

Excessive protein loss through the gastrointestinal tract has been associated with a variety of diseases, including intestinal lymphangiectasia, Crohn disease, Menetrier disease, amyloidosis, and intestinal fistula. The resulting hypoproteinemia can be a serious clinical problem.

Tc-99m human serum albumin, In-111 transferrin, and Tc-99m dextran have all been successfully used to scintigraphically confirm a protein-losing enteropathy. In-111 chloride binds in vivo to serum proteins, most notably transferring similarly to Ga-67, and abdominal imaging can be used to visualize the protein leak. Serial abdominal images show radiotracer collection in the small bowel in the first 30 minutes within increasing amounts over 24 hours (Fig. 11-32). None of these radiopharmaceuticals are available commercially in the United States.

SUGGESTED READING

Bunker SR, Lull RJ, Tanasescu DE, et al: Scintigraphy of gastrointestinal hemorrhage: superiority of 99mTc red blood cells over 99mTc sulfur colloid. AJR 143:543-548, 1984.

Camilleri M, Hasler W, Parkman HP, et al: Measurement of gastrointestinal motility in the GI laboratory. Gastroenterology 115:747-762, 1998.

Castronovo FP, Jr: Gastroesophageal scintiscanning in a pediatric population: dosimetry. J Nucl Med 27:1212-1214, 1986.

Datz FL: Considerations for accurately measuring gastric emptying. J Nucl Med 32:881-884, 1991.

Diamond RH, Rothstein RD, Alavi A: The role of cimetidine-enhanced Tc-99m pertechnetate imaging for visualizing Meckel's diverticulum. J Nucl Med 32:1422-1424, 1991.

Emslie JT, Zarnegar K, Siegel ME, et al: Technetium-99m-labeled red blood cell scans in the investigation of gastrointestinal bleeding. Dis Colon Rectum 39:750-754, 1996.

Fahey FH, Ziessman HA, Collin MJ, et al: Left anterior oblique projection and peak-to-scatter ratio for attenuation compensation of gastric emptying studies. J Nucl Med 30:233-239, 1989.

Heyman S: Pediatric nuclear gastroenterology: evaluation of gastroesophageal reflux and gastrointestinal bleeding. In Freeman LM, Weissman HS (eds): Nuclear Medicine Annual. New York, Raven Press, 1985.

Klein HA, Wald A: Esophageal transit scintigraphy. In Freeman LM, Weissman HS (eds): Nuclear Medicine Annual. New York, Raven Press, 1985.

Marianai G, Boni G, Barreca M, et al: Radionuclide gastroesophageal motor studies. J Nucl Med 45:1004-1028, 2004.

Maurer AH, Kevsky B: Whole-gut transit scintigraphy in the valuation of small bowel and colon transit disorders. Sem Nucl Med 25:326-338, 1995.

Sfakianakis GN, Haase GM: Abdominal scintigraphy for ectopic gastric mucosa: a retrospective analysis of 143 studies. AJR Am J Roentgenol 138:7-12, 1982.

Tougas G, Eaker EY, Abell TL, et al: Assessment of gastric emptying using a low fat meal: establishment of international control values. Am J Gastroenterology 95:1456-1462, 2000.

Winzelberg GG: Radionuclide evaluation of gastrointestinal bleeding. In Freeman LM (ed): Freeman and Johnson's Clinical Radionuclide Imaging, vol. 3. New York, Grune & Stratton, 1986.

Ziessman HA: Keep it simple—it's only gastric emptying. In Freeman LM (ed): Nuclear Medicine Annual. Philadelphia, Lippincott Williams & Wilkins, 2000.

Ziessman HA, Fahey FH, Atkins FB, Tall J: Standardization and quantification of radionuclide solid gastric-emptying studies. J Nucl Med 45:760-764, 2004.

Zuckier LS: Acute gastrointestinal bleeding. Sem Nuclear Medicine 33:297-311, 2003.

CHAPTER 12

Infection and Inflammation

Early identification and localization of infection is critical for the appropriate and timely selection of therapy. Computed tomography (CT), magnetic resonance imaging (MRI), and ultrasonography are often first-line imaging methods for detection and localization of infection. These methods are not always successful in finding the site of infection, particularly if the patient has no localizing symptoms or signs and if there is no focal fluid collection or morphological change. Postsurgical or posttherapeutic anatomic changes can make detection problematic.

Although developed in the early 1970s as a tumor-imaging agent, gallium-67 citrate (Ga-67) was noted to have an infection-seeking property. It remained the only infection-imaging radiopharmaceutical available until leukocytes labeled with indium-111 (In-111) were approved for clinical use in the mid-1980s. The next advance was radiolabeling leukocytes with technetium-99m (Tc-99m), with its better image quality and lower patient radiation.

Today, both In-111- and Tc-99-radiolabeled leukocytes are successfully used for infection scintigraphy. However, in vitro radiolabeling of leukocytes has drawbacks. Because of the time required for radiolabeling, reinfusion of the cells typically cannot be accomplished until 3–4 hours after their initial withdrawal. There is also concern for the potential transmission of bloodborne infections. Recently, a monoclonal antibody against surface antigens on granulocytes, Tc-99m fanolesomab (NeutroSpec), has been approved for clinical use. F-18 fluorodeoxyglucose (FDG) also has a potential role in infection imaging. New radiopharmaceuticals with various other mechanisms of uptake (e.g., peptides, cytokines) are under investigation (Box 12-1, Table 12-1).

PATHOPHYSIOLOGY OF INFLAMMATION AND INFECTION

Inflammation is a response of tissues to injury that attracts cells of the immune system, specialized serum proteins,

---

Box 12-1 Radiopharmaceuticals for Infection Imaging

CLINICAL USE

Gallium-67 citrate
Indium-111 oxine-labeled leukocytes
Technetium-99m HMPAO-labeled leukocytes
Tc-99m fanolesomab (NeutroSpec)
Tc-99m sulesomab (LeuTech) (approved in Europe)
F-18 fluorodeoxyglucose

INVESTIGATIONAL

Nonspecific IgG immunoglobulins
Tc-99m ciprofloxacin (Infecton)
Chemotactic peptides (interleukin-8)
Liposomes
Anti-E-selectin
Lymphocytes

Table 12-1 Inflammation Terminology

Mast cell	Tissue cell with basophilic granules containing vasoactive amines and heparin. Degranulates in response to injury
Prostaglandins, leukotrienes	Family of unsaturated fatty acids, components of most cell membranes. Responsible for induction of pain, fever, vascular permeability, chemotaxis of neutrophils
Vasoamines	Vasoactive amines that cause increased capillary permeability (e.g., histamine, 5-hydroxy-tryptamine, produced by mast cells, basophils, and platelets)
Kinin system	Series of serum peptides sequentially activated to cause vasodilation and increase permeability
Complement	Cascading sequence of serum proteins, activated directly or via antigen–antibody interaction
C3a and C5a	Stimulate release by mast cells of their vasoactive amines known as anaphylotoxins
Opsonization	C3b attached to particle promotes sticking to phagocytic cells because of their C3 receptors. Antibody, if present, augments this by binding to Fc receptors.
CRP	Acute phase protein made in liver, appears in serum within hours of tissue damage or infection. Binds to phosphorylcholine on bacterial surface, fixes complement, promotes phagocytosis.
Polymorphonuclear leukocyte (PMN)	The major mobile phagocytic cell, whose prompt arrival in tissues plays a vital part in removing invading bacteria
Monocyte	Precursor of tissue macrophages (MAC) responsible for removing damaged tissue and microorganisms. Tissue macrophages are an important source of inflammatory cytokines.
Lysosomal enzymes	Bactericidal enzymes released from the lysosomes of neutrophils, monocytes, macrophages
Inflammatory cytokines	Inflammatory response is coordinated by several cytokines produced by various cell types, including TNF-α, IL-6, and IL-1. All have many functions (e.g., initiating changes in vascular endothelium which promote leukocyte entry into an inflammatory site). They induce acute phase response and tissue repair.
Chemotaxis	C5a, C3a, leukotrienes and chemokines stimulate PMNs and monocytes to move into tissues. Movement towards the site of inflammation is called chemotaxis
Chemokines	Polypeptides that play a role in chemotaxis and regulation of leukocyte trafficking, e.g., interleukins (e.g., IL8).
Adhesion and cell traffic	Change in expression of endothelial surface molecules, induced by cytokines, cause PMNs, monocytes, and lymphocytes to adhere to vessel walls. These adhesion molecules and the molecules they bind fall into well-defined groups (selectins, integrins).
T-lymphocytes	Undergo blast transformation if stimulated by antigens, occurs in most infections. By releasing cytokines such as IFNλ, T cells greatly increase the activity of macrophages.
Clotting system	Intimately bound up with complement and kinins because of several shared activation steps. Blood clotting is a critical part of the healing process
Fibrin	The end product of blood clotting and in tissues, the matrix into which fibroblasts migrate to initiate healing.
Fibroblast	Tissue cell that migrates into the fibrin clot and secretes collagen.

Modified with permission from Playfair JHL and Chaim BM: Immunology at a Glance, ed. 7, Malden, MA, Blackwell Publishing, 2001.

and chemical mediators to the site of damage. Infection implies the presence of microorganisms. Although infection is almost always associated with inflammation, the reverse is not always true. The inflammatory reaction is triggered by the products of tissue injury which can also result from trauma, foreign particles, ischemia, and neoplasm. Infection can be present without inflammation, as in severely immunosuppressed patients.

The inflammatory response results in regionally increased blood flow, increased vascular permeability, and emigration of leukocytes out of the blood vessels into the tissues (chemotaxis). The plasma carries various proteins, antibodies, and chemical mediators that modulate the inflammatory response at the site of infection (Fig. 12-1, Table 12-1).

RADIOPHARMACEUTICALS

Gallium-67 Citrate

Ga-67 was developed initially as a bone-seeking radiopharmaceutical, found use as a tumor-imaging agent, and later was found to have infection-seeking properties. In the 1970s, Ga-67 was the mainstay of infection scintigraphy for over a decade. Although subsequently superceded by radiolabeled leukocytes in many clinical settings, Ga-67 still has important utility in selected clinical situations.

Chemistry and Physics

Gallium is a group III element in the Periodic Table (*see* Fig. 1-1) with atomic structure and biological behavior similar to iron (ferric ion). The radionuclide Ga-67 is cyclotron produced. It decays by electron capture, emits a spectrum of gamma rays (93, 185, 288, 394 keV), and has a physical half-life of 78 hours (Table 12-2).

Mechanism of Uptake

The radiopharmaceutical Ga-67 citrate circulates in plasma bound to the protein transferrin. The Ga-67 transferrin complex is transported to the inflammatory site because of locally increased blood flow and vascular permeability (Box 12-2). Localization at the site of infection is to a large extent secondary to its ferric ion-like properties.

Sites of inflammation contain iron-binding compounds (e.g., lactoferrin released by leukocytes) and siderophores elaborated by bacteria. After migration to an inflammatory site, neutrophils release large amounts of lactoferrin. Ga-67, with a higher binding affinity for lactoferrin than transferrin, localizes at the site of inflammation by

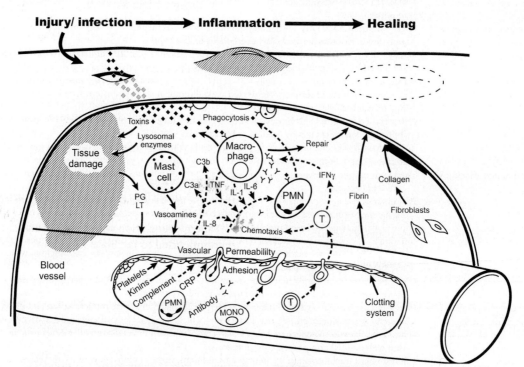

Figure 12-1 Pathophysiology of inflammation. This simplified schema illustrates the body's response to tissue injury or infection. Permeability of the vascular endothelium plays a central role in allowing blood cells and serum components access to the tissues. Antibodies and lymphocytes amplify or focus these primary mechanisms. If inflammation persists beyond a few days, macrophages and lymphocytes play an increasing role. See Table 12-1 for explanations of inflammation terminology. (Modified with permission from Playfair JHL and Chaim BM: Immunology at a Glance, ed. 7, Malden, MA, Blackwell Publishing, 2001.)

dissociating from transferrin and binding to lactoferrin. There is lesser Ga-67 uptake by bacterial siderophores.

Pharmacokinetics and Distribution
Ga-67 clears slowly from the blood pool. At 24, 48, and 72 hours after injection, approximately 20%, 10%, and 5%, respectively, of the tracer is still bound to plasma

Table 12-2 Physical Characteristics of Gallium-67 (Ga-67), Indium-111, (In-111) and Technetium-99m (Tc-99m)

Radionuclide	Half-life (hr)	Photopeak (keV)	Relative abundance of photons (%)
Ga-67	78	93	41
		185	23
		288	18
		394	4
In-111	67	173	89
		247	94
Tc-99m	6	140	89

Box 12-2 Mechanisms of Localization of Infection-Seeking Radiopharmaceuticals

Radiopharmaceutical	Mechanism
Gallium-67 citrate	Vascular permeability, binding to lactoferrin
Leukocytes	Diapedesis and chemotaxis
Nonspecific IgG antibodies	Increased vascularity, nonimmunological
Antigranulocyte monoclonal antibodies	Antibody-antigen binding to activated leukocytes
Chemotactic peptides	Binding to activated leukocytes
Tc-99m ciprofloxacin	Binds to living bacteria
Liposomes	Increased vascular permeability

proteins. It becomes firmly bound at the site of infection by 12–24 hours. Of the injected dose, 15–25% is excreted via the kidneys by 24 hours. Although some further renal excretion occurs, the colon then becomes the major route of excretion. Total body clearance is slow, with a biological half-life of approximately 25 days.

The distribution of Ga-67 is widespread (Table 12-3). Soft-tissue uptake outlines the body. Liver has by far the highest uptake, perhaps because of its metabolism of transferrin and lactoferrin (Figs. 12-2 and 12-3). Uptake is normal in the bone marrow and bone, and to a more variable extent in the spleen, salivary, and lacrimal glands. Lacrimal glands, salivary glands, and the breasts all elaborate lactoferrin. Inflammatory or stimulatory processes in these organs increase production and result in increased Ga-67 uptake, (e.g., increased uptake is seen in the salivary glands in Sjögren's syndrome, the lacrimal glands in sarcoidosis [Fig. 12-4A], and the breast during lactation [Fig. 12-5]).

Ga-67 distribution can be altered by an excess of carrier gallium and whole-body irradiation. Excess ferric ion from multiple blood transfusions and recent gadolinium exposure, a MRI contrast agent, also may alter biodistribution by saturation of the protein-binding sites. The resulting Ga-67 scan may look more like a bone scan (Fig. 12-6).

Imaging Characteristics
Ga-67 is not an optimal radionuclide imaging agent. It emits four photopeaks ranging from approximately 100 to 400 keV, all with relatively low abundance (Table 12-2). The lower-energy photons result in a high percentage of scatter relative to usable photons. The higher-energy photons are difficult to collimate and are not efficiently detected by present-day thin gamma camera crystals. To maximize detection, the three lower photopeaks (93, 185, and 300 keV) are usually acquired.

Methodology
Box 12-3 describes a standard Ga-67 infection imaging protocol.

Patient preparation with laxatives and enemas has been recommended to facilitate more rapid bowel clearance. Evidence for its effectiveness is limited. In many clinics,

Table 12-3 Normal Distribution of Radiopharmaceuticals Used for Infection Imaging

Radiopharmaceutical	Liver	Spleen	Marrow	Bone	Gastro-intestinal	Genito-urinary	Lung
Gallium-67 citrate	***	*	*	*	***		
Indium-111 oxine leukocytes	**	***	**				*
Technetium-99m HMPAO leukocytes	**	***	**		**	**	*
Antigranulocyte monoclonal antibodies	**	*	***		**		
Nonspecific IgG antibodies	***	**	**		*	*	*

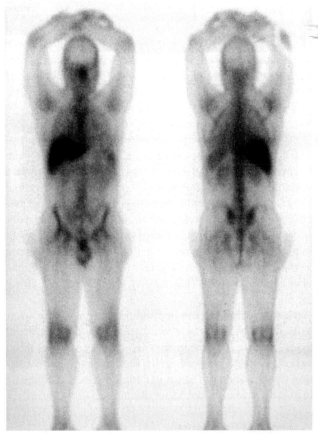

Figure 12-2 Normal gallium-67 distribution (male). Imaging at 48 hours after injection shows highest uptake in the liver, followed by bone and bone marrow. Lesser uptake is seen in the spleen, scrotum and nasopharyngeal region. Mild uptake is noted in the kidneys, and some intestinal clearance is noted. Inflammatory arthritic changes are present in the knees.

they are prescribed as needed. Vigorous bowel cleansing has been reported to cause mucosal irritation and inflammation, which may result in increased Ga-67 uptake.

The usual administered adult dose for planar imaging is 185 MBq (5 mCi), although sometimes higher doses of 278 MBq (7.5 mCi) are administered if single-photon emission computed tomography (SPECT) imaging is anticipated. This dose is lower than that typically used for tumor imaging (10 mCi [370 MBq]), where the radiation dose is of lesser concern.

Whole-body imaging or limited-spot imaging may be done as clinically indicated. A medium-energy collimator is standard. Images are usually acquired at 48 hours, which allows time for background clearance and an improved target-to-background ratio. Imaging at 24 hours may be useful in patients with suspected abscess where early diagnosis allows for prompt intervention. Imaging the abdomen at 24 hours can also help in differentiating physiological bowel clearance from infection. Abdominal

activity not seen at 24 hours but seen at 48 hours likely is due to normal bowel clearance and not a site of acute infection. However, 24-hour images are not standard and the usual approach, when this question arises, is to give laxatives and obtain delayed imaging at 72–96 hours.

Normal Scintigraphy

Diffuse lung uptake of moderate degree is often present at 24 hours but usually clears by 48 hours. The kidneys and bladder are seen during the first 24 hours after tracer injection owing to normal renal clearance. Subsequently, biological clearance is through the large bowel. By 48–72 hours, the kidneys are normally only faintly visualized.

The organ with the greatest Ga-67 uptake at 48-hour imaging is the liver. Lesser uptake is seen in the spleen. Bone and bone marrow can be seen throughout the axial and proximal appendicular skeleton (*see* Figs. 12-2 and 12-3). Other normal sites of more variable uptake are the nasopharynx, the lacrimal and salivary glands, and the breast. The latter depends to some extent on the phase of the woman's hormonal cycle (*see* Fig. 12-3) and is particularly prominent postpartum (*see* Fig. 12-5). Thymus uptake is normal in children (Figs. 12-7 and 12-8). The scrotum, testes, and female perineum may have some uptake.

Postoperative sites may have Ga-67 uptake for 2–3 weeks. Ga-67 can be seen in sterile abscesses associated with frequent intramuscular injections (e.g., insulin injection sites) and iron-depot injections. Increased salivary gland uptake occurs after local external beam irradiation or chemotherapy.

Dosimetry

The highest radiation absorbed dose (rad) from Ga-67 is to the large intestine, 3.7 cGy/185 MBq (3.7 rads/5 mCi). Slow transit accounts for the high radiation dose. The marrow receives 3.5 cGy (rads) and the liver 2.2 cGy (2.2 rads). The whole-body dose is 2.2 cGy/185 MBq (2.2 rads/5 mCi) (Table 12-4).

Radiolabeled Leukocytes

Radiolabeled leukocytes have been used for three decades for detection of infection and inflammation. Both In-111 oxine and Tc-99m HMPAO labeled white blood cells are in current clinical use.

Leukocyte Physiology

Leukocytes are the major cellular components of the inflammatory and immune response that protect against infection and neoplasia and assist in the repair of damaged tissue. Nucleated precursor cells differentiate into mature cells within the bone marrow. The normal blood leukocyte count of $4.5–11.0 \times 10^6$ cells/mm^3 includes granulocytes (neutrophils, 55–65%; eosinophils, 3%; and

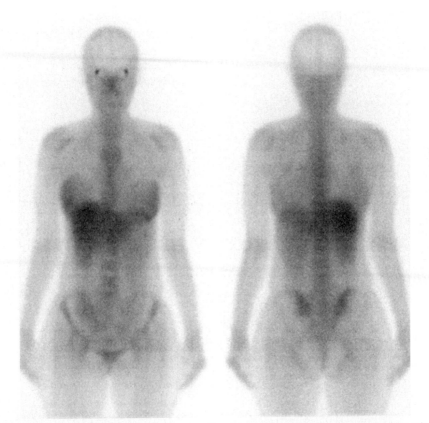

Figure 12-3   Normal gallium-67 distribution (female). Distribution at 48 hours is similar to the male in Fig. 12-2, except for the addition of breast uptake. In this case, there is also more prominent but normal lacrimal uptake and bowel activity.

basophils, 0.5%), lymphocytes (25–35%) and monocytes (3–7%). Leukocytes spend a small part of their short lifespan in the peripheral blood, using it mainly for transportation to sites of need.

Neutrophils circulate in the peripheral blood for 5–9 hours. They respond to an acute inflammatory stimulus by migrating toward an attractant (chemotaxis) and enter tissues between postcapillary endothelial cells (diapedesis) (*see* Fig. 12-1). They phagocytose the infectious agent or foreign body and enzymatically destroy it within cytoplasmic vacuoles. These actions are inhibited by exposure to corticosteroids or ethanol. Leukocytes survive in tissues for only 2–3 days.

At any one time, only 2–3% of *neutrophils* reside in the circulating blood. The rest are distributed in a "marginated" pool that is adherent to vascular endothelial cells in tissues: 90% are in the bone marrow, the rest are in the spleen, liver, lung, and, to a lesser extent, the gastrointestinal tract and oropharynx. These marginated cells can be marshaled into the circulating pool by various stimuli, including exercise, epinephrine, or exposure to bacterial endotoxin. *Basophils*, also granulocytes, release histamine, serotonin, and leukotrienes in inflammation, and they are involved in allergic responses. *Eosinophils* are particularly increased with parasitic infections.

Lymphocytes arrive at inflammatory sites during the chronic phase of an inflammatory response. *Monocytes* act as tissue scavengers, phagocytosing damaged cells and bacteria and detoxifying chemicals and toxins. At sites of inflammation, monocytes transform into tissue *macrophages*.

Indium-111 Oxine Leukocytes

In 1976, McAfee and Thakur first radiolabeled leukocytes with In-111 8-hydroxyquinoline (oxine). Many investigations over the years have confirmed the radiopharmaceutical's clinical utility. The scintigraphic images reflect the distribution of white blood cells

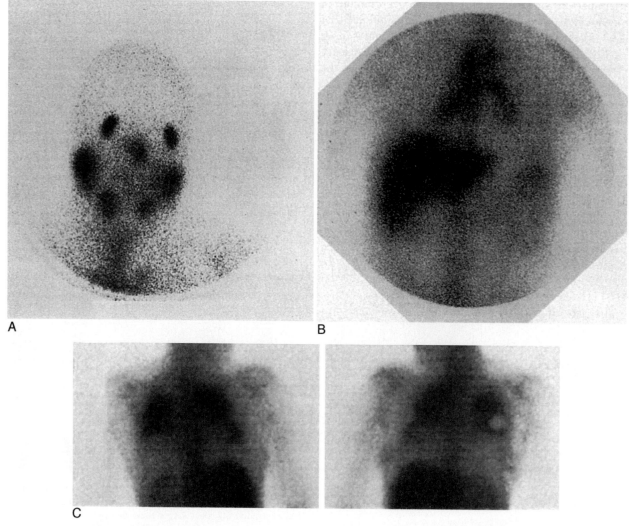

Figure 12-4 Sarcoidosis. **A,** Panda sign. Prominent increased uptake in the lacrimal, parotid and submandibular salivary glands. Nasal uptake is also prominent. **B,** Lambda sign. Paratracheal and hilar nodal uptake seen with early active sarcoidosis. **C,** Parenchymal pulmonary uptake. Upper lobes diffusely involved.

within the body, as well as localization at the site of infection or inflammation.

Indium is a group III element in the Periodic Table (*see* Fig. 1-1). The radionuclide In-111 is cyclotron produced. It decays by electron capture, emits two gamma photons of 173 and 247 keV (*see* Table 12-2), and has a physical half-life of 67 hours (2.8 days).

Oxine (8-hydroxyquinolone) is a lipid-soluble complex that chelates metal ions such as indium. As described in the next section, labeling leukocytes with oxine cannot be done in plasma. Alternatives to oxine have been developed that allow for labeling in plasma (e.g., tropolone and mercaptopyridine-N-oxide [MERC]), but they are not approved by the Food and Drug Administration (FDA).

Fifty mL of venous blood ensures sufficient numbers of radiolabeled leukocytes, although adequate labeling can often be accomplished with 20–30 mL, which is important for children. Careful handling is required to avoid damaging the cells, which otherwise might result in loss of their ability to migrate or even their viability. Proper labeling does not adversely affect normal physiological function, and the radiolabel usually remains stable in vivo for over 24 hours.

The higher the serum leukocyte count, the more likely that labeling efficiency will be high. Ideally the patient's leukocyte count should be >5000/mm^3, although diagnostic scintigraphy can often be performed with patient counts as low as 3000/mm^3.

Because In-111 is cyclotron produced, it usually must be ordered the day prior to cell labeling. Radiolabeling should be performed in a well-equipped laboratory with a laminar flow hood. The in vitro labeling procedure

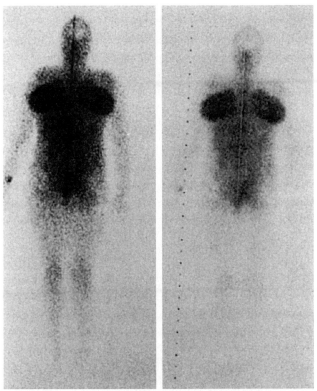

Figure 12-5 Postpartum gallium-67 breast uptake. The increased production of lactoferrin results in prominent postpartum breast uptake. Although some uptake is normal in the non-lactating female (*see* Fig. 12-3), it is considerably less and quite variable, dependent on the normal hormonal cycle. Two intensity settings are shown.

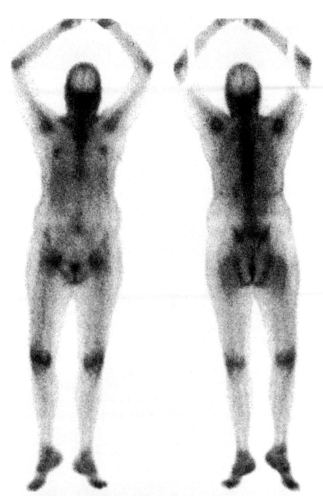

Figure 12-6 Abnormal gallium-67 distribution. This patient received chemotherapy the day before administration, an unusual situation and likely the cause of these findings. Almost no uptake is seen in the liver, the organ normally having greatest Ga-67 uptake. This has also been reported in patients with multiple blood transfusions or recent gadolinium contrast administration with MRI.

requires a minimum of 2 hours. Lacking facilities and trained personnel, most hospitals send the patient's blood to an outside commercial pharmacy for radiolabeling. Thus, it may be 3–4 hours before the cells are reinfused. The longer the interval between blood withdrawal and reinfusion, the higher the likelihood is that the cells will lose viability.

Details of the radiolabeling process are described in Box 12-4. The patient's withdrawn blood is allowed to settle, and the majority of the erythrocytes are removed. In-111 oxine indiscriminately labels granulocytes, lymphocytes, monocytes, platelets, erythrocytes, and also plasma transferrin. Thus the plasma must be separated and removed from the cells by centrifugation to ensure preferential cell labeling. It is kept for later resuspension of the leukocytes before reinfusion.

The leukocyte pellet is suspended in normal saline and incubated with In-111 oxine. The lipid solubility of the In-111 oxine complex allows it to diffuse through cell membranes. Intracellularly, the complex dissociates. Oxine diffuses back out of the cell, whereas In-111 binds to nuclear and cytoplasmic proteins.

Pure granulocyte preparations have been radiolabeled; however, they require elaborate density gradient separation techniques and have not shown a clear clinical advantage. Thus, they are not generally used.

Standard quality control measures (e.g., testing for sterility and pyrogenicity) cannot be performed because of the need for prompt reinfusion after labeling to ensure cell viability. However, the final radiopharmaceutical preparation is examined for abnormal morphology, clumping, and excessive red cell contamination. The final preparation contains predominantly radiolabeled granulocytes, lymphocytes, and monocytes, but there will also be 10–20% platelets and erythrocytes. The percent of labeling efficiency is routinely determined (*see* Box 12-3). Typical labeling efficiency ranges from 75–90%. When it is <50%, the cells should probably not be reinfused.

The ultimate test of viability of leukocytes is their in vivo function manifested by a normal distribution

---

Box 12-3 Gallium-67 Citrate Imaging: Protocol Summary

PATIENT PREPARATION

No recent barium contrast studies

RADIOPHARMACEUTICAL

Gallium-67 citrate, 185 MBq (5 mCi) injected
  intravenously

INSTRUMENTATION

Camera: Large-field-of-view gamma camera
Photopeak: 20% window over 93 keV, 185 keV, and
  300-keV photopeaks
Collimator: Medium energy

IMAGING PROCEDURE

24-hr images (optional): Site of suspected infection if
  early intervention considered; abdominal images may
  be helpful for interpreting activity seen at 48 hours
48-hr images: Whole body imaging, including head and
  extremities, unless the site of suspected infection is
  limited to one site, e.g., hip prosthesis
Delayed 72- to 96-hr images of abdomen as indicated
  to differentiate intraabdominal infection from normal
  bowel clearance; laxatives or enemas as needed
SPECT of the abdomen, pelvis, or chest as indicated

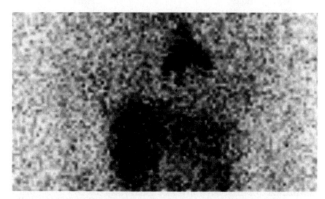

Figure 12-7 Thymus uptake of Ga-67. This child's malignant lymphoma responded to chemotherapy. On this follow-up Ga-67 study, the coronal SPECT cross-sectional slice shows thymus uptake. Thymus uptake may be seen normally in children.

within the body and their ability to detect infection. If the infused leukocytes become nonviable, as might result from an interval greater than 4 hours between labeling and reinfusion, increased liver and lung uptake is typically seen on scintigraphy. With excessive erythrocyte and platelet labeling, blood pool is prominent.

After infusion of the radiolabeled leukocytes, no significant elution of the In-111 from the leukocytes occurs.

The effective half-life of clearance from the blood circulation is 7.5 hours.

Initial distribution after reinfusion is seen in blood pool, lungs, liver, and spleen. Lung activity is the result of cellular activation from in vitro cell manipulation. By 4 hours after reinjection, lung activity and blood pool normally decrease, although not always completely (Fig. 12-9). By 24 hours, blood-pool activity is not normally present. Persistent blood pool at 24 hours indicates a high percentage of labeled erythrocytes or platelets.

At 24 hours, the most intense uptake is seen in the spleen, followed by the liver and then the bone marrow (see Fig. 12-9). Neither genitourinary nor bowel activity is normally seen. Table 12-3 compares this normal organ distribution of radiolabeled leukocytes with other infection-seeking scintigraphic agents.

The spleen receives the highest radiation-absorbed dose, approximately 15–20 cGy/18.5 MBq (15–20 rads/500 µCi) in adults, but up to 30–50 cGy (rads) in small children (Table 12-4). In addition to gamma emissions, In-111 emits low-energy conversion and Auger electrons of 0.6–25.4 keV with a short range in tissue that can damage labeled cells. Neutrophils are not typically damaged; however, because lymphocytes are more radiosensitive and longer-lived, there is a theoretical concern for possible mutagenic and oncogenic effects. Data are limited. The high splenic radiation dose is the reason In-111 leukocytes are rarely used in children.

Imaging Methodology

A typical imaging protocol for In-111 oxine leukocytes is detailed in Box 12-5. Both the 173- and 247-keV photopeaks are acquired. A medium-energy collimator is used. Whole-body imaging is routine, although high-count spot images and SPECT are acquired when needed.

Images are routinely acquired 18–24 hours after radiopharmaceutical injection (Box 12-6). This allows sufficient time for leukocyte localization and blood pool clearance. Further delayed images do not often give additional information. Earlier imaging (e.g., at 4 hours) is less sensitive than 24 hours for detecting infection but may occasionally be useful for urgent diagnosis (e.g., an abscess that requires prompt intervention).

Four-hour imaging is mandatory for the localization of inflammatory bowel disease because the inflamed mucosal cells slough, become intraluminal, and move distally. Twenty-four hour images may provide misleading and erroneous information as to the site of inflammation. Fixed activity between 4- and 24-hour images would suggest an abscess as a complication of the inflammatory bowel disease.

In some cases, diagnostic accuracy is improved by performing an additional scintigraphic study for direct correlation using a different radionuclide with a different mechanism of uptake. In current practice, the most common one is a Tc-99m sulfur colloid (Tc-99m SC)

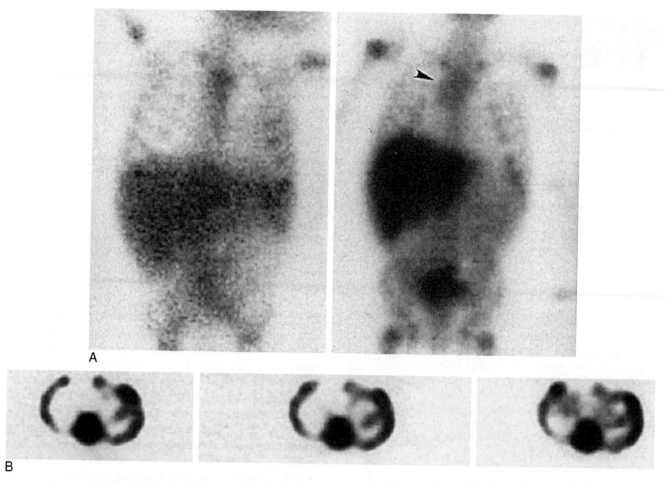

A

B

Figure 12-8   Gallium-67 uptake in heart in myocarditis and thymus. A 20-month-old child received azathioprine and steroids for treatment of idiopathic myocarditis. **A,** *Left,* Pre-therapy planar image of the chest showed no abnormal uptake. *Right,* Post-therapy planar image shows prominent uptake by the thymus (*arrowhead*). **B,** In contrast to the planar study, the pretherapy SPECT study showed myocardial uptake (best seen on middle image). Three sequential transverse slices through the myocardium are shown.

Table 12-4   Radiation Dosimetry for Ga-67 Citrate, In-111 Oxine and Tc-99m HMPAO Leukocytes (WBCs)

Organ	Ga-67 citrate cGy/185 MBq or rad/5 mCi	In-111 oxine WBCs cGy/18.5 MBq or rad/500 μCi	Tc-99m HMPAO WBCs cGy/370 MBq or rad/10 mCi
Bladder wall			**2.8**
Large intestine	**3.7**		**3.6**
Liver	2.2	2.66	1.5
Bone marrow	3.5	1.99	1.6
Spleen	1.8	**20.00**	2.2
Ovaries	1.5	0.20	0.3
Testes	1.0	0.014	1.9
Total body	2.2	0.37	0.3

WBCs, White blood cells.
Target organ dose is in bold.

bone-marrow scan. Dual-isotope studies require special attention to the imaging characteristics of the radionuclides (e.g., photopeaks, half-lives, downscatter, the relative administered doses, and the camera's capability for simultaneous multichannel acquisition).

The problem of downscatter or upscatter should be considered. One approach is to perform the Tc-99m scan first because of its shorter half-life. By 24 hours, 94% of the Tc-99m activity will have decayed. Blood required for In-111 leukocyte labeling could be drawn prior to injection of the Tc-99m tracer and the In-111 radiolabeled cells reinfused after acquiring the Tc-99m scan. In-111 leukocyte scintigraphy would be acquired the next day.

An alternative approach is to acquire both studies simultaneously, using a dual-isotope acquisition technique. This approach ensures identically positioned images for direct comparison. One approach to minimize upscatter from Tc-99m is to acquire only the upper 247-keV photopeak of In-111. Alternatively, one could

Box 12-4 Radiolabeling Autologous Leukocytes with Indium-111 Oxine

PREPARATION

Patient's peripheral leukocyte count should be greater than 5000 cells/mm^3.

PROCEDURE

1. Collect autologous blood:
   Draw 30 to 50 ml into an ACD anticoagulated syringe using a 19-gauge needle.
2. Isolate leukocytes:
   Separate red blood cells (RBCs) by gravity sedimentation and 6% Hetastarch, a settling agent.
   Centrifuge the leukocyte-rich plasma (LRP) at 300 to 350 *g* for 5 min to remove platelets and proteins.
   A white blood cell (WBC) button forms at the bottom of the tube.
   Draw off and save the leukocyte-poor plasma (LPP) for later washing and resuspension.
3. Label leukocytes:
   Suspend WBCs (LRP) in saline (includes granulocytes, lymphocytes, monocytes, and some RBCs).
   Incubate with In-111 oxine for 30 min at room temperature and gently agitate.
   Remove unbound In-111 by centrifugation. Save wash for later calculation of labeling efficiency.
4. Prepare injectate:
   Resuspend 500 µmCi In-111 leukocytes in saved plasma (LPP).
   Inject via peripheral vein within 2 to 4 hr.
5. Perform quality control:
   Microscopic examination of cells.
   Calculate labeling efficiency:
   Assay the cells and wash in dose calibrator.
   Labeling efficiency = $C/([C + W] \times 100\%)$
   C, activity associated with the cells; *W*, activity associated with the wash.

acquire a narrow window for the lower 173-keV photopeak. Downscatter of In-111 into the Tc-99m window is not a significant problem because of the low activity of In-111 (500 µCi) used compared to Tc-99m (20 mCi).

Image Interpretation

Activity outside the expected normal distribution of leukocytes suggests infection (Figs. 12-10 to 12-16). Focal uptake equal to or greater than that of the liver is typical for an abscess. Activity equal to the liver generally signifies a clinically important inflammatory site; activity less than bone marrow suggests a low-level inflammatory response.

One should keep in mind interpretive pitfalls and potential false-positive and false-negative findings with leukocyte scintigraphy (Box 12-7). Leukocytes may accumulate at sites of inflammation without clinical infection (e.g., intravenous catheters; nasogastric, endogastric, and drainage tubes; tracheostomies; colostomies; and ileostomies). Unless very intense, this uptake should not be considered abnormal. Uninfected postsurgical wounds commonly show faint uptake for up to 2 weeks. If uptake is intense, persists, or extends beyond the surgical wound site, infection should be suspected (Fig. 12-12). Low-grade uptake may be seen at healing bone-fracture sites.

Activity seen within the abdomen may be due to a variety of causes not due to infection and thus have the potential for misinterpretation. These include pseudo-aneurysm, noninfected hematomas, and accessory spleens (Fig. 12-17). Renal transplants normally accumulate radiolabeled leukocytes.

Even intraluminal intestinal activity can be the result of swallowed or shedding cells that occur with herpes esophagitis, pharyngitis, sinusitis, pneumonia, or gastrointestinal bleeding (Fig. 12-18). Very rarely, tumors have uptake.

Technetium-99m HMPAO Labeled Leukocytes

Leukocytes labeled with Tc-99m have a number of advantages over In-111 leukocytes (Table 12-5). Being generator produced, Tc-99m is available when needed. The radiation absorbed dose to the patient is much lower, which is particularly important for pediatric patients. The greater activity that can be administered results in a higher photon yield and better image quality. The more optimal Tc-99m photopeak results in superior image quality. This all potentially translates into improved infection detectability.

The element technetium is in group VIIB of the Periodic Table (*see* Fig. 1-1). The radionuclide Tc-99m is generator-produced from molybdenum-99. It decays by isomeric transition, emits one gamma photon of 140 keV (*see* Table 12-1), and has a physical half-life of 6 hours.

Tc-99m hexamethyl-propylene-amine oxime (Tc 99m HMPAO; Ceretec, Mediphysics) was initially approved by the FDA for cerebral perfusion imaging. HMPAO is lipophilic, allowing it to cross cell membranes. In the cerebral cortex, after crossing the blood–brain barrier, it is taken up intracellularly in cortical cells. Intracellularly, Tc-99m HMPAO changes into a hydrophilic complex and becomes trapped, bound to the mitochondria and the nucleus. This observation led to the development of a labeling technique for leukocytes using Tc-99m HMPAO.

With Tc-99m HMPAO labeled leukocytes, the colon is the organ receiving the highest radiation dose (3.6 cGy/370 MBq [3.6 rads/10 mCi]), followed by the bladder and spleen (2.2 cGy/MBq [2.2 rads/10 mCi])

4 hours   ## 24 hours

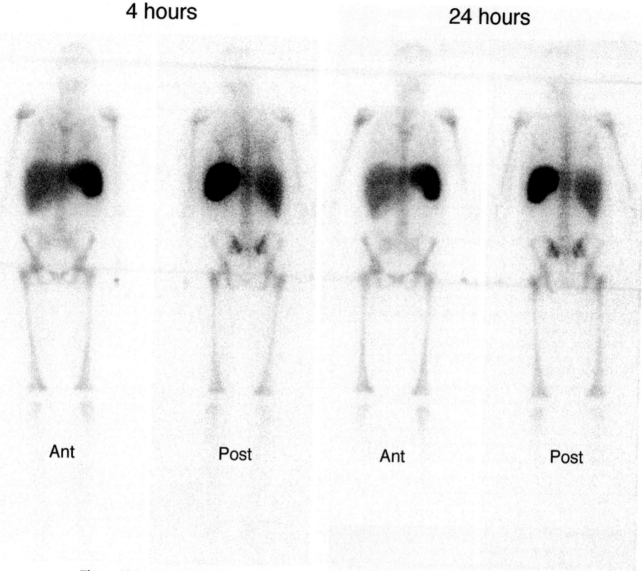

Ant   Post   Ant   Post

Figure 12-9   Normal distribution of indium-111 oxine leukocytes at 4 and 24 hours. Anterior and posterior whole-body images. The highest uptake is seen in the spleen, followed by the liver, then the bone marrow. No intestinal or renal activity is present which is normal. The 4-hour images show some lung uptake that resolves by 24 hours. There is no other apparent change in distribution between 4 and 24 hours.

(*see* Table 12-4). Unlike In-111, there is no concern regarding potential direct radiation damage to leukocytes.

The methodology for leukocyte radiolabeling with Tc-99m HMPAO was described in 1986 and is very similar to that used for labeling leukocytes with In-111 oxine. In contrast to In-111 oxine, Tc-99m HMPAO leukocyte labeling can be performed in plasma. HMPAO preferentially labels granulocytes, a potential advantage for imaging acute purulent processes. The radiolabeling process does not adversely affect leukocyte function. The FDA views Tc-99m HMPAO–labeled leukocytes as an acceptable alternative use of an approved radiopharmaceutical.

The biological half-life of Tc-99m HMPAO labeled leukocytes in blood is shorter than that of In-111 oxine leukocytes (4 hours versus 6 hours) due to the slow elution of the Tc-99m HMPAO from circulating labeled cells.

Tc-99m HMPAO–labeled leukocytes distribute in the body similar to In-111 oxine leukocytes, with localization in the spleen, kidney, and bone marrow (Fig. 12-19). Early lung uptake similar to that seen with In-111 oxine occurs but also decreases by 4 hours. Unlike In-111-oxine–labeled cells, Tc-99m HMPAO leukocytes are partially cleared by the hepatobiliary and renal systems with excretion of a secondary hydrophilic complex, which also occurs with Tc-99m HMPAO cerebral perfusion

Box 12-5   Indium-111 Oxine Leukocyte Scintigraphy: Protocol Summary

RADIOPHARMACEUTICAL

In-111 oxine in vitro labeled leukocytes, 500 µCi (18.5 MBq)

INSTRUMENTATION

Camera: Large field of view
Windows: 20% centered over 173 and 247 keV photopeaks
Collimator: Medium energy

PATIENT PREPARATION

Draw 50 ml of blood. Radiolabel cells in vitro (Box 12-3)

PROCEDURE

Inject labeled cells intravenously, preferably by direct venipuncture through a 19-gauge needle. Contact with dextrose in water solutions may cause cell damage.
Imaging at 4 hr may be helpful to diagnose an acute abscess and is critical in localizing inflammatory bowel disease.
Perform routine whole body imaging at 24 hr.
Acquire anterior abdomen for 500k counts, then other images for equal time. Include anterior and posterior views of the chest, abdomen, and pelvis, and spot images of specific areas of interest (e.g., feet) for a minimum of 200k counts or 20 min.
Perform SPECT in selected cases.

Box 12-6   Optimal Imaging Time for Infection-Seeking Radiopharmaceuticals

Radiopharmaceutical	Time (hr)
Gallium-67	48
Indium-111 leukocytes	24
Nonspecific IgG antibodies	10–24
Antigranulocyte monoclonal antibodies	1–6
Technetium-99m HMPAO leukocytes	1–4
Chemotactic peptides	1–4
Technetium-99m nanocolloids	1
Fluorine-18 fluorodeoxyglucose	1

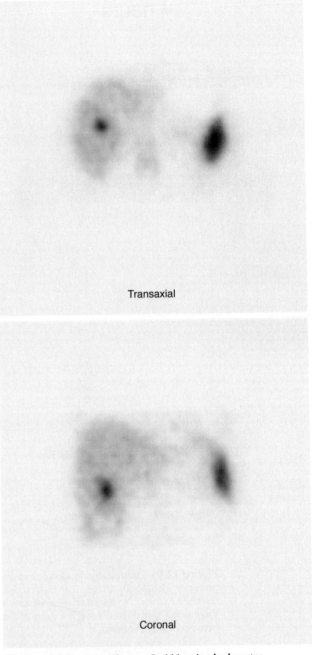

Transaxial

Coronal

Figure 12-10   Liver abscess: In-111 oxine leukocytes. Transverse (*above*) and coronal (*below*) cross-sectional SPECT slices with focal uptake of leukocytes in the right lobe of the liver. An abscess was subsequently drained.

Imaging Methodology

The imaging methodology is somewhat different for Tc-99m HMPAO than for In-111 oxine labeled leukocytes because of its shorter physical half-life and its hepatobiliary and urinary clearance. A detailed protocol is described (Box 12-8). Imaging of the abdomen should be performed between 1 and 2 hours after reinfusion in order to avoid hepatobiliary and urinary clearance (*see* Box 12-5). Four-hour imaging is preferable for peripheral extremities.

imaging. The kidneys and bladder may be seen by 1–2 hours after injection. The gallbladder is visualized in 4% of patients at 1 hour and in about 10% by 24 hours. Biliary clearance may be seen as early as 2 hours and bowel activity is routinely visualized by 3–4 hours and increase with time.

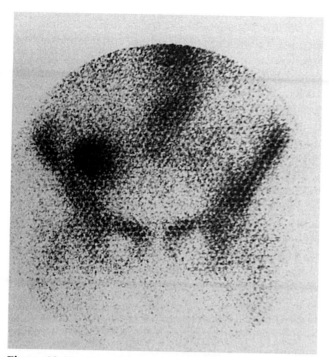

Figure 12-11 Intra-abdominal abscess: In-111 oxine leukocytes. Anterior view of pelvis. Focal uptake in the right lower quadrant caused by a perforated appendix with abscess formation.

Considerable blood-pool activity is commonly seen because of the early imaging period of Tc-99m HMPAO leukocytes compared to In-111 oxine leukocytes, which may complicate interpretation, particularly in the chest. The high count rate of Tc-99m allows for better SPECT quality than In-111. Delayed imaging up to 24 hours may be useful on occasion (Fig. 12-20).

Image Interpretation

The discussion under In-111 oxine leukocytes applies here. The only difference is the biliary and genitourinary excretion of the Tc-99m HMPAO. Uptake outside that expected for normal distribution suggests infection (Fig. 12-21). Relative advantages of Tc-99m HMPAO versus In-111 oxine leukocytes are listed in Table 12-5. These will be discussed further.

Technetium-99m Fanolesomab (NeutroSpec)

Alternative infection-seeking radiopharmaceuticals have been sought that do not require cell labeling and would not have the potential for transmission of bloodborne diseases. An antigranulocyte monoclonal antibody, Tc-99m fanolesomab (NeutroSpec, Mallinckrodt), was approved by the FDA in 2004 for scintigraphy in patients with equivocal signs and symptoms of acute appendicitis.

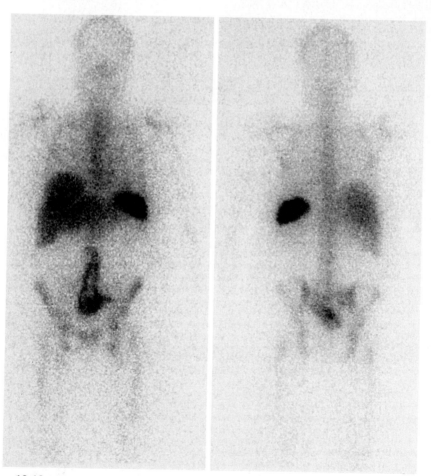

Figure 12-12 Postoperative wound infection: In-111 oxine leukocytes. Dehiscence of the incision site because of an abscess inferior and deep to incision. Note the more intense uptake inferiorly.

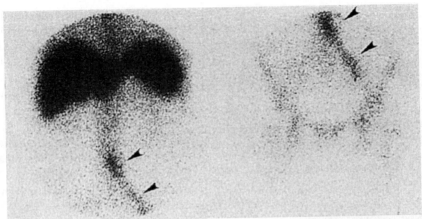

Figure 12-13   Infected aortofemoral graft: In-111 leukocytes. *Left,* Anterior abdomen. *Right,* Anterior pelvis. Abnormal uptake confirms the clinical suspicion of a surgical graft infection (*arrowheads*).

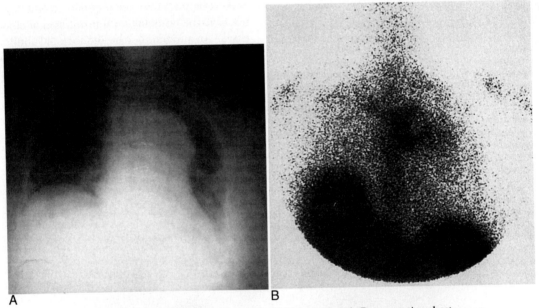

Figure 12-14   Infected thoracic aortic graft: In-111 leukocytes. **A,** Postoperative chest radiograph. **B,** In-111 oxine leukocytes localize in the aortic graft in the region of the aortic knob.

Tc-99m fanolesomab is a murine IgM monoclonal antibody that binds avidly to surface CD-15 antigens expressed on human neutrophils, monocytes, and eosinophils. Less than 5% of circulating leukocytes are monocytes or eosinophils. Therefore, uptake is primarily due to neutrophils.

Blood concentrations decrease rapidly with an initial half-life of 0.3 hours and a second phase half-life of 8 hours. At 2 hours postinjection, the liver has the highest radioactivity with 50% of the total injected dose, followed by the kidney, spleen, and red marrow. At 26–33 hours after injection, 38% is cleared through the urinary tract.

The spleen receives the highest radiation absorbed dose (2.3 rads/10 mCi or 2.3 cGy/370 MBq) (Table 12-6), approximately in the range of Tc-99m HMPAO leuko-cytes. The liver and bladder receive the next highest radiation dose.

As with all murine derived antibodies, autoimmume HAMA reactions are a concern. The incidence of human antimouse antibodies is quite low after a single adminis-tration (near zero), although detection of antibodies is dependent on the sensitivity of the assay. Limited data suggest that repeat injections result in a slightly higher incidence of about HAMA 10% but have a very low inci-dence of clinical side effects.

The usual adult administered dose is 10–20 mCi (370–740 mBq). In investigational studies, dynamic imaging was acquired, starting at the time of injection. Initially, ten 4-minute images were acquired. The patient voids and static images are acquired, including

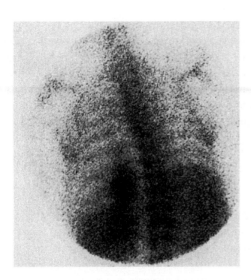

Figure 12-15   Pneumonia: In-111 leukocytes. Posterior chest view. Focal uptake in the left lower lobe. The purpose of the study was to locate the source of postoperative fever. Pneumonia was not suspected clinically. The last chest x-ray had been 10 days earlier. A subsequent radiograph confirmed the diagnosis.

supine anterior, posterior, right anterior oblique and left anterior oblique views, followed by a standing anterior image if the concern for infection is in the abdomen or pelvis. Finally, a static one-million count image is obtained. Imaging up to 90 minutes is recommended. This protocol was specific for acute appendicitis.

Image Interpretation

Normal distribution includes the blood pool, liver, spleen, bone marrow, and urinary excretion. A diagnostic abnormality is characterized by the presence of focal irregular, asymmetric uptake of radiotracer localized at the site of inflammation or infection (Fig. 12-22). The abnormal localization remains constant or increases in intensity in follow-up imaging.

Clinical Utility and Accuracy

See later section on Intra-Abdominal Infection and Table 12-9.

Technetium-99m Sulesomab (LeukoScan)

This radiopharmaceutical is commercially available in Europe. LeukoScan (Immunomedics, Morris Plains, N.J.), is Tc-99m-labeled antigranulocyte (IgG1) murine

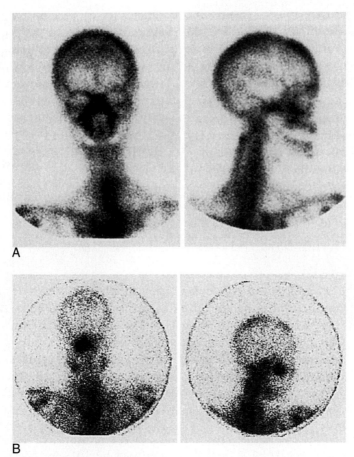

Figure 12-16   Osteomyelitis of the right maxillary sinus: In-111 leukocytes. History of bilateral sinus surgery. **A,** Bone scan shows fairly symmetrical ethmoid and maxillary sinus uptake. **B,** Indium-111 oxine leukocyte study shows uptake just right of midline in a pattern different from the bone scan, consistent with focal maxillary sinus infection, abscess, or osteomyelitis. Osteomyelitis was confirmed at surgery.

Box 12-7   Interpretative Pitfalls: False Negative and False Positive Leukocyte Scans

FALSE NEGATIVE

Encapsulated, nonpyogenic abscess
Vertebral osteomyelitis
Chronic low-grade infection
Parasitic, mycobacterial, or fungal infections
Intrahepatic or perihepatic or splenic infection
Hyperglycemia
Steroids

FALSE POSITIVE

Gastrointestinal bleeding
Pseudoaneurysm
Healing fracture
Soft tissue tumor
Swallowed leukocytes; oropharyngeal, esophageal, or lung disease
Surgical wounds, stomas, or catheter sites
Hematomas
Tumors
Accessory spleens
Renal transplant

Fluorine-18 Fluorodeoxyglucose

F-18 fluorodeoxyglucose (FDG) PET imaging is used on a clinical basis primarily for tumor imaging, and to a lesser extent, cardiac and brain imaging. A common cause for abnormal uptake not due to malignancy is that of inflammation and infection, due to glucose utilization by activated granulocytes and macrophages.

F-18 FDG PET has potential advantages over radiolabeled leukocyte studies. The study length is completed within 2 hours of radiopharmaceutical injection and PET image resolution is superior to single-photon imaging. Furthermore, the problems associated with radiolabeling leukocytes and reinfusion of blood products is eliminated.

Preliminary investigations suggest that F-18 FDG may be useful for diagnosing a variety of infections (e.g., inflammatory bowel disease, fever of unknown origin, and osteomyelitis). Although investigations have sought to use it to differentiate aseptic from septic hip prostheses, false positives are not uncommon. Radiolabeled leukocyte imaging combined with bone marrow scintigraphy is superior. For knee prostheses, the specificity is even poorer than for the hip.

Investigational Radiopharmaceuticals

There continues to be active investigation for new infection-seeking radiopharmaceuticals (*see* Box 12-1). Investigation has changed over time from developing large proteins with nonspecific uptake mechanism (IgG) to receptor specific proteins of large size (antigranulocyte antibodies) and moderate size (antibody fragments) to small receptor-binding proteins and peptides (cytokines). Some of these investigational radiopharmaceuticals are briefly discussed.

Nonspecific polyclonal immunoglobulin (Ig) G shows localization in a variety of clinical infections.

antibody Fab' fragment. Fab' fragments have less immunoreactivity than whole antibodies and a better target-to-background ratio because of their rapid renal clearance. Early clinical trials have found the accuracy of LeukoScan imaging to be equal or superior to that of In-111 leukocyte imaging particularly for musculoskeletal infection and osteomyelitis. Imaging can be performed within 1-6 hours after injection.

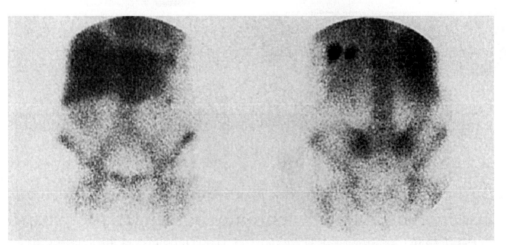

Figure 12-17   False positive In-111 leukocyte scan caused by accessory spleens. A 78-year-old woman with bacterial endocardititis had prior splenectomy. The In-111 leukocyte study was ordered to localize extra-cardiac infection. A Tc-99m SC study confirmed that the focal uptake in the left upper quadrant was due to accessory spleens (see Fig. 7-49).

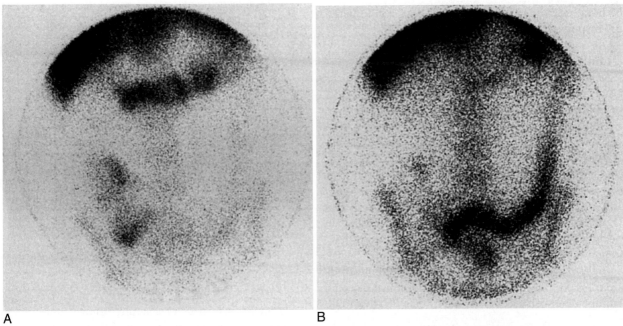

A B

Figure 12-18 False positive In-111 leukocyte study. Fever of uncertain etiology. Images obtained at 4 hours (**A**) and 24 hours (**B**). Although there is leukocyte localization predominantly to the transverse bowel at 4 hours, it is seen in the descending colon and rectum on 24-hour images. The patient had gastrointestinal bleeding on the day of the exam. The fever resolved spontaneously. The intraluminal activity was presumed due to gastrointestinal bleeding.

Accumulation is not the result of an immunological mechanism, but rather from the increased vascular permeability associated with inflammatory processes. The gastrointestinal and genitourinary systems show varying degrees of uptake. Slow blood clearance requires a multiple day imaging protocol. Preliminary data suggests good accuracy; however, there is no commercial interest in this agent.

Tc-99m ciprofloxacin (Infecton) is a Tc-99m radiolabeled fluoroquinolone broad-spectrum antimicrobial agent that binds to DNA of living bacteria. One early study has shown good general sensitivity similar to radiolabeled leukocyte studies. Of particular note, vertebral infections had increased uptake in five of six patients with negative radiolabeled leukocyte studies. This radiopharmaceutical is under investigation.

Chemotactic peptides or *cytokines* are involved in the initiation, amplification, and termination of the inflammatory response. They act through interaction with specific cell-surface receptors. Produced by bacteria, chemotactic peptides bind to receptors on the cell membrane of neutrophils, stimulating the cells to undergo chemotaxis. Analogs of these peptides have been synthesized and radiolabeled. Localization at sites of infection is rapid owing to the small size of these compounds; they easily pass through vascular walls and quickly enter an abscess. High target-to-background ratio occurs at 1 hour. Radiolabeled cytokines (e.g., interleukin-8) show promise.

Liposomes are spherical envelopes of cell membrane that have been investigated over the years for various indications. Newer improved techniques have revitalized its potential for infection imaging. A new approach is to target endothelial adhesion molecules expressed during inflammation (e.g., anti-E-selectin).

Radiolabeled lymphocytes are potentially useful for diagnosing chronic and more indolent inflammatory processes, such as rejection of kidney and heart transplants.

Table 12-5	Advantages/Disadvantages of In-111 Oxine versus Tc-99m HMPAO Labeled Leukocytes	
	In-111 oxine leukocytes	**Tc-99m HMPAO leukocytes**
Radionuclide immediately available	No	Yes
Stable radiolabel, no elution from cells	Yes	No
Allows labeling in plasma	No	Yes
Dosimetry	Poor	Good
Early routine imaging	No	Yes
Long half-life allows for delayed imaging	Yes	No
Imaging time	Long	Short
Permits dual isotope imaging	Yes	No
Bowel and renal clearance	No	Yes
Image resolution	Good	Fair

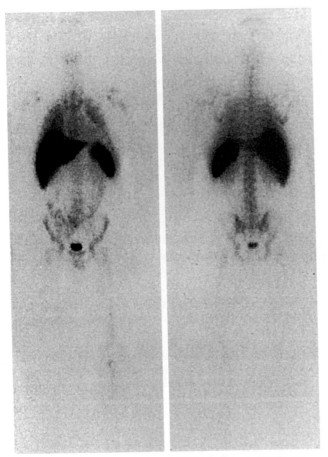

Figure 12-19 Normal Tc-99m HMPAO leukocyte distribution 4 hours postinjection. Uptake is greatest in the spleen, followed by the liver and bone marrow, similar to that seen with In-111 leukocytes in Fig. 12-9. Unlike In-111 leukocyte distribution, Tc-99m HMPAO shows bowel and urinary clearance. Low-grade diffuse pulmonary uptake is also seen. The study was performed because of suspected left knee prosthesis infection.

Only preliminary studies have been reported. Unlike neutrophils, lymphocytes are quite radiosensitive. Concerns have been expressed about the radiation effect on function, viability, and, more importantly, the potential for oncogenesis because of the lymphocytes' long lifespans.

CLINICAL APPLICATIONS FOR INFECTION SCINTIGRAPHY

Many of the factors that need to be considered in deciding which radiopharmaceutical is indicated for a specific clinical situation have been mentioned. This section focus on individual disease processes and discusses the pathophysiology of some of the more common problems, preferred radiopharmaceuticals for specific indications, and any special methodologies that should be used.

Box 12-8   Technetium-99m HMPAO Leukocyte Scintigraphy: Protocol Summary

PATIENT PREPARATION

Wound dressings should always be changed prior to imaging.

RADIOPHARMACEUTICAL

Tc-99m hexamethylpropylene amine (HMPAO) in vitro labeled leukocytes, 10 mCi (370 MBq)

INSTRUMENTATION

Camera: Large field of view; two-headed camera preferable for whole body imaging
Windows: 15%, centered over 140-keV photopeaks
Collimator: Low energy, high resolution

PATIENT PREPARATION

Draw 50 ml of blood to radiolabel cells in vitro

PROCEDURE

Radiolabel the patient's leukocytes in vitro with Tc-99m HMPAO.
Reinject labeled cells intravenously, preferably by direct venipuncture through 19-gauge needle. Contact with dextrose in water solutions may cause cell damage.

IMAGING

Imaging between one and two hours is mandatory for intra-abdominal imaging or to localize inflammatory bowel disease. Imaging at 4 hr or later may be advantageous for peripheral skeletal imaging, e.g., osteomyelitis of feet.
Whole body imaging: Two-headed camera with whole body acquisition for 30 min; 10-min spot images for regions of special interest
SPECT in selected cases

General Considerations

In-111 leukocytes have replaced Ga-67 for most indications. Ga-67 has suboptimal imaging characteristics due to its multiple high-energy photopeaks with low abundance and high scatter fraction. Intra-abdominal clearance via the bowel limits intra-abdominal diagnosis and the usual 48-hour imaging time is clinically disadvantageous. The major role for Ga-67 is for the diagnosis of pulmonary inflammatory disease such as sarcoidosis, *pneumocystis*, and drug-induced etiologies (e.g., bleomycin). Ga-67 may also be useful in the leukopenic patient (Box 12-9). It has also been successfully used for discitis in the spine and vertebral osteomyelitis.

Generally, for acute infection, the largest and most successful experience has been with radiolabeled leukocytes. Tc-99m HMPAO has distinct advantages over In-111 leukocytes (*see* Table 12-5). Being generator produced, Tc-99m is available for same-day radiolabeling, whereas In-111 is cyclotron-produced and must be ordered (and in most cases radiolabeled) the following day. Tc-99m has superior imaging characteristics and much greater activity can be administered, resulting in higher count images and better resolution. Imaging is routinely performed on the same day of administration with Tc-99m HMPAO, whereas In-111 leukocytes are usually imaged at 24 hours. The considerably lower radiation absorbed dose to the spleen of Tc-99m HMPAO makes it the agent of choice for pediatric patients.

Tc-99m HMPAO is cleared via hepatobiliary and genitourinary excretion. Abdominal imaging with Tc-99m HMPAO must be performed before intra-abdominal clearance, at 1–2 hours. Because leukocytes may take many hours to localize, detectability may be less at this early time period. Thus, In-111 labeled leukocytes are the agent of choice for intra-abdominal infection (Table 12-7), with the only exception being pediatric patients and inflammatory bowel disease.

Radiolabeled antigranulocyte antibodies have been approved for infection scintigraphy in the United States (Tc-99m fanolesomab, NeutroSpec) and in Europe (Tc-99m sulesomab, LeukoScan). Although NeutroSpec has only been approved for diagnosis of acute appendicitis, it is anticipated that it will have a much wider applicability because it does not require leukocyte radiolabeling. However, at present, data is limited for other indications.

There is concern about the sensitivity of leukocyte imaging in patients with clinical conditions or therapies that might alter leukocyte function, such as hyperglycemia, steroid therapy, chemotherapy, hemodialysis, and hyperalimentation. Data are limited.

Conflicting data exists regarding the sensitivity of In-111 leukocyte scintigraphy for detecting infection in patients receiving antibiotics. The discrepant reports may be due to the adequacy or inadequacy of treatment. Invariably many patients who have leukocyte imaging are on antibiotics.

There has also been concern that false-negative studies might occur with chronic infection. However, most investigations have found no significant difference in sensitivity for detection of acute or chronic infections. Although chronic inflammations consist largely of lymphocytes, monocytes, plasma cells, and macrophages, they also have significant neutrophilic infiltration and, at

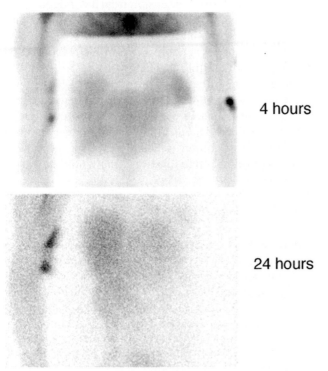

Figure 12-20 Infected arterial-venous graft imaged with Tc-99m HMPAO leukocytes. Image obtained at 4 hours (*above*) shows focal uptake within the graft on the right. Delayed image at 24 hours show increasing uptake in the same region.

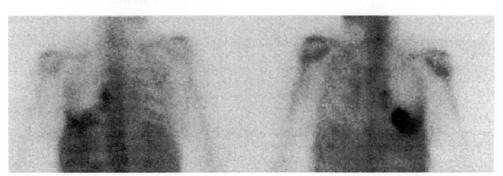

Figure 12-21 Postoperative empyema: Tc-99m HMPAO leukocytes. The infection occurred following thoracotomy for lung cancer. *Left,* Posterior view. *Right,* Anterior view.

times, frank pus. Furthermore the In-111–labeled mixed-cell population contains many lymphocytes.

Tc-99m HMPAO preferentially labels granulocytes. Thus, some chronic infections may not be detected with In-111 oxine labeled leukocytes. Ga-67 may have a role in patients with low-grade infection (e.g., fungal, protozoa).

Osteomyelitis

The histopathology of osteomyelitis during the acute phase includes neutrophilic inflammation, edema, and vascular congestion. Because of the bone's rigidity, intramedullary pressure increases, compromising the blood supply and causing ischemia and vascular thrombosis. Over several days, the suppurative and ischemic injury may result in bone fragmentation into devitalized segments called *sequestra*. Infection may spread via Haversian and Volkmann's canals to the periosteum, resulting in abscesses, soft-tissue infection, and sinus tracts.

With persistent infection, chronic inflammatory cells, including lymphocytes, histiocytes, and plasma cells, join the neutrophils. Fibroblastic proliferation and new bone formation occur. Periosteal osteogenesis may surround the inflammation to form a bony envelope, or *involucrum*. Occasionally a dense fibrous capsule confines the infection to a localized area of suppuration called a *Brodie's abscess*.

Bone infection is usually bacterial in origin. Microorganisms reach the bone by one of three mechanisms: hematogenous spread, extension from a contiguous site of infection, and direct introduction of organisms into bone by trauma and surgery.

The terminology of acute and chronic osteomyelitis is frequently confused. The word *acute* implies hematogenous spread. *Chronic osteomyelitis* is not chronic in the traditional sense. It is nonhematogenous in origin, but is an active infection with a neutrophilic inflammatory component, although with time there may be a subacute or chronic inflammatory response as well. Perhaps chronic active osteomyelitis would be better terminology.

Acute Hematogenous Osteomyelitis

In children, bone is usually infected by hematogenous spread. It usually involves the red marrow of long bones due to its relatively slow blood flow in metaphyseal capillaries and sinusoidal veins in the region adjacent to the growth plate and there is also a paucity of phagocytes (Figs. 12-23 and 12-24). The osteomyelitis is often secondary to staphylococcal skin or mucosal infection.

	Adults cGy/370 MBq or rads/10 mCi	5-year-old children cGy/ 37 MBq or rads/mCi
Table 12-6 Radiation Dosimetry for Tc-99m Fanolesomab (NeutroSpec)		
Organ		
Bladder wall	1.20	0.27
Large intestine	0.34	0.21
Liver	1.80	0.41
Bone marrow	0.38	0.11
Spleen	2.30	0.70
Ovaries	0.19	0.06
Testes	0.04	0.02
Total body	0.19	0.05

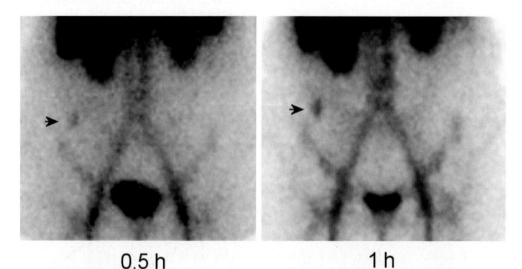

0.5 h   1 h

Figure 12-22   Acute appendicitis: Tc-99m fanolesomab (NeutroSpec). Patient with clinically uncertain but suspected acute appendicitis. The scan demonstrates focal activity in the right lower quadrant of the abdomen at 30 minutes (*arrow*), which increases in intensity at one hour. (Used with permission. Love C, Palestro CR: Radionuclide imaging of infection. J Nucl Med Technol 32:47–57, 2004.)

Table 12-7   Specific Indications for In-111 Oxine or Tc-99m HMPAO Leukocytes

In-111 oxine leukocytes	Tc-99m HMPAO leukocytes
Intra-abdominal infection	Pediatric patients
Cardiovascular infection	Inflammatory bowel disease
Diabetic mid-foot and hind-foot osteomyelitis*	Osteomyelitis of extremities including the feet in non-diabetic patients
Inflammatary bowel disease	Diabetic forefoot osteomyelitis
Hip and knee prosthesis*	
Orthopedic hardware, prior fracture, infection*	

*In conjunction with Tc-99m SC bone marrow scan.

In the adult, osteomyelitis from hematogenous spread rarely involves the long bones because red marrow has been replaced by adipose tissue (yellow marrow). It often occurs in vertebral bodies, where the marrow is cellular with an abundant vascular supply. Infection begins near the anterior longitudinal ligament and spreads to adjacent vertebrae by direct extension through the disk space or via communicating venous channels. Because the adult disk does not have a vascular supply, disk space infection is always due to osteomyelitis in an adjacent vertebra. The initiating event is usually septicemia from urinary tract infection, bacterial endocarditis, or intravenous drug abuse.

Extension from a Contiguous Site of Infection

The most common cause of osteomyelitis is direct extension from overlying soft tissue infection, which is usually secondary to trauma, radiation therapy, burns, or pressure sores. In patients with diabetes and vascular insufficiency, organisms enter the soft tissues through a cutaneous ulcer, often in the foot, causing cellulitis and then osteomyelitis.

Direct Introduction of Organisms into Bone

Direct inoculation of infection may occur with open fractures, open surgical reduction of closed fractures, or penetrating trauma by foreign bodies. Osteomyelitis may also arise from perioperative contamination of bone during surgery for nontraumatic orthopedic disorders, as in laminectomy, diskectomy, or placement of a joint prosthesis.

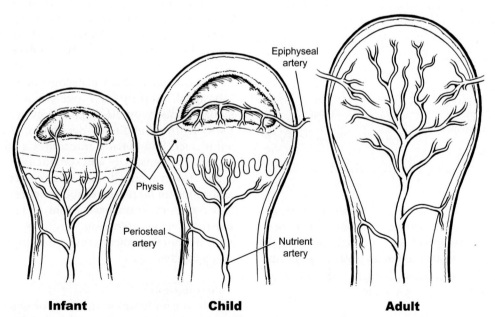

Figure 12-23   Vascular supply of long bones. In the infant and until 18 months of age, small vessels perforate the physis to enter the epiphysis. After 18 months and during childhood, the perforating vessels involute. The epiphysis and metaphysis then have separate blood supplies. Following closure of the physis, branches of the nutrient artery extend to the end of bone (adult) and the principal blood supply to the end of long bones is again from the nutrient artery in the medullary canal. The periosteal artery supplies the outer cortex, whereas branches of the nutrient artery supply the inner cortex.

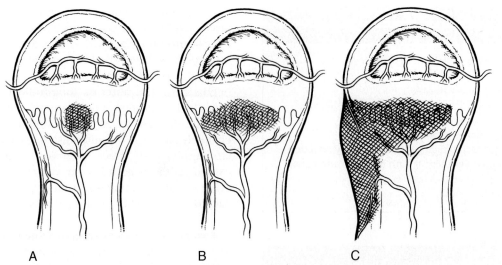

Figure 12-24 Pathophysiology of hematogenous osteomyelitis (child). **A,** Bacterial embolization occurs via the nutrient artery, and bacteria lodge in the terminal blood supply in the metaphysis. **B,** After the infection is established, it expands within the medullary canal toward the cortex and diaphysis. The physis serves as an effective barrier. **C,** The infection then extends through the vascular channels to the cortex to elevate and strip the periosteum from the cortex and periosteal new bone forms. The bond between the periosteum and perichondrium at the physis prevents extension of the infection into the joint.

Table 12-8	Diagnosis of Osteomyelitis: Accuracy of Different Scintigraphic and MRI Methods

Type of study	Sensitivity (%)	Specificity (%)
Three-phase bone scan (normal x-ray)	94	95
Three-phase bone scan (underlying bone disease)	95	33
Gallium-67	81	69
Indium-111 oxine leukocytes	88	85
Technetium-99m HMPAO	87	81
Leukocytes (vertebral)	40	90
Leukocytes + bone marrow	95	90
Antigranulocyte	92	88
Magnetic resonance imaging	95	87

Osteomyelitis initially acquired as a child or in adulthood may be manifested later as intermittent or persistent drainage from sinus tracts communicating with the involved bone, usually the femur, tibia, or humerus, or as a soft tissue infection overlying it. Signs of infection may recur after years of quiescence.

Clinical Diagnosis

Biopsy with culture is the most definitive test for the diagnosis of osteomyelitis, but this is invasive and often contraindicated. Noninfected bone may become contaminated by overlying soft tissue infection and there is risk of pathological fracture in the small bones of the hands and feet. Radiographic methods and nuclear medicine scans have become important for confirming or excluding the diagnosis (Table 12-8).

Conventional Imaging

Plain film radiography should be performed whenever osteomyelitis is suspected because it can be diagnostic. However, the characteristic changes of permeative radiolucencies, destructive changes, and periosteal new bone formation may take 10–14 days to develop and are not always specific.

MRI can detect marrow changes of osteomyelitis (i.e., low-signal intensity on T1-weighted images and high signal intensity on T2-weighted images and enhancement with gadolinium). Secondary changes such as sinus tracts and cortical interruption increase the certainty. The sensitivity and specificity is reported to be high. However, any disease that replaces bone marrow and results in increased tissue water (e.g., healing fractures, tumors, and Charcot joints) may not be distinguishable from infection. Artifacts caused by joint implants can degrade images sufficiently to make diagnosis impossible.

Scintigraphy

The best scintigraphic method for diagnosis of osteomyelitis depends to some extent on the particular clinical situation (*see* Box 12-9).

Bone Scan

In patients who do not have an associated underlying bone condition, a three-phase bone scan should be performed first. Its overall sensitivity for the diagnosis

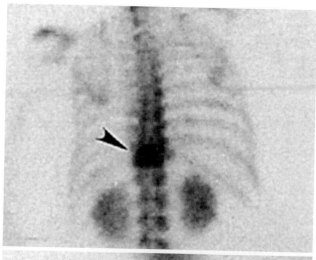

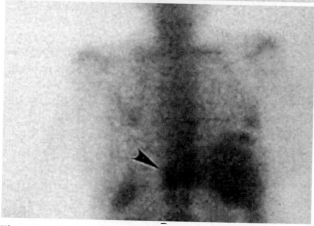

Figure 12-25   Combined Ga-67 and bone scan: confirm or exclude osteomyelitis of the spine. Fever after laminectomy raised the question of infection. Vertebral Ga-67 uptake *(bottom)* was judged to be less than that seen on the Tc-99m medronate (MDP) bone scan *(top),* and the study was interpreted as negative for vertebral osteomyelitis. The low-grade Ga-67 uptake was likely the result of reactive healing bone.

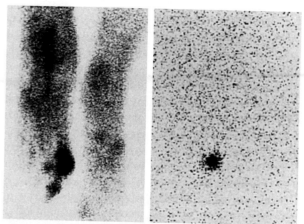

Figure 12-26   Osteomyelitis of diabetic foot: In-111 leukocytes and bone scan. Diabetes, peripheral vascular disease, cellulitis, and infection in the region of the first metatarsal. *Left,* Two-hour delayed bone scan shows marked increased uptake in the distal first metatarsal. The first two phases (not shown) were also positive. *Right,* In-111 oxine leukocyte study shows intense uptake in the same distal metatarsal. No uptake is noted in other areas of the foot that had increased uptake on the bone scan (i.e., the distal phalanx of the first toe and the second distal metatarsal).

of osteomyelitis is greater than 95%. A negative study excludes osteomyelitis with a high degree of certainty. The one exception is in neonates who on occasion may have false-negative bone scintigraphy. However, the specificity of the bone scan is poor in patients with underlying bone disease such as fractures, orthopedic implants, and neuropathic joints (30–50%) *(see* Table 12-8).

Gallium-67 Citrate

Because Ga-67 is taken up by normal bone as well as marrow, locally increased Ga-67 uptake occurs at sites of increased bone turnover, similar to that seen with a bone scan. Thus, false-positive interpretations may result in patients with underlying bone conditions. The specificity of the Ga-67 scan can be increased if interpreted in conjunction with a bone scan.

The accepted criteria for diagnosis of osteomyelitis using Ga-67 scintigraphy in conjunction with a bone scan are: (1) if Ga-67 uptake is greater than that seen on the bone scan or (2) if the Ga-67 and bone scan distribution are incongruent in distribution (Fig. 12-25). If Ga-67 uptake is less than seen on the bone scan, it is negative for osteomyelitis. A similar degree of uptake on both studies is considered equivocal for the diagnosis. However, the accuracy of the combined two studies is still inferior to that of labeled leukocytes *(see* Table 12-8).

Radiolabeled Leukocytes

The reported accuracy of radiolabeled leukocytes for diagnosis of osteomyelitis has varied considerably. Attempts have been made to improve the accuracy by interpreting the study in conjunction with a bone scan, similar to the approach used with Ga-67 imaging (Figs. 12-16, 12-26, and 12-27). However, this has not appreciably improved the overall accuracy, particularly in the problematic diabetic foot, spine, and hip and knee prostheses.

Bone Marrow Scan in Conjunction with Leukocyte Scan   An underlying assumption of leukocyte scan interpretation for osteomyelitis is that bone marrow distribution is uniform and symmetrical and that an area of focally increased uptake is diagnostic of infection. However, when marrow distribution is altered, there is potential for misinterpreting focal uptake as infection.

A solution to the problem of altered marrow distribution is to interpret the leukocyte scan in conjunction with a bone marrow scan. The Tc-99m SC marrow scan can serve as a template for the distribution of marrow in that patient. With infection, the radiolabeled leukocyte study will be discordant with the marrow scan (i.e., focal increased uptake on the leukocyte study), whereas the marrow scan will show decreased or normal uptake. This

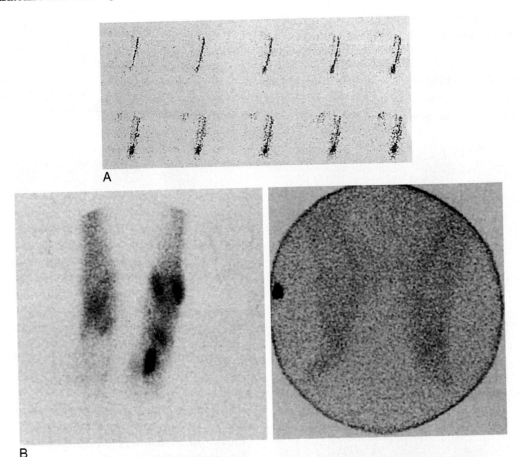

Figure 12-27 Metatarsal osteomyelitis: positive three-phase bone scan, negative In-111 leukocytes. **A,** Flow study shows increased flow in the region of the distal left mid-foot. **B,** *Left,* A 3-hour delayed image shows increased uptake by the third metatarsal. Diffuse ankle uptake is also noted. *Right,* The In-111-leukocyte study is negative for infection. Radiograph showed a metatarsal fracture.

spatial incongruity is diagnostic of infection. With no infection, the leukocyte and marrow scan will have similar distribution.

Diabetic Foot

Insensitivity of the neuropathic foot to pain often results in asymptomatic trauma, fractures, ulcers, infection, and delay in diagnosis. Foot ulcers serve as a common portal of entry for infection. The diagnosis of osteomyelitis in the setting of soft tissue infection is a common but difficult diagnostic problem in the diabetic. Radiographs and MRI are often nonspecific for infection.

The three-phase bone scan is frequently not helpful because it is so often abnormal due to overlying soft tissue infection (increased flow) (*see* Fig. 12-27), fractures, neuropathic Charcot's joints (can be three-phase positive), and degenerative changes. Although the sensitivity of the bone scan for diagnosis of osteomyelitis approaches 100%, its specificity is much poorer (*see* Table 12-8). Delayed imaging at 24 hours (fourth phase) is reported to improve accuracy, but false positives are still a problem.

Confirmation or exclusion of the diagnosis of osteomyelitis often requires leukocyte scintigraphy. However, differentiating bone infection from overlying soft tissue infection can be problematic with In-111 leukocyte because of the paucity of anatomical information on the leukocyte scan (*see* Fig. 12-26). The improved resolution of Tc-99m HMPAO leukocytes with low-level distribution in soft tissue is an advantage over In-111 leukocytes. Tc-99m HMPAO is particularly useful in the distal foot (Figs. 12-28 and 12-29).

The foot proximal to the metatarsals is more problematic diagnostically. Although red marrow is not present in the distal extremities in adults, neuropathic Charcot joints form marrow and accumulate leukocytes. Fractures may also stimulate marrow formation. Thus, marrow scintigraphy in conjunction with In-111 leukocyte imaging is important for evaluating the mid- or hindfoot of the diabetic. One approach is to acquire the leukocyte and bone marrow studies on separate days. In that case Tc-99m HMPAO would be preferable. However, an alternative approach and perhaps preferable is to do simultaneous dual-isotope leukocyte scintigraphy and bone marrow scan using In-111 oxine labeled leukocytes and Tc-99m SC for the marrow scans (Fig. 12-30).

Vertebral Osteomyelitis

The most common route of vertebral infection is hematogenous spread via the arterial or venous system. However, postoperative infections are not rare with direct implantation of microorganisms into the intervertebral disc.

Microorganisms lodge at different sites depending on patient age. Below 4 years of age, end arteries perforate the vertebral body end plates and enter the disc space producing discitis. In adults, the richest network of nutrient arterioles is localized in the subchondral region of the

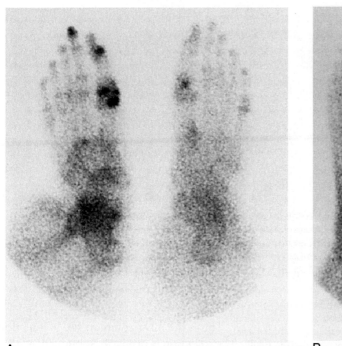
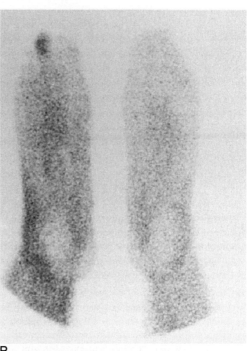

A   **B**

Figure 12-28   Osteomyelitis of distal phalanx: Tc-99m HMPAO leukocytes and bone scan. Diabetic with purulent drainage of the distal second digit of the right foot. **A,** Bone scan shows increased uptake on the distal second digit of the right. The first two phases were also positive. **B,** Tc-99m HMPAO leukocytes were positive in the distal second digit, consistent with osteomyelitis. Other uptake on the bone scan was negative on the leukocyte study.

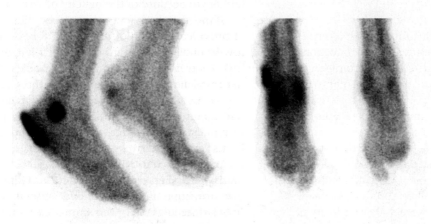

Figure 12-29   Tc-99m HMPAO soft tissue infection. Clinically ulcers of the right lateral malleolus and heal of right foot. Soft tissue infection was diagnosed, not osteomyelitis, was diagnosed with the leukocyte study. The low-grade soft tissue of Tc-99m HMPAO distribution makes it easier to differentiate osteomyelitis from soft tissue infection than with In-111 leukocytes.

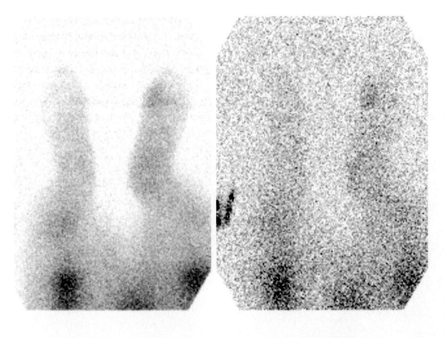

Tc-99m SC   In-111 WBCs

Figure 12-30 Combined In-111 leukocyte and Tc-99m SC studies for possible osteomyelitis of the first phalanx. Recent bunionectomy and internal fixation. The joint became infected, was treated with antibiotics, but C-reactive protein was persistently elevated and concern for osteomyelitis. Plantar images of feet. Tc-99m SC *(left)* and In-111 oxine leukocytes *(right)*. Both have similar extended pattern of uptake (concordant) in region of first MP on the left. Negative for bone infection.

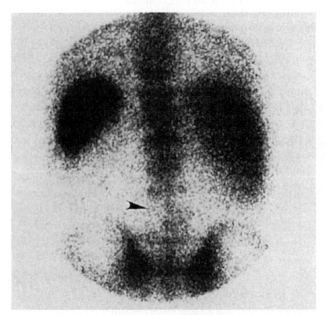

Figure 12-31 Vertebral osteomyelitis: false negative. A cold defect at L5 on indium-111 leukocyte scintigraphy. Biopsy was necessary to make the diagnosis of osteomyelitis.

vertebral body, similar to the vascular tree in the childhood metaphysis. This is the most common site of infection in the adult. The infection is primarily spondylitis with secondary spread into the disc space. The infection spreads from the anterior subchondral focus through the vertebral end plate into the intervertebral disc. Later it destroys the neighboring end plate, involves the opposite vertebral body, and finally may extend to adjacent soft tissue and result in epidural or paravertebral abscess formation.

Bone Scan

The typical pattern of discitis is increased blood flow, blood pool, and delayed uptake involving adjacent contiguous ends of adjoining vertebral bodies. With isolated osteomyelitis, the bone scan will be three-phase positive. However, blood flow and blood pool images can be difficult to evaluate in the thoracic spine because of normal cardiac, pulmonary, and vascular structures.

Leukocyte Scintigraphy

Multiple studies have now reported a high false negative rate for both In-111 oxine and Tc-99m HMPAO radiolabeled leukocytes in the spine. False-negative results occur in approximately 40% of studies. The labeled leukocyte study may be normal or there may be a photopenic or cold defect at the site (Fig. 12-31). Thus, infection cannot be differentiated from metastasis, frac-

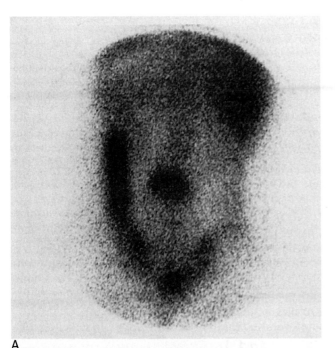

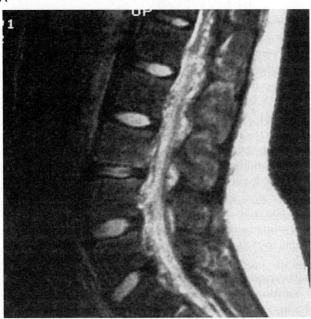

Figure 12-32 Disk space infection: Ga-67. Clinically suspected disk infection. **A,** Magnetic resonance imaging showed only a narrowed interspace with evidence of degenerative disc disease. **B,** Posterior view, prominent Ga-67 uptake in the region of the L3-4 disc space.

ture, Paget disease, surgical defects, or irradiation. The explanation for this finding is uncertain, but may be due to bone marrow thrombosis and infarction.

Ga-67 Scintigraphy

Ga-67 is probably superior to leukocyte scintigraphy for vertebral osteomyelitis. However, false positives may result due to reactive bone. To minimize this problem, Ga-67 should be done in conjunction with a bone scan using the criteria discussed previously (*see* Fig 12-25). An associated paraspinal abscess or disc infection can be also diagnosed with Ga-67 scintigraphy (Fig. 12-32).

Other Scintigraphy

F-18 FDG may have a role in this setting, although reimbursement is an issue at present. Early data suggest that Tc-99m ciprofloxacin (Infecton), still investigational, may be useful for this indication.

Infected Joint Prostheses

The infection rate after primary hip or knee replacement is only 1% and after revision surgery is less than 3%. However, when present, an infected prosthesis produces severe morbidity. Diagnosis of an infected prosthetic joint can be difficult because the symptoms and signs are often indolent. Radiographs also have poor sensitivity for early detection. Joint aspiration also has a low sensitivity for diagnosis.

Bone Scan

Characteristic bone scan findings have been described to differentiate loosening and infection of hip prostheses. In patients studied for more than 12 months after insertion of cemented total hip prostheses, diffuse uptake surrounding the femoral component suggests infection. However, this pattern is only moderately predictive. Cementless or porous coated prosthesis depend on bony ingrowth for stabilization. Ongoing new bone formation is part of the fixation process, causing periprosthetic uptake on bone scintigraphy in a variable pattern for a prolonged period, making interpretation more difficult.

Knee prostheses are a particular problem for bone scintigraphy. More than half of all femoral components and three-fourths of all tibial components show periprosthetic uptake more than 12 months after placement. Thus, for patients with cementless hip replacement or total knee replacement, bone scintigraphy is most useful when the scan is normal or when serial studies over time are available for comparison.

Ga-67 Scintigraphy

Even in conjunction with bone scintigraphy Ga-67 is only moderately accurate, reportedly 80%, in the diagnosis of infected joint prostheses.

Leukocyte Scintigraphy

The reported accuracy of leukocyte scintigraphy in combination of the bone scan imaging has been variable. Evidence strongly suggests that superior diagnostic accuracy results when the leukocyte scan is interpreted in combination with bone marrow scintigraphy. The Tc-99m

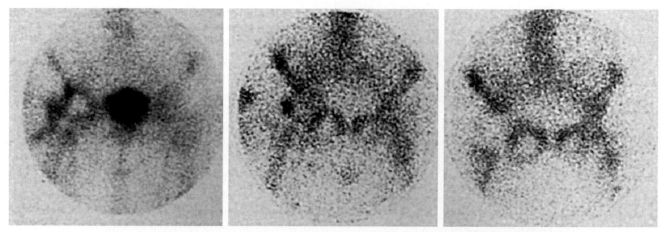

Figure 12-33   Infected hip prosthesis: In-111 leukocyte and Tc-99m SC marrow study. *Left,* Tc-99m medronate (MDP) bone scan shows increased uptake in the region of the right hip prosthesis laterally consistent with heterotopic calcification. *Middle,* Indium-111 leukocyte study shows focal intense uptake just lateral to the femoral head and more diffuse uptake within the joint space consistent with infection. *Right,* Tc-99m SC marrow study shows a normal bone marrow distribution with cold head of the femur consistent with prosthesis. The discordance of the bone marrow and In-111 leukocyte study indicates an infected prosthesis.

bone marrow scan serves as a template for the patient's normal marrow distribution. The normal distribution of marrow in the elderly population is variable. Placement of an orthopedic device inevitably results in marrow displacement in an unpredictable manner. The marrow study avoids the potential for a false-positive study, that is, interpretation of focal uptake as infection when it is merely displaced marrow distribution.

If performed on different days, Tc-99m HMPAO leukocytes can be used in conjunction with Tc-99m SC. Simultaneous dual-isotope acquisition in the identical projections is advantageous and can be done with the dual-isotope scanning In-111 oxine leukocytes and the Tc-99m SC marrow scan. Discordance of uptake on the leukocyte study and the marrow scintigraphy is diagnostic (Fig. 12-33). Accuracy is reported to be greater than 90%.

Response to Therapy
Both Ga-67 and leukocyte scintigraphy can also be useful for monitoring response to therapy (e.g., to ascertain that infection has been controlled prior to surgical replacement of a new prosthesis). Scintigraphic findings of infection should revert to normal by 2–8 weeks of appropriate antibiotic therapy.

Intra-Abdominal Infection

The diagnosis of intra-abdominal infection is often made by CT with directed interventional aspiration. However, in patients with nonlocalizing symptoms and negative conventional imaging, scintigraphy has clinical value. Gallium-67 has been used to diagnose intra-abdominal infection; however, it has numerous drawbacks, particularly normal bowel clearance and delayed imaging. In-111–oxine leukocytes have a distinct advantage (*see* Tables 12-5 and 12-7). The radiopharmaceutical is not cleared in the abdomen. Thus any intra-abdominal localization is likely due to infection. Combined data from three large series reported an overall sensitivity of approximately 90% for detection and localization of intra-abdominal infection.

Early imaging at 4 hours with In-111 leukocytes has a reduced sensitivity for the detection of infection compared to 24 hours; however, in some situations, early imaging may expedite making the diagnosis (e.g., in acutely ill patients with suspected acute appendicitis, diverticulitis, and ischemic bowel disease). In these acute illnesses, early intensive leukocyte uptake is likely due to the increased blood flow to the site of infection and the marked inflammatory response with leukocyte infiltration.

Tc-99m HMPAO label has the advantages of its superior image quality and preferential labeling of granulocytes, resulting in rapid uptake in pyogenic infections. However, its hepatobiliary and renal clearance requires imaging at 1–2 hours. A large study found that the sensitivity for detecting abdominal infection and inflammatory disease was 88% at 30 minutes and 95% at 2 hours. Delayed imaging can sometimes be helpful to confirm that the early detected abnormal activity is a fixed pattern. A shifting pattern of activity over time implies intraluminal transit of labeled leukocytes, as seen with inflammatory or ischemic bowel disease, fistula, abscess in communication with bowel, or false-positive causes (e.g., swallowed leukocytes from sinus or tracheobronchial infection) (*see* Box 12-7). Abnormal leukocyte uptake has been described in a variety of

Table 12-9	Diagnostic Accuracy of Tc-99m Fanolesomab (NeutroSpec) for Acute Appendicitis

	Percentages (95% CI)	
200-patient multicenter trial	Blinded readers	Study investigators
Sensitivity	75 (62–86)	91 (80–97)
Specificity	93 (87–97)	86 (79–91)
Accuracy	87 (82–92)	87 (81–91)
Positive predictive value	82 (69–91)	74 (62–84)
Negative predictive value	90 (84–94)	96 (90–99)

noninfectious inflammatory diseases (e.g., pancreatitis, acute cholecystitis, polyarteritis nodosa, and rheumatoid vasculitis).

Leukocyte uptake occurs in ischemic colitis (common in elderly patients), pseudomembranous colitis (antibiotic related), and bowel infarction. Inactive colitis is negative on scintigraphy.

Tc-99m fanolesomab (NeutroSpec) has recently been approved for the diagnosis of acute appendicitis when the clinical diagnosis is uncertain. A multicenter trial of 200 patients with equivocal signs and symptoms of appendicitis were investigated. The overall accuracy was good with a positive predictive value of 82% and negative predictive value of 90% (Table 12-9). Some of the false positives may have been other sites of infection. The high negative predictive value saves patients from admission or surgery.

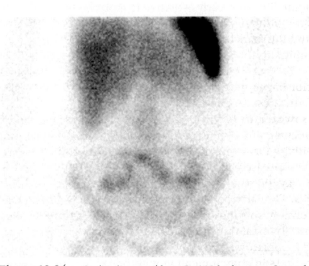

Figure 12-34   Crohn disease: 4-hour In-111 leukocytes. Several year history of regional ileitis. Two months of recurrent and worsening symptoms. Scintigraphy confirms active inflammation of ileum.

Inflammatory Bowel Disease

Both ulcerative colitis and Crohn's disease (granulomatous or regional enteritis) are characterized by intestinal inflammation that can be detected with leukocyte scintigraphy (Fig. 12-34). Scintigraphy has been used to make the diagnosis, to determine disease distribution, and to confirm relapse. Scintigraphy can aid in the evaluation of regions hard to see with endoscopy and can also monitor the effectiveness of therapy. Studies have shown good correlation between the site and amount of leukocyte uptake compared with the endoscopic and radiological localization.

Leukocyte scintigraphy can differentiate reactivation of inflammatory bowel disease from abscess formation resulting from bowel perforation. The latter is a serious clinical problem, requiring very different therapy (surgical rather than medical). Radiolabeled leukocyte uptake in an abscess is typically focal, whereas uptake in inflamed bowel typically follows the contour of the intestinal wall. In-111 leukocyte imaging can also aid the surgeon in determining if a partially obstructed bowel is the result of active inflammation or is a fibrotic stricture. In the latter case, surgery is indicated.

In-111 oxine leukocyte imaging should be performed at 4 hours rather than the usual imaging time of 24 hours because of shedding of the inflamed leukocytes into the bowel lumen from the inflammatory sites and subsequent peristalsis may result in incorrect assignment of disease to sites distal to the true lesion. Tc-99m HMPAO imaging must be performed at 1–2 hours prior to intra-abdominal hepatobiliary and genitourinary radiotracer clearance.

Comparative studies have indicated that Tc-99m HMPAO-labeled leukocytes are advantageous over In-111–oxine leukocytes to diagnose inflammatory bowel disease because of its superior image resolution enabling disease localization to specific bowel segments and better identification of small bowel disease. Accurate results with Tc-99m HMPAO leukocytes are possible by 1 hour after injection. Crohn disease and ulcerative colitis can usually be distinguished from each other by the distribution of disease activity. Rectal sparing, small bowel involvement, and skip areas suggest Crohn disease, whereas continuous colonic involvement from the rectum without small bowel involvement suggests ulcerative colitis.

Renal Disease

Ga-67 has been used to diagnose diffuse interstitial nephritis and localized infection, but delayed imaging must be performed because of its clearance through the urinary tract during the initial 24 hours after injection. Renal parenchymal infection such as pyelonephritis or diffuse interstitial nephritis (Fig. 12-35), lobar nephronia (focal interstitial nephritis), and perirenal infections (Fig. 12-36) have been diagnosed with Ga-67. However, with renal or hepatic failure and iron overload, renal uptake is increased without infection.

For the most part Ga-67 has been superceded by leukocyte imaging Tc-99m DMSA and, importantly, biopsy. Radiolabeled leukocytes also accumulate at sites of acute pyelonephritis, focal nephritis (lobar nephronia), and renal

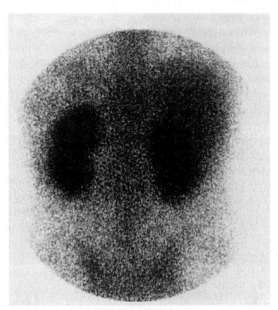

Figure 12-35 Interstitial nephritis: Ga-67. Bilateral intense renal gallium-67 uptake is seen at 48 hours (posterior view). Normal uptake is seen in the liver, bone, and bone marrow.

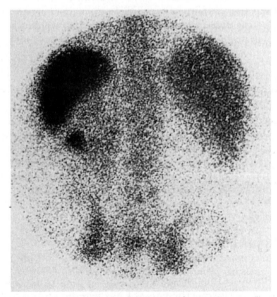

Figure 12-36 Perirenal abscess: Ga-67. Fever and pain developed after renal stone removal and nephrostomy. Focal increased Ga-67 uptake is seen just inferior to the spleen and adjacent to the left kidney, consistent with an abscess.

or perirenal abscess. However, In-111–labeled leukocytes have limited utility for evaluation of renal transplants because all exhibit uptake, regardless of the presence or absence of clinically significant disease or rejection.

Cardiovascular Disease

In-111–labeled leukocytes are reported not to be highly sensitive for detecting subacute bacterial endocarditis. The vegetative lesions contain high concentrations of bacteria, platelets, and fibrin adherent to damaged valvular endothelium, but relatively few leukocytes. However, it occasionally can be useful and SPECT may be helpful. Leukocyte uptake occurs in acute myocardial infarction and cardiac transplant rejection, but leukocyte scintigraphy is used for making these diagnoses.

Infection of arterial prosthetic grafts (e.g., femoropopliteal and aortofemoral) is associated with significant morbidity and mortality. Ultrasound, CT, and MRI are often unable to distinguish infection from aseptic fluid collections around the graft. Prompt diagnosis of graft infection is critical but often delayed because of their indolent and insidious course. Radiolabeled leukocytes can detect surgical prosthetic graft infection (Fig. 12-14). In-111 has a theoretical advantage of having no blood pool distribution, a potential problem with Tc-99m HMPAO. However, early imaging with Tc-99m HMPAO at 5 minutes, 30 minutes, and 3 hours has been shown to be quite accurate for confirming the diagnosis. Infected grafts have persistent uptake.

Pulmonary Infections

Pulmonary uptake of radiolabeled leukocytes should be interpreted cautiously. Low-grade diffuse uptake has been associated with a variety of noninfectious causes, including atelectasis, congestive heart failure, and adult respiratory distress syndrome, and therefore should not be considered diagnostic of infection.

Focal intense uptake is likely to be due to infection (*see* Fig. 12-16). Tuberculosis and fungal infections may be detected by In-111 leukocytes, but with a generally lower sensitivity than Ga-67.

Ga-67 citrate accumulates in virtually all types of pulmonary infections and inflammatory diseases, including pneumonia, lung abscess, and tuberculosis. However, the usual clinical role for Ga-67 is for the most part in more chronic diseases, such as sarcoidosis (*see* Fig. 12-4), idiopathic pulmonary fibrosis, *Pneumocystis carinii* (*see* Fig. 12-37), and for therapeutic drug-induced pulmonary disease (Boxes 12-10 to 12-12).

Sarcoidosis

Sarcoidosis a chronic granulomatous multisystem disease of unknown etiology characterized by an accumulation of T-lymphocytes, mononuclear phagocytes, and non-

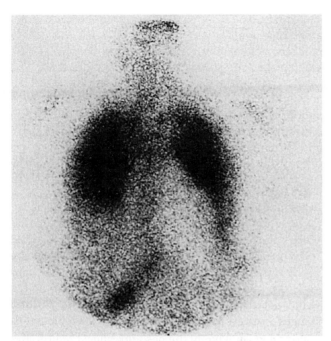

Figure 12-37   *Pneumocystis carinii*-Ga-67. Diffuse intense homogeneous, as seen in this study, or diffuse heterogeneous uptake is typical of this infection. The characteristic pattern is different from that of most other common pulmonary infections in AIDS patients.

Box 12-10   Scintigraphic Diagnosis of Osteomyelitis in Different Clinical Situations

Normal x-ray: three-phase bone scan
Neonates: three-phase bone scan; if negative, Tc-99m HMPAO
Suspected osteomyelitis in non-marrow-containing skeleton (distal extremities): bone scan + leukocyte study
Suspected osteomyelitis in bone marrow-containing skeleton (hips and knees): marrow scan + leukocyte study
Suspected vertebral osteomyelitis: gallium-67

Box 12-11   Ga-67 Uptake in Interstitial and Granulomatous Pulmonary Diseases

Tuberculosis
Histoplasmosis
Sarcoidosis
Idiopathic pulmonary fibrosis
Pneumocystis carinii
Cytomegalovirus
Pneumonoconioses (asbestosis, silicosis)
Hypersensitivity pneumonitis

Box 12-12   Therapeutic Agents Associated with Gallium-67 Lung Uptake

Bleomycin
Amiodarone
Busulfan
Nitrofurantoin
Cyclophosphamide
Methotrexate
Nitrosourea

---

caseating epithelioid granulomas. The lungs are the organ most commonly involved. Manifestations include hilar and mediastinal adenopathy, endobronchial granuloma formation, interstitial or alveolar pulmonary infiltrates, or pulmonary fibrosis.

Systemic symptoms such as weight loss, fatigue, weakness, malaise, and fever are common (40%). Pulmonary disease predominates. However, disease can involve any organ of the body, most commonly the liver and spleen. Extrapulmonary manifestations of the skin, eyes, heart, central nervous system, bones, and muscle are not rare. Central nervous system and cardiac involvement when present may lead to death.

The initial presentation is usually pulmonary and one-half of patients present with complaints of dyspnea and dry cough. However, as many as 20% are asymptomatic and have only an abnormal chest radiograph at initial detection. The clinical course is variable. Spontaneous resolution occurs in about one-third of patients. Another 30–40% have a smoldering or progressively worsening course, 20% develop permanent loss of lung function, and 5–10% die of respiratory failure.

There are four types of x-ray findings (Box 12-13): no abnormality (type 0), bilateral hilar adenopathy (type I), bilateral adenopathy with diffuse parenchymal abnormalities (type II), and diffuse parenchymal changes without hilar adenopathy (type III). The alveolitis of sarcoidosis is manifested on radiographs as an infiltrative process. Although patients with type I radiographs tend to have a reversible form of the disease and those with types II and III usually have chronic progressive disease, these patterns are not necessarily consecutive stages.

Diagnosis is based on a combination of clinical, radiographic, and histological findings. The chest x-ray, although characteristic, is not diagnostic because the typical bilateral hilar adenopathy may be seen with other diseases. Biopsy evidence of a mononuclear cell granulomatous inflammatory process is mandatory for definitive diagnosis. Because the lung is so frequently involved, it is the most common biopsy site, usually via fiberoptic bronchoscopy. Biopsy may be performed on any involved organ.

| Box 12-13 | Classification of Chest Radiographic Findings in Sarcoidosis |

Type	Radiographic Findings
0	Hilar and/or mediastinal node enlargement with normal lung parenchyma
II	Hilar and/or mediastinal node enlargement and diffuse interstitial pulmonary disease
III	Diffuse pulmonary disease without node involvement
IV	Pulmonary fibrosis

Other tests and methods are used to diagnose sarcoidosis. *Bronchoalveolar lavage* is an accurate method of making the diagnosis. The finding of an increase in the relative and absolute numbers of T-lymphocytes, monocytes, and macrophages in the lung is used as an indication for therapy. The serum angiotensin-converting enzyme is negative in two-thirds of patients and false-positive results are common. The *Kveim-Siltzbach test* requires intradermal injection of human sarcoid tissue. A nodule develops at the injection site in 4–6 weeks in patients with sarcoidosis and biopsy reveals noncaseating granulomas in 70–80%. This is not commonly used today.

Many patients require no specific therapy. However, those with severe active disease are often treated with glucocorticoids that suppress the activated T-cells at the disease site and the clinical manifestations of the disease. Steroids are only administered if the disease is active. The chest radiograph is not a sensitive indicator of disease activity. Bronchoalveolar lavage and Ga-67 scans are used as indicators of disease activity.

Gallium-67 Scintigraphy
Ga-67 scans are positive in most patients with active sarcoidosis. Scintigraphy has been used to assess the magnitude of alveolitis, to guide lung biopsy, and to choose the pulmonary segments for bronchoalveolar lavage. It can distinguish active granuloma formation and alveolitis from inactive disease and fibrotic changes. Increased Ga-67 uptake in the lungs is more than 90% sensitive for clinically active disease. Scans are negative in inactive cases.

Ga-67 is more sensitive than a chest radiograph for detecting early disease. Pulmonary uptake on scintigraphy can be seen before characteristic abnormalities are present on radiographs. One third of patients have normal radiographs at this stage of disease. Patients with a normal Ga-67 scan nearly always have a negative biopsy. Patients with a diagnosis of sarcoidosis and an abnormal chest radiograph, but inactive disease, have a negative Ga-67 scan. In these cases the abnormal radiograph represents past, not present, disease.

There is generally good correlation between Ga-67 lung uptake and lymphocyte content in lavage fluid. The Ga-67 scan's primary use has been to evaluate for disease activity and to guide therapeutic decisions. It is a sensitive indicator of treatment response, superior to clinical symptoms, chest radiograph, and pulmonary function tests.

Scintigraphic Patterns
In early disease the Ga-67 scan often shows bilateral hilar and paratracheal uptake (lambda sign) (*see* Fig. 12-4B). Pulmonary parenchymal uptake when present is intense and symmetrical (*see* Fig. 12-4C) and may or may not be associated with hilar and mediastinal involvement.

Patients with malignant lymphoma usually have asymmetrical hilar or mediastinal uptake, often involving the anterior mediastinal and paratracheal nodes. Although paraaortic, mesenteric, and retroperitoneal lymph node involvement may be seen in sarcoidosis, uptake is much more common in lymphoma.

Prominent uptake in the nasopharyngeal region, the parotid, salivary, and lacrimal glands is common (panda sign) (*see* Fig. 12-4C). The combination of ocular involvement (iritis or iridocyclitis) with accompanying lacrimal gland inflammation and bilateral salivary gland involvement is known as *uveoparotid fever*.

The degree of pulmonary uptake of Ga-67 is judged relative to uptake in the liver, bone marrow, and soft tissue. Lung uptake greater than liver is positive for sarcoidosis. Uptake less than soft tissue is negative. The posterior view is preferable for estimating uptake. Oblique views or SPECT can be useful for discerning mediastinal and hilar uptake or confirming pulmonary uptake when in question.

Semiquantitative indexes of Ga-67 uptake have been proposed. Although more objective quantification is desirable, uptake by normal overlying soft tissue, breasts, heart, sternum, ribs, scapulae, and spine and bone marrow complicate quantification. F-18 FDG also has prominent uptake in active sarcoidosis.

Idiopathic Interstitial Pulmonary Fibrosis
The etiology of idiopathic interstitial pulmonary fibrosis is unknown. Typically the disease follows a progression through stages of alveolitis, with derangement of the alveolar-capillary units, leading to end-stage fibrotic disease. Ga-67 uptake is seen in approximately 70% of patients. Ga-67 has been used to monitor the course of disease and response to therapy. The amount of uptake correlates with the degree of cellular infiltration, but does not predict the results of steroid treatment.

Pulmonary Drug Reactions
Some of the therapeutic drugs known to cause lung injury and result in Ga-67 uptake include cytoxan, nitrofurantoin,

bleomycin, and amiodarone (*see* Box 12-11). Contrast used for lymphangiography may cause a chemical-induced alveolitis. Ga-67 uptake is an early indicator of drug-induced lung injury, before the radiograph is abnormal.

Immunosuppressed Patients

The clinical presentation, physical findings, and radiological abnormalities in immunosuppressed patients are often obscured by an impaired inflammatory response caused by the underlying disease or therapy. Furthermore, many of the organisms causing infection (e.g., *Pneumocystis carinii, Cryptococcus,* and cytomegalovirus [CMV]) produce a minimal inflammatory response even in healthy hosts.

Immunosuppression is seen most commonly in patients with AIDS and those receiving drugs for cancer chemotherapy or organ transplantation. The diagnostic sensitivity of sonography, CT, and MRI depends on the presence of normal anatomical markers, which can be disrupted by disease or previous surgical procedures. Monitoring the effects of therapy is complicated by the slowness of response, the lack of microbiological methods for assessing response, and the need for extended courses of therapy for some opportunistic infections.

Ga-67 citrate can aid in the differential diagnosis of pulmonary disorders in immunosuppressed patients (Fig. 12-38). The patterns of Ga-67 pulmonary uptake can be classified as diffuse parenchymal, focal parenchymal, or nodal.

Diffuse Parenchymal Uptake
The first pulmonary manifestation of AIDS is often *Pneumocystis carinii* pneumonia (PCP). The chest x-ray findings are usually abnormal, with bilateral diffuse infiltrates originating from the hilum and extending peripherally. However, the radiograph may show a lobar or nodular infiltrate or be normal.

Ga-67 scans are abnormal in approximately 90% of cases. The scan is often positive before the chest radiograph becomes abnormal. The characteristic pattern in PCP infection is diffuse bilateral pulmonary uptake (*see* Fig. 12-37), uniform or nonuniform, without nodal or parotid uptake.

Increased Ga-67 uptake in an immunocompromised patient may be from other causes, including CMV infection, bacterial pneumonitis, lymphocytic interstitial pneumonitis, or the effects of various drug therapies. The greater the Ga-67 uptake, the more likely the diagnosis is PCP. Uptake at initial presentation of PCP is typically higher than that seen after the treatment of recurrences. The prophylactic use of aerosolized pentamidine therapy has resulted in atypical heterogeneous patterns of uptake.

Cytomegalovirus Infection
The radiographic appearance in *lymphoid interstitial pneumonia* may be normal or similar to that seen in PCP, viral infections, or miliary tuberculosis. Ga-67 uptake is only low-grade and diffuse without nodal uptake. This may be accompanied by ocular uptake caused by retinitis, adrenal and renal uptake, persistent colon uptake associated with diarrhea, and sometimes symmetrically increased parotid uptake.

Focal Pulmonary Uptake
This is a less common pattern typically seen with bacterial pneumonia. Corresponding infiltrates are seen on chest radiographs. Intense Ga-67 uptake in a lobar configuration in the absence of nodal and parotid uptake suggests bacterial pneumonia. When multiple sites of focal accumulation are present, aggressive infections caused by *Actinomyces, Nocardia,* and *Aspergillus* should be considered.

Nodal uptake Mycobacterium avium-intracellulare (MAI) infection, tuberculosis, lymphoma, and occasionally PCP will have nodal uptake in conjunction with pulmonary uptake. Other causes are lymphadenitis, cryptococcal infection, and herpes simplex. Infection with MAI causes widespread disease in 25–50% of AIDS patients and requires more aggressive therapy than that used for tuberculosis. Patchy lung uptake with hilar and nonhilar nodal (axillary, inguinal) uptake suggests MAI.

Negative Ga-67 Uptake
The absence of Ga-67 uptake in conjunction with a negative chest radiograph excludes pulmonary infection with a high degree of certainty. When the chest x-ray findings are positive, particularly in a patient with deteriorating

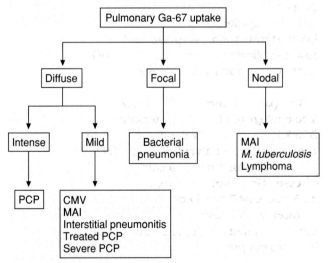

Figure 12-38 Diagnostic decision tree: pulmonary Ga-67 uptake in the immunosuppressed patients. *Ga,* Gallium; *MAI,* mycobacterium avium-intracellulare; *PCP,* pneumoocystis carinii pneumonia; *CMV,* cytomegalovirus.

respiratory status, but Ga-67 is negative, Kaposi's sarcoma must be considered.

Intracerebral Infection

The differential diagnosis of an intracerebral mass in an AIDS patient includes infection, most commonly toxoplasmosis and malignancy, most commonly lymphoma. Generally Tl-201 has been used for this purpose. Increased uptake greater than contralateral brain or scalp is consistent with malignancy and low or no uptake is characteristic of inflammatory disease.

Abdominal and Pelvic Infections

In-111-labeled leukocytes are superior to Ga-67 for diagnosing intestinal infection because of normal Ga-67 intestinal clearance. Occasionally abnormal uptake will be noted incidentally when pulmonary disease is being assessed. In the immunosuppressed patient, proximal small bowel uptake occurs with the protozoon infection *Cryptosporidium.* When stool cultures are negative for *Salmonella* or *Shigella,* diffuse colonic uptake that does not change with time is probably the result of CMV infection or antibiotic-induced colitis. The findings of eye, adrenal, esophageal, and low-grade pulmonary uptake increases the certainty of CMV. Multifocal activity (e.g., paratracheal and bowel) is indicative of mycobacterial infection.

Malignant External Otitis

This life-threatening infection occurs in diabetics secondary to *Pseudomonas.* Increased Ga-67 uptake can differentiate this disease from other less serious causes such as therapy-resistant external otitis. With malignant otitis, increased uptake is seen in the temporal bone on both bone scans and Ga-67 scans. The bone scan can establish the initial diagnosis. Ga-67 scan is useful for evaluating the effectiveness of therapy.

Fever of Unknown Origin

Fever of unknown origin is defined by clinicians as a temperature of at least 38.3°C that occurs on more than three occasions, remains without a diagnosed cause for at least 3 weeks, and results in at least 7 days of hospitalization. For patients who have not had recent surgery, Ga-67 is a sensitive test for uncovering the source of the fever. In addition to localizing acute infection, Ga-67 can detect chronic and indolent infections, granulomatous infections, and even tumor sources of fever. However, postoperative patients with fever are better served with In-111-labeled leukocytes because

fever is most commonly caused by an acute infection. Additionally In-111 leukocytes do not have the bowel clearance problem of Ga-67 to confound intra-abdominal interpretation.

SUGGESTED READING

Blockman D, Knockaert D, Maes A, et al: Clinical value of 18F fluoro-deoxyglucose positron emission tomography for patients with fever of unknown origin. Clin Infect Dis 32:191–196, 2001.

Coleman RE, Datz FL: Detection of inflammatory disease using radiolabeled cells. In Sandler M, Coleman RE, Wackers FJTh, et al (eds): Diagnostic Nuclear Medicine, ed. 4, Baltimore, Lippincott Williams & Wilkins, 2003.

Datz FL, Taylor AT Jr: Cell labeling: techniques and clinical utility. In Freeman and Johnson's Clinical Radionuclide Imaging, ed. 3, Grune & Stratton, 1986.

McAfee JG, Samin A: In-111 labeled leukocytes: a review of problems in image interpretation. Radiology 155:221–229, 1985.

Meller J, Koster G, Liersch, et al: Chronic bacteria osteomyelitis: Prospective comparison of F-18 FDG imaging with a dual-headed coincidence camera and In-111 label led autologous leucocyte scintigraphy. Eur J Nucl Med 29:53–60, 2001.

Merkel KD, Brown ML, Dewanjee MK, Fitzgerald RH Jr: Comparison of indium-labeled-leukocyte imaging with sequential technetium-gallium scanning in the diagnosis of low-grade musculoskeletal sepsis. J Bone Joint Surg 67A:465–476, 1985.

Oyen WJG, Boerman OC, van der Laken CJ, et al: The uptake mechanism of inflammation- and infection-localizing agents. Eur J Nucl Med 23:459–465, 1996.

Palestro CJ, Kim CK, Swyer AJ, et al: Total-hip arthroplasty: Periprosthetic Indium-111-labeled leukocyte activity and complementary Technetium-99m-sulfur colloid imaging in suspected infection. J Nucl Med 31:1950–1955, 1990.

Palestro CJ, Kipper SL, Weiland F, et al: Osteomyelitis: diagnosis with 99mTc-labeled antigranulocyte antibodies compared with diagnosis with 111In-labeled leukocytes—Initial experience. Radiology 223:758–764, 2002.

Palestro CJ, Mehta HH, Patel M, et al: Marrow versus infection in the Charcot joint: indium-111 leukocyte and technetium-99m sulfur colloid scintigraphy. J Nucl Med 39:346–350, 1998.

Palestro CJ, Thomas MB: Scintigraphic evaluation of the diabetic foot. In Leonard M. Freeman (ed). Nuc Med Annual 2000. Philadelphia, Lippincott Williams & Wilkins, 2000.

Peters AM, Danpure HJ, Osman S, et al: Clinical experience with 99mTc-hexamethylpropylene-amineoxime for labeling leucocytes and imaging inflammation. Lancet 2525:946–948, 1986.

Rennen HJ, Boerman OC, Oyen WJ, et al: Specific and rapid scintigraphic detection of infection with 99m Tc labeled interleukin-8. J Nucl Med 42:117–123, 2001.

Rypins EB, Kipper SL, Weiland F, et al: 99mTc Anti-CD 15 monoclonal antibody (LeuTech) Imaging improves diagnostic accuracy and clinical management in patients with appendicitis. Ann Surg 235:232–239, 2002.

Nuclear medicine has imaged the central nervous system (CNS) for decades. Before the development of computed tomography (CT) in the 1970s, nuclear medicine brain scans were the only noninvasive method for diagnosing diseases of the brain including tumors, strokes, and vascular anomalies. Although magnetic resonance imaging (MRI) and CT are the most commonly utilized brain-imaging modalities today, nuclear medicine offers unique diagnostic information based on imaging physiology. Single photon emission tomography (SPECT) and positron emission tomography (PET) can visualize physiologic changes of disease before anatomic changes can be detected. Numerous radiopharmaceuticals have been used and some clinically important SPECT and PET agents are listed in Box 13-1.

Cerebral Anatomy

Knowledge of brain anatomy is critical in understanding patterns of disease and image interpretation. The brain consists of the two cerebral hemispheres above the tentorium and the cerebellum below in the posterior fossa. The regions or lobes of the brain are illustrated in Figure 13-1. The frontal lobe extends back to the central sulcus with the parietal lobe just posterior to it. The occipital lobe is most posterior, below the parieto-occipital sulcus. The temporal lobes are below the lateral fissure. Within these lobes, key functional centers or regions have been identified, which are important when trying to assimilate clinical changes with anatomical and functional images (Fig. 13-2).

Studies such as dynamic radionuclide brain flow and brain death exam allow visualization of the vascular supply of the brain to a limited degree (Figs. 13-3 and 13-4). Even more important for image interpretation is familiarity with the cerebral regions these vessels supply (Fig. 13-5).

Box 13-1 Brain SPECT and PET Radiopharmaceuticals Used Clinically

Radiopharmaceutical	Radionuclide Photopeak (keV)
Blood–brain barrier	
Tc-99m glucoheptonate	140
Tc-99m DTPA	
Brain perfusion	
I-123 iodoamphetamine (IMP)	159
Tc-99m HMPAO *(Ceretec)*	140
Tc-99m methyl cysteinate dimer (ECD)	140
Metabolism	
F-18 fluorodeoxyglucose (FDG)	511
Brain tumor imaging	
Thallium-201	69–83, 167 (10%)
Tc-99m sestamibi	140
F-18 FDG 511	
Cisternography	
In-111 DTPA	173, 247
Tc-99m DTPA	140

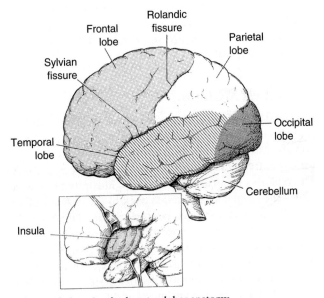

Figure 13-1 Cerebral cortex lobar anatomy.

Radiopharmaceuticals

Radiopharmaceuticals can be divided into those that do and those that do not cross the blood-brain barrier (BBBB). The first radionuclide brain scan agent, used in

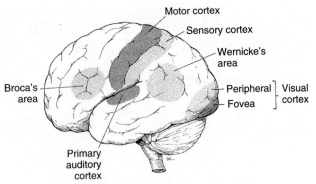

Figure 13-2 Motor, sensory, visual, speech, and auditory functional and associative centers of the brain.

the 1970s, was Tc-99m pertechnetate. It did not normally cross the intact BBB. Accumulation in the choroid plexus and salivary glands and slow blood pool clearance made interpretation difficult. Tc-99m diethylenetriaminepentacetic acid (DTPA) and Tc-99m glucoheptonate, renal radiopharmaceuticals, were subsequently used and did not have those problems. Uptake in the brain only occurred if there was disruption of the BBB (e.g., with tumor and stroke). The sensitivity for detecting disease was quite good, ranging from 80% for stroke and 85% for brain tumors. However, with the advent of CT in the 1980s, the use of BBB studies declined markedly.

Currently, functional nuclear medicine imaging studies rely on PET and SPECT radiopharmaceuticals, which cross the BBB and reveal details not seen by CT or MRI. Of course, the anatomy seen on CT and MRI is much more detailed than the structures seen with SPECT or PET, but many structures can be visualized (Fig. 13-6). Different categories of radiopharmaceuticals can be used to evaluate regional cerebral perfusion (rCBF), brain metabolism (e.g., regional glucose metabolism, rCGM), or neurotransmitter receptor binding. Indications for nuclear medicine evaluation of the CNS are listed in Box 13-2.

Over a quarter of a century ago, PET imaging began with the brain. Unlike other functional imaging tests such as functional MRI (fMRI), PET offers the ability to precisely measure or quantitate not only the one parameter being studied, but also global changes in flow and metabolism. The physical properties of common PET radionuclides used in the CNS are described in Table 13-1. F-18 fluorodeoxyglucose (F-18 FDG) is the only agent approved by the U.S. Food and Drug Administration (FDA) and is available on a clinical basis. However, an extensive array of radiopharmaceuticals targeting metabolism, blood flow, and neurotransmitters are under investigation. Some are listed in Box 13-3.

The clinical availability of PET technology is only a recent phenomenon, and most clinical nuclear

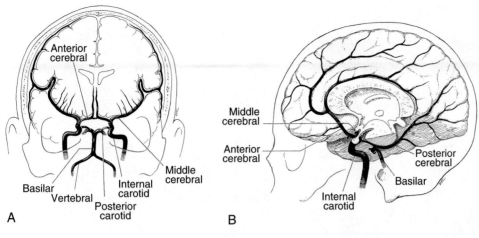

A

B

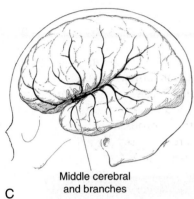

C

Figure 13-3   Cerebral arterial anatomy.   **A,** Coronal section shows circle of Willis and course of the middle and anterior cerebral arteries. Internal carotids divide at the base of the brain (circle of Willis) into the anterior and middle cerebral arteries.   The middle cerebral artery runs laterally in the sylvian fissure, then backward and upward on the surface of the insula, where it divides into branches to the *lateral* surface of the cerebral hemisphere and to portions of the basal ganglia.   **B,** Midline sagittal view shows distribution of anterior, middle, and posterior cerebral arteries.   The anterior cerebral artery supplies the cerebrum along its *medial* margin above the corpus callosum and extends posteriorly to the parietal fissure as well as to the anterior portion of the basal ganglia.   Vertebral arteries fuse into the basilar artery, which branches at the circle of Willis into the two posterior cerebral arteries supplying the occipital lobe and the inferior half of the temporal lobe.   **C,** Left lateral view shows distribution of the middle cerebral artery over the cerebral cortex.

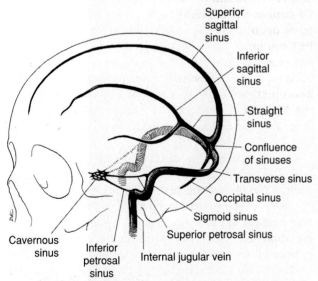

Figure 13-4   Cerebral venous anatomy.   The superior sagittal sinus runs along the falx within the superior margin of the interhemispheric fissure.   The inferior sagittal sinus is smaller, courses over the corpus callosum, and joins with the great vein of Galen to form the straight sinus, which drains into the superior sagittal sinus at the confluence of sinuses (torcular Herophili) at the occipital protuberance.   Transverse sinuses drain the sagittal and occipital sinuses into the internal jugular vein.

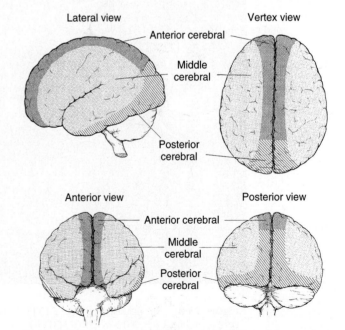

Figure 13-5   Regional cerebral cortex perfusion of the anterior, middle, and posterior cerebral arteries.

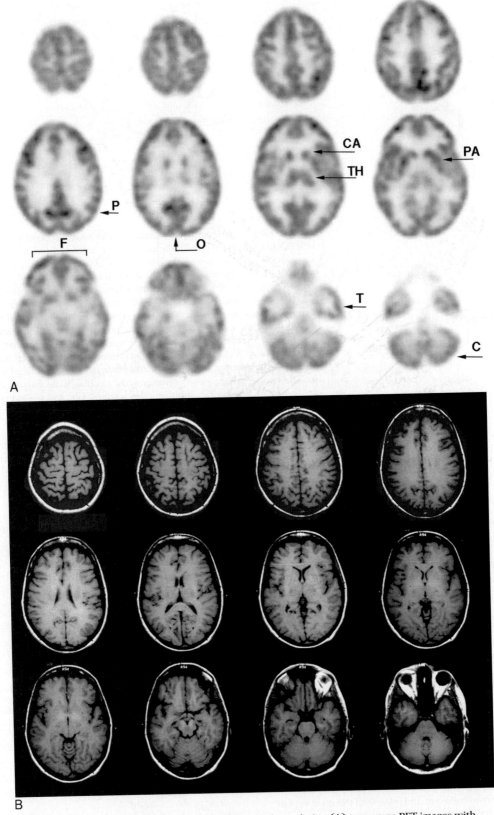

Figure 13-6 Normal distribution of F-18 FDG. High-resolution (**A**) transverse PET images with corresponding levels on T1-weighted MRI (**B**).

Continued

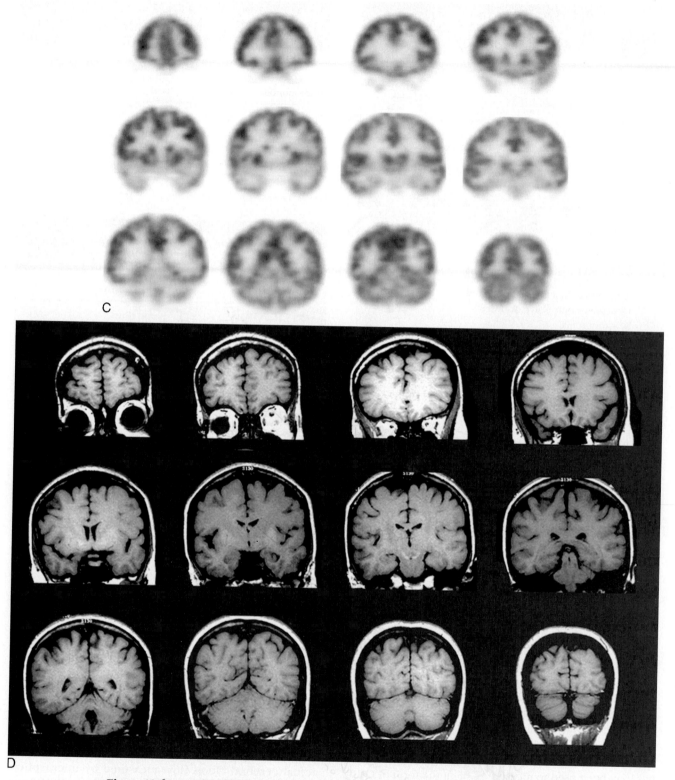

C

D

Figure 13-6, cont'd   Coronal PET **(C)** and comparable T1-weighted MRI **(D)**. *F,* Frontal lobe; *T,* temporal lobe; *P,* parietal lobe; *O,* occipital lobe; *C,* cerebellum; *Th,* thalamus; *Ca,* caudate; *PA,* putamen.

Box 13-2   Clinical Indications for Cortical Cerebral Scintigraphy

Dementia
  Alzheimer's disease
  Lewy body disease
  Pick's disease
  Multi-infarct dementia
  Acquired immunodeficiency syndrome–dementia
    complex
Epilepsy
Stroke
Transient ischemia attacks
Head trauma
Movement disorders
  Parkinson's disease
  Huntington's chorea
Psychiatric disorders
  Attention deficit disorder
  Obsessive-compulsive disorder
  Schizophrenia
Brain death
Tumor imaging

Table 13-1   Positron Emission Tomography Radionuclides

Radionuclide	Half-life (min)	Imaging photo peak (keV)	Maximum beta-energy (MeV)
Fluorine-18	110	511	0.635
Carbon-11	20	511	0.970
Nitrogen-13	10	511	1.2
Oxygen-15	2	511	1.7

Box 13-3   Positron Emission Tomography Radiopharmaceuticals

Compound	Application
O-15 H$_2$O	Blood flow
O-15 O$_2$	Oxygen metabolism/flow
O-15 or C-11 carboxyhemoglobin	Blood volume
C-11 methionine	Amino acid metabolism
C-11 methylpiperone	Dopamine receptor activity
C-11 carfentanil	Opiate receptor activity
C-11 flunitrazepam	Benzodiazepine receptor activity
C-11 scopolamine	Muscarinic cholinergic receptors
C-11 ephedrine	Adrenergic terminals
F-18 fluorodeoxyglucose (FDG)	Glucose metabolism
F-18 fluoro-L-dopa	Presynaptic dopamine system
F-18 fluorothymidine (FLT)	DNA synthesis

medicine brain studies utilize SPECT gamma camera technology. SPECT radiopharmaceuticals are lipophilic, cross the intact blood–brain barrier, and are ideally labeled with Tc-99m. There is no SPECT radiotracer equivalent to F-18 FDG for measuring metabolism. SPECT agents generally reflect blood flow changes because cortical rCBF is closely linked to the oxygen demands of the brain and usually approximates metabolism. Areas with more synaptic activity require greater blood flow. Activational studies can therefore target areas of the brain showing increased flow when activated by a certain task. In many ways, the SPECT images are similar to the F-18 FDG PET images. Like F-18 FDG, a similar pattern of increased gray matter to white matter differential is seen.

Cerebral Blood Flow Radiopharmaceuticals

Studying rCBF patterns can help diagnose disease. Many inert, freely diffusible radiotracers have been developed, which closely approximate rCBF as measured by microsphere injection techniques. The positron emitter O-15 has long been used to measure rCBF in the form of O-15 labeled water (O-15 H$_2$O). Inhaled O-15 can be used to measure oxygen extraction and metabolism. Many technical demands are created by the short half-life of O-15 (2 minutes), including rapid imaging, continuous radiotracer input flow, and an onsite cyclotron. It should also be noted that although accurate quantitation is possible

with PET, arterial sampling and even sometimes arterial injections are needed for true quantitation.

The noble gas xenon-133 (Xe-133) is best known as a ventilation lung scan agent. However, once in the lungs, it rapidly travels throughout the body and readily diffuses across the BBB. Given its high extraction efficiency, the perfusion pattern correlates better with actual cerebral blood flow measured by microsphere techniques than the other currently available SPECT perfusion agents. It is cleared quickly from the body, allowing for multiple acquisitions as might be needed in activational studies. However, this rapid clearance also makes Xe-133 technically demanding to use. Another limitation of Xe-133 is the lower-energy gamma photons

(80 keV) and a high scatter fraction, which both contribute to poor image quality. Xe-133 is a valuable research tool, providing an inexpensive and noninvasive approach to quantitate rCBF.

The lipophilic amines derivative iodine-123 isopropyl iodoamphetamine (I-123 IMP or Spectamine) localizes in the brain by temporarily binding to amphetamine receptors. With an extraction ratio greater than 90%, I-123 IMP reasonably approximates rCBF. Imaging must be done rapidly, usually within 1 hour, as it is not fixed in the neurons but washes out. This allows for interesting imaging possibilities, as abnormal but viable ischemic regions will show "redistribution" like a thallium-201 cardiac stress test (Fig. 13-7). No longer clinically available, I-123 IMP has been replaced by the Tc-99m agents, which have better dosimetry and imaging characteristics.

Technetium-99m rCBF Radiopharmaceuticals

Currently, the neutral, lipophilic Tc-99m labeled hexamethylpropyleneamine oxime (Tc-99m HMPAO) and ethyl cysteinate dimer (Tc-99m ECD) are used clinically. Favorable characteristics of these two agents include high first-pass extraction across the BBB, close correlation with rCBF, and desirable 140 keV gamma photons. However, both slightly underestimate true rCBF, especially at high flow states. Unlike O-15 water, Xe-133, and I-123 IMP, the Tc-99m perfusion agents are relatively fixed in the neuron. Therefore, delayed imaging shows what the perfusion pattern looked like at the time of injection. If injected during an epileptic seizure, perfusion abnormalities can be seen hours after seizure resolution.

In practice, the distribution of Tc-99m HMPAO and Tc-99m ECD is slightly different might be difficult to compare directly in serial patient studies. Tc-99m HMPAO accumulates more in the frontal lobes, thalamus, and cerebellum, whereas Tc-99m ECD shows higher affinity for the parietal and occipital lobes. Most clinicians use the agent with which they are most familiar.

Tc-99m HMPAO (Tc-99m Exametazime or Ceretec) was first introduced in the mid-1980s. Originally available as a kit requiring use within 30 minutes of radiolabeling, stabilizers have since been added allowing a 4-hour shelf-life following the addition of the radiolabel. Tc-99m HMPAO has a good first-pass extraction of roughly 80%, with 3.5-7.0% of the injected dose localizing in the brain within 1 minute of injection. Once across the BBB, it enters the neuron and becomes a polar hydrophilic molecule remaining trapped inside the cell. However, some of the radiopharmaceutical may be present in different isomeric forms, which do not remain trapped. Although up to 15% of the dose washes out in the first 2 minutes, there is little loss over the next 24 hours. SPECT image acquisition can be done anywhere from 15 minutes to 2 hours after injection. Excretion is largely renal (40%) and gastrointestinal (15%).

Tc-99m ECD (Tc-99m Bicisate, Neurolite) is a neutral lipophilic agent that passively diffuses across the BBB like Tc-99m HMPAO. Once prepared, the Tc-99m ECD dose is stable for 6 hours. Like Tc-99m HMPAO, it also underestimates true rCBF. It has a first-pass extraction of 60-70%, with peak brain activity reaching 5-6% of the injected dose. The blood clearance is more rapid than Tc-99m HMPAO, resulting in better brain-to-background ratios. At 1 hour, less than 5% of the dose remains in the blood, compared to over 12% of a Tc-99m HMPAO dose.

Once inside the cell, the mechanism of Tc-99m ECD retention differs from Tc-99m HMPAO, as it involves enzymatic de-esterification forming polar metabolites unable to cross the cell membrane. However, there is a slow (roughly 6% per hour) washout of some labeled metabolites. Although images may be superior to Tc-99m HMPAO 15-30 minutes after injection, they may be suboptimal if imaging is delayed. Almost 25% of the brain activity has cleared if imaging is delayed 4 hours.

Glucose Metabolism—F-18 FDG

The brain is an obligate glucose user, and F-18 FDG is a glucose analog allowing accurate assessment of regional glucose metabolism (rCGM). F-18 FDG is able to cross the blood–brain barrier utilizing glucose transporter systems and enters the neuron. After rapid phosphorylation by hexokinase-1, F-18 FDG is metabolically trapped and cannot proceed further along the glucose metabolism pathway. F-18 FDG PET, with a resolution of 4-5 mm, is superior to the 7 mm of SPECT. Approximately 4% of the administered dose is localized to brain. By 35 minutes after injection, 95% of peak uptake is achieved. Urinary excretion is rapid with 10-40% of the dose cleared in 2 hours. In addition to reflecting rCBF as a marker of glucose metabolism, F-18 FDG can be used to determine tumor viability. With its 110-minute half-life, F-18 FDG does not require an expensive onsite cyclotron. As PET technology enters mainstream medicine, costs (including the price of the dose) continue to drop.

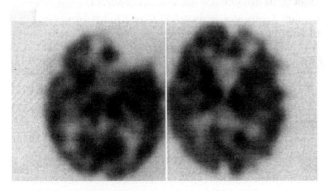

Figure 13-7   Type I-VI are described in Table 13-5.

Normal Distribution of rCBF and rCGM Agents

As blood flow relates to brain activity, the greater than 2:1 differential in blood flow of gray matter to white matter seen on SPECT and PET scans is not surprising. Lesions in the white matter often can not be detected or even differentiated from cerebrospinal fluid (CSF) spaces on PET or SPECT. Close correlation with MRI or CT is necessary for identifying white matter changes and enlarged ventricles.

It is important to be familiar with normal radiopharmaceutical distribution and the factors that can alter that pattern. Typically, activity is fairly evenly distributed between the lobes of the brain. However, this is dependent on the conditions at the time of injection. For example, bright lights will increase occipital lobes activity, falsely causing the frontal lobes to appear decreased. Therefore, conditions must be carefully controlled. Having intravenous access in place well before the dose is injected helps decrease stimuli. The patient should be in a quiet, dimly lit room, with eyes usually kept open.

The normal distribution of SPECT and PET agents also changes with age. In children, there is a relative decrease in perfusion to the frontal lobes. This increases over time, reaching an adult level by about 2 years of age. In adults, global activity decreases with age, and this decrease is more prominent in the frontal regions. Utilizing comparison age-matched normal databases and computer programs that quantitate rCBF may help improve not only sensitivity but specificity given these changes.

Methodology

Imaging protocols will vary greatly depending on the specific instrumentation used. However, it is safe to say that when SPECT is being performed in the brain, more heads are better than one. Dedicated triple-head gamma cameras are increasingly rare but yield the best results if available. A dual-headed camera creates images superior to a single-headed SPECT camera. Patient positioning is just as important as the equipment used. The heads of the camera must come as close to the patient as possible or resolution is lost. In heavy patients and those whose shoulders get in the way, the posterior fossa may not be seen. A protocol for Tc-99m cerebral perfusion SPECT imaging is given in Box 13-4. The SPECT images may be processed using filtered back projection, although newer systems offer iterative reconstruction. A filter is applied to smooth the image. In general, filters can be sampled and modified for each patient in the postprocessing stage to achieve an optimal image.

PET imaging with F-18 FDG provides higher resolution than SPECT imaging with the technetium-labeled perfusion radiopharmaceuticals. Resolution can be optimized by acquiring images with septa in front of

---

Box 13-4   SPECT Cerebral Perfusion Imaging: Protocol Summary

PATIENT PREPARATION

None.

RADIOPHARMACEUTICAL

20 mCi technetium-99m HMPAO (Ceretec) or Tc-99m ECD (Neurolite)

INSTRUMENTATION

Camera: triple-headed SPECT or dual headed SPECT
Collimators: ultra-high resolution parallel hole
Computer setup: SPECT acquisition parameters
    Matrix size: 64 × 64
    Zoom: 2
    Rotation: step and shoot
    Orbit: circular
    Angle step size: 3 degrees
    Stops: 40 per head
    Time per stop: 40 sec (total time, 1600 sec or 27 min)

IMAGING PROCEDURE

Prepare dose according to package insert. Note shelf life.
Begin IV or tape butterfly in place; make patient comfortable in quiet, dimly lit room; inject; eyes open; begin scanning in 15 minutes to 2-3 hours later
Position patient so that brain is entirely within field of view of all detectors
Position collimators as close as possible to patient's head
Record radius

PROCESSING

Filtered back projection or iterative reconstruction
Filter: Hamming, 1.2 high-frequency cutoff
Attenuation correction: $0.11\ cm^{-1}$

---

the detectors (two-dimensional [2-D] mode). The septa minimize scatter. Many sites prefer the higher count rate three-dimensional mode, which does not use septa. Although resolution is lowered by scatter, many camera systems have done away with 2-D mode for the brain. A sample protocol is listed in (Box 13-5). Like SPECT studies, the patient should be injected in a quiet, dimly lit room. The patient should remain undisturbed during the uptake period. Postprocessing protocols typical use iterative algorithms rather than filtered back projections.

Dosimetry

The dosimetry of cerebral radionuclide imaging depends on the radiopharmaceutical utilized. A comparison of several agents is given in Table 13-2.

Box 13-5   PET Imaging Protocol

PATIENT PREPARATION

Fast 4-6 hours, avoid carbohydrates, maintain normal blood glucose.

Check blood glucose. If <180–200, continue.

Elevated glucose: consider rescheduling, administer insulin, recheck, delay 2 hours.

Inject in quiet, dimly lit room, eyes open.

Wait 35-45 minutes

RADIOPHARMACEUTICAL

5-15 mCi (185–555 MBq) F-18 fluorodeoxyglucose (F-18 FDG)

INSTRUMENTATION

Dedicated PET or PET-CT camera

Coincidence camera

IMAGING

Attenuation correction scan: gadolinium rods or CT

Acquisition: 7 min per bed position for one bed position

PROCESSING

Iterative reconstruction, automated software

CLINICAL APPLICATIONS OF CEREBRAL PERFUSION IMAGING

Dementia

As our population ages, dementia has an increasing impact on our society and healthcare systems. Patients may display differing clinical symptoms (e.g., short- or long-term memory loss, loss of judgment, personality changes, and loss of other higher cortical functions). The functional decline can occur rapidly over months or slowly over years. The mental changes must be differentiated from the normal decline in memory and decreased ability to learn new things that accompany aging. However, the clinical diagnosis is often difficult and delayed, and MRI may not reveal changes such as atrophy until the end stages of disease.

Dementia is a manifestation of many diseases, not all primarily of the brain (Box 13-6). Only about 10% of dementias, such as those caused by vitamin B_{12} or thyroid hormone deficiency, are treatable. However, with better understanding of the diseases underlying dementia, new therapies are being developed. For example, the cholinesterase inhibitors have shown some stabilizing effects in patients with AD, occasionally even reversing perfusion trends seen on SPECT scans. As treatments are developed, early diagnosis will likely be more critical.

SPECT and PET can help diagnose the etiology of dementia much earlier than clinical criteria or MRI. Studies have shown that combining clinical diagnosis

Table 13-2   Absorbed Radiation Doses

Dose	Tc-99m HMPAO Rads/20 mCi (cGy/740 MBq)	Tc-99m ECD Rads/20 mCi (cGy/740 MBq)	F-18 FDG Rads/10 mCi (cGy/370 MBq)	Tl-201 Rad/2mCi
Brain	0.5			
Lens and retina	0.5			
Heart			1.5	
Lung		0.2	0.6	1.0
Liver	1.1	0.2	0.6	
Spleen			1.4	1.1
Gallbladder	3.8	4.0		
Kidney	2.6	0.5	0.7	
Large bowel	1.6	1.1		2.4
Bladder	0.9	2.2	4.1	
Testes	0.1	0.3		
Ovaries	0.5	0.6		1.0
Red marrow				1.0
Total body	0.3	0.2	0.2 0.4	0.4

Box 13-6   Causes of Dementia

Alzheimer's disease
Parkinson's disease
Lewy body disease
Multi-infarct dementia
Pick's disease
Progressive supranuclear palsy
Creutzfeldt-Jacob disease
Huntington's chorea
Multiple sclerosis
Vitamin B_{12} deficiency
Endocrine disorders (hypothyroidism)
Chronic infection (tuberculosis, syphilis)
Human immunodeficiency virus (HIV) encephalopathy
Alcohol and drugs

---

with perfusion findings on SPECT raises the positive predictive value compared to either method alone. PET has equal or better results in comparison with SPECT. Some investigations report that PET has a sensitivity and specificity of 94% and 73%, respectively.

Although PET has higher sensitivity and higher resolution than SPECT, the overall patterns seen in disease are similar for both rCGM and rCBF. Certain perfusion patterns have been recognized that are characteristic for different types of dementia. In general, these types of dementia can be characterized as posterior, frontotemporal, or vascular. The posterior dementias include AD, Lewy body disease, and dementia of PD. The frontotemporal dementias include Pick's disease and primary progressive aphasia. There is some overlap of vascular dementia and frontotemporal dementia. Multi-infarct dementia tends to display a generalized decrease in activity.

Posterior Dementias

AD is the most common of the dementias. It is estimated that nearly 10% of the population over 65 and 50% of those over 85 are affected. Diagnosis can be definitively made at autopsy or by the rarely performed brain biopsy with pathological samples showing characteristic neurofibrillary tangles and amyloid plaques. Originally described as a dementia of a relatively young person (presenile dementia), it is now recognized that many older people originally thought to have multi-infarct dementia actually have AD. On the other hand, 25% of those thought to have AD clinically were found to have other etiologies at autopsy.

Imaging findings vary with the stage of disease, but characteristic patterns are well established in AD for both PET and SPECT. Early disease tends to involve the superior parietotemporal cortex manifested as hypometabolism/hypoperfusion (Fig. 13-8A). Although the classic examples are

symmetric, AD is often rather asymmetric, especially in the early stages (Fig. 13-8B). As the disease progresses, it involves the frontal cortices, although parietal and temporal lobe involvement usually remains greater. It may be more difficult to diagnose very elderly patients and end-stage patients because the imaging pattern may be more of a generalized nonspecific decrease in cortical uptake (Fig. 13-8C). However, sparing of the occipital visual cortex, somatosensory and motor cortex, basal ganglia, thalamus, and cerebellum is the norm (Fig. 13-9).

The strength of FDG PET may be in differentiating which patients with so-called mild cognitive impairment (MCI) will progress on to actual AD. MCI patients have deficits on mini-mental status testing but do not meet probable AD criteria. Approximately 15% of MCI patients progress to AD per year. PET studies have shown that MCI patients with parietal and temporal hypoperfusion were much more likely to go on to AD than those without the pattern. Identification of patients in the presymptomatic or early phases of AD will be crucial for therapy in the future.

New PET radiopharmaceuticals are being investigated that bind to amyloid, muscarinic receptors, nicotinic receptors, and components of the cholinergic system. Correlation with genetic factors influencing AD will be ongoing. Recent developments have shown a strong link between scintigraphic perfusion patterns and certain genes, including the E4 allele of the apolipoprotein E gene in AD. The other diseases that affect the posterior regions of the brain often overlap with each other and with AD. These include Lewy body disease (dementia with Lewy bodies or DLB) and Parkinson's disease (PD). Roughly 30% of PD patients will develop dementia. Diagnosis of the dementia may be complicated clinically by depression. DLB is second only to AD among dementias caused by neurodegenerative disorders rather than by vascular etiologies. Pathological specimens of PD patients show Lewy body intracellular inclusions in the midbrain. In DLB, these Lewy bodies are found in the cerebral cortex. Clinically, these DLB patients often demonstrate a fluctuating dementia, falls, some Parkinsonian symptoms, such as tremor and visual hallucinations. It is likely that DLB and PD are related as part of a spectrum of disease. Movement disorder patients who later develop dementia are considered to have PD, whereas DLB patients are those who develop the movement disorder at the same time or later than dementia. FDG PET and SPECT perfusion agents images can confirm DLB by showing changes in the posterior cortical regions. The pattern is often similar to AD but tends to involve the occipital lobes to a greater extent (Fig. 13-10). The involvement of the primary visual cortex can explain the visual hallucinations. Another deviation from the AD patterns may be preservation of hippocampal activity in DLB but with

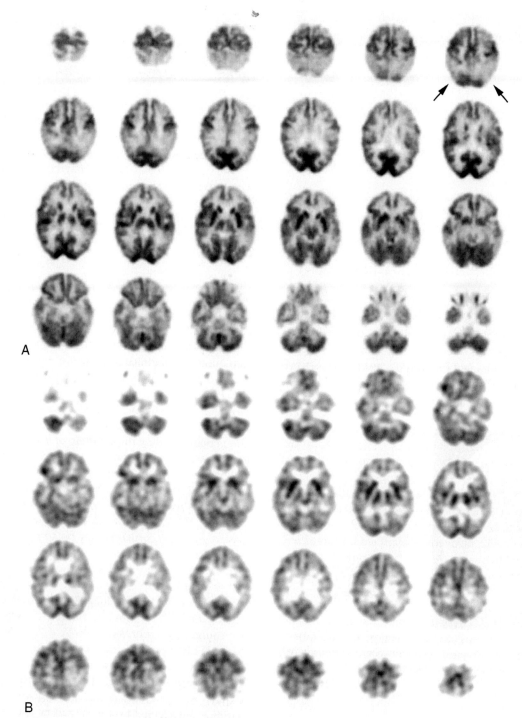

Figure 13-8   Alzheimer's disease. **A,** Transaxial PET images reveal decreased perfusion to the temporal parietal cortex beginning high in the posterior parietal region with sparring of the basal ganglia, thalamus and cerebellum. **B,** Tc-99m HMPAO SPECT show that while Alzheimer's is classically described as a symmetrical process, it may be quite asymmetric, as seen in the left posterior parietal region.

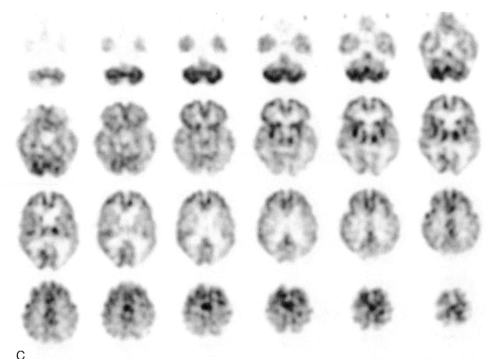

C

Figure 13-8, cont'd **C,** As Alzheimer's becomes more severe it is more diffuse on this SPECT study.

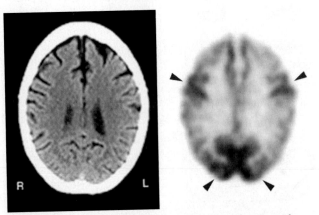

Figure 13-9 Alzheimer's disease on PET-CT. A patient with moderately advanced Alzheimer's shows hypometabolism not only in the posterior parietal and temporal regions but involvement now extends anteriorly. Sparring of the occipital region and sensory motor cortex is clear (*arrowheads*).

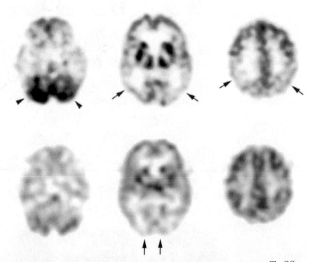

Figure 13-10 Comparison of posterior dementias on Tc-99m HMPAO. *Top row:* Alzheimer's disease generally begins near the superior convexity and involves the parietal and temporal regions laterally (*arrows*), sparing the occiput and cerebellum (*arrowhead*). *Bottom row:* Lewy body disease involves the medial occipital region (*arrows*) and usually has more caudal extension than Alzheimer's.

possibly greater involvement of the cerebellum. The imaging pattern of dementia in PD is also similar to AD with the exception of greater occipital involvement and more mesial temporal sparing. As depression (which often occurs in PD) can be confused with dementia, it is important to note these depressed PD patients can show decreased prefrontal and caudate activity rather than the posterior pattern so typical of dementia. However, other patterns have been described.

Frontotemporal Dementia

The frontotemporal dementias (FTD) are a diverse group of diseases that involve the frontal and temporal lobes (Fig. 13-11). Clinically, patients show varying presentations. Aphasia occurs with temporal lobe abnormalities

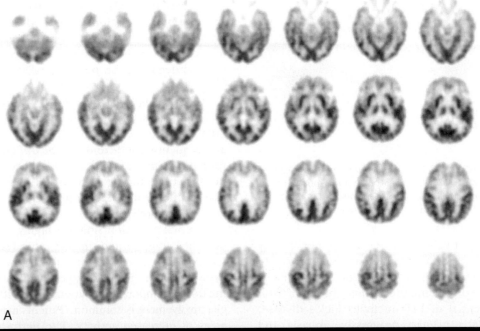

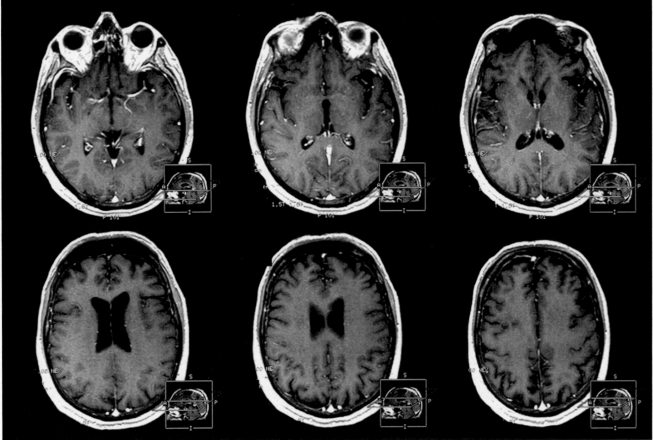

Figure 13-11   Frontotemporal dementia sparing posterior parietal regions. **A,** Frontal hypometabolism on PET can be due to many causes and changes visible long before MR shows atrophy or signal changes. **B,** Post-contrast T1-weighted MR shows no atrophy and other MR sequences were unremarkable.

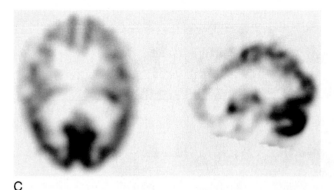

C

Figure 13-11, cont'd C, Pick's disease is rare. It classically shows frontal hypoperfusion with a sharp anterior to posterior cutoff, but the findings are somewhat nonspecific and other causes for decreased frontal activity must be considered.

and frontal lobe involvement results in personality changes, including loss of judgment and inappropriate behavior. In FTD, memory loss is often secondary or absent as opposed to being the primary problem as in AD. The differential of FTD includes Pick's disease, semantic dementia, primary progressive aphasia, and familial FTD. Pick's disease is the classic but rare FTD showing frontal and anterior temporal neuronal degeneration (Fig. 13-11C). Pick bodies are sometimes found but amyloid plaques, neurofibrillary tangles and Lewy bodies are absent. Severe atrophy on MRI is not visualized until much later than the perfusion and metabolic changes of SPECT and FDG PET.

Decreased perfusion and metabolism in the frontal and temporal lobes may be seen in diseases other than those in the FTD group. These include cocaine abuse, depression, progressive supranuclear palsy, spinocerebellar atrophy, amyotrophic lateral sclerosis, and very rarely in AD as an isolated finding. More commonly, decreased frontal and temporal rCBF and rCGM is secondary to a vascular process. Focal cortical defects, abnormalities on MRI, and areas of scintigraphic asymmetry should raise the level of suspicion for a vascular degenerative process.

Vascular Dementia

In vascular dementia, MRI often shows changes such as focal white matter lesions (subcortical encephalomalacia) and tiny cortical infarcts, which may not be visible on a SPECT or FDG PET study. However, because AD can overlap with vascular etiologies, PET or SPECT may be ordered in a patient with nonspecific vascular changes on MRI or with multi-infarct dementia. A strong frontal predisposition may be present in vascular dementia which must be differentiated from expected age-related decreases. Often, the generalized decrease in rCGM or rCBF seen in the vascular dementia patient is difficult to differentiate from severe Alzheimer's (Fig. 13-12). Sometimes small disruptions in the cortical ribbon or

subcortical defects such as in the thalamus can be seen. At other times, a regional decrease is seen that clearly correspond to regions supplied by main arterial branches such as the MCA. At times, when other causes for dementia such as Alzheimer's disease are excluded, vascular dementia may be left as a diagnosis of exclusion.

HIV Encephalopathy and AIDS-Dementia Complex

Early clinical signs of human immunodeficiency virus (HIV) and acquired immunodeficiency syndrome (AIDS) are frequently subtle and may be difficult to distinguish from depression, psychosis, or focal neurological disease. Because treatment (e.g., with AZT) can improve cognitive function, early detection is helpful. Findings on CT and MRI are not specific.

Cerebral perfusion SPECT is highly sensitive for AIDS-dementia complex and shows a typical scintigraphic pattern of patchy, multifocal cortical and subcortical regions of hypoperfusion. These changes occur most frequently in the frontal, temporal, and parietal lobes, although basal ganglia involvement is common. Patients may also have focal areas of increased activity. The perfusion pattern can improve with therapy. A similar brain perfusion pattern has been described in chronic cocaine and polydrug users.

Stroke and Cerebrovascular Disease

Although MRI and CT are now preeminent modalities for diagnosing stroke, there is a renewed interest in assessing patients with cerebrovascular disease with PET and SPECT to determine the role of therapeutic intervention. Nuclear medicine studies are frequently positive earlier than CT and may show characteristic cortical defects (Fig. 13-13). Functional imaging offers the ability to visualize and quantitate rCBF and rCGM, which can assess parameters of disease not seen on structural imaging. PET and SPECT can help determine which patients are at risk for stroke, most likely to benefit from intervention, and even predict stroke recovery. Relationships such as distant neuronal activity loss (diaschisis), neuron recruitment, and recovery through neuronal plasticity can be studied (Fig. 13-14).

The role of functional imaging in the acute stroke is evolving. The temporal development of a stroke has been studied. In the very early hours, tissue oxygen metabolism is maintained in the face of markedly reduced rCBF. This mismatch or "misery perfusion" implies viable tissue could be rescued, and the area at risk may be larger than seen on MRI. This is especially important in the periphery, or penumbra, of the affected area. PET and SPECT may play a part in determining who should get thrombolytic therapy, predicting recovery, and determining the amount of tissue at risk. Eventually, as the ischemia progresses, damage to vessels may result in excessive or "luxury perfusion,"

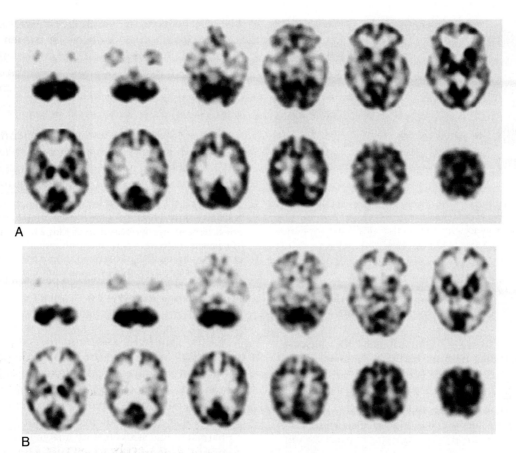

Figure 13-12   Vascular dementia, often shows a frontal predisposition similar to other FTD. **A,** Vascular dementia may be more diffuse as seen in this patient and difficult to differentiate from other etiologies including severe Alzheimer's. **B,** Slow progression was seen in this patient clinically and on a repeat scan 5 years later.

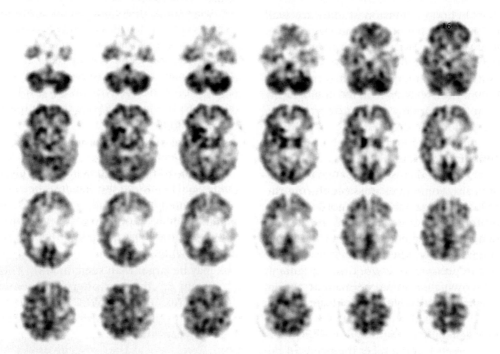

Figure 13-13   Left parietal middle cerebral artery cortical stroke. HMPAO SPECT shows significantly decreased perfusion to the region including subcortical structures.

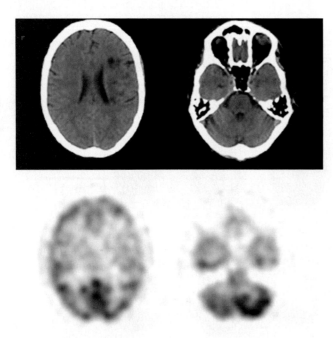

Figure 13-14   Crossed cerebellar diaschisis. *Top row,* A sub cortical stroke in the left parietal region on CT is subtle on SPECT as the gray matter where HMPAO localizes is not heavily involved. No abnormality is seen in the cerebellum on CT. *Bottom row,* One type of distant stroke effect not seen on CT is revealed on the Tc-99m HMPAO SPECT. Hypoperfusion of the contralateral cerebellum or crossed cerebellar diaschisis is seen.

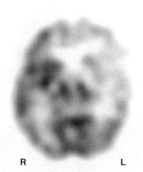
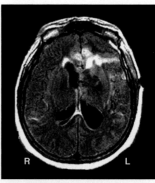

Figure 13-15   *Left,* HMPAO SPECT performed after a carotid balloon occlusion injection shows severe left middle cerebral artery territory hypoperfusion identifying a high risk for stroke. The patient underwent permanent left carotid occlusion using gradual occlusion with a Selverstone clamp rather than bypass. *Right,* This gradual occlusion was not sufficient to protect the patient and the patient did indeed suffer a stroke seen on CT in the same distribution as the SPECT.

obscuring the early findings seen with Tc-99m HMPAO.

Carotid artery balloon occlusion studies are well established in the assessment of vascular reserve. These studies are used in patients who may require permanent internal carotid artery occlusion such as for treatment of intracranial aneurysm. An intravenous injection of Tc-99m HMPAO is done in the angiography suite at the time of internal carotid artery balloon occlusion. The balloon is deflated after 1 minute. Imaging is done once the catheter has been removed. A cerebral arteriogram can show which patients have an intact Circle of Willis and cross-filling. WADA neurological testing is also sometimes possible during the temporary occlusion. Amobarbitol infused into the carotid is used to predict speech and memory function. However, up to a 20% decrease in morbidity and mortality can be seen by adding a Tc-99m HMPAO SPECT scan to the preoperative workup. Patients at risk for stroke following a planned permanent arterial occlusion are easily identified with a significant drop in perfusion to the occluded side on SPECT images. Carotid bypass is generally warranted in these patients as the remaining vessels can not meet the needs of the side that will be occluded (Fig. 13-15).

SPECT can help assess suspected ischemia and stroke risks in the cases of transient ischemic attacks (TIAs) and vascular diseases like atherosclerosis and Moyamoya. Previously, I-123 Spectamine was used to show reversibility of a region of ischemia (Fig. 13-7). The vascular reserve of patients can be assessed by a pharmacologic stress test by imaging after vasodilatory response to increased CO_2 caused by acetazolamide (Diamox), a carbonic anhydrase inhibitor and antihypertensive agent. Vasodilation following intravenous administration of 1 gram of Diamox leads to an increase in rCBF. Although global blood flow is increased, abnormal vessels cannot dilate and blood is shunted away. This will accentuate any abnormality and better demonstrate territories at risk for infarction (Fig. 13-16). It is important to compare the resting state to the stress state. Change may be best assessed with semiquantitative analysis of cortical activity. Xe-133 may have superior sensitivity to Tc-99m HMPAO, although it is not frequently used clinically.

Brain Death

Diagnosis of brain death is primarily clinical. Accuracy and speed in making the diagnosis become critical when organ donation is considered and life support systems must be used. Clinical diagnosis may be difficult due to the specific criteria necessary to make the diagnosis of brain death, as follows:

1. The patient must be in deep coma with total absence of brainstem reflexes or spontaneous respiration.
2. Potentially reversible causes such as drug intoxication, metabolic derangement, or hypothermia must be excluded.
3. The cause of the brain dysfunction must be diagnosed (e.g., trauma, stroke).

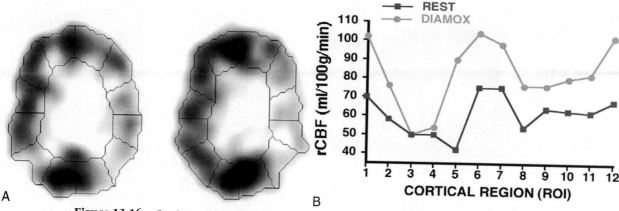

Figure 13-16   Semiquantitative analysis of ischemia with Diamox SPECT. **A,** Tc-99m HMPAO SPECT before Diamox (*left*) shows mild left parietal hypoperfusion. After Diamox (*right*), the brain shows increased activity in response to vasodilation with the exception of the left parietal defect and the decreased activity from ischemia is even more apparent. **B,** Cortical ROI boxes are drawn like a clock numbered from 1 o'clock to 12 o'clock to generate rCBF curves. In this patient, the post-Diamox curves are increased relative to rest perfusion with the exception of a dip from 2 o'clock to 4 o'clock. This signifies an area at high risk for infarction because it is unable to respond to the vasodilation.

4. The clinical findings of brain death must be present for a defined period of observation (6–24 hours).

Confirmatory ancillary tests are used by clinicians to increase certainty, but the diagnosis of brain death is still primarily a clinical one. An isoelectric electroencephalogram (EEG) by itself does not establish brain death, and at least one repeat study is required. In the patient with intoxication from barbiturates and other depressive drugs or with hypothermia, the EEG may be flat, even though cerebral perfusion is still present and recovery is possible.

Lack of blood flow to the brain is diagnostic of brain death. Edema, softening, necrosis, and autolysis of brain tissue lead to increased intracranial pressure. As pressure rises, eventually it prevents intracranial perfusion. This can be demonstrated with four-vessel arteriography, but the test is invasive and unnecessary.

The radionuclide brain death study is usually performed when the EEG and clinical criteria are equivocal. It is simple, rapid, and can be performed at the bedside. Scintigraphy is not affected by drug intoxication or hypothermia. An abnormal radionuclide angiogram showing no cerebral perfusion is more specific for brain death than an isoelectric EEG.

Radiopharmaceuticals

Brain death can be diagnosed using a radionuclide flow study alone because the lack of intracerebral blood flow is diagnostic. Technetium-labeled radiopharmaceuticals are used to assess dynamic flow. Tc-99m DTPA was often used because it is cleared rapidly from the blood, allowing a repeat study if necessary. However, optimal technique is mandatory and interpretation may be diffi-

cult. Visualization of normally draining veins can be helpful (Fig. 13-17).

Tc-99m HMPAO and Tc-99m ECD studies are easier to interpret and are now preferred (Fig. 13-18). Flow images can be obtained but are not necessary, because delayed images will show the fixed presence or absence of brain uptake, requiring flow to the brain. If no CBF is present, no cerebral uptake will occur. Planar images are adequate, and SPECT is not necessary to diagnose brain death.

Methodology

A scalp tourniquet has been suggested for studies utilizing Tc-99m DTPA to minimize flow through the external carotid arteries, facilitating image interpretation of brain perfusion. However, a tourniquet is contraindicated in children, because it could increase intracranial pressure. Adults also probably do not require a tourniquet, because peripheral scalp activity can be differentiated from cerebral perfusion. An adequate radiopharmaceutical dose of 10–20 mCi (370–740 MBq) and good bolus are required to ensure a diagnostic flow study. Images of the injection site can be performed to ensure the dose was adequate and not infiltrated. The radionuclide angiogram protocol for CBF is used in brain death (Box 13-7).

Image Interpretation

Diagnostic findings of brain death include the lack of intracranial arterial flow or major venous sinuses on subsequent static images (Tc-99m DTPA). Flow to both common carotid arteries is seen to the level of the base of the skull. No visualization of the brain is seen with Tc-99m HMPAO. Often the "hot nose" sign is seen as increasing intracranial perfusion diverts

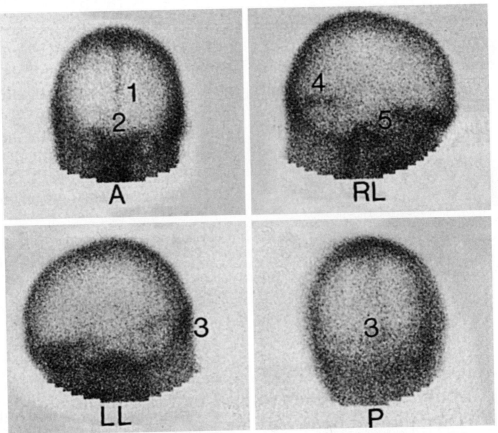

Figure 13-17 Normal delayed Tc-99m DTPA planar images. (*A*) Anterior, (*RL*) right lateral, (*LL*) left lateral, and posterior projections. The superior sagittal sinus (*1*) is seen on anterior and posterior views. The floor of the frontal sinus (*2*), confluence of sinuses (*3*), transverse sinuses (*4*), and sphenoid sinus (*5*) are faintly seen.

intracranial blood flow into external carotid circulation, resulting in relatively increased flow to the face and nose. This pattern is nonspecific and can also be seen in internal carotid artery occlusion without brain death. Faint visualization of the venous sagittal or transverse sinus in the absence of intracranial perfusion is also sometimes seen on Tc-99m DTPA scans. Due to such factors as variable anatomy, delayed images may be difficult to interpret. Furthermore, flow images may be inadequate due to poor bolus technique or computer malfunction. There-fore, Tc-99m DTPA is clearly less desirable than Tc-99m HMPAO.

Epilepsy

Intractable or medically refractory seizures may require surgery for therapy. Precise seizure localization often requires a combination of scalp EEG, MRI, magnetoencephalography (MEG), and nuclear medicine imaging for evaluation. These noninvasive studies are important in directing the invasive intracranial EEG grid placement in the operating room and determining therapeutic options. Although MRI often reveals abnormalities at the site of seizure foci, such as mesial temporal hippocampal sclerosis, it is rare for structural imaging to fully visualize the actual extent of the abnormally activated neurons by structural imaging. EEG remains critical in seizure localization, but is often inconclusive.

PET and SPECT have very important roles in such seizure evaluation. In the ictal state, activated foci show increased activity, representing increased rCBF and glucose metabolism. Interictal images, however, show normal or decreased activity. In the postictal state, activity is changing and may show areas of increased and decreased activity. Clinical knowledge of the seizure status is essential and is best accomplished with continuous monitoring. In addition, as patients may have more than one type of seizure, it must be determined if the seizure of interest was occurring during the ictal state.

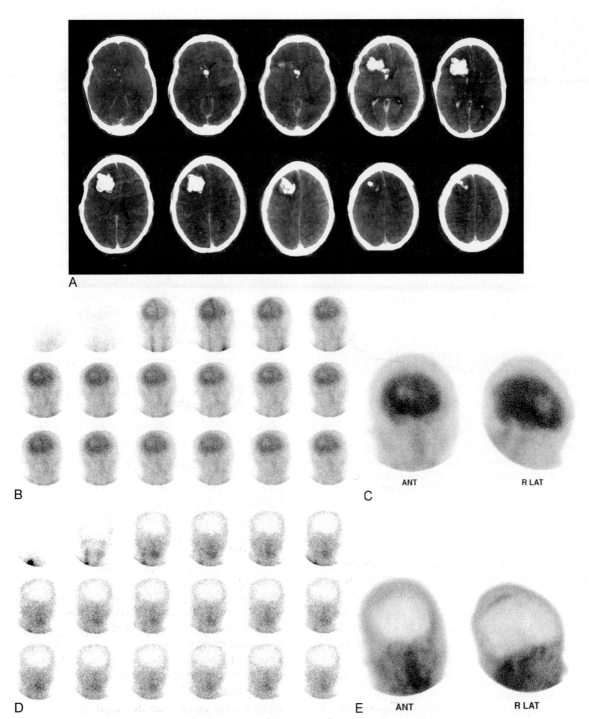

Figure 13-18   Brain death evaluation. **A,** CT images of a head trauma victim show a right frontal parenchymal hemorrhage extending into the ventricles. **B,** Tc-99m HMPAO exam to evaluate for brain death. The exam does not show the early arterial phase of perfusion but good cortical perfusion and venous drainage into the superior sagittal sinus and (**C**) good delayed cortical uptake although with a defect from the hemorrhage. **D,** A follow-up study 3 days later shows internal carotid arterial flow terminating below the head from brain death. **E,** This is confirmed with absent delayed cortical uptake. Any peripheral activity is due to external carotid flow.

Box 13-7   Brain Death Scintigraphy: Protocol Summary

PATIENT PREPARATION

None.

RADIOPHARMACEUTICAL

Technetium-99m HMPAO (or Tc-99m DTPA), 20 mCi (740 MBq)

INSTRUMENTATION

Collimator: high resolution, low energy. Camera setup: large-field-of-view gamma.

Window: 15% over 140-keV photopeak

Camera formatter setup: 2- to 3-sec flow images for 30 sec, then immediate and delayed static images in multiple views

Computer setup: 1-sec flow images for 60 sec (64 × 64 byte mode), then static images (128 × 128 frame mode)

IMAGING PROCEDURE

1.   Inject radiopharmaceutical as an intravenous bolus.
2.   Acquire dynamic flow study.
3.   *Immediate* 750k static images in the anterior, posterior, right lateral, and left lateral views (optional). Image injection site.
4.   Starting 2 hours after injection, acquire *delayed* 750k static images in the anterior, posterior, right lateral, and left lateral views. Vertex view if needed.

Although ictal studies are most sensitive, they are technically highly demanding and done with SPECT (Fig. 13-19). Patients must be admitted and continuously monitored off medication. Once the seizure is identified, trained personnel must inject the radiotracer within seconds of seizure onset. Although imaging can then be delayed, the patient must be able to cooperate with imaging in a reasonable amount of time. Ictal PET would not be practical given the half-life of F-18 FDG. Interictal studies are far less sensitive, although interictal PET appears to be better than interictal SPECT. Clinical knowledge of the seizure is needed to be sure that a study is truly ictal or interictal. Ictal SPECT has a sensitivity of nearly 90% in temporal lobe seizures, and the abnormal areas are generally more extensive than any structural abnormality on MRI. However, sensitivity for extratemporal seizures is much lower, on the order of 50–75%. Interictal FDG PET and SPECT is approximately 70% sensitive for seizure localization.

Tumor Imaging

The SPECT agents Tc-99m HMPAO and Tc-99m ECD are generally not useful for the detection of intracranial malignancies. Of the two agents, Tc-99m ECD may occasionally show increased activity. However, both agents usually show normal or decreased activity. Although MRI is the most sensitive method for detecting metastatic lesions, there are several situations where MRI is limited and nuclear medicine studies offer potential solutions. The most common of these is the detection of recurrent gliomas when MRI shows signal changes and enhancement, which could be due to either radiation necrosis and surgical therapy. The differentiation of intracranial lymphoma from Toxoplasmosis in immunocompromised patients is another situation where MRI is often inconclusive as both processes can show ring-enhancing lesions.

F-18 FDG PET has long played an important role in diagnosing recurrent gliomas when MRI shows nonspecific posttherapy signal changes. Evaluating changes in metabolism is a more specific way to assess intracranial tumor compared to agents relying on blood flow and BBB breakdown. Because more aggressive tumors have higher metabolic activity, glucose metabolism is increased (Fig. 13-20). F-18 FDG uptake is, therefore, related to tumor grade. Therefore, PET can help direct biopsy and grade tumors.

Primary tumors can be graded based on the amount of F-18 FDG uptake. Low-grade gliomas (WHO grade I and II) typically show uptake similar to white matter, whereas high-grade tumors (WHO grade III) are similar or increased compared to grey matter. Grade IV (glioblastoma multiforme) shows markedly increased activity compared to normal cortical grey matter. Interestingly, low-grade pilocytic astrocytomas and benign pituitary tumors can show increased F-18 FDG accumulation.

Following therapy, gliomas commonly recur. Detection of recurrent gliomas is a common problem clinically as the MRI typically shows persistent increased T2 signal changes and contrast enhancement. PET images show absent or decreased activity in the normal postoperative brain and any area of increased uptake most likely represents tumor. Direct side-by-side comparison with the MRI is critical for image interpretation, and actual fusion of PET images to the MRI is extremely helpful. In the case of high-dose radiation therapy, increased F-18 FDG activity can be seen and may persist. Although this activity is generally mild and not greater than normal cortical uptake, serial images to look for any areas of increasing activity may be necessary to exclude early recurrence. Recurrences are often more aggressive with intense radiotracer accumulation.

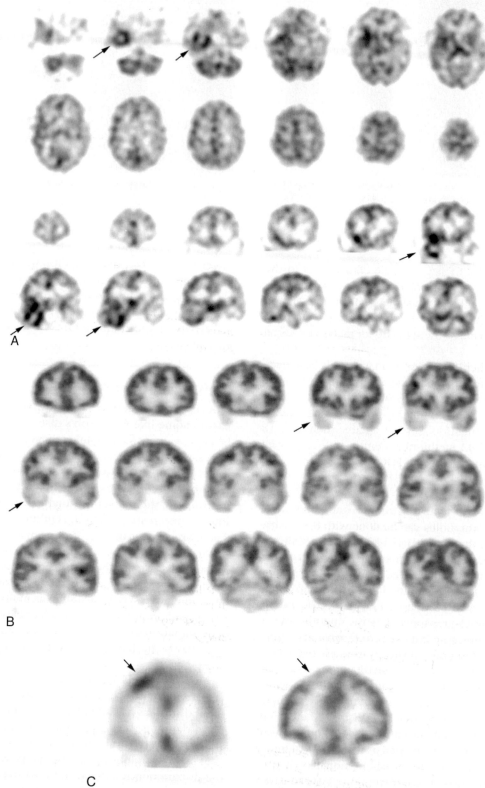

Figure 13-19   Seizure imaging. **A,** Ictal HMPAO SPECT axial (*top*) and coronal (*bottom*) images reveal increased perfusion to the right temporal region from an active seizure. **B,** The abnormal temporal region is a subtle area of hypometabolism on the Interictal FDG PET. **C,** A second patient ictal SPECT demonstrates hyperperfusion in the right parasagittal region (*left*) which is an area of hypometabolism on interictal PET (*right*) from a seizure focus.

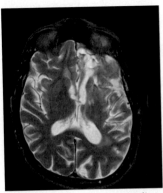
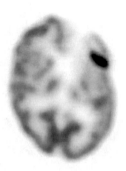

Figure 13-20   Recurrent gliomas may be difficult to detect on MRI. T2-weighted MRI shows posttherapy signal changes (*left*). The recurrent tumor is seen as an intense focus on the FDG PET (*right*).

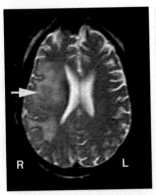
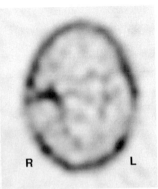

Figure 13-21   Intracranial lymphoma. A mass is seen in a patient with AIDS on the T2-weighted MRI (*left; arrow*) with the Tl-201 SPECT showing intense tumor uptake (*right*).

Although FDG PET is a valuable clinical tool in the workup of many types of malignancy outside of the CNS, nearly two thirds of intracranial metastatic lesions are not seen on PET due to the high background activity. Therefore, MRI remains the standard for metastatic lesion detection.

Numerous other PET radiopharmaceuticals have been made which image aspects of metabolism other than glucose, such as DNA synthesis, protein synthesis, and fat metabolism. Although limitations often persist in low-grade tumor evaluation, several agents such as F-18 thymidine and C-11 methionine demonstrate improved sensitivity and specificity over FDG.

SPECT Tumor Imaging

SPECT evaluation of recurrent gliomas and differentiating intracranial lymphoma can be done with the cardiac imaging agents thallium-201 (Tl-201) and Tc-99m sestamibi (Fig. 13-21). These agents have shown accumulation in several tumor types. Tl-201 is a potassium analog. Its distribution depends on blood flow, BBB breakdown, and metabolic activity with uptake by the Na^+/K^+ pump. Tc-99m sestamibi is transported by the endothelial cell to the mitochondrial activity. There is some accumulation of Tc-99m sestamibi in the choroid plexus, which may make it less than ideal in some tumors.

The procedure for SPECT tumor imaging involves imaging approximately 20–30 minutes following injection of 2–4 mCi (74–148 MBq) of Tl-201 or 20 mCi (740 MBq) Tc-99m sestamibi. Occasionally, a 2-hour delayed Tl-201 acquisition may be helpful as the abnormal tumor tissue would be expected to washout more slowly than normal brain or areas of BBB disruption. Visual analysis typically shows uptake equal to or greater than the scalp or the contralateral side in tumors. There is some overlap in the appearance of malignant and infectious processes. An intracranial abscess, for example, often has increased activity. Because infections usually have lower uptake than malignancies, quantitative analysis may help improve specificity. A region of interest (ROI) is drawn around the abnormal uptake and compared to the contralateral normal. Delayed images may improve sensitivity as the tumor retains activity and the background clears.

Movement Disorders

Movement disorders consist of a wide variety of diseases. Some like Parkinson's disease (PD) have diminished movement states while others like chorea produce excessive movement. PD is the most familiar disorder, affecting approximately 1.5% of people over 65 and 2.5% of those over the age of 80. As the dopaminergic neurons in the substantia nigra degenerate, patients experience resting tremor, rigidity, and bradykinesia. There are three groups of Parkinsonian syndromes: idiopathic PD, secondary PD (due to disease such as Wilson's disease or other extrinsic agents such as carbon monoxide poisoning and neuroleptic drugs), and neurodegenerative syndromes such as multisystem atrophy (MSA) and progressive supranuclear palsy (PSP). Clinical differentiation of idiopathic PD from etiologies such as MSA may be difficult when patients do not respond to L-dopa therapy.

The ability of PET to image the dopaminergic system in patients with Parkinson's disease and other movement disorders has been known for decades. The corpus striatum is the key to understanding PD in imaging studies. The striatum consists of the lentiform nucleus (putamen and globus pallidus) and caudate nucleus. As the dopaminergic striatal neurons degenerate, effects downstream in the globus pallidus can be imaged. Diagnosis hinges on the ability to discriminate anterior from posterior changes. Generally, it is not possible to separate the components of the lentiform nucleus into the putamen and globus pallidus by PET. Over the course of the disease, PD affects the posterior striatum first and moves anteriorly: posterior putamen first, then anterior putamen, then finally the caudate nucleus. It is estimated that there is a 2–10% decrease in striatal activity per year in PD.

PET has largely been a research tool in movement disorders, utilizing expensive agents such as (F-18) 6-fluorodopa. Now, many new agents help study different components of the dopamine neurotransmitter system (Fig. 13-22). These radiopharmaceuticals are grouped based on the location or mechanism of dopamine metabolism they image. The classic agent, F-18 dopa, enters the dopamine metabolism pathway early as an analog of L-dopa and measures dopamine neuron integrity and loss. However, F-18 dopa tends to underestimate loss. Other agents target the vesicular monoamine transporter type 2 (VMAT2), presynaptic membrane dopamine transporter (DAT), and postsynaptic dopamine receptors (D2 and D1).

New tropane agents derived from cocaine have been developed to image DAT activity. These include F-18/C-11 β-CIT and SPECT agents I-123 β-CIT, Tc-99m TRODAT-1, and I-123 IACFT (ALTROPANE). These agents may detect preclinical disease and differentiate patients with Parkinson's disease from those with non-Parkinson's tremor. Patients with Parkinson's disease show decreased radiotracer binding on the symptomatic side, as well as often detecting preclinical disease on the contralateral side (Fig. 13-23).

Huntington's Chorea

The hereditary disorder Huntington's chorea, also called Huntington's disease, usually manifests itself between ages 35 and 50 years, and inevitably progresses to uncontrollable choreiform movements and dementia. The caudate and putamen are deficient in the inhibitory neurotransmitter gamma-aminobutyric acid

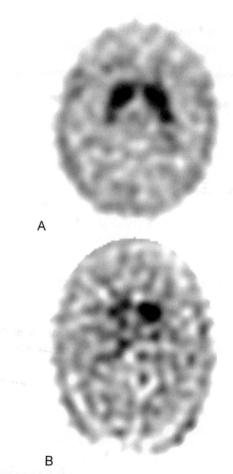

A

B

Figure 13-23   Dopamine metabolism. **A,** Normal distribution of an experimental dopamine transporter agent, I-123 Altropane, has high striatal uptake relative to cortex. **B,** Parkinson's disease demonstrates diffusely low striatal activity on the more severely affected right side. Partial loss is seen on the left, sparing the left caudate. This reflects the progression from unilateral to bilateral involvement as well as from the posterior striatum forward. (Courtesy of Dr. Robert Licho and Boston Life Sciences, Inc.)

(GABA) and in glutamic acid decarboxylase. Although the disease can begin asymmetrically, symmetrical involvement eventually develops. Both PET and SPECT imaging can show decreased uptake in the caudate nucleus, which often precedes the basal ganglia atrophy seen on CT.

Head Trauma

Tc-99m HMPAO SPECT is more sensitive than CT in detecting abnormalities in patients with a history of closed traumatic brain injury. SPECT can detect the changes earlier, particularly in patients with minor head injuries. In addition to evidence of acute injury in the

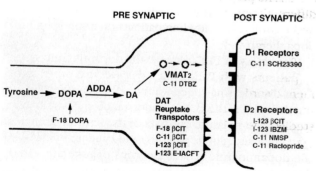

Figure 13-22   Dopamine neuron production and metabolism. The sites of PET and SPECT agent uptake are shown. *AAAD,* Aromatic amino acid decarboxylase; *VMAT$_2$,* vesicular monoamine transporter type 2; *DAT,* dopamine reuptake transporter.

form of coup and contrecoup rCBF deficits, SPECT studies can demonstrate residual flow defects in patients with remote trauma, often in the temporal lobes. In one study, SPECT showed rCBF defects in 80% of patients with head trauma versus 55% on CT and 45% on MRI. With minor head injuries, 60% showed deficits on SPECT and only 25% on CT.

Psychiatric Diseases

The role of PET and SPECT imaging in psychiatric disease is uncertain. Although frontal lobe hypometabolism and hypoperfusion have been described in schizophrenia, the findings are nonspecific. Studies in patients with depression have yielded conflicting results, although patients with depression and metabolic disturbances usually have normal perfusion. Limited studies in patients with obsessive-compulsive disorder, mostly with PET, have shown increased metabolism in the orbital region of the frontal cortex and caudate nuclei. Presently, functional scintigraphy may be of most value in identifying underlying organic disease in patients with psychiatric disease.

CISTERNOGRAPHY

Study of cerebrospinal fluid (CSF) dynamics using radiotracers has been used for many years to diagnose a site of CSF leakage, to determine shunt patency, and to manage hydrocephalus. Although CT and MRI are now often used, radionuclide cisternography can still play an important role because of the unique physiologic information it provides. To be effective, close coordination with structural imaging studies and detailed knowledge of the clinical problem are necessary.

An understanding of normal CSF dynamics is important for image interpretation. CSF is secreted by ventricular choroid plexus and, to a lesser extent, from extraventricular sites. Normally, CSF drains from the lateral ventricles through the interventricular foramen of Monro into the third ventricle (Fig. 13-24). With the additional CSF produced by the choroid plexus of the third ventricle, it then passes through the cerebral aqueduct of Sylvius into the fourth ventricle and then leaves the ventricular system through the median foramen of Magendie and the two lateral foramina of Luschka. The CSF then enters the subarachnoid space surrounding the brain and spinal cord. Along the base of the brain, the subarachnoid space expands into a number of lakes called *cisterns*. The subarachnoid space extends over the surface of the brain. The CSF is absorbed through the pacchionian granulations of the pia arachnoid villi into the superior sagittal sinus.

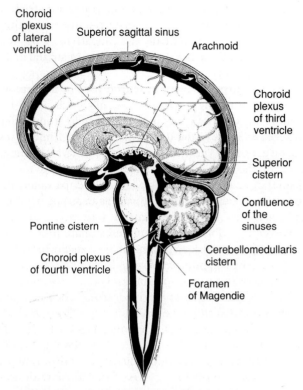

Figure 13-24   Flow dynamics of cerebral spinal fluid (CSF). Originating in lateral ventricle choroid plexus, CSF flows through the third and fourth ventricles into the basal cisterns, moves over the convexities, and finally is reabsorbed in the superior sagittal sinus.

Radiopharmaceuticals

Radiopharmaceuticals injected intrathecally into the lumbar subarachnoid space must meet strict standards for sterility and apyrogenicity. They should follow the flow of the CSF without affecting the dynamics, and they should rapidly clear through the arachnoid villi. The chelating agent, diethylenetriamine pentaacetic acid (DTPA), is often used in renal imaging. DTPA is ideal as it is nonlipid soluble, not metabolized, and not absorbed across the ependyma before reaching the arachnoid villi. Because imaging in cisternography studies may extend over a period of days, indium-111 DTPA (In-111 DTPA) is the agent of choice due to its longer half-life (67 hours) and reasonable imaging characteristics. Studies looking for CSF leaks may be done with Tc-99m DTPA as its improved imaging characteristics may improve sensitivity. CSF shunt patency exams often utilize Tc-99m DTPA, although In-111 DTPA is used in situations requiring extended imaging.

Methods

Proper sterile lumbar puncture technique is critical and should be done by an experienced clinician to ensure subarachnoid injection. An initial image of the injection site ensures that the radiotracer was delivered to the correct location. Early evaluation confirms dose migration up the vertebral column and a lack of excessive renal activity. Serial imaging is needed as described in the protocol in Box 13-8.

Pharmacokinetics

Radiotracer injected into the intrathecal space normally reaches the basal cisterns by 1 hour, the frontal poles and sylvian fissure area by 2–6 hours, the cerebral convexities by 12 hours, and the arachnoid villi in the sagittal sinus by 24 hours. Flow to the parasagittal region occurs through both central and superficial routes. The radiotracer does not normally enter the ventricular system because physiological flow is in the opposite direction.

Dosimetry

To some extent, the radiation absorbed dose depends on the clearance dynamics of a particular patient. The spinal cord receives the highest dose, followed by the kidney and bladder, because the radiopharmaceutical undergoes renal excretion (Table 13-3).

Table 13-3	Dosimetry for In-111 Cisternography
Organ	**Rads/500 uCi (cGy/18.5MBq)**
Total body	0.04
Kidneys	0.22
Spinal cord	
Surface	5.0
Average	1.5
Brain	
Surface	4.1
Average	0.50
Bladder	0.50
Testes	0.05
Ovaries	0.06

Clinical Applications

Hydrocephalus

Hydrocephalus is abnormal enlargement of the CSF spaces resulting from abnormalities of CSF production, circulation, or absorption (Table 13-4). MRI and CT are most often used to select patients who might benefit from intervention, whereas radionuclide cisternography is generally reserved for situations that remain unclear. When assessing hydrocephalus, it must first be known if the process is noncommunicating or communicating. Then the route of radiopharmaceutical administration and expected pattern during cisternography can be predicted and evaluated.

In noncommunicating etiologies of hydrocephalus, there is an obstruction of flow from the ventricular system into the basal cisterns and subarachnoid space. This is commonly due to a mass or congenital abnormality at or above the fourth ventricle. The diagnosis is usually made by MRI.

In communicating hydrocephalus, CSF is free to flow from the intraventricular region into the subarachnoid

---

Box 13-8   Cisternography: Protocol Summary

PATIENT PREPARATION

None.

RADIOPHARMACEUTICAL

Indium-111 DTPA, 250 µCi (9.3 MBq)

INSTRUMENTATION

Camera: large-field-of-view gamma
Collimator: medium energy

IMAGING PROCEDURE

Inject slowly into lumbar subarachnoid space using a
    22-gauge needle with the bevel positioned vertically.
Patient should remain recumbent for at least 1 hr after
    injection.
All images should be obtained for 50k counts.

IMAGING TIMES

1 hr: thoracic-lumbar spine for evaluation of injection
    adequacy.
3 hr: base of the skull to visualize basilar cisterns.
24 and 48 hr: evaluation of ventricular reflux and
    arachnoid villi resorption.
Obtain anterior, posterior, and both lateral views of the
    head at 3, 24, and 48 hr.

Table 13-4	Classification of Hydrocephalus	
Classification		**Site of obstruction**
Obstructive		
Noncommunicating		Intraventricular between lateral ventricles and basal cistern
Communicating		Extraventricular, affecting basal cisterns, cerebral convexities and arachnoid villi
Nonobstructive		
Generalized atrophy		None
Localized atrophy		None

space. The obstruction to CSF flow is extraventricular, in the basal cisterns, cerebral convexities, or arachnoid villi. Common causes include previous subarachnoid hemorrhage, chronic subdural hematoma, leptomeningitis, and meningeal carcinomatosis all leading to poor CSF movement and reabsorption. On anatomical imaging, the ventricular system is dilated out of proportion to the prominence of cortical sulci and the basal cisterns. It may be difficult to differentiate this extraventricular obstruction from nonobstructive "hydrocephalus ex vacuo," a secondary expansion of the ventricles to fill the void following neuronal tissue loss from atrophy or stroke.

Most commonly, radionuclide studies help assess those communicating hydrocephalus patients with normal-pressure hydrocephalus (NPH) to determine if the patient is likely to benefit from CSF shunting. NPH manifests clinically with progressive dementia, ataxia, and incontinence. Surgical shunting of CSF can potentially cure this cause of dementia, but not all patients improve with surgery. Predicting which patients will respond is a diagnostic problem. Radionuclide cisternography can be helpful when used in conjunction with clinical findings, such as a response (mental clearing) to CSF fluid reduction.

Cisternography Image Interpretation

Several patterns of flow can be observed after introduction of radiopharmaceutical into the intrathecal space (Table 13-5). Normal flow should not reflux into the ventricles and should move over the convexities by 24 hours (Figs. 13-25 and 13-26).

In patients with noncommunicating hydrocephalus, cisternography usually shows a normal pattern of flow up to the basal cisterns, over the convexities. No ventricular reflux is seen. However, if activity is injected into the ventricles through a ventriculostomy rather than via lumbar puncture, serial images show minimal activity in the basal cisterns.

In communicating hydrocephalus, including NPH patients, cisternography can show a spectrum of CSF flow patterns (Fig. 13-27). The common denominator is absent flow or a marked delay of activity flow up over the convexities of the brain. Ventricular reflux of activity may occur transiently or persist. Atrophy alone will cause delayed tracer movement through the enlarged subarachnoid space, sometimes with transient ventricular reflux. However, normal clearance over the hemispheres is seen by 24 hours. It has been suggested that communicating hydrocephalus patients with persistent ventricular activity and no activity over the convexities (the type IV cisternographic pattern) are most likely to benefit from shunting.

Surgical Shunt Patency

A variety of diversionary CSF shunts (ventriculoperitoneal, ventriculoatrial, ventriculopleural, lumboperitoneal) have

Table 13-5 Patterns of Cerebrospinal Fluid Flow

Type	Cerebrospinal fluid movement	Etiologies
I	Basal cistern 2–4 hr Sylvian fissure 6 hr Over convexities 24 hr Decreased activity 48 hr	Normal Intraventricular obstructive hydrocephalus (noncommunicating)
II	No ventricular activity Delayed migration over convexities	Cerebral atrophy Advanced age
IIIA	Transient ventricular activity Clearance by usual migration (often)	Intraventricular obstruction Cerebral atrophy Evolving or resolving communicating hydrocephalus
IIIB	Transient ventricular activity Clearance but not by usual migration to convexity	Communicating hydrocephalus with alternate reabsorption pathway (transependymal)
IV	Persistent ventricular activity Inadequate clearance	Communicating hydrocephalus

been used to treat obstructive hydrocephalus. Complications may include catheter blockage, infection, thromboembolism, subdural or epidural hematomas, disconnection of catheters, CSF pseudocyst, bowel obstruction, and bowel perforation.

The diagnosis of shunt patency and adequacy of CSF flow can often be made by examination of the patient and inspection of the subcutaneous CSF reservoir. When this assessment is uncertain, radionuclide studies with In-111 DTPA or Tc-99m DTPA are useful for confirming the diagnosis. Familiarity with the specific shunt type and its configuration is helpful. For example, the valves may allow bidirectional or only unidirectional flow. A proximal shunt limb consists of tubing running from

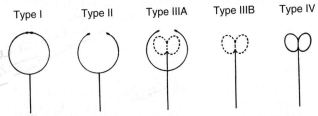

Figure 13-25 Iodine-123 Isopropyl iodoamphetamine (IMP) redistribution. *Left,* Immediate postinjection I-123 IMP transaxial SPECT image shows a cortical perfusion defect in the left frontal cortex. *Right,* Repeat SPECT 4 hours later shows much improved perfusion in a comparable transverse section, consistent with at least partially reversible ischemia.

4 Hour Images

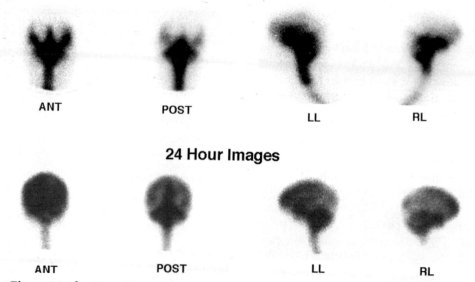

ANT   POST   LL   RL

24 Hour Images

ANT   POST   LL   RL

Figure 13-26   Normal cisternogram. Anterior and lateral images 4 and 24 hours after intrathecal radiotracer injection show normal transit up over the convexities with no ventricular reflux.

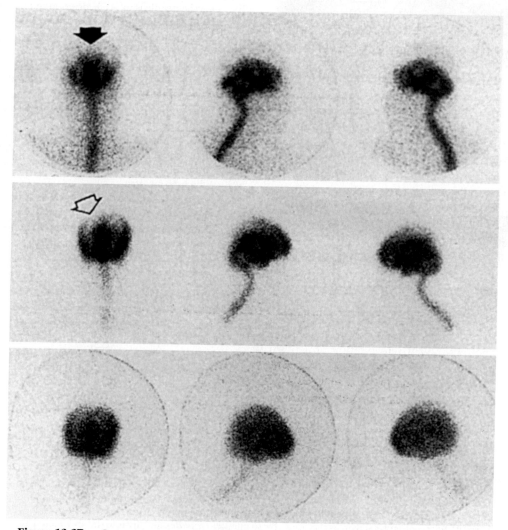

Figure 13-27   Communicating normal pressure hydrocephalus at 24 hours (*top row*), 48 hours (*middle row*) and 72 hours (*bottom row*) in anterior (*left*), right lateral (*middle*) and left lateral (*right*) projections. Ventricular reflux (*closed arrowhead*) is present, as is very delayed flow over the convexities (*open arrowhead*). The intracerebral activity at 72 hours was caused by transependymal uptake.

the ventricles into the reservoir while the distal limb carries CSF away from the reservoir into the body.

Shunt injection should be performed with aseptic technique by a physician familiar with the type of shunt in place, preferably the neurosurgeon (Box 13-9). Patency of the proximal shunt limb can sometimes be evaluated before checking distal patency. In patients with certain types of variable or low pressure two-way valves, the distal catheter is initially occluded by manually pressing on the neck. The pressure may cause injected tracer to flow into the proximal limb.

Images should show prompt flow into the ventricles followed by spontaneous distal flow through the shunt catheter (Figs. 13-28 and 13-29). The shunt tubing is usually seen. Catheters draining into the peritoneum show accumulation of radiotracer freely within the abdominal cavity.

Cerebrospinal Fluid Leak

Trauma and surgery (transsphenoidal and nasal) are the most common causes for CSF rhinorrhea. Nontraumatic causes include hydrocephalus and congenital defects. CSF rhinorrhea may occur at any site, from the frontal sinuses to the temporal bone (Fig. 13-30). The cribriform plate is most susceptible to fracture which can result in rhinorrhea. Otorrhea is much less common. Accurate localization of CSF leaks can be clinically difficult. Although glucose oxidase test strips are used to confirm CSF leak, both lacrimal and nasal secretions contain glucose, and the false positive rate may be as high as 50%.

Radionuclide studies are sensitive and accurate methods of CSF leak detection. To maximize the sensitivity of the test, nasal pledgets are placed in the anterior and posterior portion of each nasal region by an otolaryngologist and then removed and counted 4 hours later

---

Box 13-9 Shunt Patency: Protocol Summary

PATIENT PREPARATION

None.

RADIOPHARMACEUTICAL

Technetium-99m DTPA, 0.5 to 1 mCi (18.5–37 MBq), or indium-111 DTPA, 250 µCi (9.3 MBq)

INSTRUMENTATION

Camera: wide-field-of-view gamma.
Collimator: all purpose.
Computer and camera setup: 1-min images for 30 min.

IMAGING PROCEDURE

Using aseptic technique. Clean the shaved scalp with Betadine.
Penetrate the shunt reservoir with a 25- to 35-gauge needle.
Once the needle is in place, position the patient's head under the camera with the reservoir in the middle of the field of view.
Inject the radiopharmaceutical.
Take serial images for 30 min.
If no flow is seen, place the patient in an upright position and continue imaging for 10 min.
If still no flow is seen, obtain static images of 50k after 1 and 2 hr.
If flow is demonstrated at any point, obtain 50k images of the shunt and tubing every 15 min until flow to the distal tip of the shunt tubing is identified or for 2 hr, whichever is first.
To determine proximal patency of the reservoir, the distal catheter can be manually occluded during the procedure so that the radiotracer will reflux into the ventricular system.

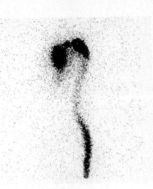 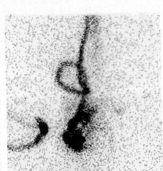 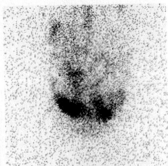

ANT Head 10 min **ANT lower ABD 30 min** **ANT lower ABD 60 min**

A

Figure 13-28 Cerebrospinal shunt patency evaluation. **A,** Ventriculoperitoneal shunt at 10 min (*left*) shows activity in the reservoir port and distal limb of the shunt moving down the neck and chest. Intraventricular activity is also seen. By 30 minutes (*middle*), activity is in the abdomen with free flow in the peritoneum (*right*).

Continued

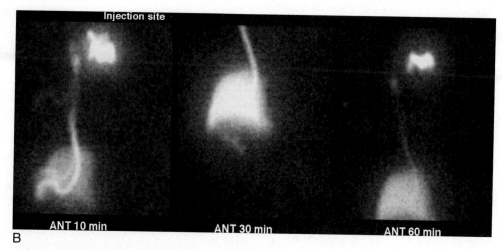

Figure 13-28, cont'd   **B,** Ventriculopleural shunt with normal radiotracer flow through the shunt into the pleural space which decreases over time.

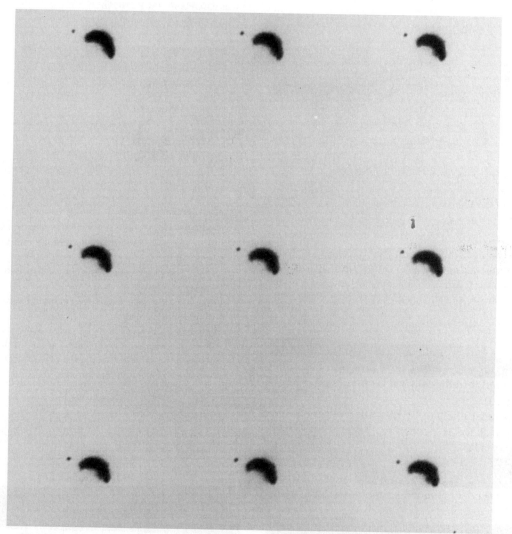

Figure 13-29   Obstructed cerebrospinal shunt. After injection of Tc-99m DTPA into the reservoir, good reflux into the ventricles is seen, consistent with patency of the proximal limb of the shunt. However, no distal drainage occurs over 60 minutes from obstruction.

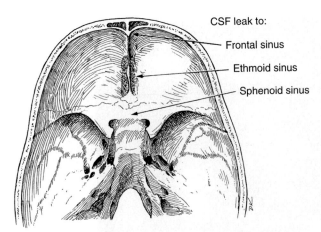

Figure 13-30   Common sites of cerebrospinal fluid leakage.

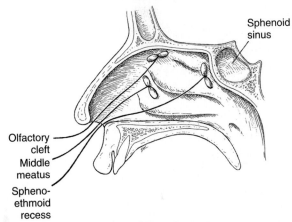

Figure 13-31   Placement of pledgets for cerebrospinal fluid leak study. The labeled cotton pledgets are placed by an otolaryngologist at various levels within the anterior and posterior nares to detect leakage from the frontal, ethmoidal, and sphenoidal sinuses.

(Fig. 13-31). A ratio of nasal-to-plasma radioactivity greater than 2:1 or 3:1 is considered positive. The radiotracer is injected intrathecally via aseptic lumbar puncture (Box 13-10).

The site is most likely to be identified during a time when heavy leakage is occurring. Often, the patient position associated with greatest leakage is reproduced during imaging. Imaging in the appropriate projection is important for identifying the site of leak; lateral and anterior imaging is used for rhinorrhea and posterior imaging for otorrhea.

Scintigraphic studies show CSF leaks as an increasing accumulation of activity at the leak site (Fig. 13-32).

Box 13-10   Cerebrospinal Fluid Leak Detection: Protocol Summary

PATIENT PREPARATION

Nasal pledgets should be placed and labeled as to location. The pledgets should be weighed before placement.

After intrathecal injection, place patient in Trendelenburg position to pool the radiotracer in the basal regions until imaging begins.

Once radiotracer reaches basal cisterns, position patient in a position that increases cerebrospinal fluid leakage.

  Rhinorrhea: incline patient's head forward and against camera face with the camera positioned in the lateral position.

  Otorrhea: obtain posterior images instead of lateral views.

RADIOPHARMACEUTICAL

In-111 DTPA, 250 μCi (9 MBq)

INSTRUMENTATION

Camera: large-field-of-view gamma
Collimator: medium energy

IMAGING PROCEDURE

Setup
Inject intrathecally 500 μCi (18 MBq) of In-111 DTPA in 5 ml of dextrose 10% in water.
Begin imaging when activity reaches the basal cisterns (1 to 4 hr).

ACQUISITION

Acquire 5 min/frame for 1 hr in the selected view, then acquire anterior, left lateral, right lateral, and posterior views.
Obtain 50k images every 10 min for 1 hr in the original view.
Remove pledgets and place in separate tubes. Draw a 5-ml blood sample.
Count pledgets and 0.5-ml aliquots of plasma.
Repeat views may be indicated at 6 and 24 hr.
Calculate the ratio of pledgets-to-plasma activity:
  pledget counts/pledget capacity divided by serum counts/0.5 ml.

INTERPRETATION

Positive for CSF leakage if the pledget/plasma activity ratio is greater than 2–3:1.

However, counting the pledgets is more sensitive than imaging for detecting CSF leaks. Pledgets are also helpful in determining the origin of the leak (anterior versus posterior).

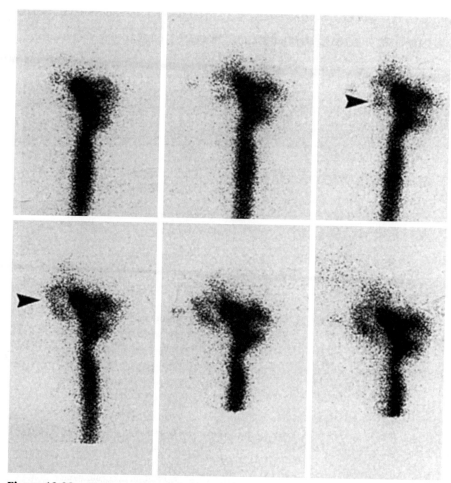

Figure 13-32   Positive radionuclide CSF leak study. In-111 DTPA left lateral views show increasing radioactivity over time originating from the nares and leaking into the nose and mouth (*arrowheads*).

SUGGESTED READING

Carmago EE: Brain SPECT in neurology and psychiatry. J Nucl Med 42:611, 2001.

Herholz K, Herscovitch P, Heiss WD: NeuroPET. Berlin, Springer, 2004.

Mountz JM, Liu HG, Deutsch G: Neuroimaging in cerebrovascular disorders: Measurement of cerebral physiology after stroke and assessment of stroke recovery. Sem Nucl Med 33:56, 2003.

Van Heertum RL, Tikofsky RS: Cerebral SPECT Imaging, ed. 2. New York, Raven Press, 1995.

Cardiac System

Radionuclides were first used in 1927 by Blumgart to investigate the circulatory system. In 1948, Prinzmetal performed the first cardiac study by injecting a subject with radiolabeled albumin and, with the use of a Geiger counter placed on the chest, recorded a time–volume curve. Modern-day clinical cardiac radionuclide imaging techniques were developed in the 1970s and 1980s. Of these, some have become routine studies used today, including myocardial perfusion scintigraphy and radionuclide ventriculography (RVG). Over the years, there have been marked advancements in instrumentation, methodologies, processing, display, and quantification.

Numerous other diagnostic studies are available to the cardiologist, such as electrocardiography (ECG), echocardiography, magnetic resonance imaging (MRI), contrast angiography, and computed tomography (CT) angiography. The continuing value of cardiac nuclear studies stems from their noninvasiveness and accurate portrayal of a wide range of functional and metabolic that predict prognosis and risk.

MYOCARDIAL PERFUSION SCINTIGRAPHY

Myocardial perfusion scintigraphy is currently by far the most commonly performed cardiac nuclear study, constituting approximately one third of all nuclear medicine procedures done annually in the United States, with substantial growth annually. Gated myocardial perfusion scintigraphy plays an important role in the diagnosis, prognosis, risk assessment, and management of heart disease.

Myocardial perfusion scintigraphy depicts two sequential physiological events. First, the radiopharmaceutical must be delivered to the myocardium. Second, a viable metabolically active myocardial cell must be present to extract the radiotracer. The scintigraphic images are a map of regional myocardial perfusion to viable myocardial tissue. If a patient has a decrease in regional perfusion due to hemodynamically significant coronary artery disease or a loss of cell viability as a result of myocardial infarction, a photon-deficient or cold region is seen on the perfusion images. All diagnostic patterns in the many diverse applications follow from these observations.

Radiopharmaceuticals

Radiolabeled potassium (K^+) was first considered for myocardial perfusion imaging because it is the major intracellular cation. Sodium (Na^+)–K^+ homeostasis is maintained as an energy-dependent process involving the Na^+–K^+ ATPase (adenosine triphosphatase) pump in the myocardial cell membrane. However, neither K^+ nor its analogs, cesium and rubidium, were found suitable for single-photon imaging because of their high-energy photons. Rubidium (Rb-82) has found use in dual-photon imaging and positron emission tomography (PET).

The first radiopharmaceutical used on a clinical basis for perfusion imaging was thallium-201 chloride (Tl-201). Tl-201 behaves physiologically much like K^+, although it is not a true K^+ analog in a chemical sense. First used for myocardial scintigraphy in the mid-1970s, it remained the only perfusion agent available until 1990. Two Tc-99m-labeled cardiac perfusion radiopharmaceuticals, sestamibi and tetrofosmin, were introduced. All three are now routinely used clinically for myocardial perfusion scintigraphy.

Thallium-201 Chloride

Chemistry

Thallium is a metallic element in the IIIA series of the Periodic Table (*see* Figure 1-1). In pharmacological doses, thallium is a poison, but it is nontoxic when used in subpharmacologic tracer doses. It is administered to the patient in the chemical form of thallium chloride.

Physics

The radionuclide Tl-201 is cyclotron produced. It decays by electron capture to its stable mercury-201 daughter with a physical half-life of 73 hours. The photons available for imaging are mercury K-characteristic x-rays in the range of 69 to 83 keV (95% abundant) and gamma rays of 167 keV (10%) and 135 keV (3%) (Box 14-1). For clinical gamma-camera imaging, a 20-30% window is centered at 69–83 keV and a 20% window at 167 keV.

Mechanism of Localization and Pharmacokinetics

After intravenous injection, blood clearance is rapid (Fig. 14-1). Tl-201 is transported across the myocardial cell membrane via the Na^+-K^+ ATPase pump. Greater than 85% of Tl-201 is extracted by the myocardial cell on first pass through the coronary capillary circulation (Table 14-1). Peak myocardial uptake occurs by 10 minutes. Approximately 3% of the administered dose localizes in the myocardium. The biological half-life is approximately 10 days.

Extraction is proportional to relative regional perfusion over a wide range of flow rates (Fig. 14-2). At very high flow rates, extraction efficiency decreases; at very low rates, it increases. Tl-201 can only be extracted by viable myocardium and does not concentrate in regions of infarction or scarred myocardium.

Box 14-1   Physical Characteristics of Thallium-201 and Technetium-99m (Sestamibi and Tetrofosmin)

Physical Characteristic	Thallium-201	Tc-99m (Sestamibi and Tetrofosmin)
Mode of decay	Electron capture	Isomeric transition
Physical half-life	73 hours	6 hours
Principal emissions (abundance)*	Mercury x-rays 69–83 keV Gamma rays 167 keV (10%) 135 keV (2.7%)	Gamma rays 140 keV (89%)

*Abundance is the percentage of time each emission type that occurs with each decay.

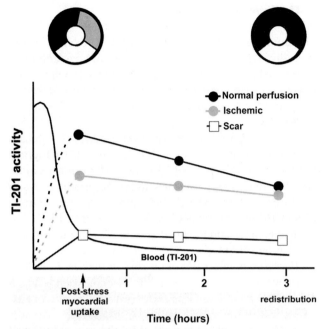

Figure 14-1   Thallium-201 pharmacokinetics: redistribution. After intravenous injection, Tl-201 clears rapidly from the blood pool. Normal stress peak myocardial uptake occurs by 10 minutes. Redistribution begins promptly after initial uptake. This is a constant dynamic exchange of thallium between the myocytes and blood pool. Normal myocardium progressively clears over 3 hours. In the presence of ischemia, uptake is delayed and reduced and clearance is slow. With infarction, there is little uptake and very little change over time. The schematic diagram relates thallium pharmacokinetics to scintigraphic findings. The ischemic region, although initially hypoperfused compared to the normal region equalizes scintigraphically at 3 hours. Modified with permission from Dilsizian V, Narula J: Atlas of Nuclear Cardiology. Philadelphia, Current Medicine, 2003.

Scintigraphy obtained early after initial uptake reflects *capillary blood flow*. After uptake, Tl-201 undergoes *redistribution*, which is a continual dynamic exchange of Tl-201 between the myocardial cell and the vascular blood pool (Fig. 14-1). As Tl-201 leaves the myocardial cell, it is replaced by Tl-201 circulating in the systemic blood pool, which is also undergoing Tl-201 redistribution. Several hours after injection, the images depict an equilibrated pattern reflecting *regional blood volume* or *myocardial K⁺ space*. This redistribution occurs after

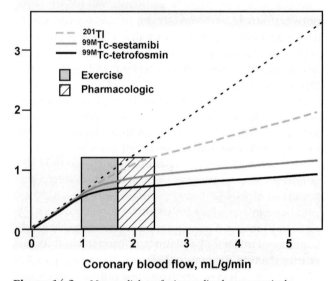

Figure 14-2   Myocardial perfusion radiopharmaceuticals: uptake relative to coronary blood flow. An ideal myocardial perfusion tracer would show a linear relationship to blood flow over a wide range of flow rates. At rest, the normal myocardial coronary low rate is 1 mL/g/min. With exercise, it can increase to 2 mL/g/min. With pharmacologic vasodilation, flow may exceed 2 mL/g/min. Tl-201, Tc-99m sestamibi and Tc-99m tetrofosmin all have extraction that is proportional to blood flow but underestimate flow at high flow rates.

Table 14-1   Pharmacokinetics of Thallium-201, Tc-99m Sestamibi, and Tc-99m Tetrofosmin

	Thallium-201	Tc-99m sestamibi	Tc-99m tetrofosmin
Chemical class/charge	Element cation	Isonitrile cation	Diphosphine cation
Mechanism of uptake	Active transport Na-K ATPase pump	Passive diffusion Negative electrical potential	Passive diffusion Negative electrical potential
Myocyte localization	Cytosol	Mitochondria	Mitochondria
Intracellular state	Free	Bound	Bound
Preparation	Cyclotron	Generator/kit	Generator/kit
First pass extraction fraction	85%	60%	50%
Percent cardiac uptake	3%	1.5 %	1.2%
Myocardial clearance	4 hr $T_{1/2}$	Minimal	Minimal
Body clearance	Renal	Hepatic	Hepatic
Imaging time after injection			
Stress	10 min	15–30 min	5–15 min
Rest	3–4 hrs	30–90 min	30 min

cardiac stress but also during a rest study. With normal perfusion, the initial capillary blood flow image and the delayed regional blood volume image are similar.

The unique pharmacokinetics of Tl-201 are the basis for the "stress-redistribution" Tl-201 imaging strategy that has been used in the detection of coronary artery disease. Regions of decreased perfusion (cold, photon-deficient) seen on early images after stress can be due to either decreased blood flow (ischemia) or to the lack of viable cells to fix the tracer (infarct). If an initial perfusion defect persists on delayed images, it depicts infarction. Those defects showing "fill-in" of Tl-201 between stress and rest are viable myocardium rendered ischemic during stress (Fig. 14-1).

Dosimetry

Tl-201 has relatively high-radiation dosimetry because of its long biological and physical half-life, thus limiting the maximum allowable administered dose to 3.5–4.0 mCi (130–150 MBq). The kidney receives the highest radiation dose (critical target organ), 5.1 rads/3 mCi (5.3 cGy/111 MBq) (Table 14-2).

Myocardial image quality is poor compared to Tc-99m agents for several reasons. The low administered dose results in a poor count rate. Thallium's relatively low photoenergy emissions (69–83 keV) compared to Tc-99m (140 keV) makes it poorly suited for modern-day gamma cameras. The lack of a distinct photopeak and its high scatter fraction further contributes to suboptimal image quality. The low count rate makes gated SPECT problematic and first-pass studies impractical.

Tc-99m Sestamibi (Cardiolite)

Tc-99m labeled sestamibi was approved by the Food and Drug Administration (FDA) for clinical use in 1990.

Chemistry

Sestamibi is a lipophilic cation and member of the chemical isonitrile family. Tc-99m is surrounded by six isonitrile ligands (chemical name: hexakis 2-methoxyisobutyl isonitrile). The radiopharmaceutical is prepared from a manufacturer-provided kit.

Mechanism of Localization and Uptake

Being lipid soluble, Tc-99m sestamibi diffuses from the blood into the myocardial cell and is retained in the region of mitochondria because of its negative transmembrane potential. The first-pass extraction fraction is lower than that of Tl-201, approximately 60% (Table 14-1). As with Tl-201, extraction is proportional to coronary flow and is underestimated at high flow rates and overestimated at low flow (Fig. 14-2).

Pharmacokinetics

After clearing rapidly from the blood, myocardial uptake is prompt, although initially obscured by high uptake in the lung and liver. Unlike the redistribution of Tl-201, the clearance half-time from the myocardium is long, and for practical purposes, this tracer remains fixed within the myocardium. This allows for an imaging time window of several hours after administration. Because of renal and biliary excretion, there is progressive clearance of liver and lung activity, thus improving the myocardium-to-background activity ratios over time. Imaging is usually begun 45–60 minutes after tracer administration for resting studies and at 30 minutes for exercise stress studies, in contrast to Tl-201 where imaging must be started at 10 minutes before redistribution has occurred.

Dosimetry

The radiation absorbed dose to the patient is relatively low because of the Tc-99m label. The colon is the critical target organ, receiving about 5.4 rads/30 mCi (5.4 cGy/1110 MBq) (Table 14-2).

Technetium-99m Tetrofosmin (Myoview)

Chemistry

This Tc-99m-labeled myocardial perfusion agent was approved by the FDA for clinical use after sestamibi in 1996. It is a member of the diphosphine chemical class [chemical name: 6,9-bis (2-ethoxyethyl)-3,12-dioxa-6,9 diphospha-tetradecane]. It is prepared from a kit.

Mechanism of Localization and Uptake

Similar to sestamibi, Tc-99m tetrofosmin is a lipophilic cation that localizes and is retained within mitochondria. Tc-99m tetrofosmin remains fixed in the heart, also similar to sestamibi.

Pharmacokinetics

Tc-99m tetrofosmin is cleared rapidly from the blood. Myocardial uptake is prompt. First-pass extraction is slightly less than sestamibi (50%) with roughly 1.2% of the injected dose taken up in the myocardium by 5 minutes after injection (Table 14-1). Extraction is proportional to

Table 14-2	Radiation Dosimetry for Tl-201, Tc-99m Sestamibi, Tc-99m Tetrofosmin		
	Tl-201⁺	**Tc-99m sestamibi**	**Tc-99m tetrofosmin**
Dose	cGy/111 MBq (rads/3 mCi)	cGy/1110 MBq (rads/30 mCi)	cGy/1110 MBq (rads/30 mCi)
Heart wall	0.3	0.5	0.5
Liver	1.1	0.8	0.5
Kidneys	**5.1**	2.0	1.4
Gallbladder	0.9	2.8	**5.4**
Urinary bladder	0.6	2.0	2.1
Colon	0.8	**5.4**	3.4
Thyroid	3.0	0.7	0.6
Testes	0.9	0.3	0.4
Ovaries	1.1	1.5	1.1
Total body	0.4	0.5	0.2

Target organ (highest radiation absorbed dose) in **boldface** type.

blood flow, but underestimated at high flow rates, similar to Tc-99m sestamibi (Fig. 14-2).

Heart-to-lung and heart-to-liver ratios improve with time because of physiological clearance through the liver and kidneys. Heart-to-liver ratios are somewhat higher for Tc-99m tetrofosmin than sestamibi, allowing for earlier imaging. After stress, imaging at 15 minutes is feasible. Rest studies can be started 30 minutes after injection.

Dosimetry

The radiation absorbed dose to the patient is similar to Tc-99m sestamibi (Table 14-2), although the package insert states that the gallbladder receives the highest dose, 5.4 rads/20 mCi (5.4 cGy/1110 MBq). The reason for the discrepancy is probably because of the variability of gallbladder filling and emptying, depending primarily on when the patient eats. Otherwise the colon would receive the highest absorbed dose.

Other Single Photon Perfusion Agents

Tc-99m teboroxime (CardioTec, Bracco) is a drug approved by the FDA in 1990, but to date has not found general clinical use, although its proponents feel that its unique characteristics will eventually make it a clinical agent. This neutral lipophilic radiopharmaceutical comes from a class of compounds referred to as boronic acid adducts of technetium dioxime (BATO). The extraction fraction is greater than Tl-201. Uptake is proportional to flow but decreases with increasing flow. Blood clearance half-time is less than 1 minute.

Myocardial clearance is extremely rapid (half-time of 5-10 minutes). Washout is proportional to regional blood flow. Redistribution does not occur. The rapid uptake and clearance dictate a very narrow window for imaging, between 2 and 6 minutes resulting in relatively poor-quality SPECT images because of low counting statistics and rapidly changing distribution.

Technetium-99mN-NOET (bis [*N*-etoxy, *N*-ethyl dithio-carbamato] nitride technetium [V] is an investigational myocardial perfusion radiopharmaceutical. It is a neutral lipophilic compound with a first-pass extraction of 75% at rest and 85% under hyperemic conditions. After passive diffusion, uptake occurs through linkage to proteins bound in the lipid membrane of myocytes. Although clearance from the myocardium is slow, it significantly redistributes over time, predominantly by differential washout. Its clinical role has not been determined.

Scintigraphic Methodology

Planar Imaging

Two-dimensional planar imaging was the standard imaging methodology used for many years. Its accuracy for the diagnosis of coronary artery disease was generally good. However, accurate localization of regional perfusion abnormalities predicts with only moderate success the coronary artery bed involved (Fig. 14-3).

Interpretation of planar images is limited by the high background, overlapping structures, and the standard three views acquired (left anterior oblique [LAO], right anterior oblique [RAO], left lateral) (Fig. 14-4). More accurate assessment of regional perfusion became increasingly important as myocardial perfusion scintigraphy was less frequently requested for diagnosis and increasingly utilized for prognosis, risk stratification, and patient management.

In current practice, planar imaging is limited to patients who are severely claustrophobic who cannot tolerate SPECT or for those who exceed weight restrictions on the SPECT imaging table. The anterior, left anterior oblique, and left lateral (or posterior oblique) projections are routinely acquired (Boxes 14-2 and 14-3). Acquisition of the stress and rest images in the same projection is critical for proper interpretation (Fig. 14-5).

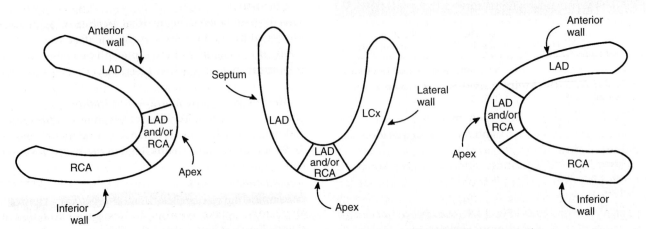

Figure 14-3 Planar scintigraphy: relationship of coronary artery vascular supply to ventricular wall segments. Anterior, left anterior oblique, and left lateral projections. *LAD,* Left anterior descending artery; *LCx,* left circumflex branch; *RCA,* right coronary artery.

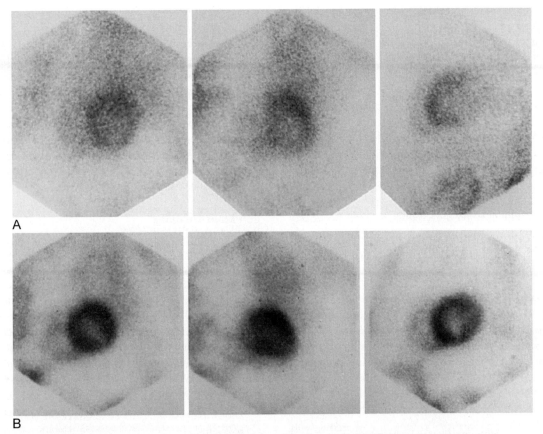

Figure 14-4   Comparison of stress Tl-201 **(A)** and Tc-99m sestamibi **(B)** planar scintigraphy in the same patient. Although the myocardium is well-visualized with both agents, the count rate with Tl-201 is less than with Tc-99m sestamibi and the target-to-background ratio is lower, accounting for its poor image quality. An attenuation artifact caused by interposition of subdiaphragmatic structures can be seen on the lateral view; the effect is greater on the Tl-201 study.

Single-Photon Emission Computed Tomography (SPECT)

SPECT has become the standard methodology for myocardial perfusion scintigraphy. The cross-sectional images have high-contrast resolution and are displayed three-dimensionally (Figs. 14-6 and 14-7), providing good delineation of the various regional myocardial perfusion beds supplied by their individual coronary arteries (Fig. 14-8).

SPECT instrumentation and methodology are discussed in some detail in Chapter 4. The acquisition and processing parameters are dictated to some extent by the specific SPECT camera and computer software employed; however, there is room for individual preference. Variations include the number and position of camera detector heads (Fig. 14-9), the choice of acquisition method (e.g., continuous versus step and shoot),

number of stops, acquisition time for each angle, and shape of orbit (e.g., elliptical or body contour versus circular). Elliptical orbits, although desirable because the camera is closer to the body, often result in unacceptable artifacts. Circular orbits are usually obtained.

Patient movement is a source of image degradation with SPECT and dictates imaging time to be as short as possible while acquiring sufficient counts for good image quality. Image acquisition usually lasts 25–35 minutes. SPECT can be obtained using a rotating single-headed gamma camera; however, multiple detectors are advantageous because a higher number of counts can be acquired in a shorter period of time. Three-headed cameras provide the highest count rate; however, two-headed SPECT cameras are the rule because of their versatility. They can be used for various other types of scintigraphic studies in the clinic.

Box 14-2   Protocol: Thallium-201 Myocardial Perfusion Imaging

PATIENT PREPARATION AND FOLLOW-UP

Patients should fast for 4 hr prior to study

EKG leads should be moved out of field of view

DOSAGE AND ROUTE OF ADMINISTRATION

3 to 3.5 mCi (111 to 120 MBq) thallium-201 chloride intravenously

TIME OF IMAGING

10 min after radiopharmaceutical administration

SPECT IMAGING ACQUISITION PARAMETERS

Collimator: low energy general-purpose parallel hole

Photopeak: 20% window centered at 80 and 167 keV

Patient position: supine, left arm raised

Rotation orbit: circular or elliptical

Matrix: 64×64 word mode

Arc and framing: 64 views, 180° (45° RAO, 135° LPO), 20 seconds per view

SPECT RECONSTRUCTION PARAMETERS*

Filter: Butterworth; cutoff 0.5 and order 8

Attenuation correction: review with and without correction

Reconstruction technique: filtered backprojection or iterative reconstruction

Image format: transaxial short axis, horizontal and vertical long axis

PLANAR IMAGING

Collimator: low-energy, general purpose, parallel hole collimator

Photopeak: 20% window centered at 80 and 167 keV

Image acquisition: anterior, 45° left anterior oblique (LAO), and left lateral for 10 min each

Acquire rest and stress images in identical projections

*Choice of SPECT acquisition and reconstruction parameters is influenced by the equipment used.

Box 14-3   Protocol: Tc-99m Sestamibi and Tetrofosmin Myocardial Perfusion Imaging

PATIENT PREPARATION

Fasting for 4 hours

DOSE AND ROUTE OF RADIOPHARMACEUTICAL ADMINISTRATION

10 to 30 mCi (370 to 1110 MBq) intravenously, see individual protocols below

SPECT IMAGING PROTOCOL

1-Day rest/stress imaging

   Rest: 370 MBq (10 mCi); imaging at 30 to 90 min

   Stress: 1110 MBq (30 mCi); imaging at 15 to 30 min

2-Day rest/stress or stress/rest imaging: 1110 MBq (30 mCi)

SPECT ACQUISITION PARAMETERS

Patient position: supine, left arm raised (180° arc)

Rotation: counterclockwise

Matrix: 128×128 word mode

Image/arc: 64 views (180°, 45° right anterior oblique, 135° left posterior oblique)

SPECT RECONSTRUCTION PARAMETERS*

Ramp filter

Convolution filter: Butterworth

Attenuation correction: review images with and without correction

Oblique angle reformatting: short axis, vertical long axis and horizontal long axis

Gated SPECT

   ECG synchronized data collection: R wave trigger 8 Frames/cardiac cycle

PLANAR IMAGING PROTOCOL

Collimator: High-resolution

Window: 20% centered at 140 keV

For single-day rest and stress studies give 370 MBq (10 mCi) at rest and image at 30 to 60 min

Rest studies: Begin imaging at 60 to 90 min after tracer injection

Obtain anterior, 45 left anterior oblique (LAO), and left lateral images

Obtain 750,000 to 1 million counts per view

Wait 4 hours and give 1110 MBq (30 mCi) with repeat imaging at 15 to 30 min

Stress studies: Begin imaging at 15 to 30 min after tracer injection

Obtain stress and rest images in identical projection

*Choice of SPECT acquisition and reconstruction parameters is highly influenced by the equipment used. Protocols should be established in each nuclear medicine unit for available cameras and computers.

Because the heart lies in the anterior lateral chest and considerable cardiac attenuation results in the posterior projections, SPECT is often acquired over a 180-degree arc from the left posterior oblique (LPO) to the right anterior oblique (RAO) projection. The left arm is positioned above the head to prevent attenuation. A two-headed camera with the detectors at 90 degrees takes maximum advantage of the 180-degree acquisition (Fig. 14-9). The higher count rate of the multiple

ANT   LAO   RAO

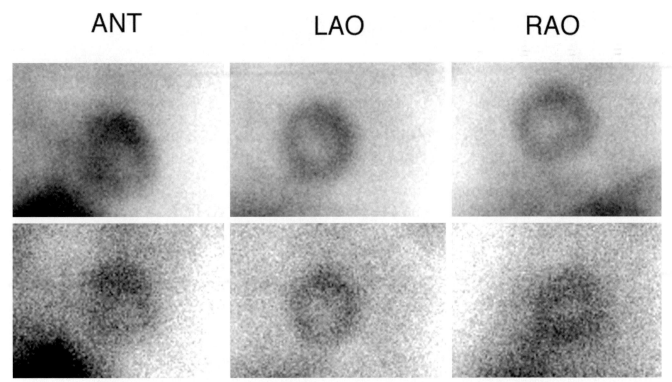

Figure 14-5   Planar stress and rest Tc-99m sestamibi scintigraphy. The rest images are considerably noisier because of the lower administered dose (8 mCi) compared to the stress images (25 mCi). The images should be acquired so that the three planar views (anterior, left anterior oblique, left lateral) are identical for optimal comparison. This study was interpreted as normal.

detectors makes possible the use of high-resolution collimators.

Filtered backprojection has been the standard method used for cross-sectional image reconstruction; however, with faster computers, iterative reconstruction techniques are increasingly available and used. Software filters are chosen to optimize image quality by optimizing the trade-off between high-frequency noise and lower frequency oversmoothing.

Unlike other SPECT displays with axial transverse, sagittal, and coronal slices, the heart is cut along its long and short axes (Figs. 14-10 and 14-11). This has become the standardized method for CT, MRI, and echocardiography. These SPECT cross-sectional images more clearly depict the regional perfusion of the myocardium as it relates to the coronary artery supplying blood to that region (Box 14-4) and permits visual estimation of the degree and extent of the perfusion abnormality (Fig. 14-12). Various different qualitative and quantitative methods have been used.

Gated SPECT

The high count rate available from 20–30 mCi (740–1110 MBq) of Tc-99m sestamibi or tetrofosmin and multidetector systems makes it a feasible and common practice to per-

form ECG gating. Gated SPECT adds a cinematic three-dimensional display of the contracting myocardium. Data collection is triggered from the R-wave of the ECG and arrhythmic beats are filtered out of the data collection cycle. The cardiac cycle is typically divided into eight frames, less than the 16 usually used for planar radionuclide Tc-99m labeled erythrocyte ventriculograms, because of limitations related to computer memory. The eight frames limit, to a mild degree, the temporal resolution (pinpointing end-diastole and end-systole) and thus the accuracy of ejection fraction calculation. Edge-detection software programs automatically draw endocardial and epicardial regions of interest for ejection fraction calculation and wall thickening analysis.

Diagnosis and Evaluation of Coronary Artery Disease

A recurrent theme in nuclear medicine is that of enhancing diagnostic information by applying an interventional maneuver to alter organ function, often while testing functional reserve. Stress cardiac myocardial perfusion scintigraphy and radionuclide ventriculography are elegant examples of this principle.

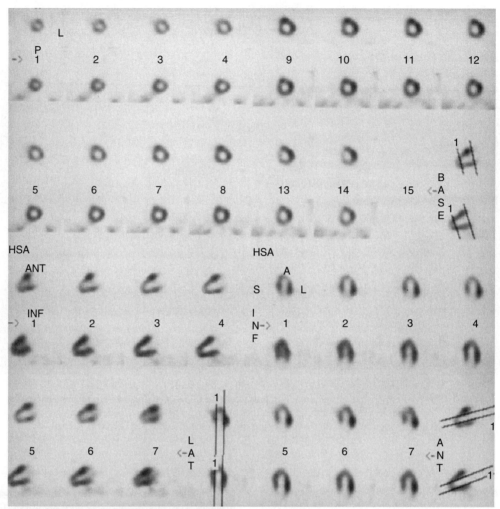

Figure 14-6   Normal SPECT stress thallium-201. Short-axis (*top four rows*), vertical long-axis (*bottom left*), and horizontal long-axis views (*bottom right*).The top row for each slice orientation is the immediate poststress study and the bottom row shows the 3-hour delayed images.

Physiology of Ischemia

Under resting conditions, coronary artery stenoses of up to 90% are not usually associated with a perfusion abnormality (Fig. 14-13). The myocardial oxygen demand is low and blood flow adequate. By increasing cardiac work, exercise stress increases the demand for oxygen and increased blood flow. Maximum exercise can increase coronary flow by three to five times by coronary dilation.

Coronary flow reserve across a fixed mechanical stenosis is limited. If exercise is vigorous, myocardium in the watershed of a coronary artery with a hemodynamically significant stenosis becomes ischemic. Regionally reduced blood flow results in less delivery and localization of the myocardial perfusion radiopharmaceutical. This is seen on scintigraphic images as a relatively cold defect in the ischemic region surrounded by normal blood flow in the adjacent normal regions of the heart (Fig. 14-A1 [see color insert]).

Coronary angiographic laboratories generally consider stenoses of greater than 70% to be clinically significant based on the rapid falloff in flow reserve augmentation above this level (Fig. 14-13). However, the anatomical degree of stenosis has a poor correlation with flow reserve and the degree of ischemia. Other factors affect the functional significance of an anatomical circumferential narrowing (e.g., the length, shape, and location of a stenotic lesion). Thus functional imaging of myocardial perfusion scintigraphy is often needed to evaluate the clinical significance of a known stenosis, particularly in the range of 50–70%.

Cardiac Stress Testing

Cardiac stress testing with ECG monitoring is an intervention that has been used for years by the cardiologist to diagnose coronary artery disease. A prerequisite of intervention is that the degree of stress must be sufficient to unmask underlying

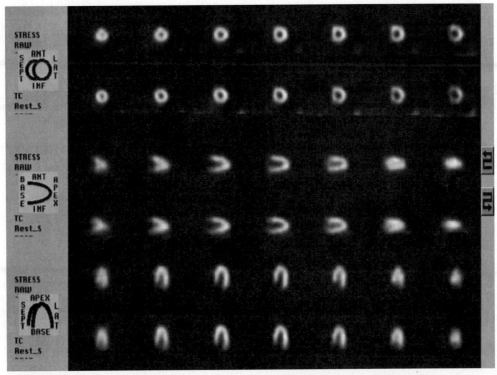

Figure 14-7   Normal SPECT stress and rest Tc-99m sestamibi. Note the excellent visualization of the left ventricular myocardium. The more proximal short-axis views (*top rows, far right*) demonstrate decreased uptake in the region of the membranous septum.

abnormalities (Box 14-5). *Graded treadmill exercise* is the standard method for cardiac stress testing. Exercise increases cardiac work load and oxygen demand. The treadmill study allows for assessment of the patient's functional cardiac status by directly monitoring exercise tolerance, heart rate, blood pressure, and ECG response to graded exercise. Indications and contraindications for cardiac stress testing are listed in Box 14-6.

Exercise-induced myocardial ischemia produces characteristic ST-T segment depression on ECG caused by alterations in sodium and potassium electrolyte flux across the ischemic cell membrane. The adequacy of exercise is judged by the degree of cardiac work. Heart rate and blood pressure provide such an indication. Patients achieving >85% of the age-predicted maximum heart rate (220 − age = maximum predicted heart rate) are considered to have achieved adequate exercise stress. The heart-rate/blood-pressure product, METS (metabolic equivalents), and length of exercise (minutes) are other indicators used to judge the adequacy of exercise. Failure to achieve adequate exercise is the most common reason for a false negative stress test (Box 14-7).

Most cardiologists perform cardiac treadmill exercise in their offices. Although it provides clinically useful diagnostic and functional information necessary to man-

age patients, the overall accuracy of the cardiac treadmill exercise test for the diagnosis of coronary artery disease is modest, in the range of 75%, with numerous false negatives and false positives. Specificity is particularly poor in women, in patients with resting ECG ST-T changes, left ventricular hypertrophy, bundle branch block, and patients on digoxin. These patients often require myocardial perfusion scintigraphy to confirm or exclude the diagnosis of coronary artery disease.

Stress Perfusion Scintigraphy

The combination of stress testing with myocardial perfusion imaging is a commonly performed nuclear medicine study. The overall accuracy for the diagnosis of coronary artery disease is considerably higher for stress myocardial perfusion imaging than the exercise treadmill study. SPECT provides valuable information on the degree and severity of coronary artery disease that allows for risk assessment, prognosis, and better patient management.

Exercise Stress Testing

Patients are requested to fast for 4-6 hours prior to the test to minimize splanchnic blood distribution and exercise or pharmacologic stress-induced gastric distress. Cardiac medications may be held depending on

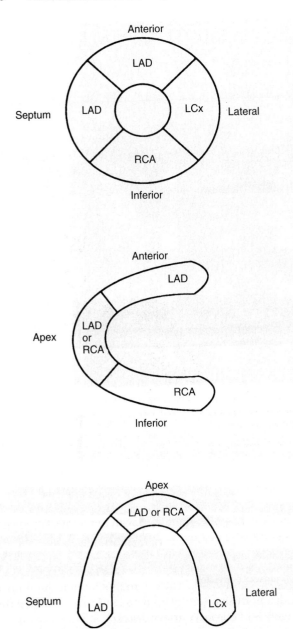

Figure 14-8 SPECT schematic correlation of myocardial wall segments and vascular supply. Short-axis, vertical long-axis, and horizontal long-axis SPECT views. *LAD*, Left anterior descending artery; *LCx*, left circumflex branch; *RCA*, right coronary artery.

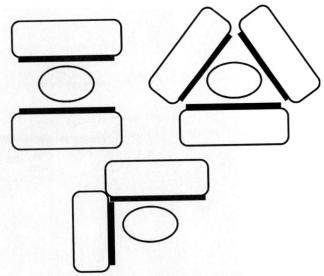

Figure 14-9 Two- and three-head gamma camera detector configurations. A common configuration with the two-headed systems is with the heads at right angles to each other (lower). Thus, maximal count rate is achieved over a 180-degree rotation. Three-heads allow for an even higher count rate and are typically acquired over a 270- to 360-degree rotation.

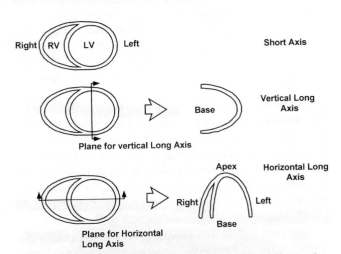

Figure 14-10 Processing SPECT to obtain short and long axis cross-sectional cuts. Schematic diagram displays the standard orientation along the short and long axis of the heart.

the indication for the stress test, whether for diagnosis or to determine the effectiveness of therapy (Box 14-8). Beta-blockers may prevent achievement of maximum heart rate and nitrates or calcium channel blockers may mask or prevent cardiac ischemia, limiting the test's ability to detect coronary disease. On the other hand, assessing the adequacy of drug therapy in blocking ischemia requires the patient to remain on the medication. A negative test while the patient is taking cardiac medications augurs well from a prognostic standpoint. The decision is left to the discretion of the referring physician.

In addition to a standard 12-lead ECG baseline evaluation and continuous monitoring during the test, an intravenous line with a keep-open solution is placed. Graded treadmill exercise is performed (Fig. 14-14) according to a standardized protocol, such as Bruce protocol (Table 14-3). When the patient has achieved maximal exercise or peak patient tolerance, the radiopharmaceutical is injected. Exercise is continued for another 1-2 minutes to ensure adequate uptake reflecting the perfusion pattern at peak stress. Early discontinuation of exercise may result in tracer distribution reflecting perfusion at submaximal exercise levels. Box 14-9 lists reasons for

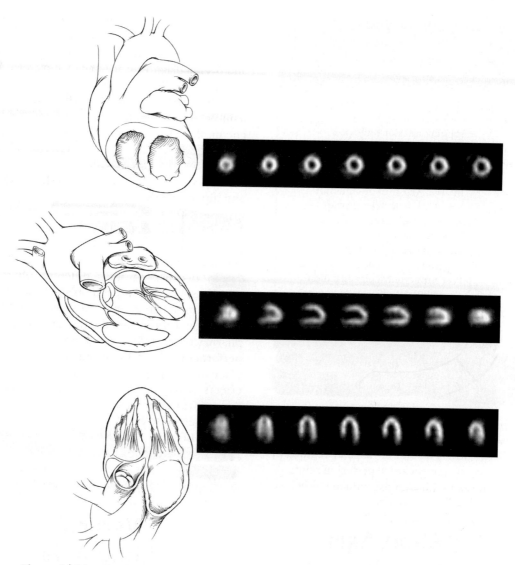

Figure 14-11 Standard display of SPECT cross-sectional images correlated with cardiac anatomy. The planes are cut along the short and long axis of the heart, top (short-axis), middle (vertical long axis), bottom (horizontal long axis). The left ventricle is best seen due to its greater myocardial mass; the right ventricle is less well seen and the display emphasizes the left ventricle. Atria are not visualized.

terminating exercise. Many of these are manifestations of ischemia and others are due to underlying cardiac or pulmonary decompensation.

Some patients cannot perform exercise treadmill stress because of medical problems such as pulmonary disease or lower extremity musculoskeletal problems. Alternative approaches to exercise stress have been used, including isometric handgrip (Box 14-10). However, pharmacologic stress is the usual alternative to exercise.

Pharmacologic Stress Testing

Pharmacologic stress with dipyridamole (Persantine), adenosine (Adenoscan), or dobutamine is used in up to

40% of patients referred for stress myocardial perfusion studies.

Dipyridamole and Adenosine

Mechanism of Pharmacologic Effect Both adenosine (AdenoScan, Fujisawa) and dipyridamole (Persantine, Bristol-Myers Squibb) are potent coronary vasodilators capable of producing a threefold to fourfold increase in normal coronary blood flow. Adenosine is normally endogenously produced in coronary endothelial cells. When released intravascularly, it activates coronary receptors that produce vasodilation. Dipyridamole exerts its pharmacologic effect by blocking the reuptake mechanism of adenosine and raising endogenous adenosine

Box 14-4 Scintigraphic Patterns for Specific Vascular Distributions: Stenosis and Obstruction

Coronary Artery	Scintigraphic Perfusion Defects
Left anterior descending	Septum, anterior wall, apex
Left circumflex	Lateral wall, posterior wall, posterior inferior wall, apex
Right coronary	Inferior wall, posterior inferior wall, right ventricular wall
Left main coronary	Anterior wall, septum, posterolateral wall
Multiple-vessel disease	Multiple vascular bed perfusion defects
	Post stress ventricular dilatation and increased Tl-201 lung uptake

blood levels. Adenosine and dipyridamole are used interchangeably, although they have somewhat different infusion protocols (Boxes 14-11 and 14-12), incidence of side effects (Table 14-4), and methods to reverse side effects.

Because coronary vessels with significant stenoses cannot increase blood flow to the same degree as normal vessels, vasodilator stress results in vascular regions of relative hypoperfusion on myocardial perfusion scintigraphy, similar to that seen with exercise-induced ischemia.

Unlike exercise, this method is not a test of ischemia, but rather of coronary flow reserve. Regardless, comparative studies have shown similar scintigraphic patterns and overall diagnostic accuracy for exercise and pharmacologic stress.

Patient Preparation Both adenosine and dipyridamole are antagonized by drugs and food containing chemically related methylxanthines, such as theophylline and caffeine (Fig. 14-15). They must be discontinued for 24 hours prior to the study since they may counteract the effectiveness of vasodilation (Box 14-8). Adenosine and dipyridamole can cause bronchospasm, thus these drugs should not be used in patients with a history of severe bronchospastic disease.

Methodology The technical details for dipyridamole and adenosine infusion protocols differ (Box 14-11 and 14-12) because of their different pharmacokinetics (Table 14-5). Both are administered as slow infusions of 4-6 minutes. A mild increase in heart rate and mild reduction in blood pressure confirm the drug's pharmacologic effect. Some protocols have the patient perform mild exercise during infusion (e.g., walking in place or handgrip isometric stress) to decrease the side effects of hypotension and dizziness and to minimize liver activity seen on scintigraphy by diverting the blood flow to leg muscles.

Side Effects Mild nausea, dizziness, headache, and flushing are common with adenosine and Persantine (Table 14-4). Approximately 20–35% of patients experience chest pain, although it is usually not ischemic in

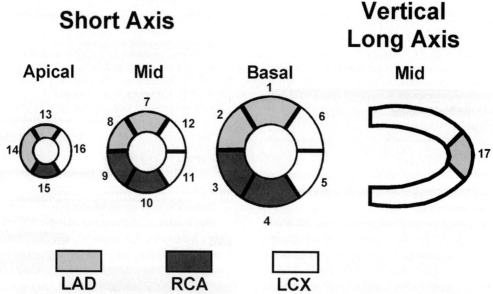

Figure 14-12 Standardization of SPECT myocardial segments. This is the method recommended and published in *Circulation* and the *Journal of Nuclear Cardiology* in an attempt to standardize the regions of the myocardium into 17 regions for all cardiac imaging. The diagram also correlates coronary artery anatomy with regional perfusion. However, some computer software systems use a different number of regions. (Modified with permission from Cerqueira MD, Weissman J, Dilsizian V, et al: J Nucl Card 2:240–245, 2002.)

origin. Rarely a coronary steal syndrome may produce true ischemia. Dyspnea more commonly occurs with adenosine and A-V conduction blocks are seen exclusively with adenosine. If ECG ST-T depression occurs during infusion, it is diagnostic for coronary disease.

With adenosine, no antidote is required to reverse side effects. The infusion is simply terminated. Because of adenosine's short half-life in serum (less than 10 seconds), conduction blocks or other adverse symptoms resolve promptly. However, because the action of dipyridamole is often prolonged due to its 20-30 minute serum half-life, aminophylline is required to

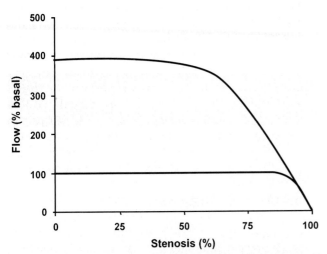

Figure 14-13   Relationship between blood flow and severity of coronary stenosis. At rest, myocardial blood flow is not reduced until a coronary stenosis approaches 90%. It then begins to drop off. However, with increased rates of coronary blood flow produced by exercise or pharmacologic stress, less severe stenoses (50-75%) cause reduced coronary flow.

Box 14-5   Exercise Testing: Rationale and Endpoint Measures

PHYSIOLOGIC RATIONALE

Physical exercise increases cardiac work
Increased work increases myocardial oxygen demand
Normal coronary arteries dilate and flow increases
Stenotic vessels cannot dilate and flow reserve is limited
Myocardial ischemia is induced

MANIFESTATIONS OF MYOCARDIAL ISCHEMIA

Electrocardiogram: Ion flux across cell membrane is impaired, produces ST segment depression on ECG
Myocardial perfusion imaging: Decrease in regional flow produces cold defect area on scintigraphy
Radionuclide ventriculography: Regional wall motion abnormality and/or fall in LVEF

Box 14-6   Stress Testing: Indications and Contraindications

INDICATIONS

Diagnosis of coronary artery disease
Evaluation of known coronary disease; location and extent of ischemia
Determine the cause for change in symptom pattern in patients with known coronary artery disease
Evaluate the effectiveness of medical therapy
Risk stratification post-myocardial infarction
Preoperative evaluation for major noncardiac surgery in patient with known coronary disease
Assessment after percutaneous transluminal coronary angioplasty or coronary artery bypass grafting
Guide to rehabilitation therapy

CONTRAINDICATIONS

Acute myocardial infarction
Unstable angina
Severe tachyarrhythmias or bradyarrhythmias
Uncontrolled symptomatic heart failure
Critical aortic stenosis
Acute aortic dissection
Pulmonary embolism
Poorly controlled hypertension

Box 14-7   Reasons for Failing to Achieve Adequate Exercise

Poor general conditioning, low exercise tolerance
Poor motivation
Arthritis, other musculoskeletal problems
Lung disease
Peripheral vascular disease
Medications (beta-blockers)
Angina
Arrhythmia
Cardiac insufficiency

Box 14-8   Drugs That Interfere with Stress Testing: Recommended Withdrawal Interval

Drug	Withdrawal Interval
EXERCISE	
Beta-blockers	72 hr
Calcium channel blockers	48-72 hr
Nitrates (long acting)	12 hr
PHARMACOLOGIC	
Aminophylline	36 hrs
Caffeine	24 hrs

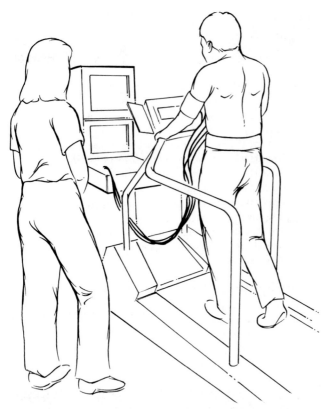

Figure 14-14   Treadmill exercise. Treadmill graded exercise with ECG, blood pressure, and heart rate monitoring.

Table 14-3   Treadmill Exercise Stress Test

Stage	Duration (min)	Total time	Speed (mile/h)	Grade (%)
STANDARD BRUCE PROTOCOL				
1	3	3	1.7	10
2	3	6	2.5	12
3	3	9	3.4	14
4	3	12	4.2	16
5	3	15	5.0	18
6	3	18	6.0	20
MODIFIED BRUCE PROTOCOL				
1	3	3	1.7	0
2	3	6	1.7	5
3	3	9	1.7	10
4	3	12	2.5	12
5	3	15	3.4	14
6	3	18	4.2	16
7	3	21	5.0	18

The modified Bruce starts with the same speed as the standard Bruce, but with no slope, followed by slight increase in slope, and then in speed. This protocol is suited for elderly patients or patients where one anticipates difficulties with physical performance.

Box 14-9   Indications for Terminating a Stress Test

Patient's request
Inability to continue due to fatigue, dyspnea, or faintness
Moderate to severe chest pain
Dizziness, near syncope
Pallor, diaphoresis
Ataxia
Claudication
Ventricular tachycardia
Atrial tachycardia or fibrillation
Onset of second- or third-degree heart block
ST segment depression >3 mm
Decrease in systolic blood pressure from baseline
Increase in systolic blood pressure above 240 mm Hg or diastolic above 120 mm Hg

Box 14-10   Cardiac Stress Tests: Exercise and Nonexercise

LEG EXERCISE

Treadmill
Bicycle ergometer

OTHER CARDIAC STRESS TESTS

Isometric handgrip exercise
Cold pressor test
Esophageal pacing

PHARMACOLOGIC STRESS

Dipyridamole, adenosine, dobutamine

Box 14-11   Dipyridamole Pharmacologic Stress: Protocol

Time from Start of Infusion (min)	Protocol
	Obtain baseline ECG and blood pressure; report at 1-min intervals
0–4	Administer dipyridamole 0.56 mg/kg for 4 min intravenously
6–8	Inject radiopharmaceutical intravenously 3–4 min after dipyridamole infusion
20	Begin imaging at 14 minutes after dipyridamole infusion completed
Optional as a routine or as needed for adverse symptoms	Administer 75 to 100 mg aminophylline *slowly* by intravenous injection

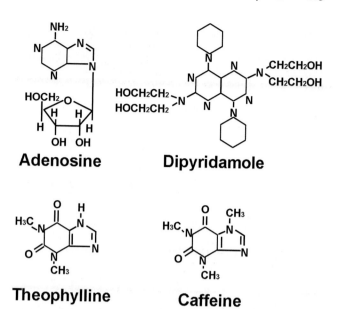

Figure 14-15 Close chemical relationship of adenosine and dipyridamole to theophylline and caffeine.

Box 14-12 Adenosine Pharmacologic Stress: Protocol

Time from Start of Infusion (min)	Protocol
	Obtain baseline ECG and blood pressure; report at 1-min intervals
0-6	Administer adenosine 0.14 mg/kg/min for 4-6 min intravenously
3	Inject radiopharmaceutical intravenously at 3 min from *start* of infusion
9-10	Begin imaging 3 minutes after adenosine infusion completed

Table 14-4 Adverse Effects: Adenosine and Dipyridamole

Adverse effect	Adenosine	Dipyridamole
Flushing	37%	3%
Dyspnea	35	3
Chest pain	25	20
Gastrointestinal symptoms	15	6
Headache	14	12
Dizziness	9	12
A-V block	8	2
ST-T wave changes	6	8
Arrhythmia	3	5
Hypotension	2	5
Bronchospasm	0.1	0.15
Myocardial infarction	0.0001	0.05
Death	0	0.5

Table 14-5 Comparison of Pharmacologic Myocardial Stress Agents

	Adenosine	Dipyridamole	Dobutamine
Half-life	<10 sec	30-60 min	2 min
Mean time to peak coronary flow velocity	55 sec	6.5 min	10 min
Onset of action	seconds	2 min	1-2 min
Side effects requiring medical intervention	0.6%	16%	5%

reverse its side effects. Some clinics routinely administer aminophylline at the end of dipyridamole stress to prevent and terminate its common side effects.

Accuracy Comparative studies have reported similar accuracy for detection of significant coronary disease for adenosine and dipyridamole compared to exercise-stress SPECT myocardial perfusion scintigraphy. The disadvantage is the lack of information on functional cardiac status provided by exercise.

Dobutamine

For patients unable to exercise but with contraindications to dipyridamole and adenosine (e.g., asthma), dobutamine can be used as an alternative.

Mechanism of Action This synthetic catecholamine acts on alpha- and beta-adrenergic receptors producing inotropic and chronotropic effects that increase cardiac work. In normal coronary arteries, this results in increased blood flow. In the face of significant stenosis, regional flow does not increase, resulting in scintigraphic patterns similar to that seen with exercise and pharmacologic stress.

Methodology The infusion begins with 5 µg/kg/min infused for 3 minutes, then increased to 10 µg/kg/min for another 3 minutes and increased by that amount every 10 minutes until a maximum of 40 µg/kg/min is achieved. The radiopharmaceutical is injected one minute after the maximal tolerable dose and the dobutamine infusion continued for at least 1 minute.

Accuracy Dobutamine perfusion imaging is reported to have accuracy similar to exercise or dipyridamole/adenosine stress. The major limitation is the frequent

Method	Radiopharma-ceutical	Rationale
2-day	Tc-sestamibi/ tetrofosmin	Obesity, image quality
1-day	Tc-sestambi/ tetrofosmin	Image quality, efficiency
1-day	Tl-201	Time tested, viability
Dual-isotope	Tl-201 and Tc-sestamibi/ tetrofosmin	Image quality, viability, logistics

Box 14-14   Advantages and Disadvantages of Tc-99m Sestamibi/ Tetrofosmin for Myocardial Perfusion Imaging

ADVANTAGES

Higher count rates; better quality SPECT images and gated SPECT possible

Higher energy photons; fewer attenuation artifacts

Simultaneous assessment of perfusion and function

First-pass assessment of right and left ventricular function possible

DISADVANTAGES

No redistribution

Lung uptake not diagnostic

Less extraction at hyperemic flows

Less sensitive than Tl-201 for viability assessment

occurrence of side effects (e.g., chest pain and arrhythmias) and the inability of many patients to tolerate the maximum required dose.

One- and Two-Day Protocols

Various different stress perfusion imaging protocols are used, depending on the radiopharmaceutical used, patient size, logistics of the clinic, and preference of the physicians (Box 14-13).

Thallium-201

Originally, a two-day protocol was used for Tl-201, with separate rest and stress injections. It was soon appreciated that Tl-201 redistributes, allowing for assessment of both stress and rest perfusion following a single injection on the same day. After stress, initial images are obtained at 10–15 minutes and delayed images at 3 hours (Box 14-2, Fig. 14-B [see color insert]). Although the new Tc-99m radiopharmaceuticals are increasingly used for myocardial perfusion scintigraphy, Tl-201 is still preferred by some because of its lesser liver and bowel activity that can adversely impact interpretation. It is also used for the diagnosis of myocardial viability, discussed later.

Tc-99m Sestamibi and Tc-99m Tetrofosmin

Because these radiopharmaceuticals do not redistribute or washout significantly from the myocardium over time, two separate injections are required. A summary of the advantages and disadvantages of Tc-99m sestamibi and tetrofosmin compared to Tl-201 are listed in Box 14-14. Several different approaches have been used.

One-Day Both rest and stress studies can be performed on the same day. The patient receives a lower administered dose for the first study (8–10 mCi [266–370 MBq]) and a several-fold higher dose (25–30 mCi [925–1110 MBq]) for the second study. The most common approach is to do the rest study first followed by the stress study. The lower dose study is more susceptible to attenuation effects similar to that seen with Tl-201. The second study commences approximately 1.5 hours later to allow time for decreased background activity biological clearance and decay (Fig. 14-C [see color insert]).

Two-Day Tissue attenuation can be marked in large patients and can result in image poor quality, particularly with the lower dose study. A 2-day approach minimizes this problem allowing administration of the maximum dose (25–30 mCi) for both studies. This approach is most commonly used in obese patients.

Dual Isotope This approach takes advantage of the different photopeaks of the Tc-99m agent (140 keV) and Tl-201 (69–83 keV) (Fig. 14-A1 [see color insert]). Simultaneous acquisition (rest Tl-201 and stress Tc-99m sestamibi or tetrofosmin) is desirable for efficiency reasons; however, it is not practical because downscatter of Tc-99m into the Tl-201 window is significant. Thus, the Tl-201 rest study is performed first using 3.0–3.5 mCi (110–130 MBq), followed by the stress study, using 20–30 mCi (740–1110 MBq) of the Tc-99m agent. Upscatter of the higher energy Tl-201 photons (167 keV) is minimal because of their low abundance (10%).

The dual isotope protocol has two advantages. The study can be completed more rapidly than Tc-99m protocols because imaging begins earlier, soon after injection for the rest study and no delay is required before starting the stress study. Another advantage is that Tl-201 can provide information on viability (hibernating myocardium).

Image Interpretation

Coronary Anatomy and Myocardial Perfusion

Although the anatomy of the coronary circulation varies in its details, the distribution of the major vessels is reasonably predictable (Fig. 14-16, Box 14-4). The *left anterior descending* coronary artery serves most of the septum and the anterior wall of the left ventricle. Its diagonal branches course over the lateral wall and septal perforators penetrate into the septum. The *left circumflex* coronary artery and its marginal branches serve the lateral and posterior walls. The *right coronary artery* and its posterior descending branch serves the right ventricle, the inferior portion of the septum, and portions of the inferior wall of the left ventricle.

The apex may be perfused by branches from any of the three main vessels.

Quality Control of SPECT Acquisition

Patient Motion   Movement of the patient during the study can degrade image quality. A review of raw acquisition data should be routine. This is best done by displaying all image projections in an endless loop cinematic rotating display. Greater than 2-pixel deviation can adversely affect image quality.

Another method for confirming motion is to review the "sinogram" display. Each projection image is stacked vertically. Each is compressed, with maintenance of the count density distribution in the X-axis but minimization of the count density distribution in the Y-axis. Because the heart is not in the center of the camera radius of rotation, the position of the left ventricle in the stacked frames varies sinusoidally. Any significant motion will be seen as a break in the sinogram (Fig. 14-17).

If there is significant motion, the study should ideally be reacquired. If this is not possible, motion correction programs are available with most camera computer systems. However, these programs correct only in the vertical axis.

Image Quality   Camera quality control is critical and discussed in Chapters 3 and 4. Image quality may be poor due to insufficient activity in the heart, due either to low dose (e.g., if much of the dose was inadvertently injected and retained subcutaneously) or the result of

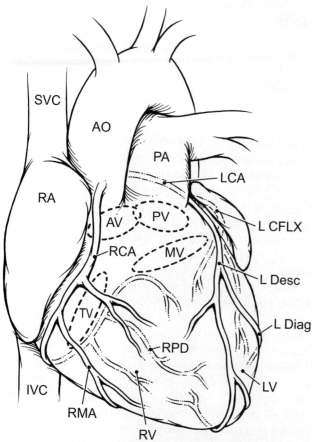

Figure 14-16   Normal distribution of the coronary arteries. The left main coronary artery is only 0–15 mm in length before dividing into the left anterior descending and left circumflex arteries. Important branches of the left anterior descending artery are the diagonal and septal branches. The left circumflex artery (LCFx) has obtuse marginal branches. The right coronary artery (RCA) originates separately and has important branches that include the posterior right ventricular branches, the posterior descending artery (PDA). "Dominance" refers to which coronary artery (RCA or LCFx) supplies the diaphragmatic surface of the left ventricle and posterior septum by giving rise to the posterior descending and posterior left ventricular branches. In 85% of patients the RCA is dominant, in 7–8% the LCFx is dominant and in 7–8% there is balanced circulation between the two. Right posterior descending (RPD), right marginal branch artery (RMA).

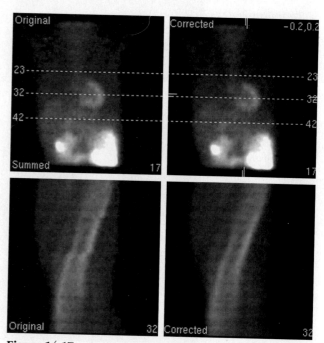

Figure 14-17   Sinogram to detect for motion. Projection images are stacked vertically. Because the heart is not in the center of the camera radius of rotation, the position of the left ventricle in the stacked frames varies sinusoidally. Any significant motion will be seen as a break in the sinogram. Note the horizontal break in the mid-sinogram (*left*). The motion corrected (*right*).

soft tissue attenuation (discussed later). The presence of free Tc-99m pertechnetate will increase background and degrade image quality.

Normal Myocardial Perfusion Scintigraphy

Rest SPECT Images Normal myocardial perfusion rest images with Tl-201 and Tc-99m sestamibi/tetrofosmin show similar uniform uptake throughout the left ventricular myocardium (Figs. 14-5 and 14-6), although the Tc-99m agents usually have superior image quality. The right ventricle is seen to a lesser extent because of its smaller myocardial muscle mass. Right ventricular hypertrophy results in increased uptake (Fig. 14-18). Atria are not visualized.

On short-axis SPECT views, the left ventricle has a doughnut appearance. The lateral wall usually appears to have more uptake than the anterior or inferior wall. Decreased uptake is seen near the base of the heart in the region of the membranous septum (Fig. 14-6). The valve planes have an absence of uptake, giving the heart a horseshoe or U-shaped appearance on long-axis (coronal and sagittal) SPECT slices. The normal myocardium appears thinner at the apex ("apical thinning"). Mild lung uptake is seen. Increased resting lung uptake occurs in heavy smokers, patients with underlying lung disease, and those with congestive heart failure (Fig. 14-19).

Stress SPECT Images Normal myocardial perfusion images obtained after exercise or pharmacological stress are not strikingly different in distribution from those obtained at rest; however, there are differences. The cardiac target-to-background ratio of the stress images is higher due to increased cardiac uptake. Right ventricular uptake is often relatively increased, but still considerably less than the left ventricle. With treadmill exercise, less activity is seen in the liver because of diversion of blood flow from the splanchnic bed to leg muscles. Assessing the degree of uptake in the liver can serve as an internal quality control check on the adequacy of exercise. Pharmacological stress with adenosine and dipyridamole stress results in considerable liver activity.

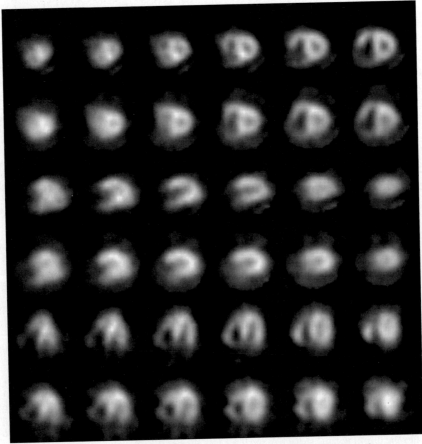

Figure 14-18 Right ventricular hypertrophy. Patient with interstitial fibrosis and severe pulmonary hypertension. Stress and rest Tc-99 sestamibi show prominent uptake in a hypertrophied right ventricle.

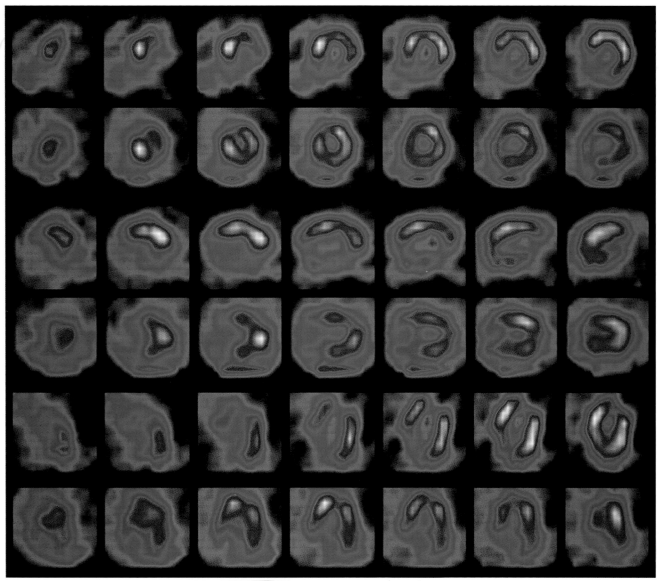

Figure 14-A   1, Inferior wall ischemia.   Exercise Tc-99m sestamibi/rest Tl-201 myocardial perfusion. Marked hypoperfusion of the entire inferior wall and inferior apex post-stress, which normalizes on rest images consistent with a large region of severe ischemia.

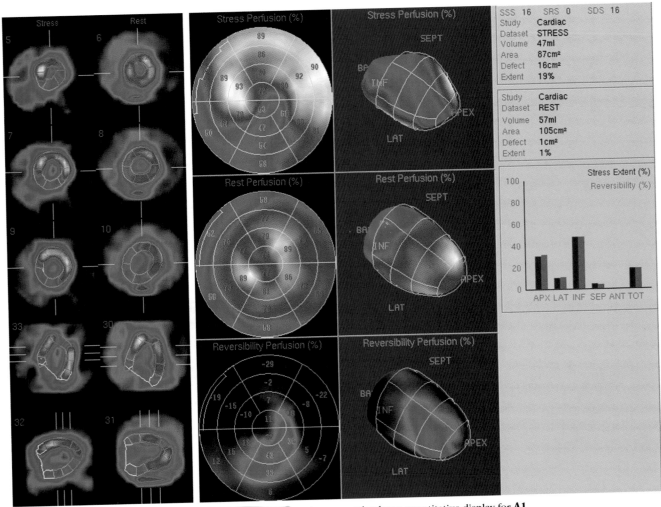

Figure 14-A   2. Inferior wall ischemia: polar map and volume quantitative display for **A1**. The reversibility perfusion (%) box shows the extent and severity of the reversible perfusion defect as a polar map and three-dimensional volume display. At the right, the stress extent (%) and reversibility (%) are shown in graph form.

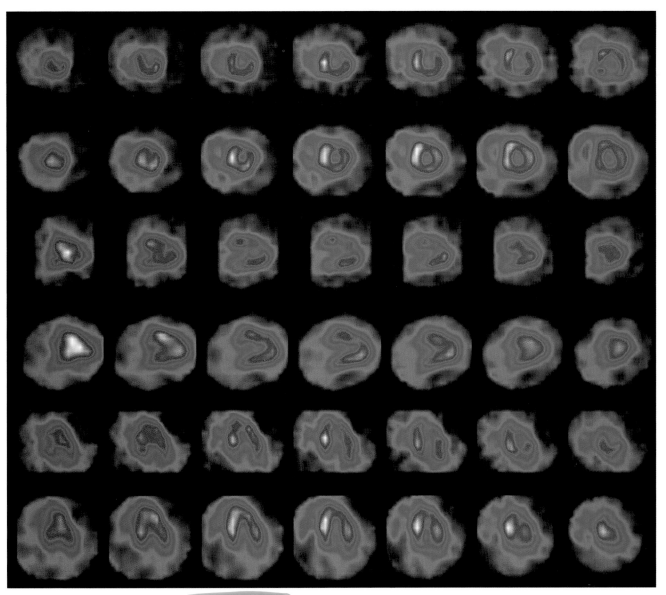

Figure 14-B 1, Anterior wall ischemia. Postexercise and 3-hour delayed Tl-201 myocardial perfusion. Stress induced hypoperfusion is seen in the anterior wall extending to the apex. At rest, there has been near complete redistribution consistent with moderate ischemia of a moderate sized region. This subjective evaluation can be compared to the quantitative display in **B2**.

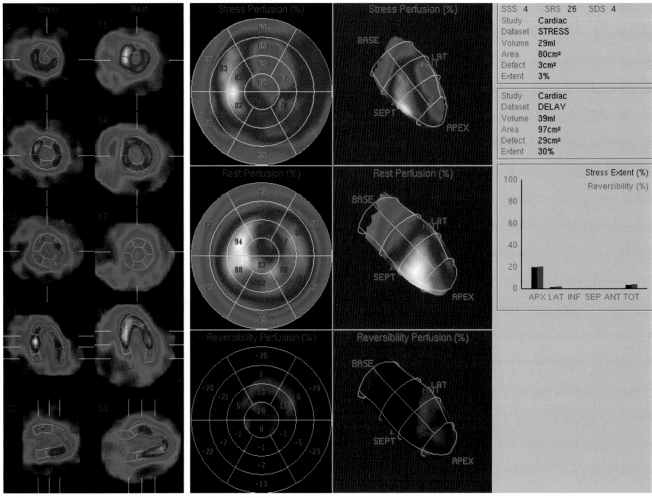

Figure 14-B 2, Anterior wall ischemia: polar map and volume quantitative display. Reversibility of 10–13% in individual regions of the anterior lateral apical region. The graph in the right hand column displays the stress extent and reversibility percentage. This suggests a somewhat lesser degree of ischemia than the interpretation of the splash display in **B1**.

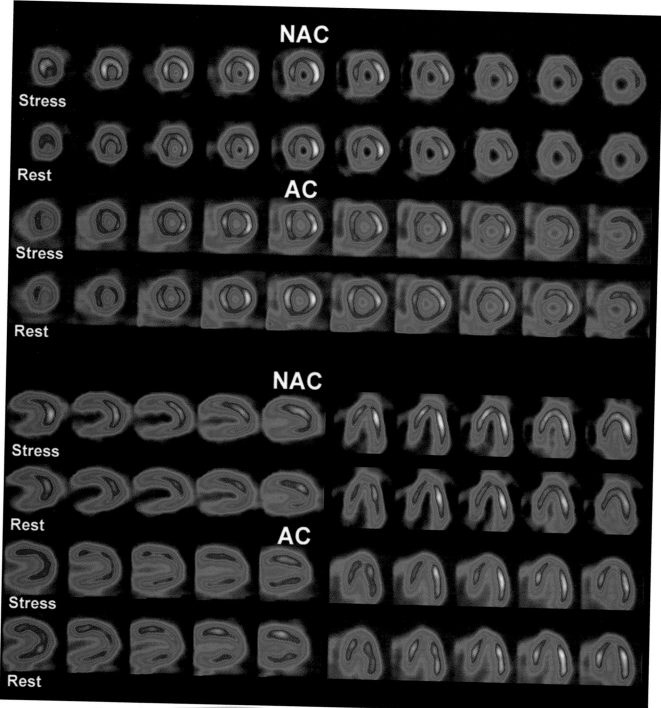

Figure 14-C   Attenuation correction: attenuation artifact. Persantine stress and rest Tc-99m sestamibi. Top two rows (stress, rest) of transverse, vertical and horizontal long axis slices are non attenuation corrected (NAC) images. Lower two rows of each section are attenuation corrected (AC). The NAC images show decreased activity in the inferior wall. With AC, the distribution of perfusion is normal. This is a normal stress myocardial perfusion study. The patient had a history of arrhythmia and some risk factors for coronary disease, but no history of angina or myocardial infarction.

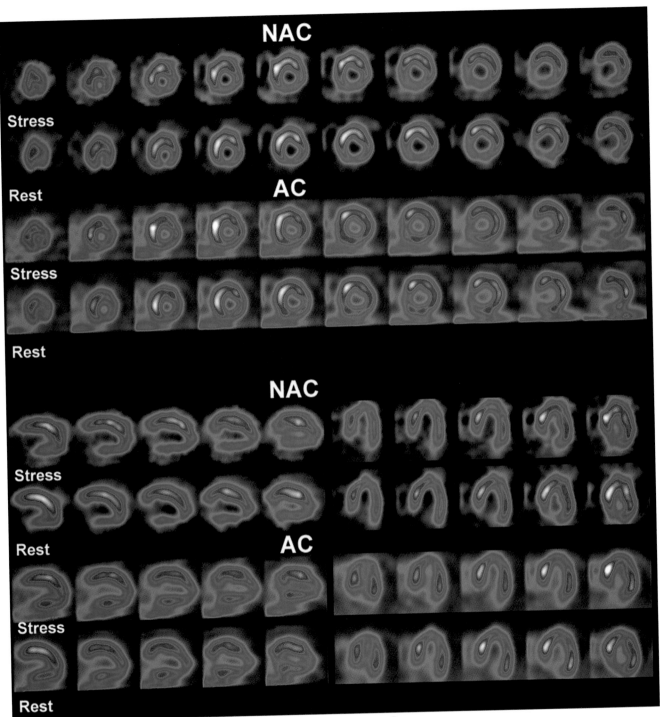

Figure 14-D Attenuation correction: inferior wall infarction. Persantine stress and rest Tc-99m sestamibi. Top two rows of transverse, vertical and horizontal long axis slices are non attenuation corrected images. Lower two rows of each section are attenuation corrected. The stress (above) and rest (below) non-attenuation corrected images show a large area of decreased activity in the inferior wall extending to the septum and lateral wall. Attenuation correction images show persistent decreased activity in the same region, although to a lesser degree. The study is consistent with large area of moderately severe infarction in the inferior wall. This patient had a history of prior myocardial infarction.

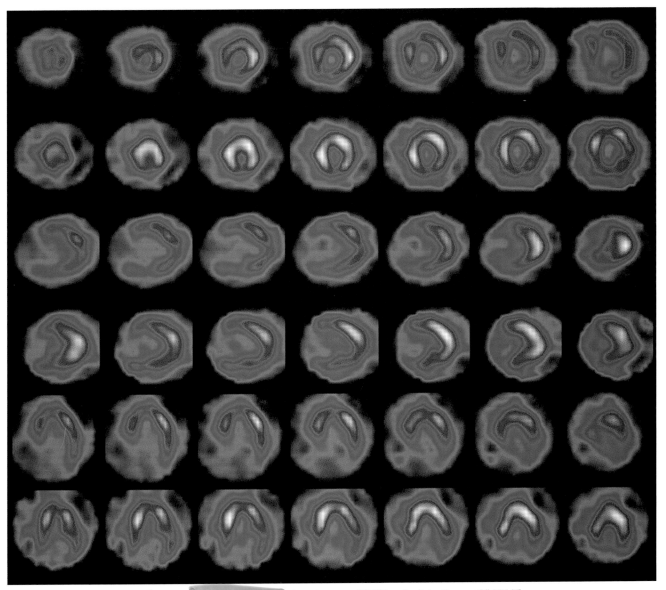

Figure 14-E   1, Multivessel ischemia. Exercise stress Tl-201 and reinjection rest Tl-201. The patient had known three-vessel coronary artery disease and poor ventricular function, and was beginning considered for coronary bypass surgery. With submaximal stress, there is reduced perfusion to the anterior, septal, and inferior walls. On delayed imaging, there is redistribution to these regions. There is a suggestion of transient ischemic dilation (TID). Stress-induced lung uptake was also seen (*see* Fig. 14-19).

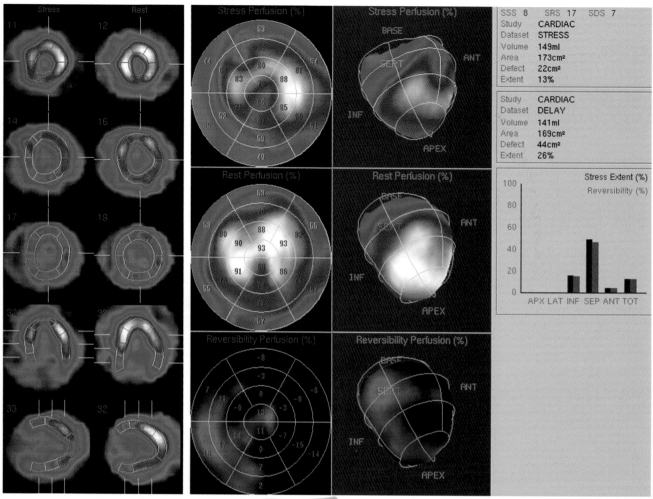

Figure 14-E 2. Multivessel ischemia: polar display. The quantitative two- and three-dimensional displays show redistribution primarily to the apex, inferior-septal and septal regions in the range of 11–17%. This display likely underestimates the degree of ischemia, when interpreted in light of submaximal exercise, TID, and exercise induced lung uptake (*see* Fig. 14-19).

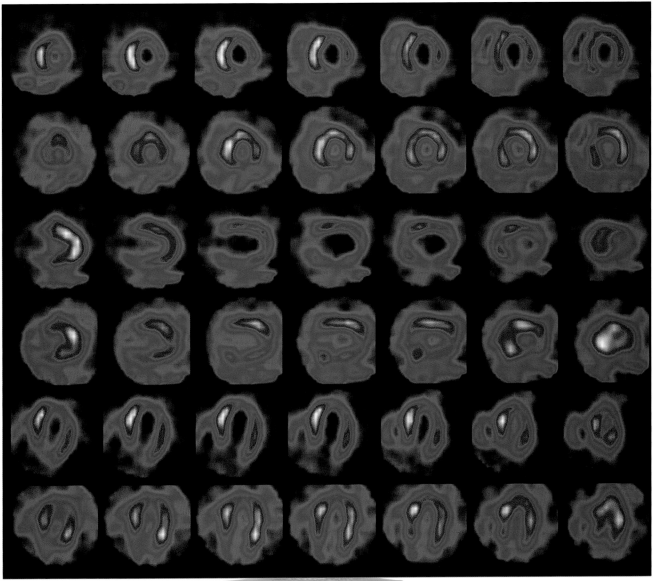

Figure 14-F 1, Anterior lateral and inferior lateral wall ischemia. Persantine stress and rest Tl-201. The stress images show hypoperfusion of the anterior lateral wall and no perfusion to the inferior wall. Rest images show definite redistribution to the anterior lateral wall but incomplete redistribution to the inferior wall.

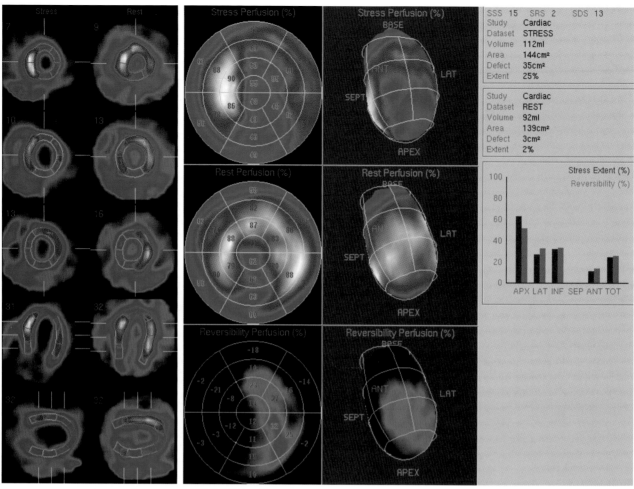

Figure 14-F 2, Lateral wall ischemia: polar and volume quantitative display. Reversibility percentage is as high as 23% to 32% in the anterior lateral and inferior lateral walls. See wall motion and thickening on Fig. 14-K.

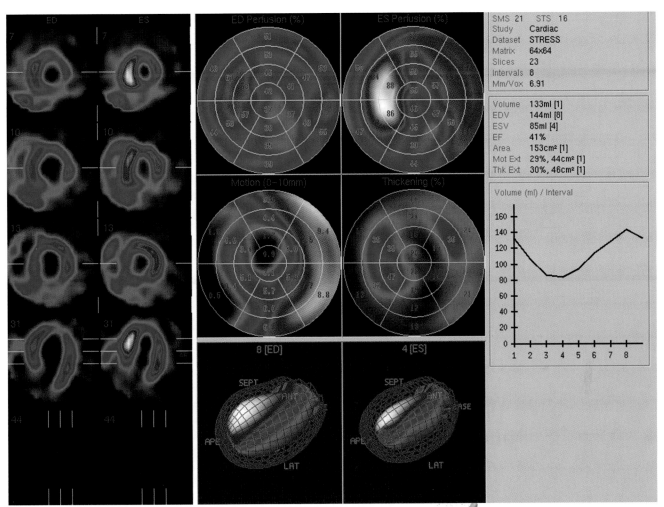

Figure 14-F 3, Lateral wall ischemia: wall motion and thickening. The images in the left column show septal thickening (manifested as brightening) and to a lesser degree anterior lateral wall thickening. There is reduced thickening in the inferior wall. The cardiac volume curve and calculated ejection fraction (41%) show diffuse hypokinesis.

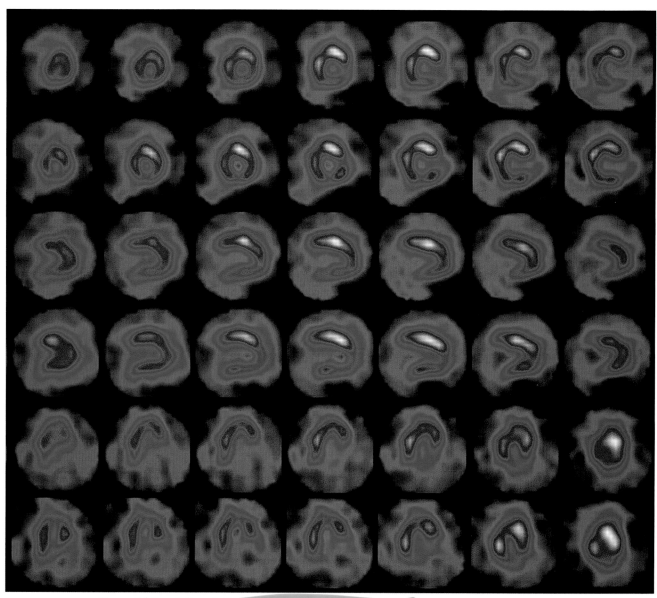

Figure 14-G   1. Lateral wall infarction and inferior lateral ischemia. Persantine stress rest Tl-201. Stress images show no perfusion of the lateral wall and reduced perfusion to the inferior wall. Rest images show no improvement in the lateral wall but improved perfusion to the inferior wall.

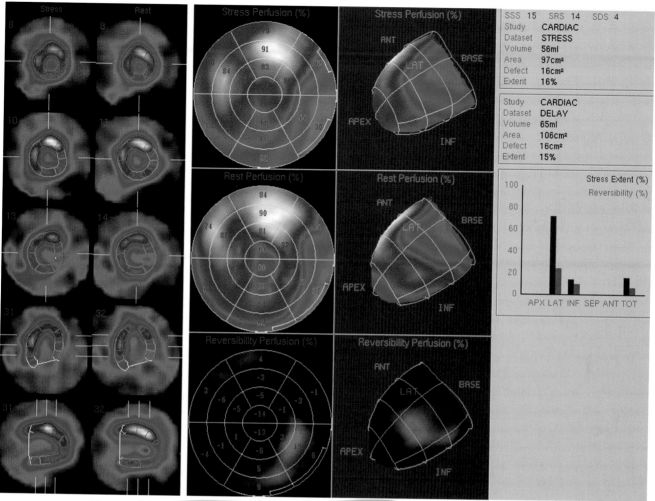

Figure 14-G   2, Lateral wall infarction and inferior lateral ischemia: polar and volume quantitative display. The reversibility percentage shows at least one inferior wall region with a 19% reversibility. The graph in the right column shows the discrepancy between the stress extent and the reversibility extent, representing the infarcted lateral wall.

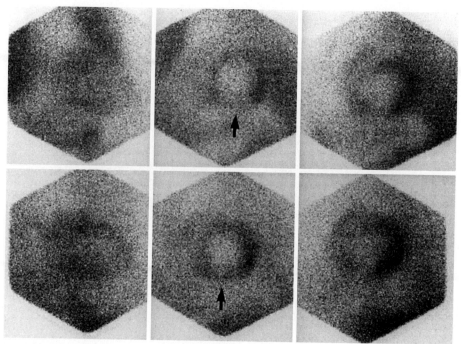

Figure 14-19   "Rest-rest" Tl-201 scintigrams: hibernating myocardium. This patient had prior myocardial infarctions and heart failure. (*Top row*) Initial rest images show decreased uptake in the septum, apex, and anterior wall. The lung shows marked uptake, compatible with congestive heart failure. (*Bottom row*) On the 4 hour delayed rest images, tracer has accumulated to a variable degree in all areas of initial abnormality. The inferoapical defect on the left anterior oblique view has filled in almost completely (*arrows*). Consistent with chronic ischemia (hibernating myocardium), not myocardial infarction.

Planar Imaging   The appearance of the heart depends to some extent on the patient's habitus and the orientation of the heart in the chest (e.g., vertical or horizontal). The heart has a variably circular or ellipsoid shape in different views (Figs. 14-4 and 14-5). The right ventricle is not usually seen on planar studies with Tl-201 but is often seen with Tc-99m agents. When present, lung uptake is easily appreciated on planar imaging (Fig. 14-19) or the raw projection (planar) images of SPECT (Fig. 14-20).

Attenuation Artifacts   Different patterns of soft tissue attenuation are seen in males and females.

Males typically have decreased activity in the inferior wall (Figs. 14-4, 14-C, 14-D [see color insert]). This is due to *diaphragmatic attenuation*, meaning attenuation by subdiaphragmatic organs interpositioned between the heart and gamma camera. The amount of attenuation effect is dependent on patient's size, shape, and anatomy.

Females often have relatively decreased activity in the anterior wall, apex, or lateral portion of the heart, secondary to breast attenuation, dependent on the size and position of the breasts (Fig. 14-21B). Women also have subdiaphragmatic attenuation, but breast attenuation is dominant. Anterior attenuation can be seen occasionally in large males.

Other causes of soft tissue attenuation include excessive adipose tissue or muscle hypertrophy and inability to raise the left arm during imaging because of arthritis, fracture, or lymphedema. Attenuation artifacts can be anticipated by routinely reviewing the cinematic rotating raw data display (Fig. 14-21A). Attenuation artifacts are generally worse for Tl-201 studies because of the lower photon energy, but are routinely seen with Tc-99m agents (Fig. 14-4).

Myocardial perfusion artifacts due to breast or subdiaphragmatic attenuation seen at both stress and rest could potentially be misinterpreted as myocardial infarction. Alternatively, if the breasts are in somewhat different positions for the two studies, this might be interpreted as ischemia. Effort should be made to ensure similar breast position for both sets of images (e.g., both studies with or without bra or breast binder).

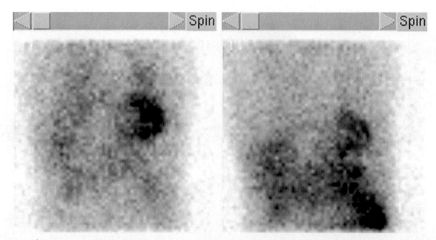

Figure 14-20   Stress-induced Tl-201 lung uptake. The lung uptake is caused by stress-induced cardiac decompensation and is usually associated with three vessel coronary artery disease. This patient also had transient ischemic dilation (see Fig. 14-E1 [see color insert]).

Attenuation Correction   Many SPECT computer systems now have attenuation correction capability for cardiac studies, although some controversy exists regarding its utility. A transmission map is acquired, often with a gadolinium-153 gamma source rotating around the patient. Some systems allow simultaneous acquisition of emission and transmission data. Hybrid SPECT-CT systems use an x-ray tube source for the transmission map to correct for attenuation (Figs. 14-C and 14-D [see color inserts]). When attenuation correct images are obtained, nonattenuation-corrected images should still always be reviewed. Misregistration of the emission and transmission images is a potential problem with the hybrid SPECT-CT systems. Scatter correction methods are on some camera computer systems; however, most require further validation.

Gated SPECT is routine in many nuclear medicine clinics (Figs. 14-22 to 14-24). The gated SPECT is typically performed poststress. It can be helpful in differentiating attenuation artifact from infarction. With good wall motion and myocardial thickening, the decreased activity is likely due to attenuation. Prone imaging has also been used to differentiate attenuation affect from infarction.

Extracardiac Uptake
Myocardial perfusion radiopharmaceuticals are taken up in all cellular, metabolically active tissues in the body except for the brain, in which they do not cross the normal blood brain barrier. Structures accumulating Tl-201 or Tc-99m sestamibi/tetrofosmin that may be in the field of view are the thyroid, salivary glands, skeletal muscle, and kidneys. Prominent liver uptake is usual in rest and with pharmacologic stress studies. Gallbladder and intestinal activity are commonly seen.

Activity from the liver and bowel may cause scatter into the inferior and adjacent walls of the heart, increasing the apparent uptake, which can complicate interpretation. Focal hot subdiaphragmatic activity adjacent to the heart can also produce apparent cold defects due to filtered backprojection reconstruction artifacts.

All three radiopharmaceuticals are taken up in benign and malignant tumors, thus incidental uptake in a known or unknown tumor is not rare (Fig. 14-25) and should be noted and reported when present.

Diagnostic Patterns in Coronary Artery Disease
Diagnosis of Ischemia and Infarction   Terms used to characterize the status of myocardium (e.g., ischemia, infarction, hibernating, stunned) are defined in Box 14-15. The diagnostic schema presented in Table 14-6 uses the appearance of the scans on the stress and rest (or redistribution) studies to characterize myocardial perfusion as:

1. Normal: no defects noted on either image set (Figs. 14-5 and 14-6)
2. Ischemia: cold defects on poststress images that fill in on delayed images (Figs. 14-A, 14-B, 14-E, 14-F [see color inserts], 14-26)
3. Infarction: defects that remain "fixed" between the image sets (Figs. 14-27 and 14-G [see color insert])

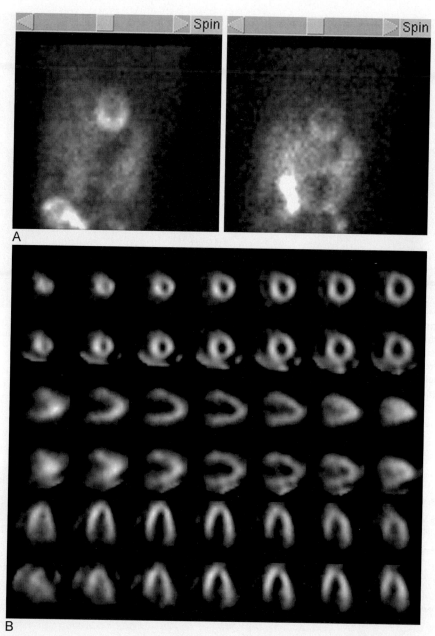

Figure 14-21   Breast attenuation. **A,** Single raw data acquisition projection of a cinematic display at stress (*left*) and rest (*right*) illustrates the artifact produced by breast attenuation. Note the apparent decreased activity in the upper portion of the heart. **B,** The SPECT cross-sectional slices of the same patient show moderate anterior wall attenuation best seen on the short axis and vertical long axis views.

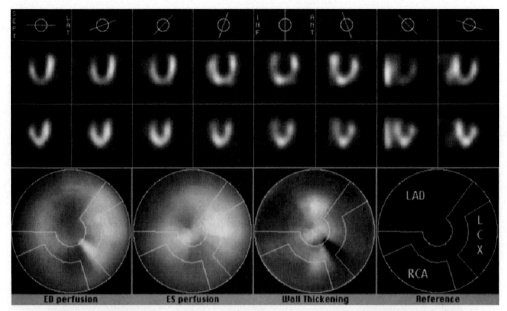

Figure 14-22 Wall motion, thickening, and bulls-eye analysis. End-diastolic and end-systolic perfusion from different reconstructed projection angles. This bull's eye display portrays perfusion at end-systole and end-systole as well as wall thickening on gated SPECT. The top row of images represents end-systole and the bottom row end-diastole. An area of relatively diminished tracer uptake inferolaterally corresponds with decreased wall thickening (*dark area*) on the bull's eye display.

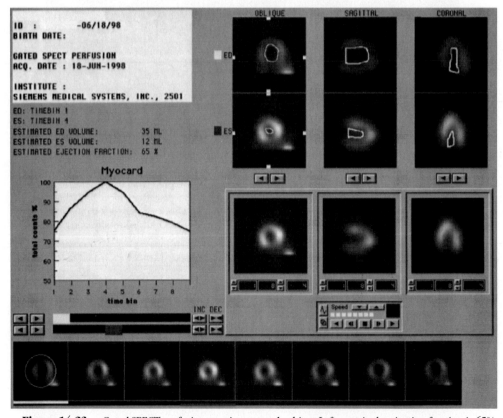

Figure 14-23 Gated SPECT perfusion scan in a normal subject. Left ventricular ejection fraction is 65%.

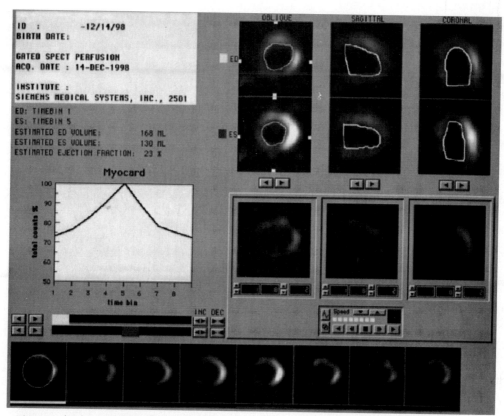

Figure 14-24   Gated SPECT in a patient with coronary artery disease. Decreased tracer uptake is seen in multiple wall segments. The left ventricular cavity is dilated with an estimated end-diastolic volume of 168 ml. The LVEF is 23%.

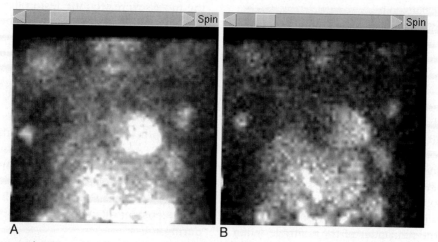

Figure 14-25   Incidental tumor uptake on stress and rest Tc-99m sestamibi studies.
A, Bilateral breast masses are seen on the cinematic display of raw data. Diagnosis of breast cancer.
B, Thymoma.

Box 14-15   Definitions Describing the Status of the Myocardium

Term	Definition and Scan Appearance
Myocardial ischemia	Oxygen supply below metabolic requirements due to inadequate blood circulation as a result of coronary stenosis
	Photon deficient (cold defect) on stress perfusion scintigrams
Myocardial infarction	Necrosis of myocardial tissue, as a result of coronary occlusion
	Photon deficient on rest and stress perfusion and metabolic imaging studies
Transmural infarction	Necrosis involves all layers from endocardium to epicardium
	High sensitivity for detection by perfusion imaging
Subendocardial infarction	Necrosis involves only muscle adjacent to endocardium
	Lower sensitivity for detection on perfusion imaging
Myocardial scar	Late result of infarction; photon deficient on scintigraphy
Hibernating myocardium	Chronically ischemic myocardium with decreased blood flow and down regulation of contractility; reversible with restoration of blood flow
	No perfusion on rest imaging, poor ventricular contraction
	Improved perfusion on rest/rest or reinjection Tl-201 imaging
	Increased uptake by FDG metabolic imaging compared to perfusion scan
Stunned myocardium	Myocardium with persistent contractile dysfunction despite restoration of perfusion after a period of ischemia; usually improves with time
	Normal by perfusion imaging, poor ventricular contraction
	Uptake by FDG metabolic imaging

Patients may have a combination of fixed and transient defects (Figs. 14-28 and 14-G [see color insert]).

After initial assessment of the presence or absence of perfusion defects, a complete evaluation of the stress study includes assessment of the location, size, severity, and likely vascular distribution of the visualized abnormalities. Various computer quantitative methods can be used in conjunction with image analysis (Figs. 14-29, 14-30, 14-A2, 14-B2, 14-E2, 14-F2, and 14-F3 [see color inserts]).

Perfusion defects caused by coronary artery disease are more common distally, rather than at the base of the heart. A true perfusion defect should be seen on more than one cross-sectional slice. Certainty also increases with lesion size and the degree or severity of photon deficiency.

Left Bundle Branch Block (LBBB)   Stress-induced reversible hypoperfusion of the septum can be seen in patients with LBBB in the absence of angiographic coronary disease. The apex and anterior wall are not involved, as would be expected with left anterior descending coronary artery disease. The stress-induced decreased septal blood flow is thought due to asynchronous relaxation of the septum, which is out of phase with diastolic filling of the remainder of the ventricle when coronary perfusion is maximal. This scintigraphic abnormality is not seen with pharmacologic stress, thus dipyridamole or adenosine stress is indicated for patients

with LBBB and probably also for patients with ventricular pacemakers.

Poor Prognostic Findings on Perfusion Scintigraphy
Multiple Perfusion Defects   The presence of perfusion defects in more than one coronary artery distribution area points to multiple vessel disease. The more perfusion defects and the larger their size, the worse is the prognosis.

Not all significant coronary artery stenoses are seen on perfusion scintigraphy. Stress-induced ischemia of the most severe stenotic lesion limits further exercise and thus other stenoses may not be seen scintigraphically. Because interpretation is based on relative perfusion of adjacent walls, multiple vessel disease may be underestimated. Three-vessel balanced disease may not be seen at all. Two findings described later are highly associated with multivessel disease.

Transient Ischemic Dilatation   Although the normal response of the heart is to dilate during stress, the SPECT acquisition is poststress. The normal heart will return to normal size promptly after exercise. Persistent dilatation poststress is abnormal and indicates multivessel disease (Fig. 14-E [see color insert]). The persistent dilatation is due to myocardial stunning during stress.

Tl-201 Lung Uptake   Tl-201 lung uptake induced by exercise is also a poor prognostic sign caused by stress-induced heart failure manifested by ventricular dysfunction, elevated left ventricular end-diastolic pressure and pulmonary capillary wedge pressure (Fig. 14-20). Lung-to-myocardial activity ratios greater than 0.5 are abnormal. Lung uptake with Tc-99m sestamibi/tetrofosmin is less reliable because of normal lung activity.

Myocardial Viability (Hibernating Myocardium)

The scintigraphic findings of regional hypoperfusion at stress and rest associated with myocardial dysfunction are usually due to myocardial infarction. However, approximately 20% of patients with these findings do not have infarction, but rather severe chronic ischemia or *hibernating myocardium* (Box 14-15, Fig. 14-31A). Although severely underperfused, the myocytes have preserved cell membrane integrity and sufficient metabolic activity to maintain cellular viability, but not contractility. Those patients with viable but hypoperfused myocardium may benefit from coronary revascularization with improvement in cardiac function and reduction in annual mortality from 16% to 3%.

Echocardiography, gated blood pool ventriculography, or gated SPECT cannot make the distinction between severe ischemia and scar because the severely ischemic segments demonstrate reduced or absent contractility. These segments are "hibernating" in a functional and metabolic sense.

Tl-201 uptake is an energy-dependent process requiring intact cell membrane integrity, thus uptake implies preserved myocardial cell viability. The magnitude of uptake correlates with the extent of tissue viability. The use of F-18 FDG to diagnose viability, considered the gold standard, is discussed later in the cardiac PET section. However, various protocols utilizing Tl-201 have been successfully used to differentiate viable or hibernating myocardium from myocardial infarction and are reviewed here. Tc-99m

Immediate poststress	Resting delayed or reinjection	Diagnosis
Normal	Normal	Normal
Defect	Normal	Ischemia
Defect	Defect (unchanged)	Infarction*
Defect	Some normalization with areas of persistent defect	Ischemia and scar*
Normal	Defect	"Reverse" redistribution

Table 14-6   Diagnostic Patterns: Stress Myocardial Perfusion

*Delayed Tl-201 imaging without reinjection may overestimate the presence and amount of infarcted area because of incomplete redistribution.

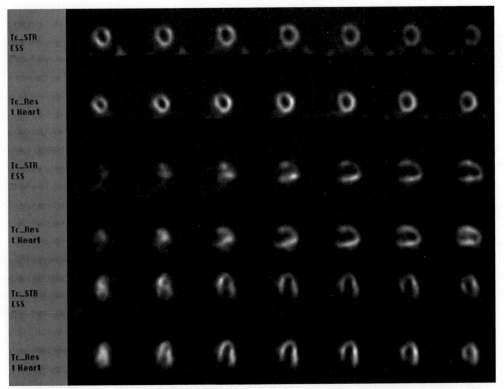

Figure 14-26   Exercise induced ischemia. SPECT stress-rest images with Tc-99m sestamibi. Decreased tracer uptake in the anterior wall is best seen on the long-axis views (*middle rows*). The defect substantially reperfuses on the resting images. This pattern indicates exercise-induced ischemia and coronary artery disease.

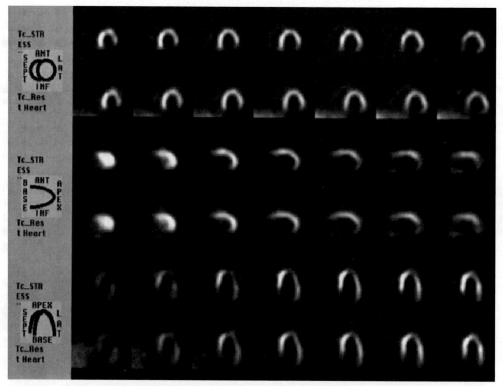

Figure 14-27   Large inferior wall infarction. SPECT images obtained at stress and rest in a patient with a history of prior myocardial infarction. A large fixed defect involving the inferior wall of the heart can best be seen on the short-axis and vertical long-axis views. No substantial change in the scintigraphic appearance is noted between the poststress and rest images.

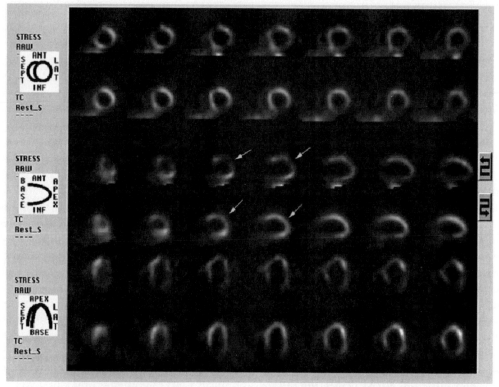

Figure 14-28   Combined ischemia and infarction. SPECT images obtained at stress and rest with Tc-99m sestamibi reveal a large perfusion defect in the anterior wall best seen on the vertical long-axis views (*arrows*) that reperfuses on rest images. A fixed perfusion defect is present in the inferior wall and is best seen on the short-axis views. This pattern of both fixed and transient defects is indicative of combined myocardial ischemia and scarring in a patient with multivessel disease.

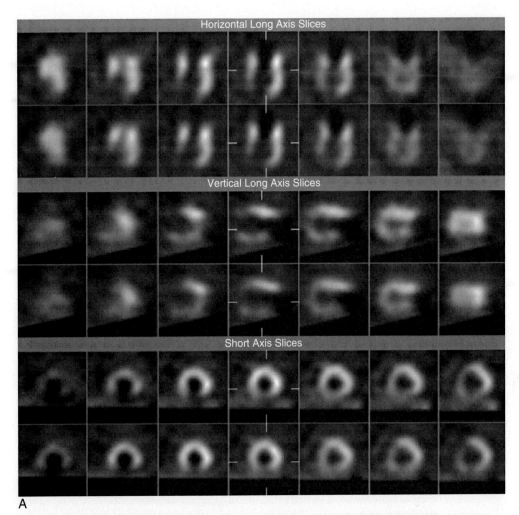

Horizontal Long Axis Slices

Vertical Long Axis Slices

Short Axis Slices

A

Figure 14-29   Three-dimensional quantitative display of myocardial infarction. **A,** SPECT images of a patient with a large fixed defect involving the apex. (The apex is at the bottom of the image on the horizontal long-axis slices and to the left on the vertical long-axis slices.) The fixed defect is seen on all three slice orientations.

Continued

sestamibi and tetrofosmin underestimate myocardial viability and are not generally useful for this purpose.

Tl-201 Protocols for Assessing Myocardial Viability   Tl-201 redistribution occurring by 3-4 hours after injection is dependent on several factors that include the presence of viable myocytes, the severity of the initial defect poststress, and the concentration and rate of decline of Tl-201 in the blood (*see* Fig. 14-1). Various protocols have been used to detect viable myocardium based on an understanding of these pharmacokinetics.

Late Redistribution Imaging   One approach is to allow additional time for redistribution to occur (e.g., 8 to even 28 hours after the stress Tl-201 injection). Severely ischemic myocardium, with slow uptake and clearance, requires a longer time to redistribute.

Improvement in uptake has good positive predictive value for identifying regions with potential functional improvement. However, the negative predictive value is suboptimal because of poor image quality caused by a low count rate from radiotracer decay and biological clearance from the body. Acquisition time can be increased to improve the count rate; however, this increases the likelihood of patient motion.

Tl-201 Reinjection   This approach assumes that the lack of redistribution is the result of a low Tl-201 blood level. To increase the blood level, Tl-201 is reinjected (usually 50% of the initial dose) after the redistribution images are complete and then repeat images are obtained 15–20 minutes later (Fig. 14-32, Fig. 14-E [see color insert]). Alternatively, some protocols routinely

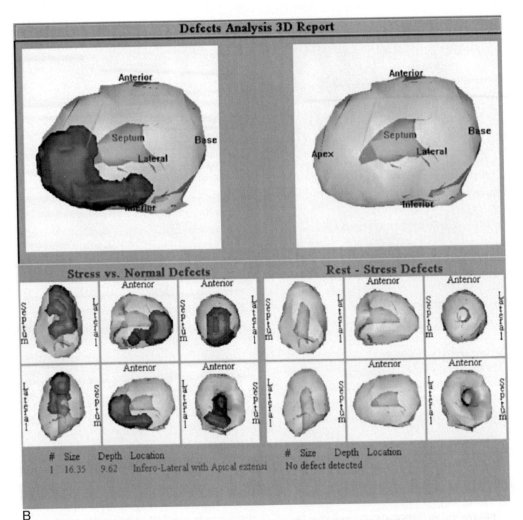

Figure 14-29, cont'd **B,** Three-dimensional quantitative analysis of the images from **A** reveals the large apical and inferior defect when the stress scintigrams are compared with a normal data set *(left images).* The left set of images compares the patient's data to a reference data set, and the right set compares post-stress with rest testing. The fixed nature of the scintigraphic defect is illustrated on the right. No differences are detected between rest and stress views.

reinject Tl-201 prior to the usual redistribution images. Definite uptake is predictive of improvement in regional left ventricular function after revascularization. The presence of a severe persistent Tl-201 defect after reinjection identifies areas with a very low likelihood for improvement in function.

One rationale for using Tl-201 for the rest study in dual-isotope studies is the opportunity to get next day imaging, with or without reinjection, in order to determine viability of a fixed defect.

Rest-Rest Tl-201 Redistribution When viability, not inducible ischemia, is the clinical question, a rest-rest study may be all that is needed *(see* Fig. 14-19). The history of such a patient is that of known coronary artery disease, prior myocardial infarction, and ventricular dys-

function, being considered for bypass surgery. In the region of infarction, considerable viable chronically ischemic myocardium may exist. The clinical question is whether there is enough viable myocardium to justify revascularization. After tracer injection at rest, images are obtained 15 minutes later, which reflect regional blood flow. Significant uptake on repeat rest images 3–4 hours later reflects viability and likely benefit from revascularization.

Stunned Myocardium
After a transient period of severe ischemia followed by reperfusion, there may be a state of delayed recovery of regional left ventricular function. This is called *stunned myocardium* (Fig. 14-31B). The ischemic episode may be single, multiple, brief, or prolonged, but not severe

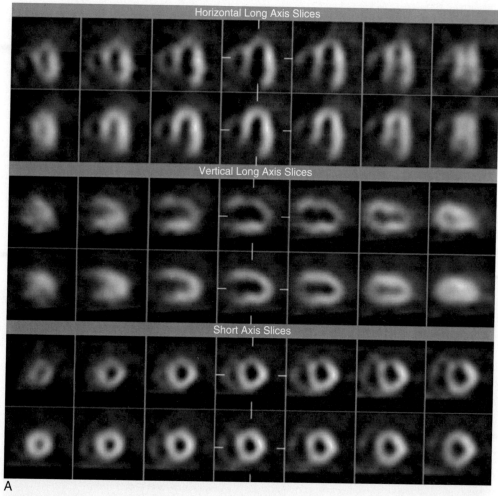

Figure 14-30   Three-dimensional quantitative display: ischemia. **A,** SPECT images at stress and rest in a patient with a large reversible defect involving the anterior wall with extension to the apex. The defect is best seen on the vertical long-axis (*middle row*) and short-axis views. The rest images are normal.

Continued

enough to cause necrosis. Tissue in the affected perfusion watershed is viable and accumulates radiopharmaceutical immediately after reperfusion. The uptake of tracer indicates viability, but the myocardial segment may be akinetic or stunned. If the segment is only stunned and not infarcted, wall motion will improve with time.

Stunning may be seen after thrombolysis or angioplasty in patients who have had acute coronary occlusion. Stress-induced transient ischemic dilation, stress-induced Tl-201 lung uptake, and poststress gated SPECT Tc-99m sestamibi/tetrofosmin ventricular dysfunction are all manifestations of stunned myocardium.

Reverse Redistribution

Worsening of a perfusion defect or the development of a new defect on Tl-201 redistribution images compared with immediate poststress images is called *reverse redis-*

tribution. It may also be seen with Tc-99m agents. The reported causes are numerous and the clinical and diagnostic importance uncertain.

Reverse redistribution has been reported in severe coronary artery disease, perhaps caused by differential washout between normal and diseased areas. It is also seen in some patients after infarction and after successful thrombolytic therapy producing patency of the infarct-related artery. If the latter situation, it is thought to be due to imbalance in tracer delivery (perfusion) versus the ability of stunned myocardium to retain the tracer, leading to a high differential washout rate from the infarct zone compared with periinfarct myocardial tissue.

However, reverse redistribution is neither sensitive nor specific for coronary disease. There are reports of reverse redistribution in a variety of seemingly unrelated

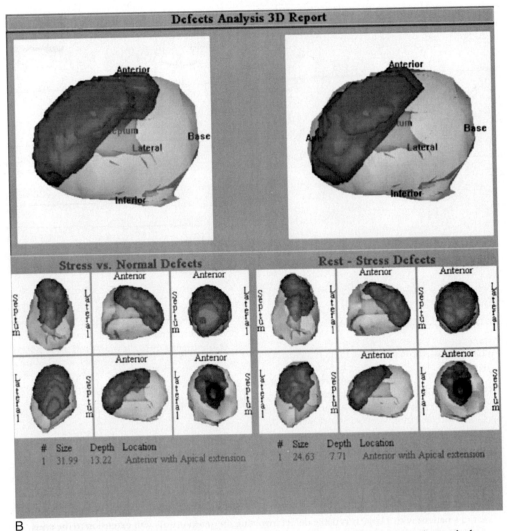

Figure 14-30, cont'd   **B,** Three-dimensional quantitative analysis of the images in **A** reveals the large stress-induced defect when the patient's images are compared with a normal reference data set (*left images*). The transient nature of the defect is illustrated in the images on the right where the rest and stress images from the patient are compared. The three-dimensional analysis demonstrates the extent of abnormality comparing the defect versus the normal reference data set (*left*) and nicely shows the reversibility (*right*).

clinical situations such as after bypass surgery, postcardiac transplantation, with Wolff-Parkinson-White syndrome, sarcoidosis, Kawasaki disease, and Chagas' disease.

Quantitative Analysis

A number of techniques are available for quantitative analysis of myocardial perfusion scans. These techniques typically use a normal database that provides a reference for the expected range of relative regional uptake and/or washout rates. A commonly used method is the *polar map*. Relative perfusion is presented in a two-dimensional "bull's-eye" display that is generated by mapping of circumferential profiles obtained from the short-axis SPECT views, with the apex at the center of the display and the base of the ventricle at the periphery (Figs. 14-A2, 14-C, 14-F2, 14-G2, [see color inserts] and 14-19).

New approaches to quantitative analysis include three-dimensional quantitative displays of regional perfusion, difference displays in perfusion between rest and stress, as well as quantitative analysis of wall motion and wall thickening (Figs. 14-A2, 14-C, 14-F2, 14-G2, [see color inserts], and 14-19). Wall thickening derives from regions of interest placed systematically around the myocardium (Figs. 14-22 to 14-24 and 14-H [see color insert]) and the left ventricular ejection fraction (LVEF) is obtained by measuring

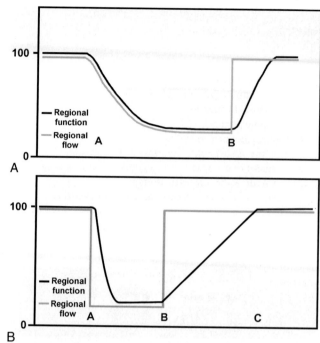

Figure 14-31   **A,** Hibernating myocardium (chronic ischemia) develops over time due to chronic hypoperfusion and causes regional wall motion dysfunction (A). When perfusion is reestablished by surgical intervention, myocardial function returns, but gradually (B). **B,** Stunned myocardium is often due to an acute ischemic episode such as thrombosis (A), which when relieved with, for example, angioplasty (B), results in prompt reperfusion. Functional recovery is considerably delayed (C). Modified with permission from Dilsizian V and Narula J. Atlas of Nuclear Cardiology, Current Medicine, Philadelphia, 2003.

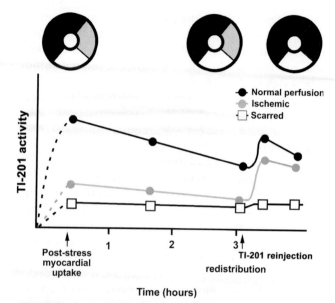

Figure 14-32   Pharmacokinetics of Tl-201 reinjection to diagnose hibernating myocardium. During routine Tl-201 imaging, delayed images may show a persistent fixed perfusion defect in a region of severe or chronic ischemia. Low blood levels of Tl-201 do not allow for adequate redistribution of Tl-201 to the myocardium. Augmenting the Tl-201 blood levels permits greater myocardial uptake and scintigraphic evidence for redistribution and thus viable myocardium. Modified with permission from Dilsizian V and Narula J. Atlas of Nuclear Cardiology, Current Medicine, Philadelphia, 2003.

the change in size of the ventricular cavity through the cardiac cycle (Figs. 14-23A and 14-24) using edge detection algorithms.

The quantitative approach has some potential pitfalls, including problems of misregistration with the reference data set, use of data sets generated from other laboratories on equipment different from that used in the patient's examination or on different patient populations, and lack of uniformity in the amount of exercise or stress achieved. Nonetheless, the use of quantitative methods has become standard practice.

Sensitivity and Specificity

Coronary angiography has been the gold standard for determination of myocardial perfusion scintigraphy accuracy. However, the estimated angiographic percent coronary stenoses often do not correlate well with their functional severity determined by coronary flow reserve. The amount and degree of coronary disease is often underestimated by angiography. Furthermore, a true physiologic decrease in blood flow may sometimes

be seen in the absence of a fixed coronary stenosis due to small vessel disease or metabolic defects.

The reported sensitivity of stress myocardial perfusion imaging has ranged from 70% to 95% and the specificity from 50% to 90%. This wide range is due in part to differences in study populations. If patients with known multiple-vessel disease and prior myocardial infarction are included in the study population, the sensitivity will be predictably high. If only younger subjects with suspected but not proven disease are studied, sensitivity will be lower. Sensitivity for patients achieving adequate exercise will be higher than if it is reported for all patients studied.

Specificity (negative imaging results in patients without disease) is particularly difficult to determine. Although causes for false-positive examinations for coronary artery disease include cardiomyopathy, valvular heart disease, and myocarditis, the problem of specificity is more complex. In most institutions, the decision to perform coronary angiography is based on the myocardial perfusion scan. When a noninvasive test is accepted as being clinically effective for diagnosis and risk stratification, its results strongly influence whether coronary angiography is done. If only patients with abnormal or equivocal myocardial perfusion scans are sent for catheterization, the specificity of myocardial scintigraphy in the "proven" population will be predictably low. Most patients with normal studies will not have had the gold standard test and thus the angiographic referral population is very statistically biased.

Analysis of the results of many studies over the years suggests that myocardial perfusion scintigraphy has sensitivity and specificity in the range of 87% and 80%, respectively.

Because true specificity cannot be determined, the concept of "normalcy rate" has been developed. The *normalcy rate* is determined in a group of patients with a low likelihood of coronary artery disease, based on Bayesian analysis using age, sex, symptom classification, cholesterol, and results of noninvasive stress testing. The normalcy rate is defined as the frequency of normal test results in patients with a low likelihood of coronary disease. Normalcy rates of greater than 90% have been reported for SPECT myocardial perfusion scintigraphy.

Other than observer and test performance, an interesting and important observation in following patients over time is that people with normal stress perfusion scans, even if the results are false negatives based on anatomical angiographic criteria, have a better prognosis than those with scintigraphic evidence of ischemia. The myocardial perfusion scan is a physiological test and the ultimate gold standard is the outcome of the patient.

Prognosis and Risk Stratification

Although diagnosis continues to be an important indication for SPECT myocardial perfusion imaging, increasingly common indications for stress myocardial perfusion imaging are risk stratification and prognosis (Boxes 14-16 and 14-17).

Acute Ischemic Syndromes

Chest Pain in the Emergency Room   More than 5 million patients present to the emergency room with chest pain each year in the United States. Half are admitted to the hospital. Ultimately only 5% are diagnosed with myocardial infarction. Clinical decision-making requires triage of patients into risk categories based on the probability of infarct or unstable angina and risk assessment (Fig. 14-33). SPECT perfusion imaging can provide information critical to this decision-making process (Fig. 14-34). The accuracy of diagnosis of acute ischemic syndromes is highest when the radiopharmaceutical is injected during pain, although good accuracy is obtainable for several hours thereafter.

Tl-201 is not used to diagnose acute ischemic syndromes because the radiopharmaceutical requires imaging promptly after injection. Tc-99m sestamibi or tetrofosmin can be injected in the emergency room and the patient transferred for imaging when initial evaluation and stabilization is complete. Because the radiopharma-

---

Box 14-16   Prognosis and Risk Stratification: Indications

Acute ischemic syndromes
    Chest pain in the emergency room
    Myocardial infarction
    Unstable angina
Chronic ischemic syndromes
    Known or suspected coronary artery disease
Assessment of coronary bypass grafts and angioplasty
Assessment of thrombolytic therapy
Assessment of percutaneous coronary intervention

Box 14-17   Indicators of Adverse Outcome and Prognosis: SPECT Perfusion Imaging

Increased lung to heart ratio after stress
Transient left ventricular cavity dilatation after exercise
Multiple and large reversible defects
Multiple and large irreversible defects
Reversible perfusion defects at low level exercise

---

ceutical is fixed and does not redistribute, delayed imaging reflects blood flow at the time of injection. Negative SPECT studies are highly predictive of a good prognosis. Cardiac events occur in less than 1.5% of patients compared to a 70% incidence in those with a positive study. SPECT has a higher sensitivity than serum enzymes or markers (e.g., troponin). Positive enzymes or markers are very specific, but require serial determination.

SPECT perfusion scintigraphy has a high sensitivity (>90%) for detection of transmural infarction immediately after the event. Diminished or absent uptake is also seen in the region of peri-infarct ischemia and edema. However, the high sensitivity decreases with time as the edema and ischemia resolve. By 24 hours after the acute event, small infarctions may not be detectable and the overall sensitivity for larger ones decreases. The sensitivity for detection is also less for nontransmural infarctions. Furthermore, an acute infarction cannot be distinguished from an old infarct.

Acute Myocardial Infarction with ST Elevation   Infarct size, left ventricular ejection fraction (LVEF), and residual myocardium at risk provide important prognostic management information. Submaximal exercise (achieving less than target heart rate) SPECT perfusion scintigraphy postinfarction can detect the presence

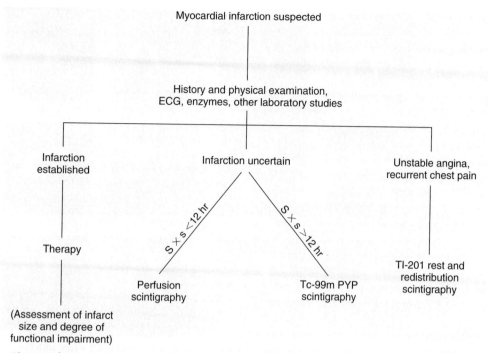

Myocardial infarction suspected

History and physical examination,
ECG, enzymes, other laboratory studies

Infarction established

Infarction uncertain

Unstable angina, recurrent chest pain

Therapy

$S \times s$ <12 hr

$S \times s$ >12 hr

Tl-201 rest and redistribution scintigraphy

(Assessment of infarct size and degree of functional impairment)

Perfusion scintigraphy

Tc-99m PYP scintigraphy

Figure 14-33   Triage of acute chest pain. Simplified schematic of potential roles for scintigraphic imaging and suspected myocardial infarction. $S \times s$, symptoms.

and extent of stress-induced myocardial ischemia. Pharmacologic SPECT scintigraphy with adenosine or dipyridamole can be safely done as early as 2 to 5 days postinfarction, earlier than the limited stress study. Evidence for ischemia warrants aggressive management (e.g., coronary angiography and revascularization). If negative, the patient can be treated conservatively.

Unstable Angina and Non-ST Elevation Myocardial Infarction   Early invasive interventional therapy is recommended for patients with high-risk indicators (e.g., positive myocardial perfusion scintigraphy). SPECT is used for the predischarge risk stratification of patients with unstable angina. Ischemia is seen in a high percentage (90%) of patients who develop subsequent cardiac events compared to those who do not have evidence of ischemia (20%).

Chronic Ischemic Syndromes

Patient Management   It is important to identify patients at high risk but with minimal symptoms whose mortality rate can be improved by coronary bypass graft surgery (Fig. 14-35). Low risk is defined as less than 1% cardiac mortality rate per year versus high risk with more than a 3% mortality. Many factors assessed by SPECT determine patient prognosis, including the extent of infarcted myocardium, the amount of jeopardized myocardium supplied by vessels with hemodynamically significant stenosis, and the severity of ischemia.

A normal stress SPECT perfusion study predicts a good prognosis, with less than a 1% annual risk of cardiac death or infarct. With abnormal SPECT, the risk of cardiac death or infarction increases. Poststress lung uptake and transient ischemic dilation suggest severe proximal LAD or multivessel disease. These findings are associated with high risk. Reduced LVEF is the strongest negative prognostic predictor.

Assessment of Coronary Bypass Surgery and Angioplasty   Because 40–60% of angiographically detected stenotic lesions are of uncertain significance, myocardial perfusion scintigraphy can stratify risk and assess which patients require revascularization. Those patients with no ischemia have low risk for cardiac events, even with left main or three-vessel disease on angiography. Successful intervention results in the elimination of transient defects caused by exercise-induced ischemia. Perfusion imaging should not be done before 6 weeks after intervention because some preintervention defects may persist.

Assessment of Thrombolytic Therapy   Tc-99m labeled perfusion agents can be given when a patient arrives at the hospital and SPECT performed after the patient is stabilized or after thrombolytic therapy. The initial resting study documents the amount of myocardium at risk. A second dose can then determine the effectiveness of therapy. Reduction in defect size correlates with vessel patency and improved prognosis

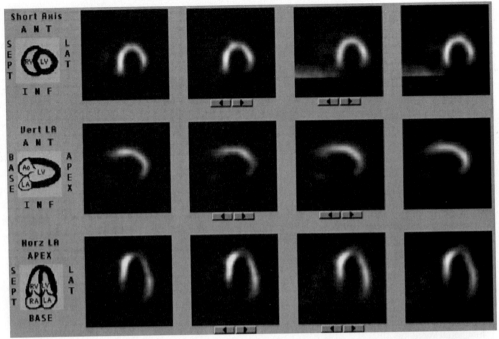

Figure 14-34 Emergency room chest pain: myocardial infarction. Resting SPECT study with Tc-99m sestamibi. Radiopharmaceutical injection given in the emergency room and imaging delayed until the patient was stabilized. The large defect involving the inferior wall of the heart is diagnostic of infarction.

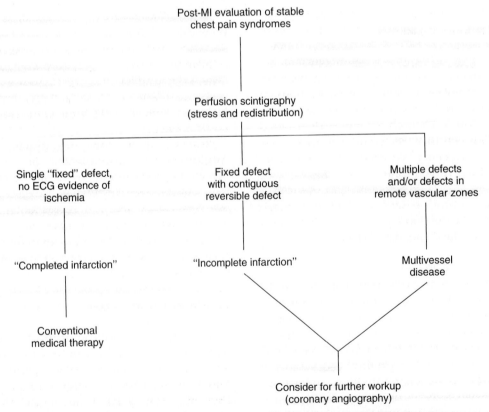

Figure 14-35 Risk stratification in chronic chest pain. Diagnostic scheme illustrating the incorporation of perfusion scintigraphy into an approach for stratifying risk after myocardial infarction. *MI*, Myocardial infarction; *ECG*, electrocardiogram.

after myocardial infarction. After recovery, stress perfusion scintigraphy can confirm therapeutic effectiveness or detect areas of residual ischemia.

After Percutaneous Coronary Intervention Symptom status and exercise ECG are unreliable indicators of restenosis. Of patients with recurrent chest pain within a month of intervention, 30% have restenosis. Because ischemia (painful or silent) worsens prognosis, stress SPECT perfusion may be useful.

After Coronary Bypass Surgery Abnormal perfusion patterns may reflect bypass graft disease, disease in the native coronary arteries beyond the distal anastomosis, nonrevascularized coronaries or side branches, or new disease. SPECT perfusion scintigraphy can determine the location and severity of ischemia and has prognostic value early and late after coronary bypass surgery. When ischemia occurs 1–12 months after surgery, the etiology is usually perianastomotic graft stenosis. Ischemia developing more than 1 year postoperatively is usually caused by new stenoses in graft conduits and/or native vessels. Exercise SPECT is strongly predictive of events.

Heart Failure: Assessment for Coronary Artery Disease Heart failure in the adult can be due to various etiologies, including hypertrophic cardiomyopathy, hypertensive or valvular heart disease, and idiopathic cardiomyopathy. Determining whether left ventricular dysfunction is due to the consequences of coronary artery disease or to other etiologies is critical for patient management. If due to coronary disease, revascularization can potentially reverse the left ventricular dysfunction.

Left ventricular dysfunction due to ischemic cardiomyopathy is the result of either a large or multiple prior myocardial infarctions with subsequent remodeling, or moderate infarction associated with considerable inducible ischemia and/or hibernation. The sensitivity of SPECT myocardial perfusion scintigraphy approaches 100% for detection of coronary disease in patients with cardiomyopathy; however, the specificity is only 50%. False-positive studies are due to perfusion abnormalities seen in many patients with nonischemic cardiomyopathy (i.e., without epicardial coronary artery disease). Some have regions of fibrosis and decreased coronary blood flow reserve, resulting in both fixed and reversible defects. More extensive and severe perfusion defects are likely to be due to coronary artery disease while smaller and milder defects are likely to occur in patients with nonischemic cardiomyopathy.

Calcium Screening Electron-beam CT and multislice helical CT measure the amount of calcium in the coronary arteries (calcium score). The risk of cardiac events is low with coronary calcium scores of 100 or less. Stress SPECT myocardial perfusion tests are positive in less than 1% of these patients. With scores between 101 and 399, risk of future cardiac events is moderate, with 12% having abnormal stress SPECT perfusion studies. Scores greater than 400 identify patients at high risk. Approximately 50% of patients have abnormal SPECT studies.

Sarcoidosis
The clinical features of myocardial involvement of the heart with sarcoidosis include dysrhythmias, conduction defects, heart failure, and sudden death. Pathologically any region of the heart can become the site of granuloma deposition. Because of the serious potential consequences of cardiac involvement, immunosuppressive therapy with corticosteroids is indicated. However, the diagnosis of cardiac involvement can be difficult. Endometrial biopsy is confirmative; however, it is an insensitive technique due to sampling error.

SPECT myocardial perfusion scintigraphy with Tl-201 and Tc-99m radiopharmaceuticals has been used to confirm or exclude myocardial involvement in patients with sarcoidosis. Perfusion defects are common in the right and the left ventricle and correlate with atrioventricular block, heart failure, and ventricular tachycardia. One successful approach has been to perform Persantine stress and rest Tc-99m sestamibi studies. In most patients with cardiac sarcoidosis, SPECT demonstrates a fixed defect. In some patients, reverse "redistribution" is noted. Ga-67 has also been used to diagnose cardiac sarcoidosis, but with lower sensitivity. Preliminary data suggest F-18 FDG PET may be useful to diagnose active cardiac sarcoidosis.

POSITRON EMISSION TOMOGRAPHY OF THE HEART

Positron emission tomography (PET) affords superior spatial resolution compared to SPECT and routine attenuation correction. The clinical use of PET for cardiac perfusion imaging is increasing, but still limited to certain centers with high volume. The most common current indication at most centers is the use of F-18 fluorodeoxyglucose (FDG) to diagnose hibernating (viable) myocardium. The use of rubidium (Rb-82) as an alternative to Tl-201 and Tc-99m SPECT for perfusion imaging is increasing because it is generator produced.

Radiopharmaceuticals for Myocardial Perfusion

In addition to the advantage of better resolution and superior attenuation correction with PET perfusion agents over SPECT, multiple serial studies can be performed within a brief period and absolute quantification of coronary flow in milliliter/gram/minute is possible. N-13 ammonia and Rb-82 are FDA-approved and reimbursable in the United States.

Nitrogen-13 Ammonia

N-13 would be the preferred PET perfusion radiopharmaceutical except that it has a very short physical half-life (10 minutes), requiring onsite cyclotron production. It decays 100% by positron (β+) emission (Table 14-7).

When injected intravenously, it clears rapidly from the circulation with 85% leaving the blood in the first minute and only 0.4% remaining after 3.3 minutes. Localization in myocardial cells is from diffusion across the capillary membrane, metabolic conversion to N-13-glutamine by glutamine synthetase, and subsequent trapping within tissues by incorporation into the cellular pool of amino acids. Thus, the N-13 label remains within the heart with a relatively long biological residence time. At physiological pH, the major form of ammonia is NH_4^+. It has a 70–80% extraction rate by myocardial cells at normal coronary flow rates.

Myocardial uptake is proportional to coronary blood flow. As with other perfusion tracers, the extraction efficiency of N-13 ammonia drops at higher flow rates. In addition to the myocardium, it is taken up by the brain, liver, and kidneys.

Technique

Ten to 20 mCi (370 MBq) of N-13 ammonia is administered intravenously and imaging typically begins 5 minutes after injection, which allows time for pulmonary background activity clearance. The long myocardial biological half-life offers some imaging timing flexibility. In the diagnosis of coronary artery disease, a second study is typically performed after pharmacologic stress (dipyridamole, adenosine, or dobutamine) with protocols similar to those described for SPECT myocardial perfusion scintigraphy (Fig. 14-36).

Radiation Dosimetry

Radiation absorbed dose to the patient is quite low compared to most clinically used radiopharmaceuticals (Table 14-8).

Rubidium-82 Chloride

Rb-82 is a generator produced positron radionuclide (Table 14-7). In the strontium-82/Rb-82 generator system (CardioGen-82, Bracco), the half-life of the Sr-82 parent is 25 days, which means that facilities using Rb-82 for myocardial perfusion imaging need to receive one new generator system each month. Thus, no onsite cyclotron or pharmaceutical production facility is required. However, the generator systems are expensive and a large volume of cardiac studies is needed to make it financially feasible. A commercial attempt to increase its clinical use provides a generator that is transported from one PET site to another. Rb-82 is increasingly being used on a clinical basis.

Rb-82 is a monovalent cation and true analog of potassium. Like thallium-201, Rb-82 is taken up into the myocardium by active transport through the Na$^+$K-ATPase pump. Its extraction is somewhat lower than that of N-13 ammonia (60%). The relative myocardial extraction and localization of Rb-82 are proportional to blood flow.

The very short half-life of Rb-82 (76 seconds) allows the performance of sequential studies before and after pharmacological interventions used for diagnostic PET myocardial perfusion scintigraphy. Rb-82 decays 95% by positron emission and 5% by electron capture. In addition to the beta particle + annihilation photons (511 keV), it emits a 776-keV gamma (15% abundance) and 1395-keV gamma (0.5% abundance).

Technique

Rb-82 (40–60 mCi) is infused intravenously over 30 to 60 seconds. Imaging is delayed for approximately 2 minutes to allow time for blood pool clearance; it is completed within 5 minutes. Imaging time is short because of rapid decay and to prevent reconstruction artifacts. About 80% of the useful counts are acquired in the first 3 minutes and 95% in the first 5 minutes. Sequential studies can be performed within 10 minutes. Rb-82 has the poorest resolution of positron radionuclides because the positrons travel about 13 mm prior to undergoing annihilation. However, image quality is superior to Tl-201 and it does not have the problems of the Tc-99 radiopharmaceuticals, (e.g., attenuation and subdiaphragmatic scatter).

Table 14-7 Cardiac Positron Radiopharmaceuticals

Mechanism	Radionuclide	Pharmaceutical	Physical half-life	Production
Perfusion	Nitrogen-13	Ammonia	10 min	Cyclotron
	Rubidium-82	Rubidium	76 seconds	Generator
	Oxygen-15	Water	110 seconds	Cyclotron
Glucose metabolism	Fluorine-18	Fluorodeoxyglucose	110 minutes	Cyclotron
Fatty acid metabolism	Carbon-11	Acetate	20 minutes	Cyclotron
	Carbon-11	Palmitate	20 minutes	Cyclotron

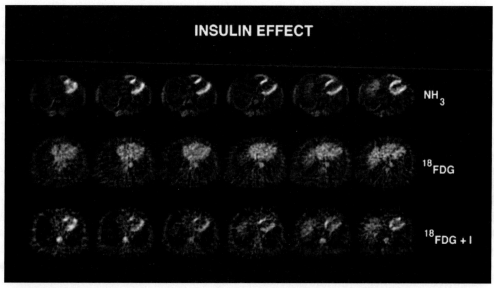

Figure 14-36   Importance of glucose loading. N-13 ammonia images (*top row*) and two sets of F-18 FDG images of a diabetic subject. The N-13 ammonia images show a large perfusion defect at the cardiac apex. The initial F-18 FDG images show essentially no myocardial uptake (*middle row*). After insulin administration, FDG accumulates in the myocardium and reveals a matched defect at the apex.

Table 14-8	Radiation Dosimetry for Fluorine-18 FDG, Rubidium-82, N-13 Ammonia		
	Fluorine-18 FDG*	Rubidum-82†	N-13 Ammonia‡
Dose	cGy/370 MBq (rads/ 10 mCi)	cGy/1480 MBq (rads/ 40 mCi)	cGy/740 MBq (rads/ 20mCi)
Heart wall	2.5	0.4	0.2
Liver	0.8	0.16	0.3
Kidneys	0.8	**2.8**	0.2
Brain	1.7		0.3
Urinary bladder	3.0		
Colon		0.4	
Thyroid	0.4	**5.6**	0.2
Ovaries	0.4	0.04	0.2
Red marrow		0.16	0.2
Effective dose	1.0	0.8	0.2

Target organ (highest radiation absorbed dose) in **boldface** type.
*, MIRD; †, IRCP; ‡, IRCP.

Dosimetry
The thyroid receives the highest radiation dose (5.6 cGy/ 1480 MBq or 5.6 rads/40 mCi) (Table 14-8), followed by the kidney (2.8 cGy/1480 MBq or 2.8 rads/40 mCi).

Oxygen-15 Water
O-15 water is ideal for quantitative regional myocardial flow measurements (ml/min/gm) because it is a freely diffusible perfusion tracer with 95% extraction by the myocardium and it is not affected by metabolic factors. Unlike other perfusion agents, extraction remains linear at very high flow rates, and therefore myocardial distribution reflects regional perfusion. However, image quality is not as good as that of other PET perfusion agents. Tracer circulating in the blood pool remains within the ventricular chamber and must be subtracted in order to visualize the myocardium. With a half-life of 2.2 minutes (123 seconds), O-15 requires an onsite cyclotron for production.

Diagnosis of Coronary Artery Disease
The two PET perfusion agents, Rb-82 and N-13 ammonia, are used clinically for the diagnosis of coronary artery disease. Cardiac PET stress tests use pharmacologic stress rather than exercise because of the short half-life of the radiopharmaceuticals. After baseline studies are obtained under resting conditions, one of the pharmacological agents is administered to challenge coronary flow reserve. The protocols are the same as in single-photon imaging. The timing of injection of the PET radiopharmaceutical is synchronized with the administration of the pharmacological agent and the desired delay after injection before the onset of imaging.

PET imaging offers superior spatial image resolution compared to SPECT and typically excellent target-to-background ratios. The scintigraphic appearance of the heart and diagnostic criteria for Rb-82 and N-13 ammonia studies are the same as for perfusion scans obtained with Tl-201 or the Tc-99m-labeled perfusion agents. Normal subjects have homogeneous uptake of the tracer throughout both the left and right ventricular myocardium. Patients with hemodynamically significant CAD but no ischemia at rest demonstrate normal resting myocardium. Perfusion defects are seen after pharmacological stress. Areas of prior myocardial infarction appear cold on both baseline and poststress images. Patients with hibernating myocardium also demonstrate persistent perfusion defects or both phases. The diagnostic patterns of ischemia and infarction are similar to SPECT (Table 14-6).

The sensitivity of PET for the diagnosis of coronary disease is high, on the order of 95%. The specificity reported in the early literature is also high. The specificity should be regarded with caution because early reports under clinical research protocols frequently use normal volunteers to determine specificity, which is very different from determining specificity in a more broadly chosen cross section of patients with and without coronary artery disease. Furthermore, there is much more limited data on the accuracy of PET than SPECT. Generally the specificity of PET is felt to be superior to SPECT because of the standard direct method of attenuation correction. Breast and subdiaphragmatic attenuation artifacts are much less of a problem with high-energy PET radiopharmaceuticals than with SPECT.

PET Metabolic Radiopharmaceutical

Fluorine-18 Fluorodeoxyglucose

F-18 FDG is a marker of myocardial glucose metabolism. The physical half-life of F-18 is 1.8 hours (110 minutes) and thus must be delivered from a regional cyclotron on a daily or twice daily basis. Only about 1–4% of the injected dose is trapped in the myocardium; however there is a high target-to-background ratio. Blood clearance of FDG is multicompartmental and takes much longer than the perfusion agents. Imaging is typically begun 45 to 60 minutes after tracer injection (10–15 mCi [370–555 MBq]) to allow maximal myocardial uptake and blood and soft tissue background clearance.

F-18 has the best resolution of all positron emitters, approaching 2 mm because most of the emitted positrons travel only about 1.2 mm prior to undergoing annihilation.

Dosimetry

The organ receiving the highest radiation absorbed dose is the urinary bladder (3.0 cGy/1480 MBq or 3.0 rads/40 mCi) (Table 14-8).

Clinical Indication

Its principal use in practice is in combination with a perfusion tracer to assess myocardial viability. Under normal conditions, most of the energy needs of the heart are met through fatty acid metabolism. However, areas of ischemia switch preferentially to glucose metabolism and have increased uptake of F-18 FDG relative to perfusion. Regional myocardial uptake of F-18 FDG reflects regional rates of glucose utilization. In the myocardial cell, FDG is

phosphorylated to FDG-6-phosphate. No further metabolism takes place, and the radiopharmaceutical stays trapped in the myocardial cell over a prolonged period.

The state of glucose metabolism in the body highly influences the amount of FDG taken up in the heart. Myocardial glucose utilization is increased by glucose administration which stimulates insulin secretion. The increased insulin levels stimulate glucose metabolism. Thus high serum glucose and insulin levels and low free fatty acids promote uptake (Fig. 14-36).

Different strategies are used to promote optimal FDG uptake. *Glucose loading* with either oral glucose (glucola) or intravenous dextrose is the most common method (Box 14-18). Serum glucose is checked to ensure euglycemia. F-18 FDG is usually injected 45–60 minutes later. Diabetics often have an attenuated increase in plasma insulin levels following glucose loading and small intravenous insulin doses are required. A more sophisticated method to ensure euglycemia, used primarily in research settings, is *hyperinsulinemic euglycemic clamping*. Glucose is infused in one arm and insulin in another. The rate is varied to optimize to euglycemia. In all three methods, F-18 FDG is infused when euglycemia is obtained, and imaging is initiated 45 minutes later.

Detection of Myocardial Viability

The combination of perfusion imaging and metabolic imaging with FDG can be of great benefit in correctly diagnosing and assessing the potential therapeutic outcome in patients with severely ischemic or *hibernating myocardium* (Table 14-9). The rationale for using FDG is that severely ischemic myocardium switches from fatty acid metabolism selectively to glucose metabolism. Thus, FDG uptake can actually be greater in the ischemic areas than in the remainder of the myocardium.

In normal subjects, perfusion and FDG uptake are matched (Fig. 14-37). The combination of matched perfusion and FDG scintigraphic defects is indicative of myocardial scarring (Fig. 14-38). The combination of a photon-deficient area by perfusion imaging that demonstrates increased FDG uptake is the scintigraphic hallmark of severely ischemic or hibernating myocardium (Fig. 14-39).

Perfusion/FDG mismatch indicates myocardial viability. In areas of flow-metabolism mismatch, the functional prognosis following revascularization is very good, with an average of 80% of such segments demonstrating contractile improvement after coronary artery bypass surgery. The matched pattern of abnormal decreased perfusion and glucose metabolism indicates a low likelihood of improved function after therapeutic intervention with only an average of 15% of such segments demonstrating contractile improvement after coronary artery bypass grafting.

Box 14-18   Protocol: F-18 FDG PET Cardiac Viability

PATIENT PREPARATION

NPO after midnight

Obtain rest myocardial perfusion scan

Serum fasting blood sugar (BS)

Nondiabetic

If BS ≤ 150 mg/dL:	50 gm oral glucose solution + regular insulin 3 units IV
If BS 151–300 mg/dL:	25 gm oral glucose solution + regular insulin 3 units IV
If BS 301–400 mg/dL:	25 gm oral glucose solution + regular insulin 5 units IV
If BS > 400 mg/dL:	25 gm oral glucose solution + regular insulin 7 units IV

At least 45 minutes after glucose loading and when BS ≤150 mg/dL, inject F-18 FDG

Diabetic

If BS ≤150 mg/dL: 25 gm oral glucose solution

If BS 151–200 mg/dL:	Regular insulin 3 units IV
If BS 201–300 mg/dL:	Regular insulin 5 units IV
If BS 301–400 mg/dL:	Regular insulin 7 units IV
If BS 401 mg/dL or greater:	Regular insulin 10 units IV

Obtain BS every 15 minutes for 60 minutes. If BS elevated, additional insulin per scale. At least 45 min after glucose loading and when BS ≤150 mg/dL, inject F-18 FDG

DOSAGE AND ROUTE OF ADMINISTRATION

F-18 fluorodeoxyglucose 0.22 mCi/kg (100 μCi/lb)

TIME OF IMAGING

After 60 minute uptake phase

PROCEDURE

PET acquisition—cardiac field of view

PROCESSING

Reconstruct along the short and long axis of the heart similar to the perfusion study

IV, Intravenously; *BS,* serum blood glucose.

Table 14-9   PET Diagnostic Image Patterns: Perfusion and Metabolic Imaging

Diagnosis	Perfusion (N-13 ammonia, Rb-82)	Glucose metabolism (FDG)
Normal myocardium	Present	Present
Ischemic myocardium	Absent or decreased	Present
Myocardial infarction	Absent	Absent

Patients with viable but severely ischemic myocardium have better survival and event outcomes from surgical revascularization than from medical management. Patients with only myocardial scarring and no ischemia do not benefit from revascularization surgery. Some may be candidates for cardiac transplantation.

Acipimox

Glucose loading and insulin administration can be time-consuming and not always effective, particularly in diabetics. As an alternative, acipimox, a nicotinic acid derivative, has been investigated and shows considerable promise. The drug, administered orally, lowers free fatty acid levels by inhibition of lipolysis and thus enhances cardiac glucose and F-18 FDG uptake. Preliminary studies are encouraging. Further investigations are necessary.

Combined Tc-99m Sestamibi and F-18 FDG Imaging

SPECT-PET cardiac studies can be acquired using specially modified gamma scintillation cameras either with high-energy collimators and appropriately shielded camera heads or, alternatively, dual-headed cameras with coincidence circuitry without a collimator. With the use of two energy windows, a simultaneous combination of Tc-99m sestamibi or tetrofosmin perfusion imaging and F-18 FDG metabolic imaging is possible.

An advantage of doing simultaneous imaging is that the data from the two radiopharmaceuticals are perfectly registered, allowing optimal comparison of the respective uptake patterns. This elegant approach uses the same diagnostic criteria described previously. Areas of

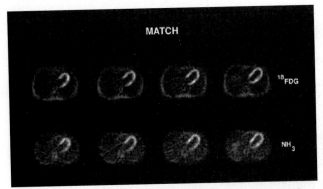

Figure 14-37 F-18 FDG and N-13 ammonia PET in a normal subject. The uniform uptake of both tracers is concordant with a normal appearance of the heart.

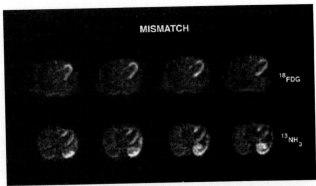

Figure 14-39 F-18 FDG and N-13 ammonia: match. Decreased uptake in the region of the septum and apex. The concordant pattern of matched abnormalities indicates myocardial scar with absence of perfusion and metabolism.

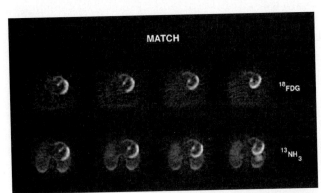

Figure 14-38 F-18 FDG and N-13 ammonia: mismatch. On the N-13 ammonia perfusion study, uptake is decreased anteroapically. The same area demonstrates good uptake by FDG. This discordant pattern indicates diminished perfusion to an area of viable myocardium. Prognosis for functional improvement after coronary artery bypass grafting is good with this pattern.

matched perfusion and metabolic abnormality are unlikely to improve (Fig. 14-40). Areas demonstrating diminished Tc-99m activity with normal or increased FDG represent ischemic but viable tissue and have a high likelihood of functional recovery after revascularization (Fig. 14-41).

RADIONUCLIDE VENTRICULOGRAPHY

Radionuclide ventriculography (RVG) or multigated acquisition (MUGA) has been used since the 1970s to evaluate global and regional right and left ventricular function. Two different methods have been used, *first-pass* studies, in which all data collection occurs during the initial transit of a tracer bolus through the central circulation, and *equilibrium* studies, in which data are col-

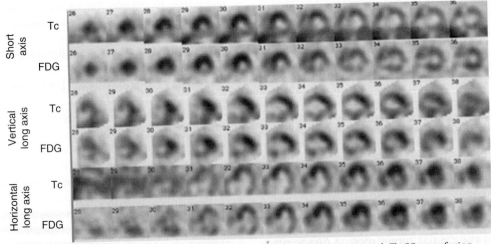

Figure 14-40 Combined Tc-99m sestamibi and F-18 FDG imaging: mismatch. Tc-99m perfusion imaging shows a large inferoapical defect that corresponds with normal uptake of FDG. This discordant pattern is indicative of ischemic but viable myocardium.

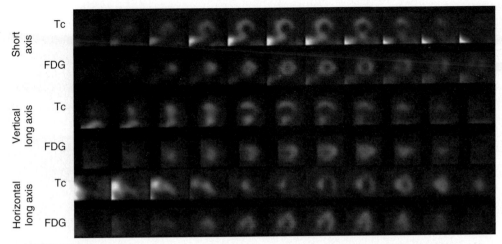

	Tc	
Short axis		
	FDG	
Vertical long axis	Tc	
	FDG	
Horizontal long axis	Tc	
	FDG	

Figure 14-41   Tc-99m perfusion imaging and F-18 FDG metabolic imaging. Simultaneously acquired study reveals matched abnormalities in the inferior wall of the left ventricle. This pattern of matched abnormalities is indicative of myocardial nonviability.

lected over many cardiac cycles using ECG gating and a tracer that remains in the blood pool. RVG can be successfully performed in most all patients and ejection fraction quantification is not dependent on mathematical assumptions of ventricular shape, as in contrast ventriculography and echocardiography.

Radiopharmaceuticals

Blood Pool Agents

The radiopharmaceutical of choice for equilibrium gated blood pool imaging is Tc-99m-labeled red blood cells (Tc-99m RBCs). Labeling may be accomplished by any of three approaches: in vivo, modified in vivo, and in vitro. These methods are described in detail in Chapter 11 (Box 11-13). Causes for poor Tc-99m red blood cell labeling are listed in Box 14-19. The modified in vivo or the in vitro method (Ultratag RBC, Mallinckrodt) are preferred because of their higher binding efficiency (85-90% for the modified in vivo method, 98% for the in vitro method).

Dosimetry

The spleen receives the highest radiation absorbed dose, 2.2 cGy/740 mBq (2.2 rads/20 mCi), followed by the heart wall. 2.0 cGy/740 mBq (2.0 rads/20 mCi). See Chapter 11 (Table 11-6).

First-Pass Agents

Any Tc-99m labeled agent may be administered as a bolus for first-pass imaging of the central circulation. Tc-99m as sodium pertechnetate is commonly used. A disadvantage

Box 14-19   Causes of Poor Tc-99m Red Blood Cell Labeling

Drug-drug interactions	Heparin, doxorubicin, methyldopa, hydralazine, contrast media, quinidine
Circulating antibodies	Prior transfusion, transplantation, some antibiotics
Too little stannous ion	Insufficient to reduce Tc (VII)
Too much stannous ion	Reduction of Tc (VII) outside of red blood cell before cell labeling
Carrier Tc-99	Buildup of Tc-99m in the Mo-99/Tc-99m generator due to long interval between elutions
Too short an interval for "tinning"	Not enough time for stannous ion to penetrate the red blood cells before addition of Tc-99m
Too short an incubation time	Not enough time for reduction of Tc (VII)

is its high residual background activity if multiple studies are required. Tc-99m DTPA is alternatively used because of its rapid renal excretion. Using Tc-99m RBCs allows combining a first pass evaluation of the right ventricle and equilibrium analysis of the left ventricle. Some institutions

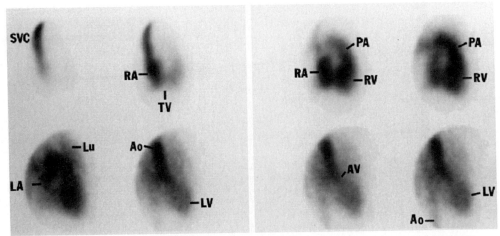

Figure 14-42   First-pass radionuclide angiogram. Cardiac structures are sequentially visualized as the bolus passes through the right side of the heart into the lungs and then returns to the left side. *Ao*, Aorta; *AV*, aortic valve; *LA*, left atrium; *Lu*, lung; *LV*, left ventricle; *PA*, pulmonary artery; *RA*, right atrium; *RV*, right ventricle; *SVC*, superior vena cava; *TV*, tricuspid valve.

perform a first-pass study with one of the Tc-99m-labeled myocardial perfusion agents in conjunction with the perfusion study.

Acquisition Techniques

First-Pass Studies

First-pass studies are obtained by injecting a compact bolus of the selected radiopharmaceutical intravenously preferably via the jugular vein. If a peripheral injection is used, the Oldendorf technique or a variation thereof is employed. The arm is held in a neutral position, and a medial vein in the basilic system is used at the antecubital fossa. Use of veins in the cephalic system should be avoided, if possible, to prevent "hang-up" of the bolus at the thoracic inlet. Injections directly through central catheters placed in the superior vena cava provide the most compact boluses. Jugular venous access is an alternative effective approach.

Data may be acquired either in rapid *frame* mode or in *list* mode, with or without ECG gating. Whichever approach is used, the goal is to obtain 16-30 frames per second while the bolus passes through the central circulation. In most patients, the total data acquisition time required is on the order of 30–60 seconds or less.

Typically a right anterior oblique view at 20- to 30-degree angulation is chosen (Fig. 14-42). This view best separates the right atrium and the right ventricle and is also one of the standard views of the left ventricle used during cardiac catheterization. It is suitable for both quantitative and qualitative analysis of biventricular function.

The major advantage of the first-pass approach is that data are collected rapidly over very few cardiac cycles. Ventricular function can be measured at peak stress during exercise ventriculography or other intervention. Right ventricular function quantification is more accurate than with equilibrium gated blood pool studies, in which there is overlap of the right and left ventricles in the RAO view and between the right atrium and the right ventricle.

The major disadvantage of the first-pass or first-transit approach is that counting statistics are low in each frame because of the count rate limitations of gamma cameras. Special *multicrystal* gamma cameras with their high count rate capability are optimally suited for first-pass studies but are not widely available. In current practice, equilibrium gated blood pool studies are performed much more frequently than first transit studies.

Equilibrium Gated Blood Pool Studies

The limited counting statistics available during any one cardiac cycle and the desirability of linking phases of the cardiac cycle to image data underlie the equilibrium gated blood pool approach to RVG. In this approach, ECG leads are placed on the patient and a gating signal that triggers the R wave of the ECG is sent to the nuclear medicine computer system (Fig. 14-43). The R wave is a useful marker because it occurs at the end of diastole and the beginning of systole. It is the largest electrical signal in the normal ECG and therefore relatively easy to detect.

The cardiac cycle is divided into 16 frames in most commercially available computer systems (Fig. 14-44). Individual frame duration is 40–50 msec. This frame rate is a compromise between optimal temporal and statistical

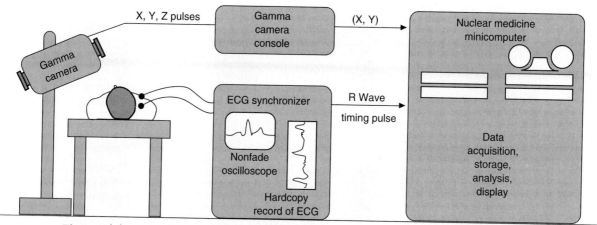

Figure 14-43   Acquisition of R-wave gated radionuclide ventriculography. A special ECG synchronizer or gating device depicts the R-wave and sends a timing pulse to the nuclear medicine computer system. This timing pulse is used to sort incoming scintillation events into a sequence of frames that spans the cardiac cycle.

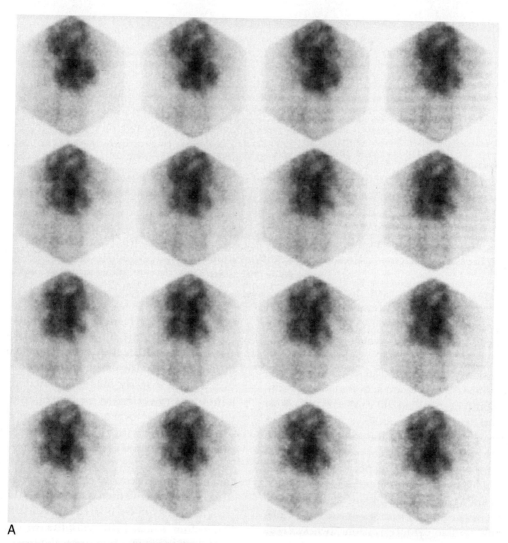

A

Figure 14-44   Sequential frames of R-wave gated MUGA study. Anterior (**A**) and the 45° left anterior oblique views (**B**). In this study, the cardiac cycle was divided into 16 frames. Note the change in size and count density of the cardiac chambers through the cardiac cycle.

Continued

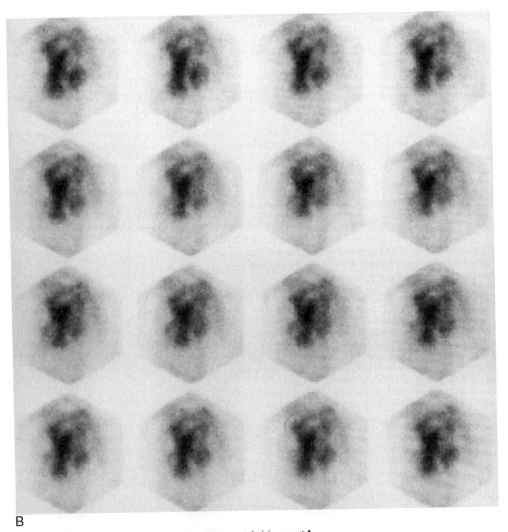

B

Figure 14-44, cont'd

data sampling. Enough frames are needed to catch the peaks and valleys of the cardiac cycle (temporal sampling), but too many frames reduce counting statistics available in any single frame (statistical sampling).

During each heartbeat, data are acquired sequentially into the frame buffers spanning the cardiac cycle. With imaging of more than 100–300 cardiac cycles, sufficient counting statistics are obtained for valid quantitative analysis and reasonable spatial resolution. Studies at rest are obtained for 250,000 counts per frame. Studies obtained during exercise or other intervention are often obtained for somewhat fewer counts per frame to capture the peak effect of the stress. Box 14-20 describes the equilibrium gated blood pool ventriculography protocol in detail.

The underlying assumption of R-wave gating is the presence of normal sinus rhythm so that data are added together from corresponding segments of the cardiac cycle over the entire time of the study. Any significant arrhythmia degrades the quality of the data and reduces the accuracy of quantitative analysis.

A rhythm strip should be obtained for every patient before the injection of a radioactive tracer to determine suitability for examination. For example, rapid atrial fibrillation with an irregular ventricular response or frequent premature ventricular contractions is a contraindication to the study (Fig. 14-45). Quantitative error may result if there are greater than 10% premature ventricular contractions or a rapid atrial fibrillation with irregular ventricular response. Recording a beat histogram throughout the study is useful (Fig. 14-46). Problems with gating include spurious signals from skeletal muscle activity, giant T waves triggering the gating device, and artifacts from

---

pacemakers. The pacemaker signal itself is usually a reliable trigger for gating.

Special computer techniques may be used to filter data from premature contractions and postextrasystolic beats, but these increase the time needed to perform a study. By the same token, elegant gated list mode data acquisition techniques have been developed to analyze separately the normal sinus beat, the premature contraction, and the postextrasystolic beat. List mode is not commonly used, in the past because of the large computer memory required, but nowadays because of the less frequent use of RVGs and the adequacy of equilibrium studies.

For studies at rest, multiple views (anterior, LAO, left lateral) are obtained to provide the most comprehensive evaluation of regional ventricular wall motion (Fig. 14-47). The exact angulation for the LAO view is determined empirically by moving the head of the gamma camera to find the view that best separates activity in the left and right ventricles for most accurate calculation of the LVEF.

Protocols for exercise RVGs have varied among institutions. Treadmill and bicycle ergometer exercise have been used. The LVEF can be determined for each stage of a graded exercise program designed to recapitulate graded treadmill stress, or more commonly a baseline

study and a single stress study during peak exercise is obtained. In addition to exercise stress, alternatives have been used, including cold pressor testing, handgrip isometric exercise, atrial pacing, and pharmacological stress. None of the alternatives have proved equal to leg exercise studies. Because of the general use of gated SPECT, exercise RVGs are performed uncommonly today.

Data Analysis and Study Interpretation

Qualitative Analysis

Comprehensive analysis and interpretation of RVGs require both qualitative and quantitative assessments (Box 14-21). Wall motion is analyzed by viewing a repetitive cinematic closed loop display on the computer screen. Ventricular contraction is inferred from "shrinkage" of the ventricular activity from diastole to systole. Failure of activity to diminish or clear along the ventricular periphery is an indication of abnormal wall motion. Septal contraction is inferred from seeing the photon-deficient area between the right ventricular and left ventricular blood pools thicken during systole.

Complete absence of wall motion is termed *akinesis*. Areas with diminished contraction are *hypokinetic*. Those demonstrating paradoxical wall motion (that is, an actual outward bulge during systole) are termed *dyskinetic*. If motion is still present but delayed compared with adjacent segments, it is referred to as *tardokinesis*. In normal subjects, all wall segments should contract, with the greatest incursion seen in the left ventricular free wall and apex. Areas of ventricular scar are typically akinetic or dyskinetic. Areas of ventricular ischemia become hypokinetic with exercise. Tardokinesis is seen with ischemia or conduction abnormalities such as bundle-branch block.

The complete qualitative or visual analysis includes an assessment of cardiac chamber size for all four cardiac chambers, assessment of overall biventricular function and regional wall motion, and assessment of any extracardiac abnormalities such as aortic aneurysms or pericardial effusions that are in the detector's field of view. Only portions of the ventricles not overlapped by other cardiac structures should be assessed on any given view. For example, on the anterior view the right ventricle usually overlaps the septum and inferior wall of the left ventricle.

Attempts have been made to use quantitative and functional or parametric images to detect abnormalities in regional wall motion. Regions of interest may be flagged along the ventricular perimeter to calculate regional ejection fractions. Fourier phase analysis and other parametric image analysis techniques are described in the following section.

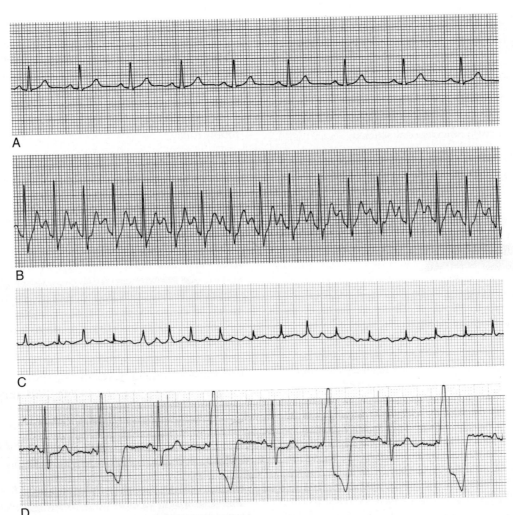

A

B

C

D

Figure 14-45   Electrocardiographic rhythm strips. Patients referred for gated radionuclide ventriculography. **A,** Normal sinus rhythm. **B,** Sinus tachycardia. **C,** Atrial fibrillation with irregular ventricular response. **D,** Ventricular premature contractions with bigeminy.

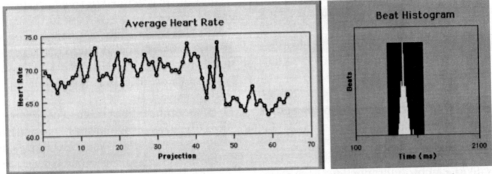

Figure 14-46   Beat histogram. The number of recorded beats for each observed cardiac cycle length are depicted. This demonstrates that the heart rate and therefore beat length varied significantly during data collection.

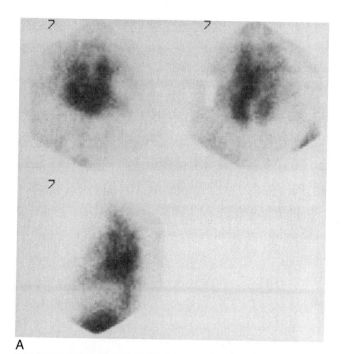

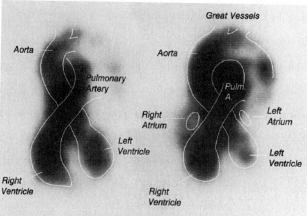

Figure 14-47   Anatomy at end-systole and end-diastole; correlation with radionuclide ventriculogram **A,** End-diastolic images from a gated radionuclide ventriculogram. Anterior (*top left*), left anterior oblique (*top right*), and left posterior oblique (*bottom*) views are the most commonly obtained. **B,** Drawings over left anterior oblique end-diastolic (*left*) and end-systolic (*right*) frames, indicating position and relationships of major structures.

Quantitative Data Analysis

Ejection Fraction

The most frequently calculated quantitative parameter of ventricular function is the LVEF, defined as the fraction of the left ventricular end-diastolic volume expelled during contraction. The underlying principle is that the left ventricular count rate at each point in the cardiac cycle is proportional to ventricular volume. The ventricular counts are determined by drawing a region of interest over the left ventricle for each frame (Fig. 14-48) of the

---

cardiac cycle and a background region, typically taken as a crescent adjacent to the left ventricular apex (Fig. 14-48). A background-corrected ventricular time–activity curve is generated (Fig. 14-49). End-diastole is the frame demonstrating the highest counts and end-systole the frame with the fewest counts.

Ejection fraction is calculated as follows:

$$\text{Ejection fraction} = \frac{\text{End diastolic count} - \text{End systolic count}}{\text{End diastolic count}}$$

The LVEF in normal subjects ranges from 55-75%. Many use 50% as a cutoff for normal. The accuracy of the LVEF calculation by RVG is considered very good, superior to that of nonnuclear techniques such as echocardiography. Numerous studies have demonstrated good correlation with contrast-enhanced left ventriculography. Most consider the RVG calculation to be the most accurate method.

The time–activity curve should be inspected in each case as a quality control measure. Theoretically, the count values at the beginning and end of the curve should be identical. In practice, the trailing frames in late diastole usually have fewer counts, owing to slight variations in the length of the cardiac cycle, even in patients with normal sinus rhythm (Figs. 14-49 and 14-50). In patients with frequent PVCs, the falloff in counts at the end of the curve is much greater. In atrial fibrillation with an irregular ventricular response, a marked falloff may occur because cardiac cycles of widely varying length are being added together. Quantitative analysis of gated data in cases with major dysrhythmias is not accurate. On cine display, a falloff in counts in later frames is seen as a flicker.

Numerous other quantitative parameters have been proposed for calculation from equilibrium gated blood pool examinations (Box 14-22). None of these can be considered as well documented and validated as the

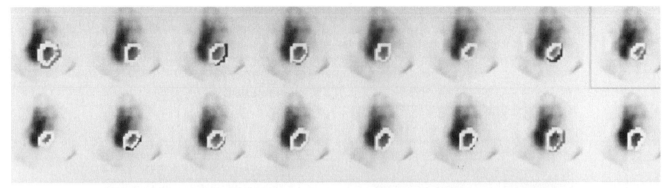

Figure 14-48 Calculation of the left ventricular ejection fraction. A region of interest is defined over the left ventricle in each frame of the cardiac cycle. A time–activity curve is then generated. The percent LVEF is calculated utilizing the end-diastolic and end systolic ventricular count rates (ED − ES) divided by (ED) × 100.

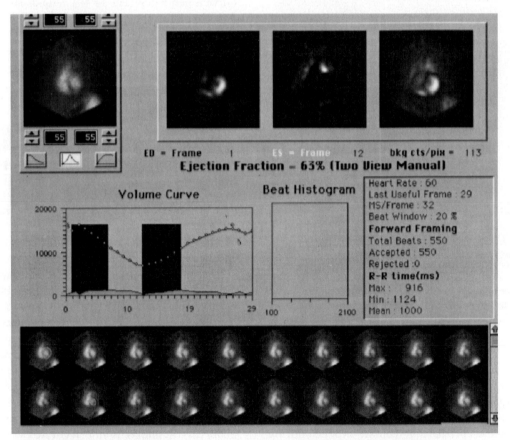

Figure 14-49 Composite computer-generated display: analysis of gated radionuclide ventriculogram. The sequential left anterior oblique views are displayed across the bottom. The end-diastolic and end-systolic regions of interest are indicated, along with the crescent-shaped background region of interest adjacent to the left ventricle at end-systole (*bottom row, second image from right*). The three parametric images in the upper right-hand corner represent ejection fraction (ES − ED), paradox (ES − ED), and amplitude. The LVEF of 63% is normal.

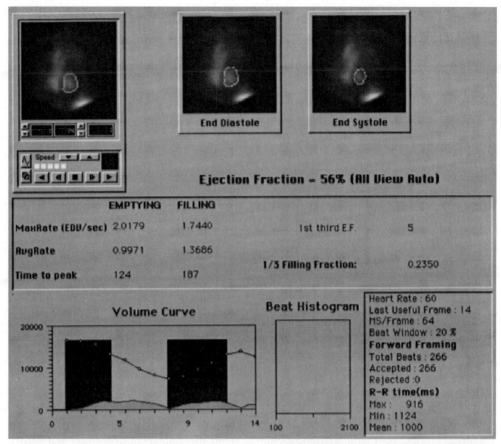

Figure 14-50   Late frame count rate loss due to sinus arrhythmia. Small changes in beat length result in fewer counts being recorded in the trailing frames of late diastole. Note how the last data point in the volume curve is lower than the one adjacent to it and the trailing end of the volume curve is somewhat lower than the beginning.

Box 14-22	**Functional Parameters Determined on Equilibrium Blood Pool Ventriculograms**

Wall motion assessment (regional and global)
End-diastolic and end-systolic ventricular volume
Stroke volume
Cardiac output
Ejection fraction (left and right ventricles)
Regurgitant fraction (stroke index ratio)
Ventricular filling and emptying rates (dV/dt) (peak and average)
Cardiac shunt quantification

LVEF. Calculation of stroke volume and cardiac output requires correction of the left ventricular count rate for soft tissue attenuation, which is subject to considerable error.

Calculation of the right ventricular ejection fraction (RVEF) from equilibrium data has problems because of overlap of chambers.

Fourier Phase Analysis

Fourier phase analysis reduces four-dimensional data into a pair of two-dimensional images. These images portray cardiac contractility (amplitude) and contraction sequence (phase) (Fig. 14-51). Simply stated, each pixel in the cardiac image can be considered to have its own cycle, having an amplitude and a characteristic temporal relationship (phase) with respect to the R wave. The amplitude image simply portrays the maximum net count variation for each pixel during the cardiac cycle. The phase image portrays the relative time delay from the R wave to the start of the cardiac cycle for that individual pixel.

If the complete cardiac cycle is taken as encompassing 360 degrees, the atria and ventricles are normally 180 degrees "out of phase" (*see* Fig. 14-51). Areas of the ventricle that contract slightly earlier in the cardiac

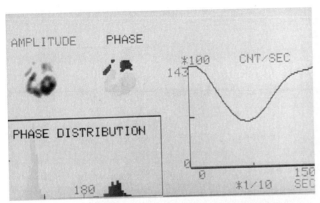

Figure 14-51   Regional ejection fraction. Calculation of regional ejection fractions from eight pie-shaped regions centered in the middle of the left ventricle. The stroke volume, paradox, and amplitude images are also illustrated.

cycle owing to the pattern of the electrical conduction down the septum and through the bundle branches are seen to be out of phase with adjacent ventricular areas.

Wall motion abnormalities are portrayed on phase images as low-amplitude areas. Regions of paradoxical motion resulting from left ventricular aneurysms, for example, are 180 degrees "out of phase" with the ventricle. Abnormal conduction patterns like those seen in Wolff-Parkinson-White syndrome or bundle-branch block cause affected areas to be out of phase with adjacent portions of the ventricle owing to premature or delayed contraction.

Amplitude and phase maps are often displayed in color to highlight the temporal sequences of cardiac chamber emptying. A dynamic color display mode can be used to demonstrate the propagating wavefront that sweeps across the ventricle during contraction, linking pixels with similar phase angles together.

Although Fourier phase analysis is elegant, the studies require exceptionally well-synchronized data to be useful for localizing abnormal conduction pathways. Amplitude and phase images are often presented automatically as part of computer analysis packages and are useful for cueing the observer to areas of abnormal wall motion.

Functional Images

The intensity of the computer display at each point in an image is determined by the number of counts recorded at that point and proportional to the amount of radioactivity in the corresponding location. By subtracting the end-systolic image from the end-diastolic image point by point, a derived functional image is created that portrays regional stroke volume. The stroke volume image may be further processed by dividing it point-by-point by the end-diastolic frame to create an "ejection fraction" image (Fig. 14-52). In these images, akinetic wall segments correspond to areas of diminished or absent intensity. In the paradox image the end-diastolic frame is subtracted from the end-systolic frame. With normal ventricular function, this leaves a void. In patients with areas of

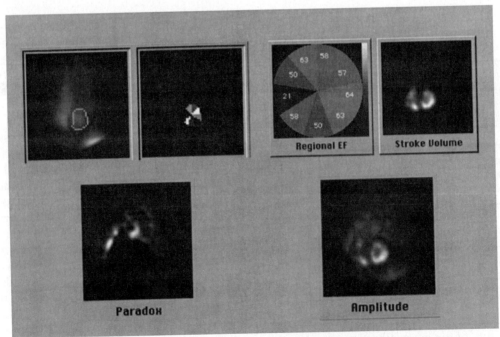

Figure 14-52   Phase and amplitude. In addition to the amplitude image that portrays cardiac contractility, the phase parametric image portrays the relative time of contraction for each pixel on the image. The atria and ventricles are normally 180 degrees "out of phase."

paradoxical ventricular wall motion, the systolic bulge is readily detected as an area of unsubtracted activity.

A complete analysis and interpretation of the RVG includes a qualitative visual assessment of the cardiac chambers and great vessels to assess their size and relationships. Visual assessment of the dynamic cinematic display is also used to analyze regional wall motion. Quantitative analysis includes at a minimum calculation of the LVEF. For specific applications other quantitative parameters such as left and right ventricular stroke volume ratios, cardiac output, ventricular volume, and rates of ventricular filling and emptying may also be calculated but require more sophisticated analysis and in some cases more sophisticated data acquisition techniques.

Clinical Applications

In the past, both myocardial perfusion scintigraphy and the RVG were used for similar indications, depending on personal preference and experience. Today, SPECT myocardial perfusion scintigraphy has become the standard radionuclide study for evaluation of coronary artery disease. RVG is reserved for specific indications. The most common clinical indication is to evaluate ventricular function and calculate an ejection fraction in patients receiving cardiotoxic drugs. This section emphasizes that indication and others review current indications, as well as a brief description of how it has been used in the past and the associated scintigraphic findings that have pertinence for specific and more general interpretation of RVGs.

Coronary Artery Disease

Many patients with coronary artery disease have normal resting ventricular function. Some will have regional motion abnormalities (Fig. 14-53). Exercise-induced myocardial ischemia can be detected with RVG. The hallmarks of ischemia are the development of a new wall

motion abnormality during exercise stress testing that was not present at rest and an ejection fraction that fails to increase or even decreases in response to exercise (Box 14-21, Fig. 14-54).

In patients able to achieve adequate levels of exercise, the technique is highly sensitive (on the order of 90%) for the detection of coronary artery disease. However, an abnormal ventricular functional response to exercise stress is nonspecific. A low LVEF is seen in many other cardiovascular diseases. Thus the specificity of the RVG for coronary artery disease is not high and varies with patient referral population (Box 14-23). In current practice, myocardial perfusion scintigraphy with gated SPECT is used to diagnose coronary artery disease.

The hallmark of an acute myocardial infarction on the RVG is that of a wall motion abnormality in the region of the infarct (see Fig. 14-53) and a reduced regional and global LVEF. Patient prognosis after acute myocardial infarction is directly linked to the degree of functional impairment. Over 75% of patients with acute myocardial infarctions have abnormal LVEFs. Patients showing a serial decline in LVEF have a significantly higher risk of mortality in the early postinfarction period. Inferior myocardial infarctions have associated right ventricular wall motion abnormalities in up to 40% of patients.

In current practice, SPECT myocardial perfusion scintigraphy is preferred over RVG for evaluation of coronary artery disease.

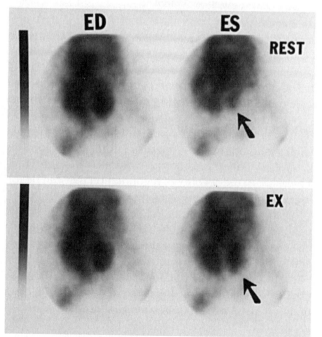

Figure 14-54   Exercise induced global hypokinesis. Note the decreased emptying of the left ventricle in response to exercise (*arrows*) compared to the rest study. *ED,* End diastolic; *ES,* end systolic; *EX,* exercise. This is characteristic of apical ischemia.

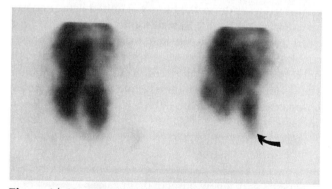

Figure 14-53   Resting apical hypokinesis due to myocardial infarction. Selected end-diastolic and end-systolic images for a patient with acute anteroapical myocardial infarction. The apex is akinetic (*arrow*). The right ventricle and other portions of the left ventricle show good contraction.

Box 14-23   Cause of Abnormal Ventricular Functional Response to Exercise

Hemodynamically significant coronary artery disease
Cardiomyopathy
Myocarditis
Valvular heart disease
Pericardial disease
Drug toxicity
Prior surgery or injury

Valvular Heart Disease

Patients with valvular heart disease can have pressure overload, volume overload, or both. The response to pressure overload from stenosis is concentric hypertrophy. The response to volume overload from insufficiency is dilatation. Pulmonary vascular hypertension and eventually congestive heart failure are the result of significant valve disease. RVG allows assessment of ventricular size and ejection fraction. Because the ejection fraction is in part determined by preload, afterload, and heart rate, resting ejection fraction cannot be used alone to assess myocardial contractility or functional reserve. Patients with valvular heart disease may have regional or global dysfunction that cannot be differentiated from coronary artery disease.

The findings regarding chamber size and function on RVG are similar to cardiac catheterization. A measurement that is easier to determine with RVG than with contrast angiography is calculation of stroke volume ratios for the left and right ventricles. With mitral insufficiency, for example, some of the blood is propelled antegrade and some regurgitates through the mitral valve during each left ventricular contraction. In normal subjects, the stroke–volume ratio between the ventricles should be 1.0 because all of the blood is propelled antegrade. Stroke–volume ratio provides a measure of the severity of regurgitation that can be followed sequentially.

The major limitation of the calculation of the stroke volume ratio from equilibrium blood pool studies is chamber overlap between the right and left ventricles and between the right ventricle and the right atrium. The exact level of the pulmonic valve is also difficult to establish in many cases. For these reasons a LV/RV ratio of 1.5 is used as the upper limit of normal, which is greater than the expected value of 1.0.

Cardiomyopathy and Myocarditis

Cardiomyopathies may be classified as congestive, hypertrophic, or restrictive. In congestive cardiomyopathies, the ventricles are typically enlarged and dysfunctional. The global ejection fraction is decreased and wall motion is uniformly poor, except that the septal and anterior basal segments are frequently spared. The hallmark of the hypertrophic cardiomyopathies is asymmetrical septal hypertrophy. Echocardiography is the diagnostic procedure of choice. The left ventricular chamber is typically small, and the LVEF is above normal. Diastolic filling is abnormal because of poor compliance of the hypertrophied myocardium.

Assessment of Cardiac Toxicity

The most common indication for RVG in current practice is to assess the potential cardiotoxic effects of noncardiac drugs. Anthracycline drugs used most commonly in the treatment of breast cancer and malignant lymphoma, such as doxorubicin (Adriamycin), produce a cumulative dose-dependent depression of left ventricular function.

Heart failure develops in 4–20% of patients who receive a cumulative dose of >500 mg/ m^2, in 18% of those receiving >550 mg/m^2, and in 36% receiving >600 mg/m^2. Acute hemodynamic decompensation may be followed by an irreversible dilated cardiomyopathy with LV dysfunction. Endocardial biopsy is diagnostic but invasive and not commonly performed.

Overt congestive heart failure is preceded by a progressive fall in the LVEF. Serial monitoring of left ventricular function can detect a change in cardiac function over time and the drug can be stopped or reduced when a reduction in LVEF is observed. The incidence of overt cardiac failure can be significantly reduced. Complete recovery may occur if therapy is discontinued at an early stage.

Both the absolute LVEF and the magnitude of fall are important. Generally, a 10% decline in LVEF to below the lower limit of normal (50%), an absolute LVEF of 40% or a 20% decline in LVEF at any level is indicative of deterioration in cardiac function.

The resting RVG is insensitive for early detection compared to endocardial biopsy. Limited data suggests an exercise RVG study in addition to rest sensitivity for detection. However, the specificity is low without serial testing. Furthermore, many of these patients are debilitated and cannot exercise adequately. Resting studies are the routine in most clinics. Noncardiac conditions can also affect the LVEF, including anemia, fever, and sepsis.

Pulmonary Disease

Right ventricular enlargement can be diagnosed with RVG. In patients with a new onset of dyspnea, the RVG can help differentiate left ventricular from pulmonary dysfunction. The demonstration of a normal left ventricular ejection fraction, wall motion, and chamber size strongly suggests a pulmonary etiology.

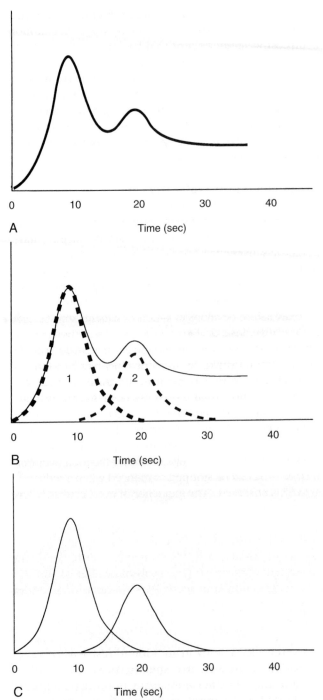

Figure 14-55 Left-to-right shunt calculation **A,** Time–activity curve obtained from a region of interest over the lungs in a patient with a left-to-right shunt. The second peak is due to early recirculation of tracer through the left-to-right shunt. **B,** The relative contributions from the initial transit and the shunt are determined from a curve-fitting technique. **C,** Initial time–activity curve and the two mathematically fitted curves. The shunt ratio (Q_p/Q_s) is calculated from the areas under these curves.

Congenital Heart Disease

Right-to-left shunts may occur due to a variety of congenital cardiac diseases. For left-to-right shunts, the central circulation is studied using the first-transit technique. Early recirculation into the right ventricle as blood flow bypasses the lung is detected with a curve-fitting technique. In brief, the lung transit curve (Fig. 14-55A) is modeled by a mathematical function called a gamma variate (Fig. 14-55B). The contribution to the time-activity curve from recirculation is taken as the difference between the total area under the time-activity curve minus the area under the gamma variate fit (Fig. 14-55C). This approach allows detection of shunts as small as 20%.

Right-to-left shunts may be detected and quantified with Tc-99m-labeled macroaggregated albumin. The ratio of tracer in the lung to tracer gaining access to the systemic circulation provides a measure of the severity of shunting. With right-to-left shunts, images show uptake with the cerebral cortex and other organs. Quantification is best done with whole-body imaging. Regions of interest can be drawn for the lungs and total body. The calculated percent shunt does not accurately reflect the real percent shunt. Greater than 10% is abnormal. Brain uptake is always seen.

Right-to-left shunts are generally given as a relative contraindication to the use of macroaggregated albumin, owing to the theoretical risk of embolizing the capillary bed of the brain. In practice, this event has not been a problem. However, it is recommended that the number of particles be reduced.

INFARCT-AVID IMAGING

Technetium-99m Pyrophosphate

Radiolabeling Tc-99m pyrophosphate (Tc-99m PYP) was originally used as a bone scan radiopharmaceutical and is prepared in the same manner. Sodium pertechnetate from a generator is added to a vial containing stannous pyrophosphate Sn (II), a reducing agent. The Tc-99m forms a chelate with the pyrophosphate molecule.

Mechanism of Localization

After cell death in acute myocardial infarction, an influx of calcium occurs and calcium phosphate complexes are formed. These microcrystalline deposits act as sites for Tc-99m PYP uptake. Some binding may also occur on denatured macromolecules. The status of the peri-infarction circulation is important in tracer uptake. Some residual blood flow is necessary to deliver the tracer to the infarct area and surrounding tissue. The tracer then diffuses into the necrotic tissue and is bound. Highest uptake is at the periphery of infarction. In large infarctions, with neither direct flow nor diffusion to the central area, no tracer is delivered and a characteristic ring or doughnut pattern is seen due to activity around the margin of the damaged area.

Methodology

Imaging is performed 3 to 4 hours after tracer administration to allow clearance from blood pool. Radioactivity retained in the circulation contributes to background blood pool activity, which can be confused with myocardial uptake; false-positive interpretations of Tc-99m PYP images could result. A further delay to allow more complete clearance should be considered if background activity remains high 4 hours after injection.

A standard protocol is described (Box 14-24). Tc-99m pyrophosphate is injected intravenously, 555–925 MBq (15–25 mCi). A high-resolution collimator should be used. Multiple planar views and/or SPECT are performed. SPECT offers greater image contrast, allowing detection of smaller abnormalities and more exact anatomical localization of infarct. In general, the technique is used only when other clinical parameters are nondiagnostic.

The sensitivity for detecting infarction is highest at 24–48 hours after the acute event. A major limitation for diagnosis of acute myocardial infarction is the delay between the time of infarction and the time of scintigram positivity. Significant uptake becomes demonstrable at 12 hours after infarction. Maximum localization occurs at 48 to 72 hours. Thereafter uptake begins to diminish as the infarcted area heals. In uncomplicated cases, the scintigram reverts to normal within 14 days. If initial images reveal diffuse activity in the region of the heart, further delay can be helpful to allow more complete clearance of tracer from the blood pool.

Scintigraphic Patterns in Acute Myocardial Infarction

Tc-99m PYP is an avid bone seeker. In normal subjects and in patients without infarction, the sternum and ribs are clearly seen, with no focal or diffuse activity in the region of the heart. Faint cardiac blood pool may be seen.

The classic scintigraphic pattern in myocardial infarction is a focal area of increased tracer uptake corresponding to the affected region of the heart. A grading system is sometimes used: zero for a normal study, 1+ for faint uptake, 2+ for uptake equal to rib intensity, and 3+ for uptake greater than rib intensity. Diagnostic confidence increases with the grade of uptake and with focal versus diffuse activity.

Complete interpretation includes assessment of location and size. Location is inferred from comparison of the relationship of the abnormal uptake to the expected location of the heart and the skeletal structures on multiple planar views or SPECT. Anterior infarctions are seen *en face* on the anterior view and project just behind the sternum on the lateral view (Fig. 14-56). Lateral wall infarcts appear as vertical curvilinear lesions on the anterior view. With progressive obliquity, the area of abnormality moves either closer to the sternum (anterolateral infarcts) or farther from the sternum (posterolateral infarcts). Inferior wall infarctions are concave upward and may have a characteristic "lazy 3" configuration if they involve the inferior septum and right ventricle.

Large infarctions, most frequently in the anterior wall of the left ventricle, may exhibit a doughnut pattern of increased uptake resulting from absence of tracer in the center of the infarct area. This pattern is associated with a poor clinical prognosis. A minimum of 3 g of tissue must be infarcted for scintigraphic detection.

Sensitivity is high for transmural or Q-wave infarctions, approximately 95%. For subendocardial infarctions, the sensitivity is considerably less, probably 65% for planar scintigraphy. Specificity is greater than 90%. Normal rib uptake may obscure small regions of uptake. SPECT can improve sensitivity and localization.

There are numerous causes of false positive Tc-99m PYP scans (Box 14-25), including diffuse activity in the cardiac blood pool misinterpreted as emanating from the myocardium, uptake in areas of chest wall trauma, in skeletal muscle that is necrotic because of prior cardioversion, and in calcifications in or near the heart. Calcifications in the costal cartilage may have uptake.

Several conditions result in diffusely increased myocardial uptake of Tc-99m pyrophosphate. The most dramatic is amyloidosis (Fig. 14-57). The tip-off to amyloid as the etiology is visualization of the entire myocardium, including the right ventricle, with quite

---

Box 14-24 Protocol: Tc-99m Pyrophosphate Infarct-Avid Imaging

PATIENT PREPARATION AND FOLLOW-UP

EKG leads should be moved out of field of view
Frequent voiding to minimize radiation dose to bladder

DOSAGE AND ROUTE OF ADMINISTRATION

740 MBq (20 mCi) Tc-99m pyrophosphate intravenously

TIME OF IMAGING

3–4 hr after radiopharmaceutical administration (may be performed at 1 hr if clinically indicated)

PROCEDURE

Collimator: low-energy, high-resolution or general purpose, parallel hole collimator
Planar images: Anterior view for 500k counts and record the length of time, 35° left anterior oblique (LAO), 70° LAO, and left lateral views for equal time
SPECT

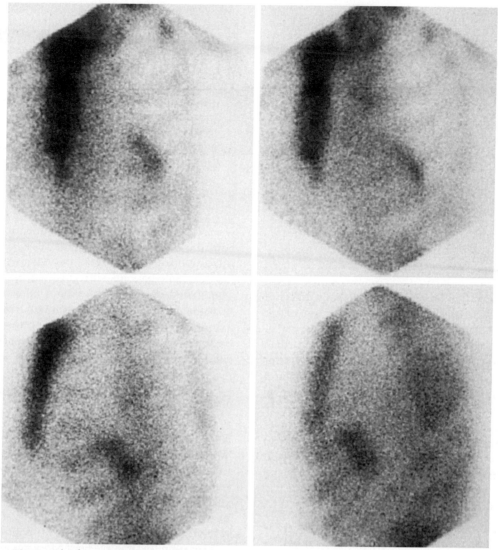

Figure 14-56   Lateral wall myocardial infarction with Tc-99m pyrophosphate uptake. The amount of myocardial uptake is greater than rib uptake and not equal to sternal uptake.

good myocardium-to-background ratio. Myocarditis, postradiation injury, and doxorubicin cardiotoxicity are all reported causes of diffusely increased myocardial uptake.

Tc-99m PYP scintigrams may remain abnormal for weeks or months after a myocardial infarction. Those scintigrams that continue to show uptake for more than 3 months correlate with a higher risk for future infarction.

The Fab′ fragment is radiolabeled with In-111 or Tc-99m. The sensitivity for detecting acute myocardial infarction is high, over 85%. A major advantage is that there is no rib uptake. A disadvantage is the slow pharmacokinetics of antimyosin antibody, which means that optimum imaging cannot be accomplished for many hours after radiopharmaceutical administration because of high background activity. Uptake may also be seen

with myocarditis, cardiac transplant rejection, and drug toxicity.

Clinical Applications and Utility

The major limitation of infarct-avid scintigraphy is its delayed positivity after the onset of symptoms. In most patients, the diagnosis is established from the history, physical examination, ECG, and serum enzyme determinations before the optimal time window for imaging. The study is used mainly when the diagnosis is uncertain (Box 14-26).

Tc-99m pyrophosphate and In-111 antimyosin antibody imaging has been used in patients with conduction system abnormalities on the resting ECG (e.g., left bundle branch block) that limited interpretation, and in patients who presented late after symptom onset when cardiac enzymes were not definitive of availability of better serum markers and imaging techniques; hot spot infarct imaging is used infrequently today. Tc-99m PYP imaging still may have a role in the diagnosis of amyloidosis.

INVESTIGATIONAL CARDIAC RADIOPHARMACEUTICALS

I-123 Meta-Iodobenzyl-Guanidine

I-123 MIBG has been used to study the adrenergic status of the heart. The heart is richly innervated and MIBG has been used to provide some interesting insights. Uptake of MIBG is blocked in patients taking drugs, such as guanethidine and cocaine, that compete for uptake into the presynaptic storage vesicles of the adrenergic system. Decreased uptake is seen after myocardial

infarction and in diabetic patients with denervated hearts. Some patients with cardiomyopathies also have diminished or absent uptake. A clinical role has not been established for MIBG, although it is being used to assess reinnervation after cardiac transplantation and to help determine prognosis in patients with dilated cardiomyopathy.

Fatty Acid Radiopharmaceuticals

Fatty acids supply the majority of the heart's metabolic requirements under normal aerobic conditions. With ischemia, energy metabolism shifts to anaerobic metabolism and the main energy substrate changes from free fatty acids to glucose metabolism. Radiolabeled fatty acids can be used to image myocardial aerobic metabolism.

PET imaging with carbon-11 palmitic acid gives information similar to perfusion agents. Myocardial time-activity curves reflect fatty acid metabolism. Decreased uptake and delayed clearance indicates ischemia. C-11 acetate also provides good images of the heart. Because of its rapid metabolism, cardiac turnover is inferred from dynamic analysis of its myocardial clearance pharmacokinetics. Controversy exists regarding the significance of the metabolic information provided. Neither agent is FDA-approved and an onsite cyclotron is required.

I-123 BMIPP (β-Methyl-p-iodophenylpentadecanoic acid) is a newly investigated single-photon branching free fatty acid radiopharmaceutical with slow metabolism; thus, it is well-suited for SPECT. With ischemia, there is decreased uptake similar to Tl-201. The uniqueness of this radiopharmaceutical is that it can demonstrate a persistent disturbance of fatty acid metabolism, even when blood flow has been reestablished, such as with unstable angina and stunned myocardium. Similar metabolic abnormalities have been described in cardiomyopathies.

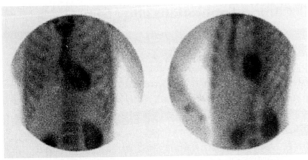

Figure 14-57   Cardiac amyloidosis. Tc-99m pyrophosphate is taken up throughout the left ventricular myocardium. Subtle uptake can also be seen in the right ventricular myocardium.

SUGGESTED READING

Books

Botvinick EH: Nuclear Medicine Self-Study Program III: Nuclear Medicine Cardiology, Topic 1-6. Society of Nuclear Medicine, 1997.

DePuey EG, Garcia EV, Berman DS: Cardiac SPECT Imaging, 2nd ed. Philadelphia, Lippincott Williams & Wilkins, 2001.

Dilsizian V, Narula J: Atlas of Nuclear Cardiology. Philadelphia, Current Medicine, 2003.

Gerson MC: Cardiac Nuclear Medicine, 3rd ed. New York, McGraw-Hill, 1997.

Zaret BL, Beller GA: Clinical Nuclear Cardiology, 3rd ed. Philadelphia, Elsevier, 2005.

Reviews

Bacharach SL, Bax JJ, Case J, et al: PET myocardial glucose metabolism and perfusion imaging: Part 1—Guidelines for patient preparation and data acquisition. J Nucl Cardiol 10:543-554, 2003.

Baird MG, Bateman TM, Berman DS: Guidelines for the clinical use of cardiac radionuclide imaging. J Am Coll Cardiol 2003.

Cerqueira MD, Weissman NJ, Disizian V, et al: Standardized myocardial segmentation and nomenclature for tomographic imaging of the heart. Circulation 105:539-549, 2002.

Freeman LM, Blaufox MD: Cardiovascular nuclear medicine, parts 1 and 2. Semin Nucl Med 19, 1999.

Hendel RC, Corbett JR, Cullom SJ, et al: The value and practice of attenuation correction for myocardial perfusion SPECT Imaging: a joint position statement from the American Society of Nuclear Cardiology and the Society of Nuclear Medicine. J Nucl Med 43:273-280, 2002.

Mieres JH, Shaw LJ, Hendel RC, et al: A report of the American Society of Nuclear Cardiology task force on women and heart disease. J Nucl Card 10:1-11, 2003.

Shelbert HR, Beanlands RB, Engel F, et al: PET myocardial perfusion and glucose metabolism imaging. Part 2—Guidelines for interpretation and reporting. J Nucl Card 10:557-571, 2000.

Publications

Arrighi JA, Soufer R: Reverse redistribution: is it clinically relevant or a washout? J Nucl Cardiol 5:195-201, 1998.

Bax JJ, Cornel JH, Visser FC, et al: Comparison of fluorine-18-FDG with rest-redistribution thallium-201 SPECT to delineate viable myocardium and predict functional recovery after revascularization, J Nucl Med 39:1481-1486, 1998.

Braunwald E, Rutherford JD: Reversible ischemic left ventricular dysfunction: evidence for the "hibernating myocardium," J Am Coll Cardiol 8:1467, 1986.

DePuey G, Parmett S, Ghensi M, et al: Comparison of Tc-99m sestamibi and Tl-201 gated SPECT, J Nucl Cardiol 6:278-285, 1999.

Hansen CL, Rastogi A, Sangrigoli R: On myocardial perfusion, metabolism and viability, J Nucl Cardiol 5:202-205, 1998.

Manrique A, Foraggi M, Vera P, et al: Tl-201 and Tc-99m MIBI gated SPECT in patients with large perfusion defects and left ventricular dysfunction: compression with equilibrium radionuclide angiography, J Nucl Med 40:805-809, 1999.

Merlet P, Pouillart F, Dubois-Rande J, et al: Sympathetic nerve alterations assessed with I-123-MIBG in the failing human heart, J Nucl Med 40:224-231, 1999.

Santana-Boado C, Candell-Riera J, Castell-Conesa J, et al: Diagnostic accuracy of technetium-99m-MIBI myocardinal SPECT in women and men, J Nucl Med 39:751-755, 1988.

CHAPTER 15

Pulmonary System

PULMONARY EMBOLISM

Pulmonary thromboembolism is a common clinical problem. Although the true incidence of clinically significant emboli is difficult to assess, pulmonary emboli have been found in up to 70% of autopsies. Some authorities have estimated an annual incidence of 650,000 cases per year with over 100,000 deaths. Untreated pulmonary embolism (PE) is frequently fatal. The mortality rate of approximately 30% can be reduced to 3–10% with anticoagulation therapy or inferior vena cava filter placement. Predisposing factors include immobilization, recent surgery, underlying malignancy, and various hypercoagulable states. In women, pregnancy and estrogen use are considered risk factors.

The clinical diagnosis of pulmonary embolism is difficult as presenting symptoms are nonspecific. The classic triad of dyspnea, pleuritic chest pain, and hemoptysis is rarely encountered. Patients often complain of shortness of breath, chest pain, and cough. Tachycardia is frequently present and, occasionally, patients present with cor pulmonale and circulatory collapse.

Arterial blood gases often show evidence of respiratory alkalosis and a low P_AO_2. However, the P_AO_2 may be normal in some patients. The plasma D-dimer is an excellent screening test with a low false-negative rate. However, it is nonspecific and can be elevated in various inflammatory conditions as well as in PE.

Pulmonary arteriography has been considered the "gold standard" for PE diagnosis with a reported sensitivity of 98% and specificity of 97%. The arteriogram offers excellent imaging resolution as well as the ability to perform direct vascular pressure measurements. However, readings vary among interpreters, particularly for distal emboli. Although the risk from the procedure is relatively low, it is an invasive test with a risk of death of approximately 0.5%. Therefore, less invasive imaging tests are more widely used.

Because there is a definite association between deep vein thrombosis (DVT) and PE, ultrasound examination of the leg veins is often indicated. Sonography has a reported sensitivity of 94% and specificity of 99% for DVT in the thigh veins but is much less sensitive for evaluating pelvic veins or the veins below the knee. The presence or absence of DVT does not determine whether or not PE is present.

Several radiographic signs of PE on chest x-ray have been described; however, these signs are rarely present. Westermark's sign is diminished vascularity in an area affected by a PE. The Fleischner sign is dilation of the pulmonary artery proximal to the embolus. Signs of infarction following a pulmonary embolus include an infiltrate from hemorrhage filling the alveolar spaces and the pleural-based Hampton's hump. The most common x-ray findings in pulmonary embolus are not specific for PE. Pleural effusions are common, present as often as 50% of the time. Infiltrates and atelectasis are also common. Normal radiographs have been described in anywhere from 12–30% of patients with PE. Although a chest radiograph is not adequate for PE diagnosis, an x-ray should always be obtained as it can identify problems that might present with similar symptoms to an embolus.

Computed tomography pulmonary angiography (CTPA) is now widely used as a method for PE diagnosis. In recent years, developments in spiral computed tomography (CT) have enabled rapid imaging techniques. The central pulmonary arteries can be visualized during contrast opacification with a fairly high degree of reliability. Acute clots and changes from chronic PE can be visualized. At the same time, CT can identify other problems and nonembolic causes for the patient's symptoms. Technical problems that make CT nondiagnostic include motion artifacts and insufficient contrast opacification. Contrast CT is often contraindicated in patients with iodinated contrast allergies or renal insufficiency.

Magnetic resonance (MR) offers the ability to image vascular structures without ionizing radiation or iodinated contrast. Currently, gradient-echo and spin-echo MR techniques are used for several vascular and cardiac applications. More powerful gradients and faster imaging sequences now allow imaging of the entire chest during a single breath-hold, and new contrast-enhanced techniques have yielded excellent pulmonary arteriography images. Preliminary results are quite good, although technical problems such as cardiac motion artifact obscuring lower lobe arteries persist. MR may play a clinical role in PE diagnosis in the future.

The ventilation perfusion (V/Q) scintigram remains an important diagnostic tool for PE. It is noninvasive, low risk, and time proven. V/Q scans are often used for patients where CT contrast is contraindicated or when patient radiation exposure is a concern, such as pregnancy. A typical CTPA protocol results in an exposure on the order of 8–10 mSv, but a V/Q scan has a fraction of the exposure at about 2 mSv.

VENTILATION PERFUSION SCINTIGRAPHY

Ventilation (V) and perfusion (Q) in the lungs are normally coupled or matched. A normal functional gradient is seen, with the lung apices receiving less perfusion and ventilation than the lung bases. Areas of the lung which are well ventilated are also normally well perfused (Fig. 15-1).

Many disease processes affect aeration. Among these are obstructive pathologies such as asthma, bronchitis, bronchiectasis, and emphysema. Acutely, the normal regional response to ventilatory causes of hypoxia is vasoconstriction, which shunts blood flow away to other aerated regions. This results in regions of reduced but matched ventilation-perfusion abnormalities and is often seen with asthma. Scarring results in matched abnormalities in chronic disease such as emphysema. Often, the chest radiograph will reveal a reason for abnormal aeration and perfusion such as an infiltrate or mass. This is often described as a "triple match" with abnormal ventilation, perfusion, and radiographic findings.

A vascular abnormality, such as pulmonary embolus, reduces pulmonary arterial perfusion. Commonly, lung parenchyma remains viable in these cases due to the bronchial arterial system. Therefore, the normal alveolar spaces will remain aerated, thus preventing infarction. Ventilation and perfusion are uncoupled or mismatched in the regions affected by the pulmonary embolus.

These physiologic parameters form the foundation for the ventilation perfusion lung scintigram. The perfusion portion of the scan uses intravenously injected microscopic particles large enough to be trapped on the first pass through the pulmonary capillary bed. When a radioactive label is attached to the particle, the distribution of microemboli can be imaged and present a picture of blood flow distribution within the lungs. To determine if a perfusion defect is the result of a ventilation abnormality rather than a primarily vascular problem, a ventilation study is done with an inhaled radiopharmaceutical (Box 15-1). By imaging pulmonary perfusion and lung ventilation, areas of matched and mismatched defects can be identified. As most mismatched perfusion defects are the result of pulmonary emboli, a diagnosis can be made with a high degree of probability.

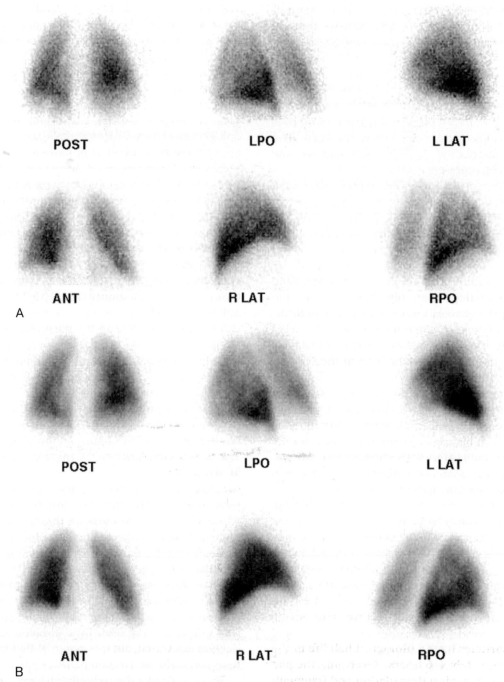

Figure 15-1 Normal V/Q scan. Ventilation (**A**) and perfusion (**B**) lung scans show homogeneous radiotracer distribution and the normal gradient of increasing activity in the bases relative to the apices.

Radiopharmaceuticals

Perfusion Radiopharmaceuticals

The diameter of a red blood cell is just under 8 μm. The capillaries are slightly larger, ranging from 7–10 μm and precapillary arterioles are on the order of 35 μm. For a perfusion agent to be trapped in the capillary bed on the first pass, the particles must be larger than capillary size. However, if the particle is too large, distribution may not fully reflect perfusion as particles become trapped in the more central arterioles rather than capillaries and precapillary arterioles.

Several different particulate agents have been used over the years. The first studies in humans were

---

Box 15-1   Ventilation and Perfusion Agents of Historical Interest

Perfusion	Ventilation
Tc-99m human albumin microspheres	**RADIOACTIVE GASES**
Tc-99m macroaggregated albumin*	Xenon-133*
	Xenon-127
	Krypton-81m
	RADIOAEROSOLS
	Tc-99m DTPA*
	Tc-99m Technegas

*Currently commercially available in the United States.

---

obtained with radioiodinated (I-131) macroaggregated albumin. Radiolabeled technetium-99m agents were subsequently introduced into clinical use. One of these, Tc-99m-labeled human albumin microspheres (Tc-99m HAM) provided rigid nondegradable particles of uniform size. However, it is no longer available in the U.S. for human use.

Tc-99m macroaggregated albumin (Tc-99m MAA) is the radiopharmaceutical used today. The preparation contains particles ranging in size from 5–100 μm. The majority (60–80%) are in the 10–30 μm range. A kit is available that contains MAA with stannous ion. Tc-99m as sodium pertechnetate is added to the reaction vial, resulting in rapid labeling of the MAA particles.

After intravenous injection into a peripheral vein, the radiolabeled particles travel through the right atrium and right ventricle where mixing occurs. They are then filtered out or trapped as they travel through the pulmonary bed. In areas of decreased or absent perfusion, correspondingly fewer particles are delivered and trapped, resulting in relatively photopenic or "cold" areas. This produces a scintigraphic map of relative perfusion in the lungs.

The MAA particles have a biological half-life in the lungs of approximately 4–6 hours. Over time, the particles undergo mechanical degradation and fragment. They may then lodge in smaller vessels but eventually gain access to the circulation where they are phagocytosed in the reticuloendothelial system. The number of particles used is an important consideration. If the dose of particles is too small, the distribution pattern in the capillary bed will not be statistically valid. A minimum of 100,000 particles is required in adults. On the other hand, injecting too many particles could theoretically obstruct a hemodynamically significant portion of the pulmonary circulation. In practice,

200,000–500,000 particles are administered. Because there are an estimated 300 million precapillary arterioles and over 280 billion pulmonary capillaries, this should result in obstruction of only a small fraction of vessels, between 0.1–0.3%. Most of these are only partially blocked.

The perfusion exam is generally very safe. Only a tiny fraction of capillaries are occluded and most of these are only partially blocked. However, certain conditions warrant reducing the number of particles. These include pulmonary hypertension, pregnancy, and right-to-left cardiac shunts. The number of particles is also reduced for neonates (10,000) and children under the age of 5 years (50,000–150,000).

Patients with pulmonary hypertension may have significantly fewer capillaries than normal. Theoretically, their condition could worsen if too many were occluded. Although significant effects are rare, the number of particles administered is often reduced to 100,000–250,000.

Patients with right-to-left cardiac shunts also require caution. The Tc-99m MAA will pass through the heart into the systemic circulation rather than remain in the lungs. The kidneys, brain, and other structures will be visualized. Although the idea of microemboli lodging in the brain is alarming, it does not seem to have clinical significance. Tc-99m MAA has been long used to diagnose right-to-left cardiac shunts and to determine their severity. This is done by calculating the amount of activity trapped in the lungs versus the amount of activity that bypasses the lungs. Investigators have also injected particles into other organs, including the brain, to study blood flow without ill-effect. Although it is prudent to decrease the number of particles to 100,000–150,000, a known right-to-left shunt is not an absolute contraindication.

When PE is a clinical consideration in pregnant patients, a V/Q exam offers the ability to diagnose the emboli with relatively low radiation to the fetus. However, the minimum radiation dose should be used. This can be accomplished by decreasing the amount of Tc-99m MAA used, but it is essential that the dose contains the minimum 100,000 particles.

When ordering the radiopharmaceutical, it must be made clear that a lower number or particles is desired and not a lower level of radioactivity. To achieve the right balance between the amount of radioactivity and the number of particles, the amount of Tc-99m pertechnetate added to the reaction vial may need to be adjusted. Because commercially available reaction vials provide for multiple doses, the radioactivity-to-particles ratio changes continuously after the initial labeling. This should be borne in mind in making dose calculations.

Ventilation Radiopharmaceuticals

Two classes of radiopharmaceuticals are available for ventilation imaging: radioactive gases and radioaerosols (Box 15-1). One aerosol, Tc-99m diethylenetriamine pentaacetic acid (Tc-99m DTPA), and one gas, xenon-133 (Xe-133), are currently available in the U.S. Comparative studies between Xe-133 and Tc-99m DTPA have not shown significant differences in overall accuracy. The choice of agent depends largely on available equipment, proper room ventilation, the frequency of chronic obstructive pulmonary disease (COPD) in the referral population, and personal preference.

Radioactive Gases

Xenon-133

The only radioactive gas available commercially is Xe-133. The physical characteristics of Xe-133 are listed in Table 15-1. Xe-133 offers superior transit to the periphery of the lung and is very sensitive for detection of COPD. The half-life of 5.27 days makes for a long shelf-life. It is available from the radiopharmacy in single- and multiple-dose vials.

The study is acquired in three phases: an initial single breath hold, equilibrium, and then washout. Xe-133 rapidly clears from the body with a biological half-life of 30 seconds during washout. Therefore, only one view (usually the posterior) is reliably obtained using a single-detector system. Although newer dual-head detector gamma cameras allow the addition of the anterior view, it is not possible to acquire the multiple views to correspond each position of the perfusion study.

Table 15-1	Comparison of Xenon-133 and Tc-99m DTPA Ventilation Agents	
	Xenon-133	**Tc-99m DTPA**
Mode of decay	Beta-minus	Isomeric
Physical half-life	5.3 days	6 hours
Biological half-life	30 seconds	45 minutes
Photon energy	81 keV	140 keV
Multiple-view imaging	No	Yes
Useful for severe COPD	Yes	+/−
Used after perfusion scan	No	No

After lung inhalation, Xe-133 equilibrates across the alveolar-capillary membrane and distributes within the body; however, it clears from the blood as it is exhaled. However, because Xe-133 is fat soluble, the radiotracer may accumulate and be retained in the liver of patients with fatty infiltration (Fig. 15-2).

There are some disadvantages to Xe-133. The low 81-keV photopeak is not optimal for the gamma camera and results in relatively low-resolution images. Ideally, ventilation images would be performed after the perfusion images in the projection most likely to give diagnostic information. However, because of its low photopeak, Xe-133 must be acquired before the Tc-99m MAA perfusion study. If performed after Tc-99m MAA, downscatter from Tc-99m would degrade the Xe-133 images and make interpretation difficult.

Being a heavy gas, Xe-133 that escapes into the room will settle out on the floor. Thus, for radiation safety, it is

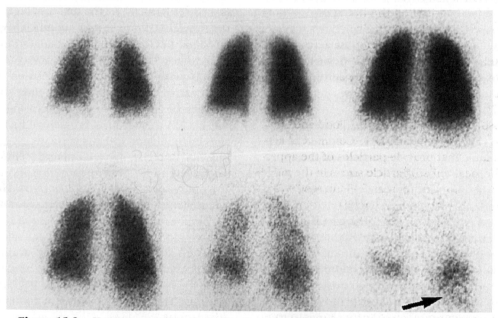

Figure 15-2 Xe-133 accumulation in the liver. Posterior ventilation images show delayed washout of xenon in the lung bases and significant xenon uptake in the region of the liver (*arrow, bottom right image*).

mandatory that the room have good airflow and safe external ventilation, and must be under negative pressure. On exhalation, the Xe-133 is directed into tubing that goes to a xeon "trap," a charcoal filter that absorbs the expired xenon and retains it until decay.

Xenon-127

The major advantage of Xe-127 is its higher photopeaks of 172 keV, 203 keV, and 375 keV. These energies are higher than that of the Tc-99m MAA perfusion agent, so the ventilation study can be done after the perfusion exam. Therefore, only patients with abnormal perfusion scans would be imaged and positioning could be optimized. However, the long physical half-life of 36.4 days poses radiation safety hazards, requiring a different xenon trap and delivery system. It is not available in the United States.

Krypton-81m

Kr-81m has a photopeak of 190 keV, which permits ventilation imaging in multiple projections following the Tc-99m MAA perfusion study. With a very short half-life of 13 seconds, Kr-81m must be continuously eluted from a rubidium-81/krypton-81m generator. Because of this short half-life, a true equilibrium is not achieved. Therefore, incomplete penetration of the alveolar spaces may limit sensitivity for the detection of COPD. The half-life of the parent, rubidium-81, is only 4.6 hours and the generator system must be replaced daily. Therefore, this expensive agent is not practical for most facilities and Kr-81 has never achieved widespread clinical use.

Radioaerosols

As an alternative to radioactive gases, various aerosolized particles have been used. The radioaerosol distribution depicts ventilation during the inhalation phase. The inhaled aerosol is deposited on the lining of the bronchoalveolar spaces. Subsequent imaging shows regional patterns of ventilation. An advantage of the aerosol technique is the ability to image in multiple views following a single dose of radiotracer because radioaerosols do not wash out rapidly like the radioactive gases.

Tc-99m DTPA

The only aerosol approved by the U.S. Food and Drug Administration (FDA) is Tc-99m DTPA. Commercial nebulizers are available that provide particles of the appropriate size. The ideal aerosol particle size is in the range of 0.1–0.5 μm. Particles greater than 2–3 μm tend to settle out in large airways including trachea and bronchi. This central airway clumping may obscure the alveolar distribution in adjacent lung and even affect the perfusion study performed later by "shining through." Clumping most commonly occurs in conditions such as asthma, COPD, or in patients unable to cooperate with deep breathing. Although this still happens with Tc-99m DTPA, it is less problematic than in the past due to technical improvements, including smaller particle size and better delivery systems. The aerosol particles cross the

membrane with a half-life of approximately 45 minutes and are cleared through the kidneys. This long residence in the lungs permits imaging in multiple views similar to the perfusion study.

Technegas

Another agent available in Europe is Technegas, Tc-99m labeled carbon particles. A Technegas generator produces very small aerosol particles (0.0005 μm) by pertechnetate combustion in argon gas. These small particles do not have the same problem of settling out and clumping in cases of turbulent flow. Technegas appears to be superior in image quality to Tc-99m DTPA but is not available in the United States.

Dosimetry

Radiation dosimetry values are listed in Table 15-2. The ventilation-perfusion lung scan will result in a low radiation exposure with either Tc-99m DTPA or Xe-133 as the ventilation agent. A 5-mCi (185 MBq) dose of Tc-99m MAA delivers just over 1 rad (1 cGy) to the lungs.

Technique

Ventilation studies are performed before the perfusion portion of the exam. The higher photopeak of Tc-99m MAA would cause downscatter into Xe-133 ventilation images if the perfusion exam was acquired first. Therefore, Xe-133 imaging is performed first. In the case of the radioaerosol Tc-99m DTPA, the radiolabel is the same as the perfusion agent, Tc-99m MAA. For both studies to be done on the same day without "crosstalk" interference with each other, the doses must be adjusted so that the second study overpowers the first (ratio of at least 3:1). The count rates achievable with the Tc-99m DTPA nebulizer are much lower than those obtained on the perfusion images. If the perfusion study was acquired first, the Tc-99m MAA dose would need to be limited. The very low dose, on the order of 1 mCi, might not result in optimal diagnostic images.

Table 15-2	Radiation Dosimetry for Ventilation-Perfusion Radiopharmaceuticals in rads/mCi (cGy/37 MBq)		
Organ	**Tc-99m MAA**	**Tc-99m DTPA**	**Xe-133**
Lung	**0.22**	0.063	0.0083
Trachea			**0.64**
Ovaries	0.007	0.012	0.001
Testes	0.008	0.008	0.001
Bladder	0.06	0.17	
Whole body	0.015	0.14	0.001

Bold type indicates critical organ.

Therefore, the ventilation study is obtained first after inhalation of 800 μCi.

Xenon-133 Ventilation

The protocol for Xe-133 is detailed in Box 15-2. A high-quality ventilation scan requires patient cooperation. Because ventilation should be optimized, patients with clinical bronchospasm should have bronchodilation therapy prior to a lung scan. The study is performed in three phases: the single-breath or wash-in phase, the equilibrium phase, and the washout phase. Severely tachypneic, uncooperative, or unresponsive patients may require protocol modification; otherwise, ventilation imaging may not be possible.

Because the location of any perfusion defects cannot be predicted, the patient is usually positioned for a posterior view. Some laboratories routinely perform both parts of the study with the patient supine. Others favor a sitting position if the patient can tolerate it. The sitting position is generally better because it permits a fuller excursion of the diaphragm and makes oblique views easier to obtain during the washout phase. Also, as chest radiographs are usually obtained in an upright position,

the best correlative information comes from comparison in similar positions.

To begin the study, a closed system must be set up with a face mask or mouthpiece. This may be difficult for some patients to tolerate. The patient is asked to breathe in and hold a single maximal inspiration of the Xe-133. An initial image is obtained for 100,000 counts, if possible, or 10–15 seconds.

The next phase of the study is the equilibrium phase. After the initial breath image is completed, the patient breathes a mixture of air and xenon at tidal volume. Two images are usually obtained for 90 seconds each. In the third phase, the patient breathes room air and the xenon is delivered to a trapping system. Three or four sequential 45-second washout images are obtained. Optional 45-degree posterior oblique images are performed.

Tc-99m DTPA

The lung ventilation protocol using Tc-99m DTPA is listed in Box 15-3. For studies with the radioaerosol Tc-99m DTPA, the radiopharmaceutical is placed in a special nebulizer system. The nose is clamped and the patient is asked to breathe through the delivery system mouthpiece until sufficient radioaerosol is delivered to the lungs. This may require several minutes. During this time, the patient may be placed in a supine position to decrease the apex to base gradient, but an erect position will improve detection of

---

Box 15-2   Protocol for Xenon-133 Ventilation Scintigraphy

PATIENT PREPARATION

None

DOSAGE AND ADMINISTRATION

10–20 mCi (370–740 MBq) inhaled

PROCEDURE

Collimator: Low-energy parallel hole
Photopeak: 20% window centered at 81 keV
Positioning: Patient seated (if possible)
    Camera centered over chest posteriorly
    If dual head camera, second head may be placed
        anteriorly
    Use tight seal face mask or mouthpiece with attached
        spirometer and intake and exhaust tubing
Acquisition:
First breath: patient exhales fully and is asked to
    maximally inspire and hold it long enough (if
    possible) to obtain 100,000 counts or 10–15 seconds
Equilibrium: obtain two sequential 90-second images
    while the patient breathes normally
Washout:
Turn system to exhaust
Obtain three sequential 45-second posterior images and
    then right and left posterior oblique images and final
    posterior image

Box 15-3   Protocol for Tc-99m DTPA Ventilation Scintigraphy

PATIENT PREPARATION

None

DOSAGE AND ADMINISTRATION

30 mCi (1110 MBq) Tc-99m DTPA in nebulizer

PROCEDURE

Collimator: Low-energy parallel hole
Photopeak: 20% window centered at 140 keV
Positioning: Place nose clamps on patient and
                 connect mouthpiece with patient
                 supine.
             Center camera over chest posteriorly
             Patient breathes continuously through
                 mouthpiece for several minutes
Acquisition: Acquire posterior image for 250k and
                 mark time
             Obtain other views for same time
             Views: Posterior, anterior, right/left
                 lateral, right/left posterior oblique,
                 anterior oblique views recommended

defects in the bases. Although 30 mCi (1110 MBq) of Tc-99m DTPA is placed in the nebulizer, only 0.5–1.0 mCi (17.5–37 MBq) is delivered to the patient. The goal is to deliver enough radioaerosol to the lung so that 200,000- to 250,000-count (200k–250k) images may be obtained in 1–2 minutes. Usually, inhalation continues until 1 mCi (37 MBq) of activity is in the lungs.

The views obtained in the radioaerosol study should be the same as those obtained in the perfusion phase. Most nuclear medicine clinics obtain anterior, posterior, right and left lateral, both posterior 45-degree oblique views. Right and left 45-degree anterior oblique views are frequently done and are especially helpful for visualizing the lingual segment and medial segment of the right middle lobe.

Tc-99m MAA

The perfusion study follows the Xe-133 or Tc-99m DTPA ventilation study. The protocol is described in Box 15-4. Immediately before injection, the syringe is inverted to mix the particles as they tend to rapidly settle out and may clump. The needle should be 23 gauge or larger to prevent fragmentation of the dose during administration. The 2- to 5-mCi (74–185 MBq) dose containing 200,000–500,000 particles is injected over the course of several respiratory cycles. Care must be taken not to draw blood back into the syringe. When this happens,

---

Box 15-4   Protocol for Tc-99m MAA Perfusion Scintigraphy

PATIENT PREPARATION

None

PATIENT PRECAUTIONS

Pulmonary hypertension: Reduce number of particles to 100,000

Pregnant patients: Adjust dose lower and observe requirement for a minimum of 100,000 particles

Right to left cardiac shunt: relative contraindication, reduce particle number

DOSAGE AND ADMINISTRATION

2–5 mCi (74–185 MBq) I.V. over several respiratory cycles with patient supine

PROCEDURE

Collimator: Low-energy parallel hole

Photopeak: 20% window centered at 140 keV

Obtain 500k to 750k counts/image

Obtain anterior, posterior, right and left lateral, right and left posterior oblique

   Right and left anterior oblique images optional but recommended

---

clots form in the syringe producing hot emboli on the lung images (Fig. 15-3). The patient is in a supine position to minimize the gravitational gradient from apex to base.

Once the injection is complete, imaging can begin immediately. The patient's position for imaging should be the same as that selected for the ventilation portion of the study. The posterior view is usually acquired for 500,000 counts, and the time noted. The remaining images can then be set for that amount of time. The fewest counts will be obtained on the lateral views, as counts are essentially coming from only the one lung next to the camera.

Image Interpretation

Perfusion Scintigram

Normal perfusion images should show homogeneous, uniform distribution of radiotracer throughout the lungs (Figs. 15-1B and 15-4B). The hilar structures are frequently seen as photopenic areas. The heart is a photopenic defect in the left base on the anterior view and more mildly decreased activity in the posterior lung. The spine and sternum attenuate activity along the midline. The pulmonary outline on perfusion images commonly appears slightly smaller than on the ventilation images. This is because of lower spatial resolution on the Xe-133 ventilation study due to lower counts.

Differences in patient positioning during radiotracer administration will cause variations in distribution due to gravity. Pleural effusions will layer out in supine patients (Fig. 15-5). It is important to know what the positioning was during imaging to assess defects from breast and soft-tissue attenuation or from an arm in the field of view. Attenuation artifacts are also common from metal such as a pacemaker. Other explanations should be sought for perfusion defects by examining the radiograph and ventilation images.

Small perfusion defects are frequently seen due to various etiologies. These may be found incidentally and are more common in smokers. Pulmonary emboli typically cause multiple moderate or large defects, most commonly in the lower lung zones. Causes for perfusion defects are listed in Box 15-5.

At times, it is necessary to determine if activity outside the lungs, such as kidney activity, is due to free Tc-99m pertechnetate or a cardiac shunt. Renal activity can be seen in both conditions or may occasionally persist following normal systemic absorption of technetium from the ventilation study. Free pertechnetate in the radiopharmaceutical preparation will also be seen as activity in thyroid and stomach. However, Tc-99m pertechnetate and other contaminants do not cross the blood–brain barrier or localize in the brain. In the case of a right-to-left shunt, Tc-99m MAA lodges in the cerebral capillary

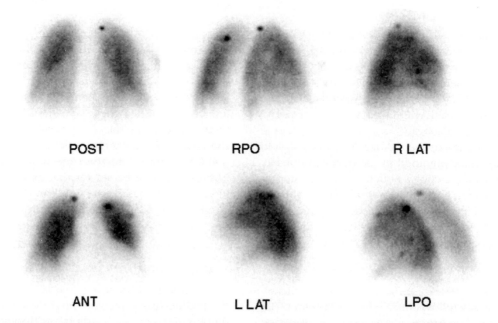

POST   RPO   R LAT

ANT   L LAT   LPO

Figure 15-3   Injected blood clot artifact with Tc-99m MAA. Blood clots formed from drawing blood back into the syringe appear as focal hot spots when they are reinjected into the patient. These have a variable appearance but can be quite large.

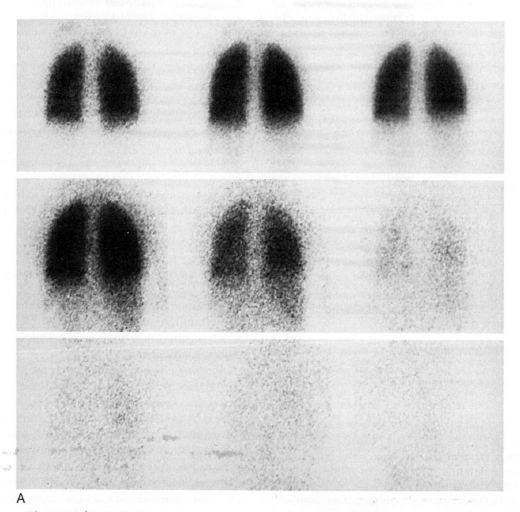

A

Figure 15-4   Xenon-133 ventilation study. **A,** The initial breath and equilibrium images are in the upper row. The sequential washout images in the middle and lower rows show no evidence of air trapping.

Continued

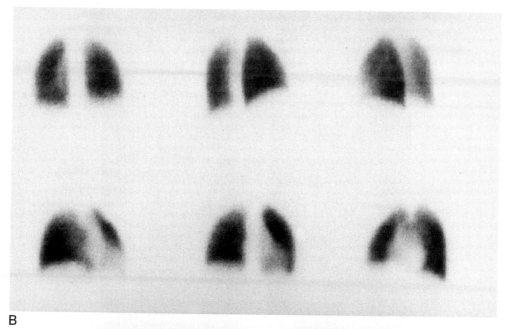

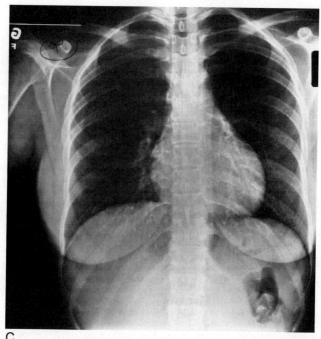

Figure 15-4, cont'd **B,** Corresponding Tc-99m MAA images show homogeneous distribution of tracer activity throughout the lungs. **C,** The chest radiograph was also normal.

circulation, and cortical uptake is diagnostic of a right-to-left cardiac shunt (Fig. 15-6). Uptake in the liver indicates colloidal impurities.

Ventilation Scintigram

The normal Xe-133 scan shows homogeneous radiotracer distribution during all three phases of the study (Fig. 15-4A). The Xe-133 initial breath or wash-in image may show

slightly less uptake compared to the equilibrium rebreathing image. The heart may be seen as a relative photopenic area in the left lung base. Washout is normally rapid with a clearance half-time of 2 minutes or less. The last washout image should have faint or no discernable activity. In an otherwise normal subject, washout may appear delayed as a result of the subject's inability to breathe comfortably through the apparatus. Occasionally, abnormal

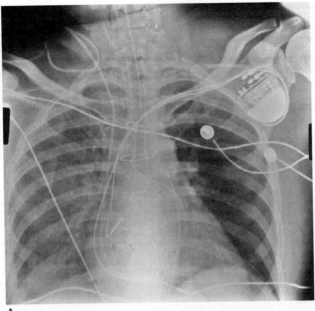

A

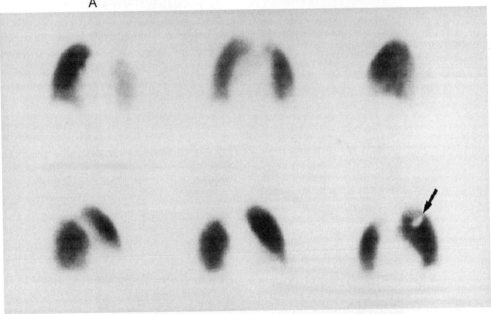

B

Figure 15-5 Pleural effusion effect. **A,** A-P chest radiograph reveals uniformly greater density in the right lung compared to the left caused by an effusion layering out posteriorly when the patient is supine. **B,** Corresponding Tc-99m MAA perfusion study shows decreased perfusion to the right lung on the posterior view (*upper left hand image*), which is not seen on the other views, tipping off the observer to the explanation for the discrepancy. The pacemaker causes a well-defined defect (*arrow*).

activity is seen in the right upper quadrant. This occurs because xenon is fat soluble and accumulates in the liver in patients with fatty infiltration of the liver.

The normal distribution of the radioaerosol Tc-99m DTPA is similar to the initial breath image of a Xe-133 study. When patients are positioned carefully, it is easy to compare these ventilation images to the multiple projections from the perfusion study. Activity may be seen in

the mouth and large airways, and swallowed activity may be seen in the trachea and stomach (Fig. 15-7).

Differential Diagnosis of Ventilation Abnormalities

The abnormal ventilation pattern varies depending on the disease process and the agent used. Abnormal Tc-99m DTPA images can show areas of absent or

Box 15-5   Causes of Perfusion Defects

PRIMARY VASCULAR LESION

Pulmonary thromboembolism
Septic, fat, and air emboli
Pulmonary artery hypoplasia or atresia
Vasculitis

PRIMARY VENTILATION ABNORMALITY

Pneumonia
Atelectasis
Pulmonary edema
Asthma
COPD, emphysema, chronic bronchitis
Bullae

MASS EFFECT

Tumor
Adenopathy
Pleural effusion

IATROGENIC

Surgery—pneumonectomy, lobectomy
Radiation fibrosis (also postinflammatory fibrosis)

decreased uptake. Xe-133 may be abnormal on any one or all three phases. The study should be interpreted as abnormal even if only one phase is abnormal. Many processes result in air trapping on the Xe-133 scan.

Asthma and COPD with bronchospasm both result in acutely decreased ventilation. The decreased ventilation, in turn, causes a reflex decrease in perfusion. In bullae, chronic bronchitis, and bronchiectasis, there is actual destruction of the bronchial walls with decreased perfusion in the affected area. Correspondingly, ventilation is decreased with delayed wash-in and air trapping with delayed clearance.

Although obstructive airway diseases, such as asthma, cause multiple matched defects, pulmonary hypertension and restrictive airway disease can cause mismatched defects. However, the typical pattern of smaller defects in the bases can usually be differentiated from that of PE, which causes multiple larger defects.

Occasionally, perfusion deficits involve predominantly one lung (Box 15-6). Although very severe asymmetric defects are often iatrogenic, other etiologies may be present. A mucous plug usually results in a matched defect sometimes involving a whole lobe or lung. A centrally located bronchogenic carcinoma or hilar mass can also cause perfusion defects, which may be matched or

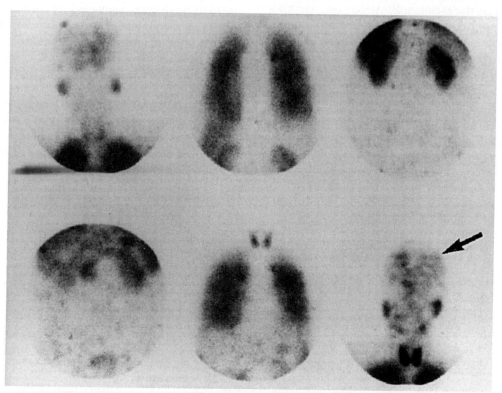

Figure 15-6   Right-to-left cardiac shunt. Tc-99m MAA images reveal abnormal uptake in the kidneys and brain from a right-to-left shunt. Free pertechnetate activity is seen in the thyroid and salivary glands but does not explain the cerebral activity.

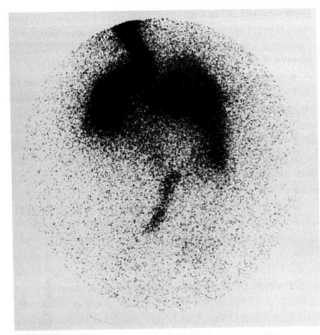

Figure 15-7 Swallowed Tc-99m DTPA. Intense uptake in the trachea and stomach may result from swallowed radiopharmaceutical.

mismatched (Fig 15-8). Although a large saddle embolus could result in a unilateral decrease in perfusion, it is very uncommon.

Often, the etiology of a ventilation and perfusion defect is found on the radiograph. Atelectasis, pneumonia, and edema from congestive heart failure are common examples. Radiographic infiltrates may be seen in PE with infarct, but pneumonia is a more common cause.

Image Interpretation for Pulmonary Embolism Diagnosis

A special set of terms has been developed for the diagnostic schemes employed in the interpretation of V/Q scans (Box 15-7). As described in the section on physiology,

perfusion defects may be matched or mismatched depending on whether or not there is a corresponding ventilatory abnormality. If Xe-133 is used, the ventilation defect may not be seen on all phases of the exam, and a defect on any phase can count as abnormal. The washout phase is most sensitive for ventilatory abnormalities and detects over 90% of defects compared to 70% for the initial single-breath image and 20% on the equilibrium view.

The distinction on whether a perfusion defect is matched or not is fundamental to V/Q interpretation. Usually, matched defects are due to nonembolic causes. Acute PE classically results in V/Q mismatch. The embolus blocks blood flow causing a perfusion defect, but the ventilation remains normal because the airway has no corresponding blockage. The likelihood of PE increases as the number of mismatched defects increases, and the greater the number of defects.

The next important concept is the difference between a *segmental* and *nonsegmental* defect. Perfusion defects caused by blockage of the pulmonary arterial tree should reflect the branching or arborization of the pulmonary

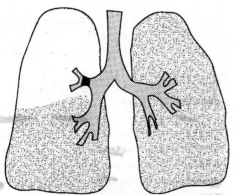 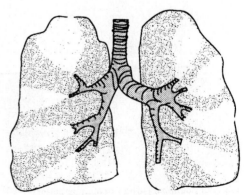

Figure 15-8 Effects of airway obstruction: Ventilation abnormalities may be due to obstructions in larger airways. This might present as a large defect (*left*) caused by bronchogenic carcinoma or mucous plugs. Constriction of smaller bronchi in asthma can also cause ventilation abnormalities (*right*).

V/Q matched defect: Both scans abnormal in same area and of equal size

V/Q mismatch: Abnormal perfusion in an area of normal ventilation or a much larger perfusion defect than ventilation abnormality

Triple-match: V/Q matching defects in a region of chest x-ray abnormality where the x-ray abnormality is of the same size or smaller than the radiographic lesion

Segmental defect: Characteristically wedge shaped and pleural based, conforms to segmental anatomy of the lung. May be caused by occlusion of pulmonary artery branches

Large: >75% of a lung segment

Moderate: 25-75% of a lung segment

Small: <25% of a lung segment

Nonsegmental defect: Does not conform to segmental anatomy or does not appear wedge shaped

| Box 15-8 | Causes of Nonsegmental Defects |

Pacemaker artifact
Tumors
Pleural effusion
Trauma
Hemorrhage
Bullae
Cardiomegaly
Hilar adenopathy
Atelectasis
Pneumonia
Aortic ectasia or aneurysm

circulation in its classic segmental pattern (Fig. 15-9). Thus, a classic segmental defect corresponds to one or more bronchopulmonary segments, is wedge-shaped, and is pleural-based. Knowledge of segmental anatomy is critical for correct interpretation. Keeping a diagram at hand for reference is useful for interpreting V/Q studies (Fig. 15-10). The term nonsegmental is reserved for abnormalities due to the patient's anatomy and those defects that do not correspond to the pulmonary segments, are not pleural-based, and do not have the classic wedge shape. Many conditions resulting in nonsegmental defects are apparent radiographically, such as pleural effusion, pneumonia, edema, and tumors. In other cases, it may be unclear if the defect could be caused by PE. Causes of nonsegmental defects are summarized in Box 15-8.

Assessment of the size of a given defect and determination of the number of defects present in each category are important for the application of the clinical diagnostic schemes. By convention, a defect is considered *large* if it equals more than 75% of the lung segment, *moderate* if it is between 25-75% of the size of a lung segment, and *small* if it is less than 25% of the segment. This may be difficult given the variable size of the different segments. Judgment is subjective and confidence increases with experience. Some authors suggest that there is no significant difference between a moderate defect and a large one. If this approach is used, interpretation is simplified.

Evaluation of the chest x-ray is essential. The chest x-ray findings can alter the final interpretation. The concept of "matching" also applies to a comparison of the perfusion exam and the chest radiograph. If a chest x-ray abnormality is in the area of a perfusion defect, it must be determined if the finding is acute or chronic. Acute radiographic abnormalities that could be associated with a PE include atelectasis, infiltrate, or effusion. A defect related to scar or tumor is not consistent with PE.

PIOPED CRITERIA

Rather than simply calling a scan positive or negative for pulmonary embolus, risk probability categories have been developed. If no perfusion abnormalities are demonstrated, the study is considered *normal*. Abnormal exams are interpreted depending on the size and number of perfusion abnormalities, as well as whether they are matched or mismatched by the ventilation study and chest radiograph, abnormal studies are categorized as either *very low* probability, *low* probability, *intermediate* probability, or *high* probability. Some physicians will use the term *indeterminate* interchangeably with intermediate, although most reserve the term indeterminate for nondiagnostic scans.

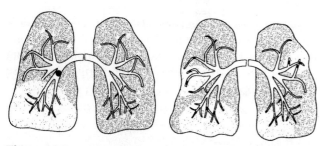

Figure 15-9 Effect of pulmonary artery branching pattern on the appearance of emboli. Emboli may be due to larger, more proximal clots (*left*) or showers of smaller clots lodging more distally (*right*). In either case, the resulting defects should be pleural-based and corresponding to the segments of the lung.

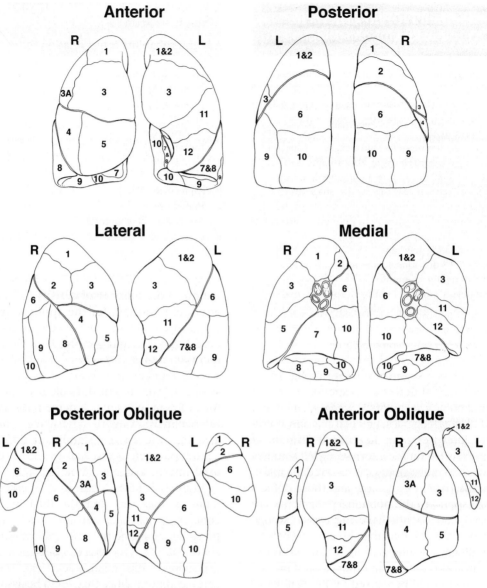

Figure 15-10   Segmental anatomy of the lungs. Upper lobe: *1*, apical; *2*, posterior; *3*, anterior. Right middle lobe: *4*, lateral; *5*, medial. Lower lobe: *6*, superior; *7*, medial basal; *8*, anterior basal; *9*, lateral basal; *10*, posterior basal. Lingula (left): *11*, superior lingual; *12*, inferior lingual.

The criteria for each of these categories have changed to some extent over time, and several diagnostic schemes have been proposed over the years. The Prospective Investigation of Pulmonary Embolism Diagnosis (PIOPED) study was a multiinstitutional study sponsored by the National Institutes of Health to assess the accuracy of V/Q scintigraphy. Patients underwent V/Q scan, chest radiograph, and pulmonary angiography. Analysis of the PIOPED study data resulted in only a few modifications to prior probability categories. Overall, this prospective study confirmed much from the published retrospective studies. The criteria listed in Box 15-9 are a summary of the widely used modified PIOPED criteria. Further modifications to the modified PIOPED criteria have been recommended by the PIOPED Nuclear Medicine Working Group (Box 15-10). However, data supporting these changes is more limited.

Normal

When the perfusion study is completely normal, the likelihood of PE is less than 5%. The likelihood of significant morbidity or mortality from PE is less than 1% (Figs. 15-1 and 15-4).

Box 15-9   Modified PIOPED Criteria for Pulmonary Embolus Diagnosis

HIGH PROBABILITY SCAN

2 or more large mismatched segmental defects or equivalent in moderate/large defects with normal x-ray

Any perfusion defect substantially larger than radiographic abnormality

INTERMEDIATE PROBABILITY SCAN

Multiple perfusion defects with associated x-ray opacities

Greater than 25% of a segment and less than 2 mismatched segmental perfusion defects with normal radiograph
 One moderate segmental
 One large or two moderate segmental
 One large and one moderate segmental
 Three moderate segmental

Solitary moderate-large matching segmental defect with matching x-ray (triple match)

Difficult to characterize as high-probability or low-probability

LOW PROBABILITY SCAN

Nonsegmental defects—small effusion blunting costophrenic angle, cardiomegaly, elevated diaphragm, ectatic aorta

Any perfusion defect with substantially larger radiographic abnormality

Matched ventilation and perfusion defects with normal chest radiograph

Small subsegmental perfusion defects

NORMAL SCAN

No perfusion defects

Box 15-10   Proposed Criteria for Very Low Probability Interpretation

Nonsegmental perfusion defect

Perfusion defect smaller than radiographic lesion

Two or more regional matched defects with normal x-ray

One to three small segmental perfusion defects

Solitary triple-match in upper lung zone or confined to single segment

Stripe sign around perfusion defect on best tangential view

High Probability

A high-probability interpretation requires identification of two or more large-segment perfusion defects with normal ventilation (mismatched) and a clear chest x-ray. These perfusion defects can also consist of a combination of defects that add up to two or more large defects, if at least one is moderate or large. For example, this might be one large and two moderate defects or four moderate defects. The perfusion defects must correspond to a bronchopulmonary segment. The high-probability category indicates the risk of pulmonary embolus is greater than 80%. The presence of a matching acute radiographic abnormality lowers the likelihood that PE is present and the study is placed in an intermediate probability category (Figs. 15-11 and 15-12).

Low/Very-Low Probability

The chance of a pulmonary embolus in a low-probability scan is less than 20%. A very-low probability category has been introduced with an estimated risk of PE at less than 10%. The updated PIOPED recommendations are largely centered on the very-low category, although actual use of the category in practice varies widely. In addition, these changes have resulted in a complicated list. The reader should start with the basics. It is helpful to remember that low-probability exams involve small defects and matched defects (Fig. 15-13). Once an exam is placed in the low-probability group, the reading can be refined to determine if very-low probability criteria apply.

Whether defects are small or large, or single or multiple, they can be called low probability. The PIOPED data found that as long as there was some perfusion in a lung field, even very extensive ventilation-perfusion matched abnormalities are low probability (Fig. 15-14). Any number of perfusion defects can be classified as low probability if they are matched by ventilation abnormalities and the chest x-ray is clear. If all the perfusion defects are small subsegmental ones (less than 25% of a segment), the exam is low probability without regard to what the ventilation images show if the chest x-ray is clear. However, if there are only one to three such small defects, the study can be called very-low probability. The very-low probability category also includes nonsegmental defects that can be attributed to structures such as the heart, vessels, or elevated diaphragm on the chest radiograph,

When the x-ray contains abnormalities, interpretation becomes more complex. Any perfusion defect with a substantially larger chest x-ray abnormality is also low probability. One way of thinking about this is to consider an infiltrate from an infarcted region of lung. The infiltrate should only be seen in areas affected by the blockage. If the infiltrate is in areas that are being

(continued on p.528)

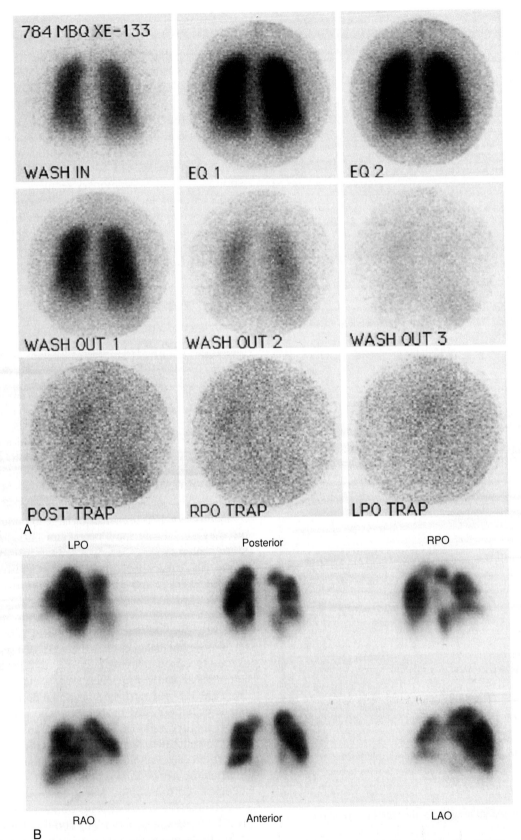

Figure 15-11 High probability V/Q. **A,** Normal posterior Xe-133 images. **B,** Corresponding Tc-99m MAA perfusion study reveals multiple bilateral large pleural-based mismatched defects. This pattern fits the high-probability diagnosis category.

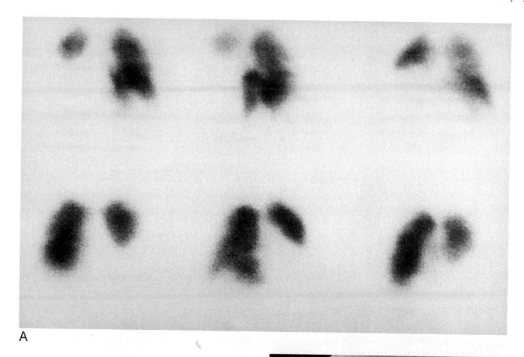

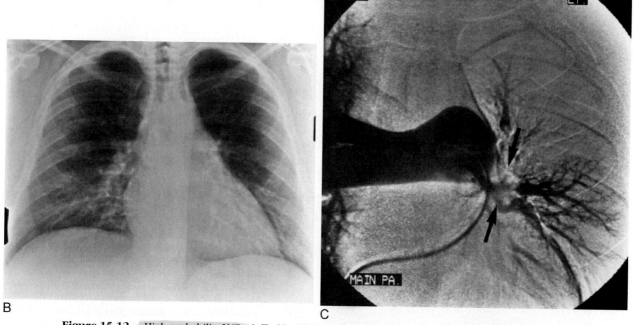

Figure 15-12 High-probability V/Q. **A,** Tc-99m MAA perfusion studies reveals absent perfusion to the left lower lobe and lingula as well as a moderate sized segmental defect in the right base and a small one in the right middle lobe. **B,** Corresponding chest x-ray was normal. **C,** Pulmonary arteriogram with injection of the main pulmonary artery shows the large left-sided clot. Some contrast is seen distal to the clot which does not completely occlude the involved arteries in this case.

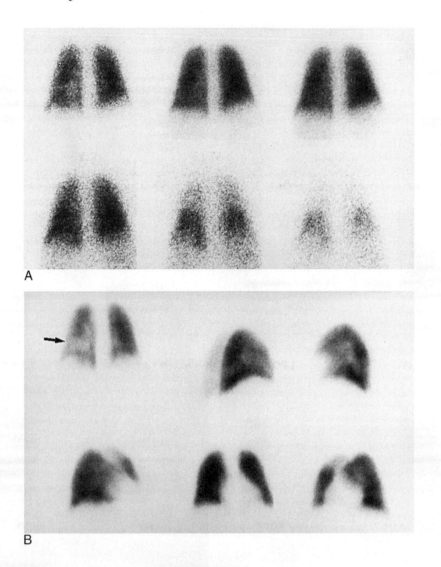

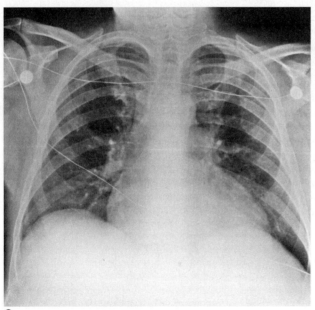

Figure 15-13   Low probability V/Q. **A,** Xe-133 ventilation images are normal on initial single breath and equilibrium images (*top row*) but bibasilar air trapping is seen on washout (*bottom row*). **B,** Tc-99m MAA shows a large area of relatively decreased perfusion in the left lower lobe (*arrow*) and a smaller area in the right base in the general area of ventilation abnormalities. **C,** The radiograph showed no abnormalities in these matched ventilation perfusion abnormalities.

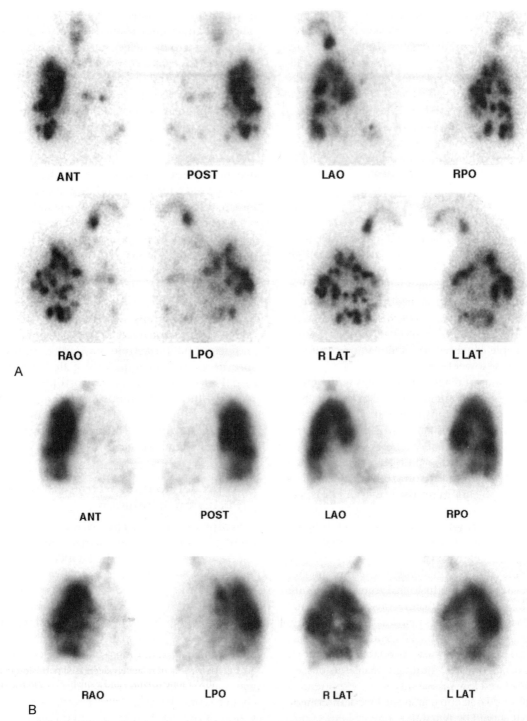

Figure 15-14   Low-probability V/Q. **A,** Tc-99m DTPA ventilation images reveal severely decreased ventilation to the right lung with essentially absent ventilation to the left lung. Significant clumping is present. **B,** Perfusion images show matching defects, although the abnormalities are less severe than the ventilation defects on the right. The clumping of the ventilation agent is seen faintly persisting.

perfused, it must be due to some other process such as pneumonia. On the other hand, a perfusion defect that is much larger than the x-ray abnormality is high probability.

Another case where the abnormal radiograph is important is the case of the so-called *triple match*. This is a segmental perfusion defect which is matched by ventilation and radiographic abnormalities. Although this combination has traditionally been placed in the intermediate category, such abnormalities in the upper lung fields are probably better categorized as low probability (Fig. 15-15).

Intermediate Probability

An abnormal study should be placed in the intermediate category if it does not meet the criteria for high or low/very-low probability groups (Fig. 15-16). A single moderate-to-large mismatched ventilation-perfusion defect is considered intermediate probability (Fig. 15-17). Also, when a matched ventilation-perfusion defect corresponds in size and shape to a radiographic abnormality (the so-called triple match), it is included in this category when located in the lower lobes.

The combinations of diagnostic findings in the intermediate category are too numerous to list. Essentially, if it cannot be placed in the low- or high-probability categories, it is intermediate probability. Theoretically, the risk of PE in the intermediate category could be anywhere between 20% to less than 80%. The actual incidence of PE in the intermediate probability category has been found to be 30–35% in retrospective and prospective studies.

Pleural effusions are a potential cause of isolated defects. How large and small effusions are categorized has changed over recent years and is still somewhat controversial. Some of the confusion is caused by the fact that PE often causes small effusions. Large effusions are rare in PE. However, large effusions obscure segmental perfusion. One report suggests that small effusions without other defects are low probability, and large effusions can be placed in the very-low probability category. However, the data is limited. Although small effusions are generally considered low probability, many experienced readers still place a large effusion in the low or intermediate category. It should be noted that a pleural effusion in PE is rarely present without other perfusion defects.

Special Signs

A number of special signs have been described to aid in V/Q scan interpretation. The *stripe sign* refers to a margin of radioactivity between a perfusion defect and the pleural surface of the lung (Fig. 15-18). Because the pulmonary circulation branches progressively toward the pleural surface, most pulmonary emboli result in pleural-based and wedge-shaped defects. The presence of activity distal to the defect suggests a parenchymal abnormality such as edema or other fluid collection is the cause rather than PE, and the exam can be placed in the very-low category. However, the stripe sign is often difficult to confirm and may be misleading. For example, if it is only seen in the lateral view, there may be overlap with normal lung.

The *swinging heart sign* refers to unusually large cardiac defects seen on lateral views when the patient has been imaged lying down and turned to the right and left for lateral views. The heart has some mobility within the chest and may compress a variable amount of tissue. This may create a confusing, changing pattern of activity depending on position.

Fluid in the pleural space can be difficult to recognize if the patient is imaged in a supine position. This fluid may layer out and can create an impression that one lung is generally hypoperfused if the effusion is asymmetric or unilateral. When patients are imaged in an upright position, fluid may collect in the major fissure in a curvilinear pattern called the *fissure sign* (Fig. 15-19). Blunting of the costophrenic angle from pleural fluid is commonly seen and positioning will alter the appearance of the effusion. Subpulmonic fluid can be missed if careful correlation with an upright radiograph is not done.

Approach to Interpreting the Ventilation-Perfusion Scintigram

A rigorous, systematic approach is needed when interpreting a V/Q scan. A summarized method of assimilating the data and applying the PIOPED criteria is outlined in Table 15-3. First, a current chest x-ray (within 24 hours) must be reviewed. Any radiographic signs of PE as well as alternative causes for the patient's symptoms such as pneumothorax or pneumonia should be sought. Any chest x-ray abnormality must be classified as acute or chronic. Acute findings such as atelectasis, infiltrates, and effusions in the area of perfusion abnormalities that may cause a triple-match V/Q defect are noted. Chronic change is unlikely to be related to PE. Cardiomegaly, elevation of the diaphragm, and hilar enlargement should be noted as they may cause nonsegmental defects.

After examining the chest radiograph, all segmental or subsegmental perfusion defects are identified on the perfusion scan and recorded by location. Decreased perfusion is considered abnormal as well as absent perfusion. The ventilation scan is then reviewed in the area of each perfusion defect. Each of these is, in turn, compared to the radiograph. If the perfusion defect has no radiographic explanation and the ventilation scan is normal, the mismatched

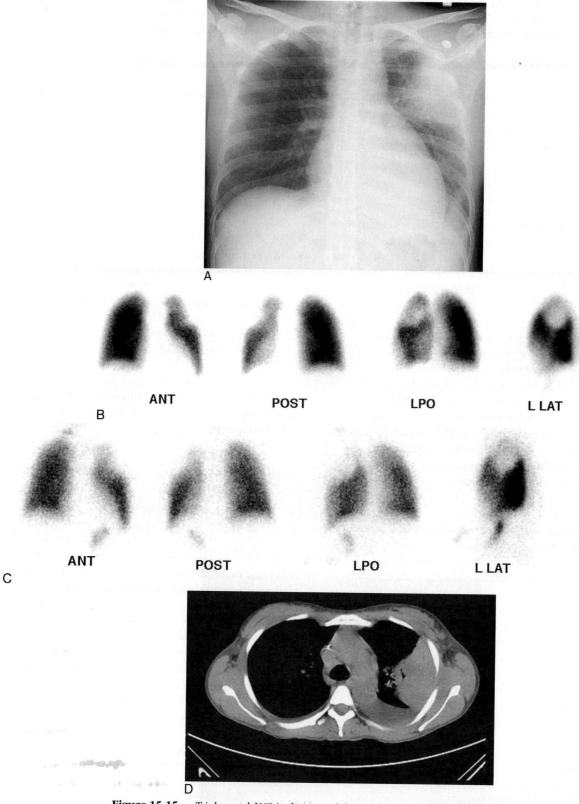

Figure 15-15   Triple match V/Q in the upper lobes. **A,** An AP radiograph raised suspicion for infarct with a large pleural-based upper-lobe wedge-shaped opacity as well as a left hazy-density from an effusion layering. **B,** Perfusion shows a large wedge-shaped perfusion defect in the left upper lobe and is seen as well as a mild overall decrease on the left corresponding to x-ray abnormalities. **C,** The ventilation images show complete matching of the abnormalities on the left. **D,** A noncontrast CT the next day also has the same left upper lobe consolidation and effusion. The clinical suspicion was low in this febrile, immunocompromised patient. The study was interpreted as low probability. The patient was later found to have aspergillosis not PE.

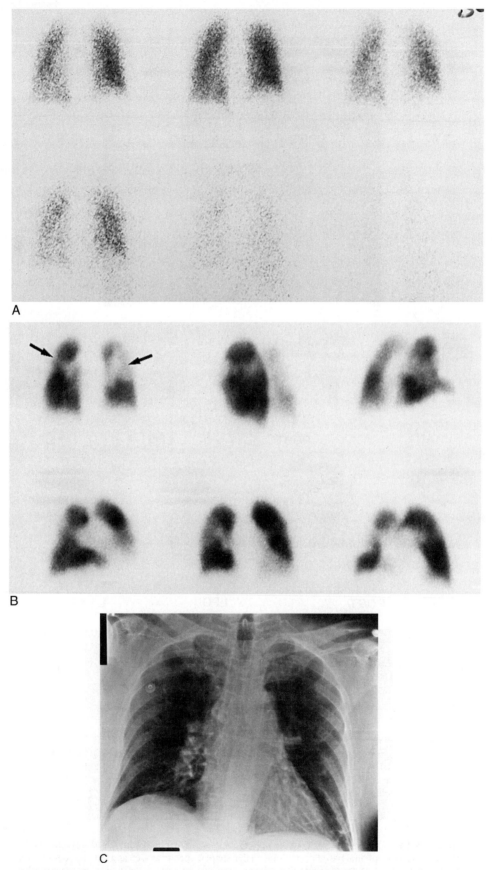

Figure 15-16 Intermediate probability V/Q. **A,** Ventilation images with Xe-133 were unremarkable. **B,** Perfusion defects are seen in the entire superior segment of the right lower lobe (*arrow*) and moderate-sized segmental defect on the left (*arrow*). **C,** The chest radiograph revealed no corresponding abnormality. The combination of one large and one moderate segmental mismatch places the study in the intermediate probability category.

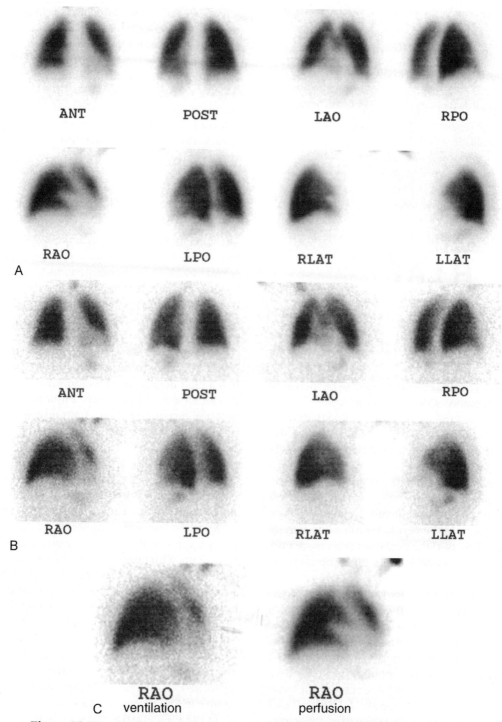

Figure 15-17   Single segmental perfusion defect. Intermediate probability V/Q. **A,** Perfusion images demonstrate a large defect in the medial segment of the right middle lobe. **B,** Ventilation was unremarkable. **C,** Close-up views show the utility of the anterior oblique view for visualizing anterior medial defects.

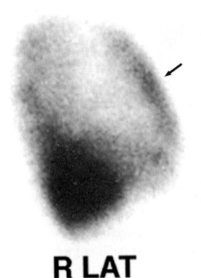

R LAT

Figure 15-18 Stripe sign. Perfusion on the right lateral view is seen anteriorly along the periphery of the lung beyond an area of decreased perfusion (*arrow*), strongly suggesting that the decreased perfusion in the upper lobe is not due to PE.

sites are candidates for PE. The likelihood of PE increases with increasing numbers of mismatched defects.

If no moderate or large segmental perfusion defects are demonstrated, attempts are made to categorize the study as low probability or less. Matched V/Q defects with no corresponding chest x-ray abnormalities have empirically been associated with a low probability of PE. If a case shows matched abnormalities with a clear chest x-ray, it is placed in the low probability category when they are numerous or in the very-low probability if there are one to three defects. If the perfusion defects are non-segmental, the study is considered to be in the very-low probability group.

When the radiograph is abnormal, the size of the abnormality is compared to the perfusion defect. If infarcted lung has resulted in an infiltrate, the perfusion defect is typically as large as or larger than the x-ray abnormality. Any perfusion defect with a *substantially* larger chest radiographic abnormality is in the low probability category. In practice, size comparisons may be difficult, and thus these criteria should be used cautiously and sparingly. Cases of triple-matched abnormalities on perfusion, ventilation, and radiographic studies could be considered intermediate probability. However, there is limited data suggesting that the chance that a pulmonary embolus is present also depends on the location of the defect. Abnormalities confined to the upper or middle lung zones less likely to be the result of an acute pulmonary embolus. Therefore, only triple-matched defects in the lower lung zones were intermediate probability, whereas such

defects in the upper and middle lung zones are low probability for PE (Table 15-4).

If the study cannot be categorized as normal, high probability or low/very-low probability, then it is placed in the intermediate probability category. When there are problems performing the ventilation scan, abnormal perfusion studies may be considered indeterminate. Also, indeterminate studies occur when posterior perfusion images cannot be obtained on portable studies performed at the patient's bedside.

Accuracy of Ventilation-Perfusion Scintigraphy

The agreement between readers for V/Q scan interpretation varies widely. Interobserver agreement is high for normal and high probability exams (90–95%). However, less agreement was seen deciding which studies should be intermediate probability or low probability (70–75%). Adherence to a strict set of criteria may help minimize variability between readers.

Clinical risk factor scores can be added to the V/Q interpretive process to improve accuracy. When clinicians had a high degree of suspicion for pulmonary embolus, the incidence of pulmonary embolus was increased to 96% among patients with a high probability. The clinical picture also had great impact among low probability exams. If the pretest suspicion for PE was high, the likelihood of PE was not less than 20% as might be expected but increased to 40%. On the other hand, when the clinical probability was low and the scintigraphic interpretation was normal or near normal, less than 2% had PE.

Another important observation from the PIOPED study is the low likelihood of an adverse clinical outcome in patients with normal and low probability scintigraphic patterns. In the study, 150 patients who had either a low probability or normal/near-normal scan but who did not undergo angiography were followed for at least 1 year. No patient had an adverse event or was readmitted for suspected PE. Some may well have had small pulmonary emboli, but none received anticoagulation therapy and the clinical course was unremarkable. This finding supports several other studies that suggest a benign clinical course in low probability cases.

In the PIOPED trial, the specificity of a high probability V/Q scan was 97% and the positive predictive value was 88%. However, the sensitivity for pulmonary embolus of a high probability scan is only 41%. This means the majority of patients with pulmonary emboli have an intermediate or low probability scan. This sensitivity is disappointing; if the criteria were relaxed, the sensitivity for PE would increase, but this would be at the expense of the specificity (Table 15-5). The high specificity of the high probability category allows initiation of antico-

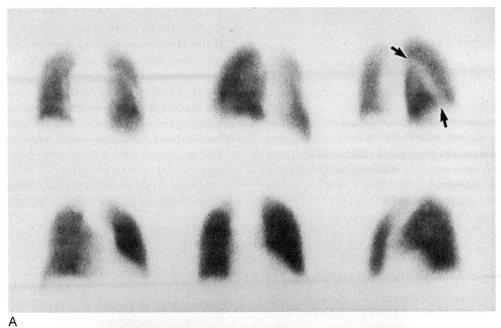

A

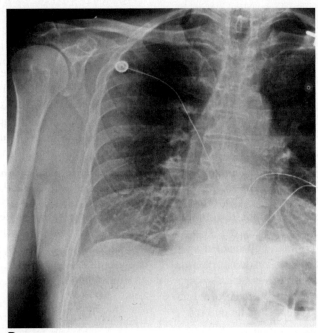

B

Figure 15-19   Fissure sign. **A,** Tc-99m MAA perfusion images show a curvilinear defect in the area of the major fissure of the right lung from the "fissure sign." **B,** Corresponding radiograph shows right costophrenic angle blunting but provides no indication of the extent of the fluid in the fissure.

agulation therapy in the appropriate clinical situation. Patients at risk for anticoagulation therapy may still require angiography.

Differential Diagnosis of V/Q Mismatches

The high probability category means there is a greater than 80% probability of pulmonary embolus. However, many processes can cause mismatched defects (Box 15-11). These can lead to false-positive readings. Of the potential causes of false-positive interpretations, or so-called PE mimics, one of the most common is an unresolved PE. Although PE typically resolves in younger patients, complete resolution is less common in the elderly. Portions of perfusion defects from pulmonary emboli may persist and remain mismatched. One study demonstrated that as many as 35% of acute emboli do not completely resolve. The positive predictive value of a high probability reading decreases from 91% in patients without prior PE to 74% in those with a history of prior PE.

The time course of defect resolution varies. After the acute event, mismatched defects generally persist for more than 24 hours. Large mismatched defects tend to decrease over time or fragment into smaller lesions in the periphery. Although exams may become normal in hours or days, abnormalities can persist for weeks or months. In fact, follow-up studies show that defects persisting at 3 months are likely to remain unresolved. After a high probability V/Q or a positive CTPA for PE, a follow-up V/Q is useful to establish a new baseline in the event that symptoms recur (Fig. 15-20). It is usually recommended that this new baseline is delayed for 3 weeks to 3 months to allow time for resolution.

Causes for mismatched defects other than PE are often discovered by taking a careful history. A patient may have a known hilar tumor, which could compress the pulmonary vessels, particularly the veins, before impacting the airway. Radiation effects and drug abuse are also common etiologies. Certain defined clinical situations may increase the possibility for septic emboli and fat emboli.

COMPUTED TOMOGRAPHY PULMONARY ARTERIOGRAPHY FOR THE DIAGNOSIS OF PULMONARY EMBOLI

Increasingly, CTPA is replacing the V/Q scan for the diagnosis of pulmonary emboli. Although the reported sensitivity of CTPA has varied greatly over recent years, from 36% to 100%, and early studies found poor detectability of subsegmental emboli. However, multidetector technology and interpretive experience have advanced rapidly. Recent multi-center data suggest that CTPA has a very high negative predictive value for pulmonary emboli, in the range of 99% (i.e., a negative study rules out pulmonary emboli). If a pulmonary vascular filling defect is seen, it is highly accurate for the diagnosis of pulmonary embolus.

The NIH-funded Prospective Investigation of Pulmonary Embolism II (PIOPED II) was initiated to determine the accuracy of CTPA for the diagnosis of PE as well as the added utility of CT venous examination of the pelvis and thighs. The results of this trial have not been reported as of this writing.

The V/Q scan has stood the test of time and remains an important diagnostic tool for the diagnosis of PE. It will continue to have an important role in patients with a history of contrast reaction, renal failure, pregnancy, and inconclusive results on CTPA.

OTHER APPLICATIONS OF VENTILATION-PERFUSION SCINTIGRAPHY

Quantitative Lung Scan

Quantification of lung perfusion and ventilation can be valuable in the preoperative assessment for operability of high-risk patients prior to planned lung resection for malignancy, dead-space lung volume reduction in severe COPD, and lung transplantation. This information is used in conjunction with respiratory spirometry (e.g., FEV_1, FVC). It can also be useful in assessing relative pulmonary perfusion before and after operations for congenital heart disease (e.g., correction of pulmonary stenosis).

Right to left lung differential function is commonly performed by acquiring the anterior and posterior views, drawing regions of interest around the right and left lungs and calculating the geometric mean to correct for attenuation (Fig. 15-22).

$$\text{Geometric mean} = \sqrt{\left(\text{counts}_{\text{anterior}} \times \text{counts}_{\text{posterior}}\right)}$$

However, the anterior and posterior views do not allow for good separation of the upper and lower lobes. Posterior oblique views allow clear separation of the upper and lower lobes (Fig. 15-23).

Adult Respiratory Distress Syndrome

The clearance of Tc-99m DTPA is significantly affected by the presence of pulmonary disease. The clearance half-time is approximately 45 minutes in healthy adults. Patients with adult respiratory distress syndrome have more rapid clearance, probably due to the rapid diffusion of Tc-99m DTPA across the airspace epithelium to the pulmonary circulation. Other conditions associated with

Table 15-3   Analysis of Ventilation Perfusion Scans

Perfusion defect(s)	Ventilation	Chest x-ray	Probability category
MODERATE TO LARGE			
≥ 2 segments (or equivalent)	Mismatch	Clear	High
< 2	Mismatch	Clear	Intermediate
	Match	Lower lung zone abnormality	Intermediate
	Match	Upper lung zone abnormality	Low
Multiple	Match	Clear	Low
SMALL (<25% OF A SEGMENT)			
> 3	N/A	Clear	Low
1–3	N/A	Clear	Very low
NONSEGMENTAL			
	N/A	Shows anatomical reason for perfusion abnormality	Very low
NONE			
	N/A	N/A	Normal

NA, Not applicable.

Table 15-4   Positive Predictive Value of Triple-Matched Perfusion Defects Based on Location

Lung zone	Defects from PE (%)	95% confidence interval
Upper	11%	3–26%
Middle	12%	4–23%
Lower	33%	27–41%

Table 15-5   V/Q Scan Sensitivity and Specificity

Probability category	Sensitivity (%)	Specificity (%)
High	41	97
High + intermediate	82	52
High + intermediate + low	98	10

increased Tc-99m DTPA clearance are cigarette smoking, alveolitis, and hyaline membrane disease in infants. This technique has not found a clear-cut clinical use.

Box 15-11   Conditions Associated with Ventilation-Perfusion Mismatch

Acute pulmonary embolus
Chronic pulmonary embolus
Other causes of embolism (septic, drug abuse, iatrogenic, fat)
Bronchogenic carcinoma (and other tumors)
Mediastinal or hilar adenopathy (with obstruction of pulmonary artery or veins)
Hypoplasia or aplasia of pulmonary artery
Swyer-James syndrome (occasional)
Postradiation therapy
Vasculitis

DETECTION OF DEEP VENOUS THROMBOSIS

Although the major thrust of this chapter is the diagnosis of PE, diagnosis of deep venous thrombi (DVT) is a related topic. Two tests no longer frequently utilized are traditional contrast venography and radionuclide venography. Radionuclide venography involved placing a tourniquet above the ankle and injecting radiopharmaceutical, Tc-99m MAA, into a small vein in the foot (Fig. 15-24). Although radionuclide venography is very sensitive above the knee, interpretation is difficult below the knee. Doppler sonography imaging in combination with various compression techniques is useful in the veins of the lower extremity above the knee. Contrast CT can be used to assess the pelvic veins. Images of the pelvis can be obtained after the pulmonary arterial imaging is completed. It may be technically difficult to time the study to achieve adequate venous opacification for diagnosis.

PIOPED II also examined utility of CTV for the pelvic and thigh veins. Preliminary reports found CTV to be 95% sensitive with a positive predictive value of 86% overall. However, the majority of lesions were found in the thighs. These would be potentially visualized by ultrasound without the exposure to ionizing radiation.

Various radiolabeled agents have been developed that bind to components of an active clot. These have included radiolabeled platelets, fibrin, and various peptides. Tc-99m apcitide (AcuTect) has been approved by the FDA for the diagnosis of DVT (Fig. 15-25). It is useful in patients with equivocal ultrasound findings or for the detection of thrombus in the calf. Tc-99m apcitide binds to a glycoprotein receptor (GpIIb–IIIa) in acute DVT.

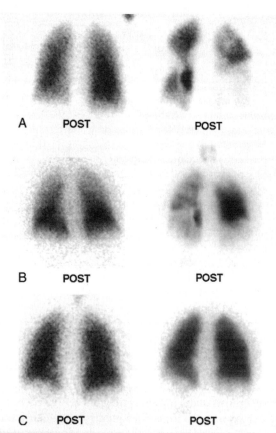

A POST POST

B POST POST

C POST POST

Figure 15-20 Resolution of PE. Normal ventilation images (*left*) and abnormal perfusion images (*right*) were obtained in the same patient at different times. **A,** The symptomatic patient had a high probability V/Q scan. **B,** Ten years later, recurrent symptoms led to another V/Q with marked mismatches. It is difficult to tell how many of these are new as no follow-up baseline study was performed after the original episode. **C,** Near complete resolution of these defects 7 days later confirms the mismatches were new and due to recurrent PE.

The protocol calls for intravenous injection of 20 mCi (740 MBq) of Tc-99m apcitide. Images of the calf, thigh, and pelvis are obtained at 10–15 minutes and 60–90 minutes. The reported sensitivity and specificity of Tc-99m apcitide varies, but is roughly 83% compared to contrast venography with a specificity of nearly 91%. It is not approved for the diagnosis of pulmonary emboli. The use of radiolabeled peptides in the diagnosis of pulmonary emboli continues to be investigated.

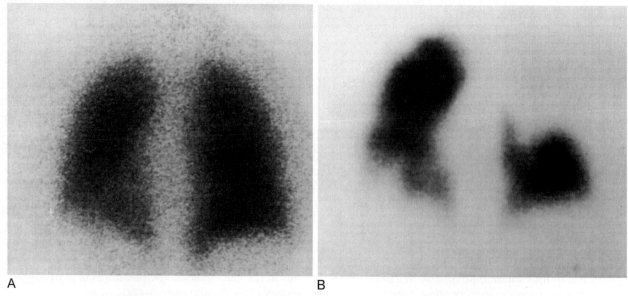

A

B

Figure 15-21 CT pulmonary arteriography. Posterior equilibrium ventilation image **(A)** and perfusion image **(B)** reveal an extensive mismatch in the left lung base and upper half of the right lung.

Continued

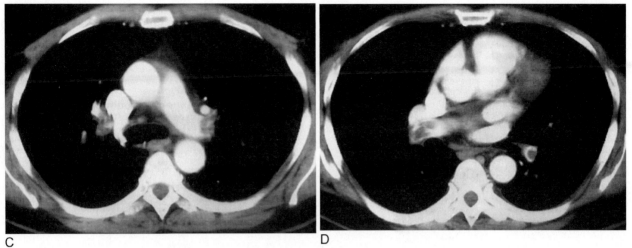

C   D

Figure 15-21, cont'd   C, Spiral CT shows contrast around a large partially obscuring clot in the left main pulmonary artery and right upper lobe pulmonary artery. **D,** Filling defects in the left descending pulmonary artery and right interlobar pulmonary artery are also present.

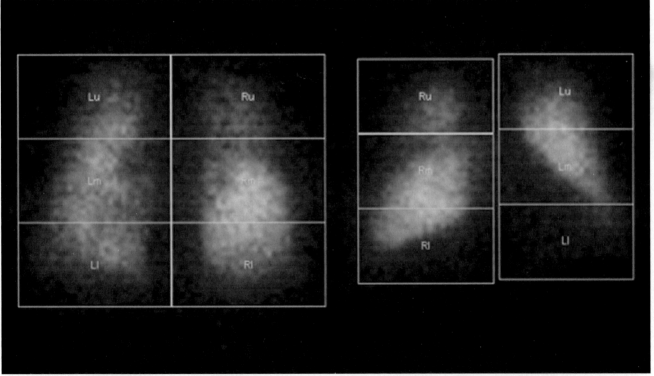

Figure 15-22   Preoperative quantitative lung scan. Anterior and posterior projections. Geometric mean quantification is performed for left to right lung differential function as well as upper, mid, and lower lung regions.

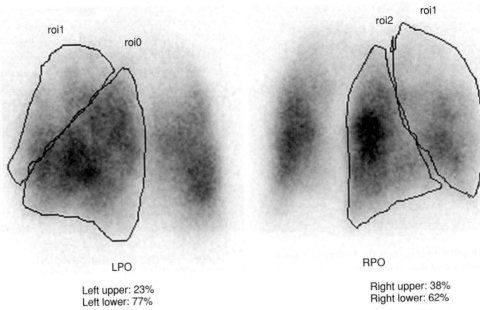

LPO

Left upper: 23%
Left lower: 77%

RPO

Right upper: 38%
Right lower: 62%

Figure 15-23   Quantitative lung scan with bilateral decreased function in the upper lobes in a patient with chronic obstructive pulmonary disease.

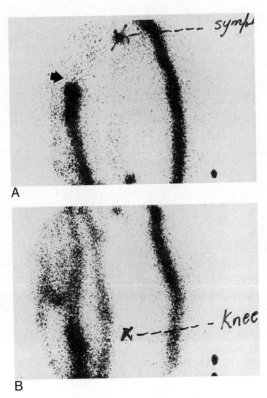

Figure 15-24   Abnormal radionuclide venogram patterns.
A, Venous obstruction (*arrow*) on the right caused by thrombus.
B, Extensive collateralization on the right indicates obstruction of the deep venous system.

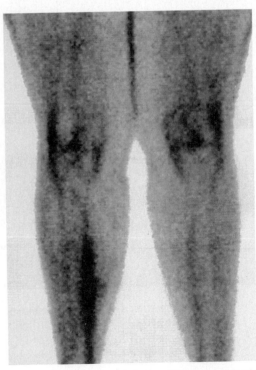

Figure 15-25   Acute thrombophlebitis with Tc-99m apcitide. Increased uptake is seen in the area of the right calf.

RECOMMENDED READING

Freeman LM, Krynyckyi B, Zuckier LS: Enhance lung scan diagnosis of pulmonary embolism with the use of ancillary scintigraphic findings and clinical correlation. Semin Nucl Med 31: 143-157, 2001.

Goldberg SN, Richardson DD, Palmer EL, Scott JA: Pleural effusion and the ventilation-perfusion scan interpretation for acute pulmonary embolus. J Nucl Med 37: 1310-1318, 1996.

Gottschalk A, Sostman HD, Coleman RE, et al: Ventilation-perfusion scintigraphy in the PIOPED study. Part II. Evaluation of the scintigraphic criteria and interpretation. J Nucl Med 34:1119-1126, 1993.

Gottschalk A, Stein P, Goodman LR, Sostman HD: Overview of prospective investigation of pulmonary embolism diagnosis II. Semin Nucl Med 32: 173-182, 2002.

Gray HW: The natural history of venous thromboembolism: impact on ventilation/perfusion scan reporting. Semin Nucl Med 32: 159-172, 2002.

Hatabu H, Uematsu H, Nguyen B: CT and MR in pulmonary embolism: a changing role for nuclear medicine in diagnostic strategy. Semin Nucl Med 32: 183-192, 2002.

Quiroz R, Kucher N, Zou KH, et al: Clinical validity of a negative computed tomography scan in patients with suspected pulmonary embolism: a systemic review. JAMA 293(16):2012-2017, 2005.

Stein PD, Henry JW, Gottschalk A: Mismatched vascular defects: an easy alternative to mismatched segmental equivalent defects for the interpretation on ventilation/perfusion lung scans in pulmonary embolism. Chest 104: 1468-1471, 1993.

Worsley DF, Alavi A: Comprehensive analysis of the results of the PIOPED study. Prospective investigation of pulmonary embolism diagnosis study. J Nucl Med 36: 2380-2387, 1995.

Worsley DF, Kim CK, Alavia A, Palevsky HI: Detailed analysis of patients with matched ventilation-perfusion defects and chest radiographic opacities. J Nucl Med 34:1851-1853, 1993.

Pearls, Pitfalls, and Frequently Asked Questions

This chapter reinforces concepts presented in this book. Every student of medicine gathers pearls of wisdom from his or her mentors that may not fit well into a didactic treatment of a subject but that are extraordinarily valuable in day-to-day practice. Likewise, we all learn to avoid pitfalls that arise in situations but that have escaped our formal education. Also, questions posed with interpretation require assembling multiple bits of information for a correct answer, and these questions never seem to be presented in quite the same way that subject material was presented didactically. By its nature, this chapter is neither comprehensive nor weighted to the relative importance of the topics.

RADIOPHARMACEUTICALS

Q: What relationship between the half-lives of a parent radionuclide and a daughter radionuclide is necessary for a generator system?

A: The parent radionuclide must have a long enough half-life to permit formulation and distribution of the generator. The daughter half-life must be reasonable for clinical application. A longer-lived parent decays to a shorter-lived daughter in all generator systems in use.

Q: How are parent and daughter radionuclides separated in generator systems?

A: Because the parent and daughter are different elements, they can be chemically separated.

Q: What is the major drawback of molybdenum-99 prepared by neutron activation?

A: When Mo-99 is prepared from Mo-98 by neutron activation, the two isotopes cannot be separated, and significant Mo-98 carrier exists in the preparation. This ultimately results in low specific concentration eluates of technetium-99m from the generator system.

Q: What is the difference between transient equilibrium generators and secular equilibrium generators?

A: In *secular equilibrium* generators, the half-life of the parent is far longer than the half-life of the daughter. If the generator system is left alone, the activity of the daughter becomes equal to that of the parent. In generator systems in which the parent half-life is 10 to 100 times that of the daughter, a condition of transient equilibrium occurs if the generator is not eluted. The point of *transient equilibrium* is defined as the time at which the ratio of the daughter and parent activities becomes a constant. Because the parent half-life is longer, the daughter appears to decay with the same half-life. The Mo-99/Tc-99m generator system is an example of transient equilibrium.

Q: What is the practical problem with having carrier Tc-99 in the generator eluate?

A: Tc-99 and Tc-99m behave identically from a chemical standpoint. Therefore, if there is excessive Tc-99 in the eluate, labeling efficiency can be impaired. For example, in a kit preparation using stannous chloride as a reducing agent, there may be unreduced Tc-99 and Tc-99m left in the preparation, with the consequent presence of radiochemical impurities in the final preparation.

Q: When is the buildup of Tc-99 at its highest?

A: Because Tc-99 has a far longer half-life than Tc-99m, the longer the interval between generator elutions, the greater the buildup of Tc-99. The first elution after commercial shipment or after a long weekend will have the highest content of Tc-99.

Q: What is the legal limit for Mo-99 in Tc-99m-containing radiopharmaceuticals?

A: The Nuclear Regulatory Commission limit is 0.15 mCi of Mo-99 activity per 1 mCi of Tc-99m activity in the administered dose.

Q: How does the ratio of Mo-99 to Tc-99m change with time?

A: In any preparation in which the radionuclidic contaminants have longer half-lives than the desired radionuclide label, the relative activity of the contaminant increases with time. This is an issue for iodine-123 preparations that have longer-lived radioiodine contaminants, as well as for the Mo-99 contamination in Tc-99m preparations.

Q: What is the purpose of stannous ion in Tc-99m labeling procedures?

A: Stannous ion is used to reduce technetium from a +7 valence state in pertechnetate to lower valence states necessary for labeling a wide range of agents. The development of this approach was a major breakthrough in nuclear pharmacy.

Q: What is Webster's rule in regard to the dose of a pharmaceutical to administer to a child?

A: It is based on the child's age: (age + 1)/(age + 7) × adult dose.

Q: What constitutes a medical event, formerly known as a misadministration of a radiopharmaceutical?

A: A *misadministration* was formerly defined by the NRC as a radiopharmaceutical given to the wrong patient, a patient receiving the wrong radiopharmaceutical, receiving the ordered radiopharmaceutical by the wrong route of administration, or the administered dose differing from the prescribed dose by greater than an allowable standard. Although these are all of concern and need discussion of quality assurance within a department and institution as well as a record of the event, the NRC now only requires reporting *medical events* where the effective dose equivalent to the patient exceeds 5 rem to the whole body or 50 rem to an individual organ or a diagnostic dose of I-131 exceeds 30 µCi.

Q: Describe the general response to the spill of radioactive material.

A: In general, the person who recognizes that a spill has occurred should notify all persons in the vicinity, and the area should be restricted. If possible, the spill should be covered. For minor spills, cleanup using appropriate disposable and protective clothing can be accomplished until background or near-background radiation levels are observed. For major spills, the source of the radioactivity should be shielded. For both major and minor spills, all personnel potentially exposed in the area should be surveyed, with appropriate removal of contaminated clothing and decontamination of skin. The radiation safety officer should be notified of all spills and has the primary responsibility for supervising cleanup for major spills and determining what reports must be made to regulatory agencies.

NUCLEAR MEDICINE PHYSICS

Pearl

Positrons are positive electrons, thus particles. With radioactive decay, an emitted positron travels 2–10 mm in tissue (depending on the radionuclide) before losing its kinetic energy, then interacting with an electron. The two particles annihilate each other and emit two 511-keV gamma photons at approximately 180-degree angles from each other. The gamma photons can be detected by positron emission tomography (PET) coincidence detectors. This conversion of mass to energy is predicted by Einstein's well-known formula: $E = mc^2$.

Q: What is the difference between x-rays and gamma rays?

A: Both x-rays and gamma rays are types of ionizing radiation. By definition, x-rays originate outside the atomic nucleus, and gamma rays originate inside the atomic nucleus. The respective energy spectra for x-rays and gamma rays substantially overlap at the high-energy end of the spectrum for all forms of electromagnetic radiation.

Q: What is the energy equivalent of the rest mass of an electron?

A: 511 keV. This is also the energy equivalent of a positron (positive electron).

Q: What is the difference between the rad, roentgen, and rem?

A: These terms are frequently confused with each other but have important distinctions. *Rad* stands for radiation absorbed dose. A rad is equal to the absorption of 100 ergs per gram of absorbing material. The rad is the traditional unit of absorbed dose. The gray (Gy) is the unit of absorbed dose in the International System of Units (SI). One gray = 100 rads.

    Rem is an acronym for *r*oentgen *e*quivalent *m*an. The rem is calculated by multiplying the absorbed dose in rads by a factor to correct for the *relative biological effectiveness* (RBE) of the type of radiation in question. The rem is the traditional unit. In the SI system, the term *sievert* (Sv) is used. One sievert = 100 rem.

    The roentgen (R) is a unit of radiation exposure. It is defined as the quantity of x-radiation or gamma radiation that produces one electrostatic unit of charge per cubic centimeter of air at standard temperature and pressure. In the SI system, radiation exposure is expressed in terms of coulombs per kilogram (C/kg). One roentgen is equal to 2.58 ¥ 104 C/kg air.

Q: Which is more penetrating in soft tissues, alpha particles or beta particles of the same kinetic energy?

A: Alpha particles have very low penetration in soft tissue because of their rapid loss of kinetic energy through interaction of their electrical charge with electrons in the tissues. Beta particles of the same respective kinetic energy of alpha particles have higher velocity, lower mass, and a single negative charge. They demonstrate significantly greater penetration in soft tissues, although penetration still is typically measured in millimeters.

Q: Define the two systems for expressing radioactive decay.

A: The traditional unit of radioactive decay is the *curie* (Ci). One curie is equal to 3.7×10^{10} disintegrations per second (dps). This number was derived from the decay rate of 1 gram of radium. (Modern measurements indicate that the actual decay rate for 1 gram of radium is 3.6×10^{10} dps.) In the SI system, decay is expressed in becquerels (Bcq). One becquerel equals one disintegration per second.

Q: How are the half-life and the decay constant related?

A: The physical *half-life* ($T_{1/2}$) of a radionuclide is defined as the time for half the atoms in a sample to decay. The half-life is expressed in units of time, typically seconds, minutes, hours, days, or years. The *decay constant* indicates the fraction of the sample decaying in a unit of time. The units of the decay constant are "per unit time" (per second, per hour). Mathematically, the half-life ($T_{1/2}$) and the decay constant (λ) are related by the following equation:

$$T_{1/2} = \frac{\ln 2}{\lambda}$$

Q: Which is longer, the biological half-life or the effective half-life?

A: The effective half-life is always shorter than either the biological half-life or the physical half-life because biological clearance and physical decay take place simultaneously. In calculation of radiopharmaceutical dosimetry, the conservative assumption is sometimes made that the biological half-life is infinite. This is probably never completely correct but simplifies calculations because the effective half-life may be taken simplistically as the physical half-life.

Q: After a photon has undergone Compton scattering, how does the energy of the scattered photon compare to the original photon energy?

A: In Compton scattering, the photon gives up energy to a recoil or Compton electron. The "scattered" photon has correspondingly lower energy. The amount of energy lost increases as the angle of scattering increases.

Q: What factors speed up or slow down radioactive decay?

A: Unlike chemical reactions, radioactive decay is a physical constant that cannot be sped up or slowed down by heating or cooling a specimen or by applying other physical or chemical influences.

Q: How many observed counts are necessary to have a percent fractional standard deviation of 5%, 2%, and 1%, respectively?

A: 400, 2500, and 10,000 counts, respectively.

Q: What is the maximum number of electrons that can occupy the outermost shell of an atom?

A: Eight.

Q: What special term is used to designate the electrons in the outermost shell of an atom?

A: They are called *valence* electrons and are responsible for many of the chemical characteristics of the element.

Q: What is the binding energy of an electron?

A: *Binding energy* refers to the amount of energy required to remove that electron from the atom. Electrons in shells close to the nucleus have higher binding energy than electrons farther from the nucleus. This energy is typically expressed in terms of electron volts (eV). Remember that the binding energy for each electron shell and subshell is characteristic for the respective element; the higher the atomic number of the element, the greater the binding energy for each shell and subshell.

RADIATION DETECTION AND INSTRUMENTATION

Q: What are some examples of the uses of ionization chambers in nuclear medicine?

A: Ionization chambers are often used in radiation survey meters and some pocket dosimeters. The radionuclide dose calibrator incorporates an ionization chamber.

Q: What is the purpose of the thallium impurity added to sodium iodide crystals?

A: The thallium is used to "activate" the sodium iodide crystal. The thallium impurity provides "easier" pathways for the return of electrons from the conduction band of the crystal to the valence bands of atoms.

Q: What is the relationship between photon energy and detection efficiency in a sodium iodide crystal?

A: For a given crystal size, detection efficiency decreases with increasing photon energy.

Q: Why do photopeaks appear as bell-shaped curves in pulse height spectra rather than as discrete spikes corresponding to the energy of the gamma ray?

A: Although gamma rays have discrete energies, the detection process is subject to statistical factors at each step of the process. The bell-shaped curve corresponding to the gamma ray photopeak reflects these statistical variations, which results in different events being measured as having slightly different energies. The better the "energy resolution" of a pulse height analyzer, the narrower the bell-shaped curve.

Q: In using a gamma scintillation camera, what does it mean to "set" the energy window?

A: Gamma cameras are equipped with pulse height analyzers that allow the operator to select a range of observed energies for accepting photons to be used in making the scintigraphic image. The "window" is usually described by giving the photopeak energy of interest and a percentage range that defines the limits of acceptance above and below the photopeak energy. A typical window for the 140-keV photon of technetium-99m is 20%, or ±14 keV.

Q: What are the causes of homogeneous flood field images in gamma camera quality control?

A: Causes include improper photomultiplier tube voltage adjustment, off-peak camera pulse height analyzer setting, crystal imperfections or damage, poor coupling of the crystal and the photomultiplier tubes, and inadequate mixing of radioactive tracer in the flood phantom.

Pitfall

Some nuclear medicine clinics use radioactivity in the patient to confirm the window setting. This can be a pitfall because scattered photons are included in the observed spectrum and can actually shift the apparent location of the photopeak. Ideally, a sample of the radionuclide to be imaged should be used for "peaking" in the gamma camera energy window.

Q: What effects do Compton-scattered photons have on scintigraphic image quality?

A: Compton-scattered photons are the enemy! Scattered photons that fall within the acceptance limits of the energy window are included in the image. They represent false data because they are recorded in a different spatial location than the origin of the primary photon. Thus Compton scattering reduces image contrast and spatial resolution. Also, Compton-scattered photons falling outside the energy window still must be processed by the gamma-camera pulse-height analyzer circuitry. These rejected events contribute to dead time and reduce the count rate capability of gamma cameras.

Q: What photons are desired in the scintigraphic image?

A: Primary (unscattered) photons that arise in the organ of interest in the body and travel parallel to the axis of the gamma-camera collimator field-of-view are the photons desired in the image. Intuitively, one may think of these as "good" photons. All other photons are "bad" photons. These include primary (unscattered) photons that arise in the object or organ of interest but travel "off axis," primary photons that arise in front of or behind the organ of interest (background photons), and all scattered photons.

Q: What is the purpose of the collimator?

A: The collimator defines the geometric field-of-view of the gamma-camera crystal. Off-axis photons, whether they are primary photons or scattered photons, are absorbed in the septa of the collimator.

Pearl

Pinhole collimators allow resolution of objects below the spatial resolution of the gamma camera through geometric magnification.

Q: What is the construction difference between a low-energy all-purpose collimator and a low-energy high-resolution collimator?

A: A high-resolution collimator has more holes that are smaller and deeper.

Q: How does poor energy resolution degrade spatial resolution?

A: Gamma cameras with poor energy resolution have reduced ability to reject scattered photons on the basis of pulse height analysis, as well as reduced ability for accurate determination of x and y coordinates for spatial localization of events.

SPECT AND PET

Pearl

Most nuclear medicine departments use 180-degree SPECT acquisition for cardiac studies and 360 degrees for imaging other organs, including the brain.

Pearl

For SPECT imaging the highest resolution collimator that provides sufficient count rate should be selected.

Pitfall

Besides equipment factors, patient motion is the most important cause of image degradation in SPECT and PET studies.

Q: What special importance does the biological half-life of a radiotracer have in SPECT imaging?

A: In SPECT imaging, data are acquired sequentially from different sampling angles. If significant biological redistribution of a radiopharmaceutical takes place between the start of data acquisition and completion, the reconstruction of tomographic images can be significantly distorted.

Q: What is a filter?

A: Filters are special mathematical functions applied to SPECT and PET data that enhance desired characteristics in the image, such as background subtraction, edge enhancement, and suppression of statistical noise. The ramp filter is designed to eliminate or reduce the star artifact.

Q: What is the star artifact in SPECT and PET reconstruction?

A: A star artifact results from simple unfiltered backprojection of a point source.

Q: What are the two basic approaches to attenuation correction?

A: The two basic approaches are the analytical or mathematical approach and the empirical approach. In the analytical approach, attenuation correction is estimated from a model of the body part under investigation. In the empirical approach, attenuation correction is accomplished by direct measurement using transmission scanning.

Pearl

One of the great advantages of SPECT and PET is the ability to perform flexible reformatting of image data in multiple image planes. For cardiac imaging, short-axis, vertical long-axis, and horizontal long-axis views of the heart are typically obtained.

Pearl

Two quick ways of assessing patient motion during SPECT imaging are to view the projection images as a cinematic closed-loop display and to create slice sinograms. In the cinematic display, patient motion is seen as a flicker from one projection image to another. On sinograms, patient motion is seen as a discontinuity in the stacked projection profiles.

Pitfall

SPECT is subject to a number of artifacts. Field flood nonuniformity can result in ring artifacts. Center-of-rotation misalignment causes loss of image resolution and if severe, ring artifacts.

Pearl

PET imaging relies on the coincidence detection of the two gamma ray photons given off simultaneously during a positron annihilation event.

Pitfall

The higher the overall count rate in PET imaging, the more likely the recording of "false" events owing to the presence of paired random events that appear to the detection circuitry as paired annihilation photons.

Pearl

The spatial resolution of PET is twice or more that of SPECT.

Pitfall

Spatial resolution in PET is limited by positron travel in soft tissue before annihilation and photon emission.

Pearl

PET imaging with transmission attenuation correction and detector sensitivity calibration allows absolute quantitative uptake determinations.

Pearl

Positron emitters, such as carbon, nitrogen, oxygen, and fluorine (as replacement for hydrogen) make possible the potential radiolabeling of any biological compound. The chemistry for developing and radiolabeling single-photon radiopharmaceuticals is usually considerably more complex.

ENDOCRINE

Q: What is the origin of lingual and sublingual thyroid tissue?
A: The main thyroid anlage begins as a downgrowth from the foramen cecum. Thyroid tissue may be seen anywhere along the tract of the thyroglossal duct from the foramen cecum to the usual location of the gland. However, with lingual thyroid tissue, there is usually a failure of normal development and no tissue in the normal location of the thyroid.

Q: What is meant by the "organification" of iodine?
A: In thyroid metabolism, iodide is oxidized to iodine and incorporated into tyrosine to form either monoiodotyrosine or diiodotyrosine. A deficiency in peroxidase, which catalyzes the reaction, is a cause of congenital hypothyroidism.

Q: What is the difference in mechanism of thyroid uptake between Tc-99m pertechnetate and radioiodine?
A: Radioiodine is taken up or extracted (trapped) by the thyroid follicular cell and organified, binding to tyrosine residues on thyroglobulin and stored in colloid of the follicle. Tc-99m pertechnetate is trapped but not organified.

Q: What has happened to the range for normal percent thyroid uptake of radioiodine in the United States over the last 50 years?
A: The normal range has dropped significantly owing to iodination of salt and the use of iodine in other foods. In many laboratories, the range was 20–45% as recently as the mid-1960s but is now 10–30% at 24 hours.

Pearl

Radioiodine is administered orally. Tc-99m pertechnetate is administered intravenously.

Pitfall

A potentially serious pitfall is to confuse microcuries with millicuries.

Pearl

The following are the approximate adult doses of I-131 and I-123 used for uptakes, scans, and therapy. Serious consequences can result from confusing these doses, particularly if a therapeutic dose is administered instead of a diagnostic dose. I-131 uptake (10 microcurie [μCi]), I-123 uptake (100 μCi), I-123 scan (400 μCi), I-131 scan (50 μCi), I-131 therapy for Graves' disease (10 millicuries [mCi]), and thyroid cancer (75–200 mCi).

Q: What is the normal distribution of radioiodine and Tc-99m pertechnetate?
A: Radioiodine is taken up by the thyroid, salivary glands, stomach, and excreted by the kidneys. Tc-99m pertechnetate has identical uptake and clearance, except that it is not organified, and thus remains in the thyroid for a considerably shorter time.

Q: Which are common causes of falsely low thyroid uptakes?

A: Patients taking thyroid hormones, iodine-containing drugs, or recent administration of intravenous iodine containing radiographic contrast.

Pearl

Synthroid should be discontinued for 4 weeks prior to a thyroid uptake or scan and Cytomel 2 weeks prior. CT intravenous iodine contrast agents should not have been received within 6–8 weeks.

Q: Which drugs are used clinically to block unwanted thyroid uptake of radioiodine, such as from administered diagnostic I-131 MIBG (metaiodobenzylguanidine) or therapeutic I-131 Bexxar (tositumomab)?

A: Iodine as supersaturate potassium iodide (SSKI) or perchlorate, a nonvalent ion, that competitively binds iodine trapping.

Q: What is the difference between and thyroid scan and thyroid uptake?

A: A thyroid uptake is usually a nonimaging study using a gamma-detector probe, whereas a thyroid scan results from gamma-camera imaging.

Pearl

Swallowed activity from salivary secretions on radiopertechnetate scans occasionally remains in the esophagus and can be confusing. The nature of the activity is readily established by having the patient drink water, followed by reimaging of the thyroid gland.

Q: How can a thyroid uptake test differentiate the two most common causes of thyrotoxicosis, Graves' disease and subacute thyroiditis? Why?

A: In the initial phase of subacute thyroiditis, thyroid hormones are released from the inflamed gland causing thyrotoxicosis. Due to pituitary feedback, TSH is suppressed. Radioiodine or Tc-99m uptake requires TSH stimulation. Thus, the uptake of radioiodine or Tc-99m pertechnetate is low or suppressed. With Graves' disease, TSH is suppressed; however, the gland is autonomous and the uptake is high.

Q: What is the mechanism of action of antithyroid drugs propylthiouracil (PTU) and methimazole (Tapazole)?

A: Both PTU and methimazole are thiourea antithyroid drugs that block the organification of iodine.

Q: What medical conditions are associated with an increased incidence of paragangliomas (pheochromocytomas)?

A: Both forms of multiple endocrine neoplasia type II are associated with pheochromocytoma, as are von Hippel-Lindau disease and neurofibromatosis.

Pitfall

Autonomous nodules are not synonymous with toxic nodules. Patients with small autonomous nodules (less than 3 cm in diameter) are most often euthyroid. The incidence of thyroid cancer in a patient with a single cold nodule is 15–20%, a multinodular goiter, 5%, and a hot nodule, less than 1%.

Q: Which radiopharmaceutical is used most commonly to localize a clinically diagnosed parathyroid adenoma? Describe its characteristic and diagnostic pharmacokinetics.

A: Tc-99m sestamibi is taken up by both thyroid and hyperfunctioning parathyroid tissue; however, it is typically cleared faster by the thyroid, thus the rationale for early (15 minutes) and delayed (2 hour) imaging. At early imaging uptake in the thyroid is dominant, whereas a hyperfunctioning parathyroid may not be apparent, or may be seen as focal hot uptake, particularly if adjacent to the thyroid. On delayed imaging, only the parathyroid uptake is dominant.

Pearl

The most common false positive for parathyroid scanning is a thyroid adenoma. Benign and malignant tumors are other causes for false-positive scintigraphy.

BONE

Q: What are the potential impurities in technetium-labeled diphosphonate compounds, based on their biodistribution?

A: Activity in the oropharynx, thyroid gland, and stomach suggests free unlabeled Tc-99m pertechnetate. Activity in the liver suggests a colloidal impurity. Rarely, activity is seen in the gut, the result of excretion of activity through the biliary system. The mechanism is not understood. Other increased soft tissue or renal activity is usually caused by a disease process rather than tracer impurity.

Q: What percentage of the Tc-99m-labeled compounds is retained in the skeleton at the usual time of imaging?

A: In normal adult subjects, 40–60% of the injected dose is in the skeleton 2–3 hours after tracer administration.

Pitfall

The greatest pitfall in interpreting bone scans is failure to understand its inherent nonspecificity. In our zeal "not to miss the cancer," many incidental areas of abnormally increased tracer accumulation are incorrectly attributed to metastatic disease. The most common pitfalls are diagnosing areas of arthritis or prior trauma as metastases. Correlative radiographs are often indicated.

Q: Which factors favor osteoarthritis versus metastatic disease as the cause of increased activity?

A: Osteoarthritis has characteristic locations in the extremities. Because metastatic lesions are relatively rare below the proximal femurs or beyond the proximal humeri, osteoarthritis should be considered first in the elbows, wrists, hands, knees, and feet of older patients. Involvement of both sides of a joint is common in arthritis but unusual in metastatic disease. The lower lumbar spine is the most problematic area because both arthritis and metastases are common there.

Q: What is the distribution of metastatic deposits from epithelial primary malignancies in the skeleton?

A: A rule of thumb is that 80% of metastases are found in the axial skeleton (spine, pelvis, ribs, and sternum). The remaining metastases are distributed equally between the skull (10%) and the long bones (10%).

Pearl

Metastases from lung cancer are the most common cause of metastases in the distal extremities, such as the hands.

Pearl

The majority of epithelial tumor metastases localize first in the red marrow. The skeletal tracers do not localize in the tumor tissue but rather in the reactive bone around the metastatic deposits.

Pitfall

A small amount of activity is frequently seen at the injection site; this should not be confused with a metastatic lesion. Likewise, variable degrees of urinary contamination on the skin may be superimposed on skeletal structures and confused with activity caused by metastatic disease.

Pearl

In many diseases, the bone scan has a very high sensitivity for detection of bone metastases. Sensitivity is lower in tumors with a lytic rather than blastic response, such as multiple myeloma, thyroid cancer, renal cell carcinoma. The bone scan is also less sensitive for tumors that preferentially go to bone marrow, such as lymphoma.

Q: How can the radiation dose to the bladder, ovaries, and testes be reduced?

A: The radiation dose to these structures is largely caused by radioactivity in the bladder. Frequent voiding reduces the radiation dose.

Q: What factors distinguish a superscan resulting from metastatic disease from a superscan resulting from metabolic disease?

A: In the usual superscan resulting from metastatic disease, the increased uptake is restricted to the axial skeleton and the proximal parts of the femurs and humeri, the red marrow-bearing areas. In metabolic bone disease, the entire skeleton is typically affected with increased uptake seen in the extremities as well as in the axial skeleton. In some cases resulting from secondary hyperparathyroidism, increased activity will also be seen in the lung and stomach.

Pearl

Faint or absent visualization of the kidneys is one of the findings on superscans that should alert the observer. This may be misinterpreted as indicating lack of excretion of tracer through the kidneys. In cases of superscan resulting from metastatic disease, visualization of the kidneys is faint because: (1) the skeleton accumulates more tracer than usual, leaving less available for renal excretion, and (2) owing to the increased skeletal tracer uptake, the renal activity may actually fall below the gray-scale threshold. The presence of renal activity is readily established by adjusting the intensity setting window.

Q: What is the mechanism of the "flare" phenomenon?

A: In some patients treated with chemotherapy for metastatic disease, regression of the tumor burden is associated with increased osteoblastic activity, presumably caused by skeletal healing in response to chemotherapy. This can appear on skeletal scintigrams as a paradoxical increase or apparent "worsening" of the abnormal tracer uptake, which may last for up to 6 months after therapy.

Q: What is the postmastectomy appearance of the thorax?

A: With radical mastectomy, the majority of the soft tissue is removed from the corresponding anterior thorax. The ribs appear "hotter" than on the contralateral side. This is probably caused by less attenuation of rib activity by soft tissue. Note, however, that if the patient is imaged with a prosthesis in place, the rib activity may be attenuated.

Q: What factors contribute to prolonged fracture positivity on scintigrams?

A: Displaced and comminuted fractures and fractures involving joints tend to have prolonged positivity scintigraphically. Elderly patients have delayed healing.

Q: What factors favor shin splints versus stress fracture scintigraphically in the tibia?

A: Stress fractures are classically focal or fusiform. The uptake can involve the entire width of the bone or extend partially across the shaft of the bone. Shin splints are classically located along the posterior medial tibial cortex and involve a third or more of the length of the bone. In pure shin splints, a focal component should not be present and superficial linear activity runs parallel to the long axis of the bone.

Q: The three-phase bone scan is used to diagnose osteomyelitis. What are other causes for a positive three-phase scan?

A: Recent fracture, tumor, Charcot's joint, and soft-tissue infection overlying chronic noninfectious bone disease.

Pitfall

False-negative scintigrams may be seen in neonates with osteomyelitis. Neonates may even have cold lesions. False negatives may also be seen in very old or debilitated patients and in patients who have received a course of antibiotic therapy before scintigraphy is performed.

HEPATOBILIARY

Q: What are the two FDA-approved technetium-99m iminodiacetic acid analog (IDA) radiopharmaceuticals in clinical use, and how are they different?

A: Tc-99m DISIDA (disofenin) and Tc-99m mebrofenin (Choletec). The latter has better hepatic extraction, 98% versus 88%, and less renal excretion, 1% versus 9%. The higher extraction of mebrofenin is preferable in patients with hepatic insufficiency.

Pearl

Tc-99m IDA is extracted by the same cellular mechanism as bilirubin but it is not conjugated. The radiopharmaceutical then follows the path of bile through the biliary system into the bowel.

Pearl

The alternative route of excretion for Tc-99m IDA radiopharmaceuticals is via the kidneys. The amount of excretion is usually small but increases with hepatic dysfunction.

Q: What is the most important question to ask a patient before starting cholescintigraphy for suspected acute cholecystitis, and why?

A: "When did you last eat?" If the patient has eaten in the last 4 hours, the gallbladder may be contracted secondary to endogenous stimulation of cholecystokinin (CCK), and therefore radiotracer cannot gain entry into the gallbladder. If the patient has not eaten in more than 24 hours, the gallbladder may not have had the stimulus to contract and will be full of thick, concentrated bile, which may prevent tracer entry.

Pearl

It is also important to ask *what* the patient ate. The meal must have contained 10 grams of fat in order to contract the gallbladder.

Q: What are four indications for CCK infusion?

A: (1) To empty gallbladder in a patient fasting longer than 24 hours. (2) To differentiate common duct obstruction from functional causes. Delayed imaging could be used as an alternative. (3) To exclude acute acalculous cholecystitis if the gallbladder fills in a patient strongly suspected of having the disease. A diseased gallbladder will not contract, due to either acute or chronic disease. (4) To confirm or exclude chronic acalculous cholecystitis.

Q: Cholescintigraphy is a very sensitive and specific test for acute cholecystitis. In what clinical settings is there an increased incidence of false positive cholescintigraphy for acute cholecystitis?

A: In patients who have fasted less than 4 hours or more than 24 hours, those receiving hyperalimentation, and those who have chronic cholecystitis, hepatic dysfunction, or concurrent serious illness.

Q: What is the *rim sign* seen with cholescintigraphy, and what is its significance?

A: The *rim sign* is increased activity in the liver adjacent to the gallbladder fossa. This finding has been associated with an increased incidence of the complications, such as perforation and gangrene.

Pearl

Increased blood flow to the region of the gallbladder as a result of severe inflammation is sometimes seen with acute cholecystitis. In these cases, the rim sign is usually also seen.

Q: At what time after Tc-99m IDA injection is nonfilling of the gallbladder diagnostic of acute cholecystitis?

A: One hour is defined as abnormal. However, nonfilling of the gallbladder is diagnostic of acute cholecystitis if delayed images show no filling by 3 to 4 hours or 30 minutes after morphine administration.

Pearl

Delayed visualization is most commonly seen in chronic cholecystitis. It is also seen with hepatic dysfunction caused by altered pharmacokinetics, which is delayed uptake and clearance.

Q: What is the mechanism of morphine-augmented cholescintigraphy?

A: Morphine increases tone at the sphincter of Oddi, producing increased intraductal pressure. This results in bile flow preferentially through the cystic duct, if it is patent.

Q: What is the most common cholescintigraphic finding in chronic cholecystitis during routine cholescintigraphy?

A: A normal study. Less than 5% of patients with chronic cholecystitis have delayed filling. Other less common associated findings include delayed biliary-to-bowel transit time and, rarely, nonvisualization of the gallbladder or intraluminal filling defects. A reduced gallbladder ejection fraction is seen with symptomatic chromic cholecystitis.

Q: What is acute acalculous cholecystitis?

A: Acute cholecystitis without a stone occluding the cystic duct. The obstruction may be caused by debris or inflammatory changes, or the cholecystitis may be limited to the gallbladder wall because of infection, ischemia, or toxemia. This disease occurs in very sick hospitalized patients who have sustained trauma, burns, sepsis, or other serious illness and is associated with a high morbidity and mortality.

Pearl

The sensitivity of cholescintigraphy for acute *acalculous* cholecystitis is probably only approximately 75–85% compared with 98% for acute *calculous* cholecystitis.

Pearl

If the clinical suspicion for acute acalculous cholecystitis is high but the gallbladder visualizes, sincalide can be helpful diagnostically. Cholecystitis can be excluded if the gallbladder contracts. If it does not contract, the cause could be acute or chronic acalculous cholecystitis. A radiolabeled leukocyte study can confirm acute disease.

Q: The diagnosis of common duct obstruction is commonly made by sonographic detection of a dilated common duct. In what clinical situations would cholescintigraphy be useful?

A: In early acute obstruction before the duct has had time to dilate (24–48 hours), and in patients with previous obstruction or ductal instrumentation who have baseline dilated ducts. In both these situations, cholescintigraphy can be diagnostic.

Q: What are cholescintigraphic findings of high-grade common duct obstruction?

A: Prompt hepatic uptake but a persistent hepatogram without clearance into biliary ducts because of the high backpressure.

Q: What are the cholescintigraphic findings of partial common duct obstruction?

A: Retention of activity in the biliary ducts, delayed biliary-to-bowel clearance, and poor ductal clearance on delayed imaging or with sincalide.

Pearl

Delayed biliary-to-bowel transit is an insensitive and nonspecific finding for common duct obstruction. Delayed biliary to bowel clearance is seen in only 50% of patients with obstruction. On the other hand, delayed biliary-to-bowel transit may be seen in 20% of healthy subjects. It is also seen in patients pretreated with sincalide.

Pearl

Administration of sincalide will cause sphincter of Oddi relaxation, prompt biliary duct clearance and biliary-tobowel transit in patients with functional causes, but will remain abnormal in patients with partial common duct obstruction.

Pitfall

The methodology use for administering sincalide is diagnostically important. A bolus infusion may cause spasm of the neck of the gallbladder and ineffective emptying. Similarly, 1–3 minute infusions may result in poor contraction of the gallbladder in approximately one-third of normal subjects. Sincalide, 0.01–0.02 µg, should be infused slowly over 30–60 minutes.

Q: What ancillary maneuver increases the sensitivity of cholescintigraphy for detection of biliary atresia?

A: The administration of phenobarbital for 3–5 days before the HIDA activates the liver enzymes. A serum phenobarbital level should be in the therapeutic range before cholescintigraphy is started.

Q: How is the diagnosis of biliary atresia made with cholescintigraphy?

A: No clearance of Tc-99m IDA tracer is seen by 24 hours. Biliary clearance is consistent with other etiologies for neonatal hepatitis.

Q: What is the postcholecystectomy syndrome and what are common causes for it?

A: Recurrent biliary colic-like pain after cholecystectomy. Cystic duct remnant, retained or recurrent stone, inflammatory stricture, sphincter of Oddi dysfunction.

Pearl

Sphincter of Oddi dysfunction is essentially a partial biliary obstruction at the level of the sphincter without evidence of stone or stricture. Cholescintigraphy will show a pattern of partial biliary obstruction. The diagnosis is ultimately made by excluding stones or stricture with ERCP and the finding of elevated sphincter pressure with manometry.

Q: What is the difference in clinical presentation and clinical course of patients with focal nodular hyperplasia (FNH) and hepatic adenoma?

A: FNH is asymptomatic and found incidentally, whereas hepatic adenomas often present with hemorrhage can be life-threatening. Adenomas are closely associated with the use of oral contraceptives and they must be discontinued.

Q: What are the Tc-99m sulfur colloid scintigraphic findings in FNH and hepatic adenoma?

A: Hepatic adenomas do not usually show Tc-99m sulfur colloid uptake because they typically do not have Kupffer cells. FNH is associated with increased blood flow. With FNH, uptake is normal or increased in two thirds of patients; however, one third have no uptake.

Q: What are the cholescintigraphic findings in FNH, hepatic adenoma, and hepatoma?

A: FNH shows increased flow, normal uptake, and delayed focal clearance. Hepatomas are cold on early images but often fill on delayed images (2 hours). The hepatoma is functional, but hypofunctional compared with the normal liver. Hepatic adenomas do not typically have uptake.

Q: The specificity of Tc-99m-labeled red blood cells for diagnosis of cavernous hemangioma is very high. False positives are rare. What factors affect the sensitivity of the test?

A: Small size (less than 1.5 cm), attenuation (small central hemangiomas are harder to detect than superficial ones, hemangiomas adjacent to major vessels may be harder to detect), and methodology (SPECT is more sensitive than planar imaging).

Q: Which of the following statements is true in regard to the diagnosis of hemangiomas?
   a. Ultrasonography is neither sensitive nor specific.
   b. CT is not very sensitive when strict criteria are used and not specific when liberal criteria are used.
   c. MRI is sensitive, has a distinctive pattern (light bulb sign on T-2 weighted images), and is much more specific than CT or ultrasonography, although various other benign and malignant tumors may have an appearance similar to hemangioma.
   d. MRI is the method of choice for small lesions adjacent to large vessels.

A: All are true.

Q: What are the characteristic scintigraphic findings in liver hemangioma?

A: Blood flow is normal. Immediate images show a cold defect, whereas delayed images acquired 1–2 hours after tracer administration show increased uptake within the lesion compared with the normal liver, often equal to uptake in the spleen and heart. SPECT is mandatory for smaller lesions.

Q: In regard to regional intraarterial chemotherapy, which of the following statements is/are true?
   a. Hepatic arterial chemotherapy preferentially perfuses the tumor, with relative sparing of uninvolved liver.
   b. Systemic toxicity is directly related to the amount of chemotherapeutic agent that reaches the systemic circulation.
   c. The response to therapy can be predicted from Tc-99m macroaggregated albumin (MAA) hepatic arterial perfusion scintigraphy.
   d. Symptoms of drug toxicity can be easily differentiated clinically from the progression of liver metastases.

A: *a.* True. Tumor in the liver receives its blood supply primarily from the hepatic artery; the normal liver receives approximately 70% of its blood supply from the portal vein.
   b. True. For example, arteriovenous shunting will result in systemic exposure and toxicity.
   c. True. Evidence of proper catheter placement and perfusion of tumor nodules is associated with a good response to therapy.

d. False. Symptoms are identical. Only the Tc-99m MAA study can make that differentiation by determining the adequacy of perfusion and the presence or absence of extrahepatic perfusion.

Q: What is the significance of the extrahepatic perfusion seen on Tc-99m MAA hepatic arterial perfusion studies in patients receiving intra-arterial chemotherapy for liver metastases?

A: Extrahepatic perfusion of abdominal viscera, most often the stomach but also the bowel, pancreas, and spleen, is associated with a high incidence of adverse symptoms (nausea, vomiting, abdominal pain), about 45%, versus a 16% incidence of similar symptoms in patients treated identically but without evidence of extrahepatic perfusion on the Tc-99m MAA study.

GENITOURINARY

Q: What percentage of renal plasma flow is filtered through the glomerulus, and what percentage is secreted by the tubules?

A: Twenty percent of renal plasma flow is cleared by glomerular filtration and 80% by tubular secretion.

Q: Which nonradioactive drugs used to calculate glomerular filtration rate (GFR) and effective renal plasma flow (ERPF) are considered to be the reference standards?

A: Inulin for GFR and paraaminohippurate (PAH) for ERPF.

Q: Which radiopharmaceuticals are most often used clinically for measurement of GFR and ERPF?

A: Tc-99m diethylenetriamine pentaacetic acid (DTPA) for GFR. Iodine-131 orthoiodohippurate (OIH) was used for ERPF in the past. As I-131 OIH is not available commercially, Tc-99m MAG3 is currently used. However, Tc-99m MAG3 does not actually measure ERPF and a correction factor based on proportional clearance compared with I-131 OIH must be applied. Some sites report these values not as ERPF but as MAG3 clearance.

Q: What is the mechanism of renal uptake for I-131 OIH, Tc-99m mercaptylacetyltriglycine (MAG3), Tc-99m DTPA, Tc-99m dimercaptosuccinic acid (DMSA), and Tc-99m glucoheptonate (GH)?

A: Tc-99m DTPA, glomerular filtration; Tc-99m MAG3, tubular secretion; I-131 OIH, tubular secretion and glomerular filtration; Tc-99m GH, cortical binding and glomerular filtration; and Tc-99m DMSA, cortical binding.

Q: What is the percent cortical binding of Tc-99m DMSA and Tc-99m GH?

A: Tc-99m DMSA, 40–50%; Tc-99m GH, 10–20%.

Pearl

The two radiopharmaceuticals bind to the proximal convoluted tubules in the cortex.

Q: What is Webster's rule?

A: Pediatric radiopharmaceutical doses can be estimated using the formula $(age + 1)/(age + 7) \times$ adult dose.

Q: The time-to-peak activity of a renal time-activity curve (TAC) represents which of the following:
a. The end of extraction
b. The beginning of renal clearance
c. The time point at which the amount of cortical uptake of the radiopharmaceutical is equal to clearance

A: c. Uptake and clearance are occurring simultaneously over a period because of several factors that include an imperfect bolus, the percent first-pass extraction fraction of the radiotracer, the amount of recirculating radiotracer, and the normal variability of nephron function.

Pearl

Dehydration does not affect the first part of the time activity curve while later phases may be altered by many factors including dehydration and hydronephrosis.

Q: What is the proper renal region of interest (ROI) selection on the computer for the following:
a. Diuresis renography
b. Captopril renography

A: a. The ROI should include the dilated pelvis and the cortex. Because of hydronephrosis, the dilated collecting system counts predominate.
b. A whole kidney ROI is adequate if there is no pelvic retention. Lasix is often given with the radiopharmaceutical to ensure pelvicocalyceal clearance. When there is pelvicocalyceal activity, a peripheral two-pixel cortical ROI should be selected to avoid the effect of these counts on the TAC. A drop in GFR with captopril is manifested as deterioration in the cortical TAC (delayed peak and decreased function) when using Tc-99m DTPA or cortical retention when the radiotracer is Tc-99m MAG3. An identical ROI should be used for the baseline comparison study.

Q: Differential renal function is evaluated by drawing kidney and background ROIs. The relative uptake of the two kidneys after background correction is determined. Which time interval is used to calculate differential renal function for dynamic renal scintigraphy?
   a. Entire 30-minute study
   b. The 60-second flow study
   c. The time after the initial flow study
   d. Interval of 1–3 minutes

A: *d.* Because cortical uptake of the renal radiopharmaceutical is of interest, the optimal interval is after the initial flow but before the collecting system activity appears, usually 1–3 minutes. With good function, activity may be seen before 3 minute, especially in children. Radiopharmaceuticals with higher extraction also clear faster. Thus the 1–2 minute interval may be optimal overall. Ideally the clinician should review the dynamic frames to determine when calyceal clearance occurred and use the 60- to 90-second interval before that.

Q: What are the general methods for calculating absolute GFR?

A: Blood sampling, blood sampling and urine collection, and camera-based methods.

Q: At what step in the renin-angiotensin-aldosterone cascade does captopril work? In which organ does this occur?

A: Captopril blocks the conversion of angiotensin I to angiotensin II in the lungs.

Pearl

The usual captopril dose, 25 mg, although pharmacologically effective on the renal vasculature, is usually inadequate to produce peripheral vasodilation and hypotension. However, a patient may rarely develop hypotension, requiring prompt fluid administration to maintain intravascular volume and pressure.

Q: In renal artery stenosis the effect of captopril is manifested by a reduction in blood flow to the kidney that can be seen on radionuclide angiography. True or false?

A: *False.* Blood flow is not affected by captopril. If it is poor to begin with, it will remain poor. If it is normal, no change is seen. The compensatory mechanism for maintaining the glomerular filtration rate is renin dependent and results in decreased GFR after captopril administration.

Q: Which of these factors affects the accuracy of diuresis renography?
   a. State of hydration
   b. Renal function
   c. Dose of diuretic
   d. Radiopharmaceutical
   e. Bladder capacity

A: *All of the above.* Adequate hydration is required for good urine flow and adequate response to the diuretic. A full bladder may cause a functional obstruction. Intravenous hydration and urinary catheterization are strongly suggested, especially in children. Tc-99m DTPA, Tc-99m MAG3, and I-131 OIH have all been successfully used. Because of its better extraction efficiency and good image resolution, Tc-99m MAG3 is the agent of choice in renal insufficiency. Tc-99m DTPA works well in patients with good renal function. Renal insufficiency is a definite limitation to diuresis renography. The kidney must be able to respond to the diuretic challenge. Therefore the dose of diuretic must be increased in renal insufficiency, but the exact dose required is only an educated estimate.

Q: A good diuretic response rules out a partial obstruction. True or false?

A: *False.* Diuretic renography is often performed to determine the functional significance of a known partial obstruction, such as in patients with cervical or bladder cancer. A poor diuretic response indicates that intervention is indicated. With good clearance, no immediate intervention is required. Follow-up evaluations may be indicated.

Q: What is the most sensitive technique for diagnosing scarring secondary to reflux?

A: Tc-99m DMSA cortical imaging. Ultrasonography and intravenous urography have considerably lower sensitivity.

Q: How can radionuclide imaging differentiate upper from lower urinary tract infection, and why is this differentiation important?

A: With upper tract infection or pyelonephritis, Tc-99m DMSA shows tubular dysfunction, manifested by decreased uptake. This is a reversible process. With appropriate therapy, tubular will return in 3–6 months. Upper tract infection has prognostic implications because it may lead to subsequent renal scarring, hypertension, and renal failure.

Q: Why is radionuclide cystography preferable to the contrast method in most cases? What is the exception?

A: The radionuclide test is more sensitive for detection of reflux than contrast-enhanced voiding cystourethrography and results in much less radiation exposure (50- to 200-fold less) to the patient. The only exception is in the first evaluation of a male, when the better resolution of the contrast study can permit the diagnosis of an anatomical abnormality such as posterior urethral valves.

Pearl

Scintigraphy allows for calculation of bladder volumes and residuals. The residual activity in the bladder is calculated by one of two methods using a region of interest (ROI) around the bladder:

$$\text{Residual volume (ml)} = \frac{[\text{voided urine volume (ml)} \times \text{postvoid bladder counts}]}{[\text{initial bladder counts} - \text{postvoid bladder counts}]}$$

or

$$\text{Residual bladder volume (ml)} = \frac{[\text{postvoid bladder counts} \times \text{volume infused}]}{\text{initial bladder counts}}$$

Q: What is meant by "direct" versus "indirect" radionuclide cystography and which is the preferred method for detecting vesicoureteral reflux?

A: Direct cystography, that is, cystography requiring urinary tract catheterization and infusion of radiotracer into the bladder, is a more sensitive method for detecting vesicoureteral reflux. Reflux can be detected during bladder filling as well as voiding. In contrast, the indirect method, where a routine renogram is initially performed, cannot be used to detect reflux during the bladder filling stage because radiotracer is flowing through the collecting system antegrade.

Q: What is the most common developmental abnormality leading to testicular torsion?

A: The bell-clapper testis.

Pearl

The bell-clapper testis is a congenital abnormality and usually bilateral. Prophylactic surgery is performed on the asymptomatic side.

Q: What is the difference in blood supply to the testes and scrotum?

A: The testes receive blood predominantly from the testicular artery, whereas the scrotum receives its supply from the pudendal vessels.

ONCOLOGY—POSITRON RADIOPHARMACEUTICALS

Q: Which of these statements is true regarding fluorine-18 fluorodeoxyglucose (FDG) PET?
  a. F-18 FDG uptake is normally high in the brain and heart.
  b. The mechanism of F-18 FDG uptake and metabolism is identical to that of glucose.
  c. Oncology patients should fast for at least 4 hours prior to injection.
  d. Unlike glucose, F-18 FDG is excreted through the genitourinary system.

A: *a, c, d.* F-18 FDG enters the cell in a fashion similar to glucose but becomes trapped within the cell because it cannot progress further through the glucose enzymatic pathways.

Q: The most common indication for F-18 FDG PET is for the staging of lung cancer. Which of the following statements is false?
  a. The sensitivity for detection is high for tumors of 5 mm and greater in size.
  b. Sensitivity and specificity of FDG PET is higher than CT for mediastinal staging of lung cancer.
  c. False negatives may be seen with hyperglycemia.
  d. False negatives may occur with bronchoalveolar carcinoma.

A: *a.* The sensitivity for detection is reduced for tumor size less than 8–10 mm.

Q: The sensitivity of FDG PET is high for detection of many malignancies. For which of the following tumors is the sensitivity of FDG PET not high?
  a. Colorectal cancer
  b. Melanoma
  c. Hepatocellular carcinoma
  d. Renal cell carcinoma
  e. Lymphoma

A: FDG PET has poor sensitivity for primary hepatocellular carcinoma, renal carcinoma, as well as prostate cancer. This is less true of metastatic disease than primary tumors.

Pearl

For thyroid cancer imaging, I-131 is more sensitive than F-18 FDG for well-differentiated papillary or follicular thyroid carcinoma. In patients who have been treated with I-131 and have a negative I-131 whole-body scan on follow-up evaluation but have an elevated serum thyroglobulin, F-18 FDG PET has good sensitivity for detection of malignancy. The reason is that in this setting, the tumor has dedifferentiated into a higher grade malignancy.

Q: What are the advantages of CT PET over PET alone?
  a. Automated hardware and software fusion for anatomical localization
  b. Diagnostic CT at the same time as the PET scan
  c. CT is used for more rapid attenuation correction
  d. Eliminates false positive interpretations

A: *a, c.* Diagnostic CT (*b*) often requires contrast. Furthermore, to minimize radiation dose to the patient, 80 mA is commonly used, which reduces diagnostic quality. CT PET reduces false positives, but does not eliminate them (*d*).

Pearl

With CT PET, misregistration due to patient motion, respiratory motion, organ movement (bowel) can introduce potential false positive interpretations. PET is acquired at normal tidal volume breathing. CT with PET may be acquired with breath-hold or shallow breathing, leading to artifacts due to errors in anatomical registration and attenuation correction.

Q: What are some limitations of FDG PET in tumor staging?

A: PET imaging does not detect microscopic metastases, tumor involvement in local lymph nodes may be obscured by activity in an adjacent tumor, concurrent infection/inflammatory processes may cause false positives, and sensitivity for intracranial metastases is low.

Q: What are limitations of tumor restaging by PET?

A: Posttherapy effects of surgery, chemotherapy, and especially radiation therapy may cause increased F-18 FDG uptake, which can be confused with activity from active tumor. Even patients scheduled for imaging after an appropriate delay after therapy may require follow-up imaging. If activity is diminishing, this helps confirm a benign process.

Pearl

The usual recommended FDG PET imaging time to evaluate response therapy after chemotherapy is 3 weeks, but at least 2–3 months for radiation therapy. It is not always possible from a clinical standpoint to follow these guidelines, but an awareness of the potential problem is critical for interpretation.

Q: What is the role of F-18 FDG PET in differentiating infection from tumor in a patient with AIDS and numerous parenchymal lung abnormalities on CT?

A: The use of PET is very limited as it can not differentiate infection from tumor, as both can show intense radiotracer uptake.

Pearl

PET can help direct biopsy to the most metabolically active area of a mass to help avoid sampling areas of necrosis.

Q: Which is the best modality for the detection of osseous metastases?

A: It depends. MRI is highly sensitive and often detects lesions not seen on bone scan as it can visualize changes in the marrow and does not depend on secondary reactive cortical bone changes to develop. Bone scan, on the other hand, can image the whole body in a cost-effective manner. It is very useful in tumors with sclerotic metastases. PET scanning with F-18 FDG is more sensitive than bone scan for more aggressive lytic tumors. At times the two modalities complement each other by detecting different lesions in the same patient. F-18 sodium fluoride PET is a very sensitive bone scan agent and some feel that it may replace Tc-99m MDP imaging. Each of these methods is more sensitive than CT or radiographs.

Q: What are some differences between nonattenuation-corrected PET images and attenuation-corrected images?

A: The noncorrected image has a very different appearance than the corrected image. Structures near the surface appear more intense as fewer photons are attenuated before hitting the detector. This explains why the skin looks like it is outlined with a charcoal pencil. The air-filled lungs are also intense. Because fewer counts are seen in central areas, lesions may be missed. For accurate quantification (SUV), the attenuation corrected images must be used.

Q: What is the most significant type of scatter experienced in PET?

A: Compton scatter is most common in the energy range of PET (511 keV). It is particularly a problem with three-dimensional (3-D) mode (no septa) acquisition. 3-D is highly sensitive and faster than two-dimensional, but also accepts more scatter counts which causes reduced image quality.

ONCOLOGY—SINGLE PHOTON RADIOPHARMACEUTICALS

Q: What is the mechanism of gallium-67 uptake in tumors?

A: Ga-67 binds to serum iron transport molecules such as transferrin, which transports the Ga-67 to the tumor. Ga-67 enters the extracellular fluid space via the tumor's leaky capillary endothelium. It is bound to the tumor cell surface by transferrin receptors and then transported into the cell, where it binds to proteins such as ferritin and lactoferrin, which are in increased concentration in tumors.

Q: Ga-67 uptake is normally seen in which of the following organs: salivary glands, lacrimal glands, thymus, spleen, breast, heart?

A: Salivary gland and lacrimal gland uptake is normal and variable. Thymus uptake may be seen normally in children, especially after they have received chemotherapy. The spleen has uptake, but it is low level. Breast uptake is variable and is most prominent post-partum. Heart visualization is not normal, but may occur with myocarditis or pericarditis.

Pitfall

Surgical wounds normally have increased uptake for 1–2 weeks postoperatively, and faint activity may remain for 3–4 weeks. Focal bone uptake may be seen after bone marrow biopsy. Increased bone uptake may also be seen wherever there is increased bone turnover, such as fractures, orthopedic hardware, arthritis.

Q: For which malignant diseases has Ga-67 been found most clinically useful for diagnosis, staging, and restaging?

A: Hodgkin's disease, malignant lymphoma, hepatoma, and melanoma. However, F-18 FDG has to a large extent replaced Ga-67 for this purpose.

Q: Which of the following statements is associated with Hodgkin's disease and which with non-Hodgkin's lymphoma?
  a. Orderly contiguous spread of lymph node involvement in young patients
  b. Multicentric disease with a highly variable clinical course and a high incidence of extranodal tumor involvement
  c. Mediastinal masses are common
  d. Abdominal involvement of mesenteric and retroperitoneal nodes is common
  e. High cure rate
  f. Variable clinical course that can be indolent or rapidly lethal

A: Hodgkin's disease: *a, c, e;* non-Hodgkin's lymphoma: *b, d, f.*

Pearl

Prior to the availability of FDG PET, Ga-67 was used in patients with Hodgkin's disease and malignant lymphoma posttherapy masses to differentiate residual tumor or fibrosis, necrosis, or scarring.

Pitfall

A pretherapy Ga-67 study is important for proper evaluation of the posttherapy Ga-67 study. The pretherapy study ensures that the tumor site is gallium-avid.

Q: Technetium-99m sestamibi has been used for determination of malignancy of breast masses detected with mammography or by palpation. Which of these statements is true?
  a. Its accuracy is higher for palpable than for non-palpable masses.
  b. Its sensitivity is poor for lesions less than 1 cm in size.
  c. Fibroadenomas are always negative.
  d. It is particularly useful in patients with dense breasts or those with architectural distortion, such as previous surgery, radiation therapy, and breast implants.

A: *a, b, d.* Fibroadenomas are a common cause for false positives.

Q: Which of the following statements are true of In-111 capromab pendetide (ProstaScint)?
  a. Murine monoclonal antibody against a prostate-specific membrane antigen expressed by more than 95% of prostate adenocarcinomas.
  b. Its main indication is for localization of soft tissue metastases after prostatectomy in patients with a rising PSA and negative bone scan.
  c. Elevated human murine antibody (HAMA) titers are observed in 50% of patients.
  d. SPECT is mandatory for the pelvis.

A: *a,b,d.* HAMA elevations are seen in less than 10% of patients.

Pearl

The membrane specific antigen that In-111 ProstaScint localizes to is not PSA but rather prostate specific membrane antigen (PSMA), a glycoprotein expressed by prostate epithelium, which is not expressed on any other adenocarcinomas.

Pearl

Adverse reactions occur in 4% of patients receiving ProstaScint. They are usually minor. The incidence of adverse affects with a second injection is only 5%, thus it can be used diagnostically a second time.

Pearl

Although In-111 ProstaScint is useful for detecting soft-tissue metastases, it is not particularly sensitive for detecting bone metastases. The bone scan is more sensitive.

Pearl

ProstaScint accumulation in the prostate bed in a patient treated with radioactive seed placement is nonspecific. Uptake in the surgical bed following prostatectomy is highly suspicious for recurrent tumor.

Q: Which of the following are true statements regarding In-111 OctreoScan?
  a. It is a somatostatin receptor imaging agent.
  b. The sensitivity for all neuroendocrine tumors is very high.
  c. Highest uptake is seen in the spleen and kidneys.
  d. Only neuroendocrine tumors have somatostatin receptors.
A: *a, c.* Although its sensitivity for detection of most neuroendocrine tumors is very high, it has a poorer sensitivity for insulinomas and medullary carcinoma of the thyroid. Somatostatin receptors are found on a variety of nonneuroendocrine tumors, including astrocytomas, meningiomas, malignant lymphoma, and breast and lung cancer.

Q: In which melanoma patients is sentinel node lymphoscintigraphy indicated and why?
A: Patients with a primary lesion less than 1 mm in thickness are at low risk of recurrence and have a good prognosis. Patients with a primary lesion thickness greater than 4 mm are at high risk for metastatic adenopathy and distant metastases. Lymphoscintigraphy is indicated for patients with primary lesions greater than 1 mm and less than 4 mm thickness.

Q: What information does sentinel node lymphoscintigraphy provide in patients with intermediate-thickness malignant melanoma?
A: Sentinel node lymphoscintigraphy can pinpoint the sentinel node for the surgeon, which can be localized easily at surgery with a gamma probe. After immunohistochemical staining of tissue from this lymph node, the presence of metastases can be determined. The results will determine which patients require further nodal bed dissection and adjuvant chemotherapy.

Q: Which radiopharmaceutical is used for melanoma lymphoscintigraphy? What is the injection methodology?
A: Filtered Tc-99m sulfur colloid is the usual agent because unfiltered Tc-99m SC does not migrate well from the site of injection. It is injected intracutaneously at four sites around the primary lesion site.

Q: In what other malignant disease, is sentinel node lymphoscintigraphy commonly performed and how is it injected?
A: Breast cancer. The method of injection varies. At some hospitals, it is injected intratumorally. However, others inject it subdermally, whereas some inject the Tc-99m SC in the periareolar region. The rationale is that all lymphatics drain to the areolar region before drainage to the axillary region. Lymphatic drainage to the internal mammary or supraclavicular nodes is occasionally detected.

Pearl

Many experts recommend using two methods to ensure optimal lymphatic transit. Massaging the site of injection vigorously after injection promotes migration of the dose.

Pearl

In patients with AIDS and an intracerebral mass, Tl-201 can differentiate tumor, usually malignant lymphoma, from inflammatory causes, most commonly toxoplasmosis. Tl-201 is not usually taken up in inflammation, but is taken up by malignant tumors. Predictive value is approximately 85%.

Q: What is the purpose of the In-111 Ibritumomab Tiuxetan (Zevalin) scan?
A: This scan assesses biodistribution of the Zevalin prior to the administration of the therapeutic Y-90 Ibritumomab Tiuxetan (Zevalin). Abnormalities that indicate therapy should not be given include excessive uptake in the lung or kidneys or activity in these organs that increases or does not decrease over time. It is normal but not mandatory to see uptake in the tumor.

Pearl

The dose of Y-90 Zevalin is adjusted based on the patient's platelet count: 0.4 mCi/kg for patients with platelets >150,000 and 0.3 mCi/kg for platelets between 149,000 to 100,000. If the platelet count is below 100,000, patients should not be treated.

GASTROINTESTINAL

Q: What is achalasia? What is the role of the esophageal transit study?

A: Achalasia is characterized by absence of peristalsis in the distal two-thirds of the esophagus, increased lower esophageal sphincter (LES) pressure, and incomplete sphincter relaxation after swallowing. It is associated with symptoms of dysphagia, weight loss, nocturnal regurgitation, cough, and aspiration. The diagnosis is confirmed by esophageal manometry. Radionuclide esophageal transit studies have a high sensitivity for making the diagnosis; however, they are most useful for evaluating the effectiveness of therapy, such as esophageal dilation.

Q: Which of the following statements in regard to reflux and aspiration studies are true or false:
   a. The milk study is a sensitive method for diagnosing gastroesophageal reflux.
   b. The milk study is a sensitive method for diagnosing aspiration.
   c. Frequent image acquisition improves the sensitivity of the milk study.
   d. The "salivagram" is a more sensitive method for diagnosing aspiration.

A: True: *a, c, d*
  False: *b*. Aspiration is seen only rarely on delayed imaging.

Q: What is the functional role of the proximal and distal stomach?

A: The proximal stomach or fundus is responsible for liquid emptying and for receptive relaxation to accommodate a large meal. The distal stomach or antrum is responsible for the grinding and sieving of solid food and solid emptying.

Q: Describe the difference in emptying patterns between solids and liquids.

A: Liquids empty exponentially. Solid emptying is biphasic, with an initial lag phase before linear emptying begins. The lag phase is due to the time required for food to be broken down into small enough pieces to allow passage through the pylorus.

Q: Which of these factors will affect the rate of gastric emptying: meal content, time of day, position (standing, sitting, lying), stress, exercise?

A: All. The gastric emptying study should be standardized for the meal, time of day, patient position, methodology of acquisition and processing. Normal values should be derived from this specific protocol.

Q: Which of the following statements are true regarding the need for variable attenuation correction of gastric emptying studies?
   a. Gastric emptying may be underestimated when an anterior acquisition alone is obtained.
   b. The characteristic pattern of attenuation effect on solid gastric emptying time–activity curve is a rise in activity after ingestion of the meal before emptying begins.
   c. The geometric mean method is considered the standard method for attenuation correction.

A: All. Both anterior and posterior acquisitions are required to correct using the geometric mean calculation (square root of the product of the anterior and posterior views).

Q: What other methods can be used as an alternative to the geometric mean method of attenuation correction?

A: Left anterior oblique method. Because the camera head is positioned roughly parallel to movement of the stomach contents, from the posterior fundus to the more anterior antrum, no mathematic correction is needed.

Q: When might the use of Tc-99m sulfur colloid offer advantages over Tc-99m red blood cells for the diagnosis of acute gastrointestinal bleeding?

A: With very rapid bleeding and vascular instability, the radiotracer can be injected and the study completed in 15–20 minutes. No radiolabeling of red cells is necessary. The patient can then go directly to angiography, potentially saving the angiographer time and contrast.

Q: List in increasing order the labeling efficiency of methods to label Tc-99m red blood cells: in vivo, in vitro, and in vivtro.

A: In vivo, 75%; in vivtro or modified in vivo, 85%; and in vitro, 98%. An in vitro commercial kit method (Ultratag) for labeling Tc-99m erythrocytes is now available and is the method of choice, particularly for gastrointestinal bleeding studies.

Q: Why is the Tc-99m red blood cell method for detecting gastrointestinal bleeding more sensitive than the Tc-99m sulfur colloid method?

A: A longer acquisition is possible, usually 90 minutes, and imaging can be performed for up to 24 hours.

Q: What are the essential criteria needed to confidently diagnose the site of active bleeding on a radionuclide study?

A: A radiotracer "hot spot" appears where there was none and conforms to bowel activity; the activity increases over time; and the activity moves antegrade or retrograde.

Pitfall

A poor label can result in gastric activity that might be construed as upper gastrointestinal bleeding or urinary activity that might be misinterpreted as a bleeding site.

Pearl

Look for thyroid and salivary gland uptake when in doubt about the presence of free Tc-99m pertechnetate.

Pearl

A lateral view of the pelvis should be routine the end of the acquisition to differentiate bladder, rectal bleeding, and penile activity.

Pitfall

Focal activity that does not move may be anatomical (e.g., kidney, accessory spleen, hemangioma, varices, aneurysm).

Pearl

Contrast angiography can detect bleeding rates of about 1 ml/min versus 0.1 ml/min for the radionuclide study.

Q: Ectopic gastric mucosa is most often seen clinically in Meckel's diverticulum. What other gastric abnormalities may contain gastric mucosa?

A: Gastrointestinal duplication, Barrett's esophagus, and a retained gastric antrum after gastrectomy. In addition, ectopic gastric mucosa may occur in gastrogenic cystis found in the pancreas, duodenum, and colon.

Pearl

The mucin cells in the stomach are primarily responsible for gastric uptake of Tc-99m pertechnetate, not the parietal cells.

Q: What is the origin of Meckel's diverticulum?

A: This most common congenital anomaly of the gastrointestinal tract results from failure of closure of the omphalomesenteric duct of the embryo, which connects the yolk sac to the primitive foregut via the umbilical cord.

Pearl

This true diverticulum (Meckel's) arises on the antimesenteric side of the bowel, usually 80–90 cm proximal to the ileocecal valve, although it can occur elsewhere.

Pearl

Gastric mucosa is present in 10–30% of all Meckel's diverticula, in 60% of symptomatic patients, and in 98% of those with bleeding.

Pitfall

A number of false-positive studies have been reported over the years in scans for Meckel's diverticula, including those of urinary tract origin (e.g., horseshoe kidney, ectopic kidney), those resulting from inflammation (e.g., inflammatory bowel disease, neoplasms), bowel obstruction (seen most often with intussusception and volvulus), and other areas of ectopic gastric mucosa.

INFECTION AND INFLAMMATION

Q: Three of four Ga-67 photopeaks are acquired for imaging. What are they and what is their abundance?

A: 185 kev (23% abundance), 300 keV (18%) and 394 keV (4%). The 91 kev (41%) is not acquired.

Q: Name the photopeaks of In-111 and their abundance that are used for leukocyte imaging.

A: 173 kev (89%) and 247 keV (94%).

Q: Which collimator should be used for Ga-67 and In-111?

A: Medium-energy collimator. A high-energy collimator can be used, although its efficiency is less and image acquisition time is longer.

Q: Image quality is not as good with Ga-67 as that achieved with Tc-99m agents for which of the following reasons?

   a.   Decreased crystal sensitivity for high-energy photons

   b.   Poor collimator efficiency

c. Scatter and septal penetration from high-energy photons

d. Multiple photopeaks

e. Low administered dose

f. High background activity

A: All except *d*. However, if the multiple photopeaks are not aligned correctly, image quality can be adversely affected.

Q: Pulmonary Ga-67 uptake is seen in which of the following diseases?

a. tuberculosis

b. histoplasmosis

c. sarcoidosis

d. *Pneumocystis carinii* infection

e. Kaposi's sarcoma

f. cytomegalovirus

g. lung cancer

h. pneumonoconioses

A: All of the above except for Kaposi's sarcoma, which is not Ga-67 avid.

Pearl

Kaposi's sarcoma is Tl-201 avid.

Q: Ga-67 is taken up by the lungs due to drug toxicity. Which drugs are the culprits?

A: Bleomycin is the most common. However uptake can be seen with cytoxin, nitrofurantoin, and amiodarone.

Q: What is the role of Ga-67 in sarcoidosis?

A: Ga-67 lung uptake is a sensitive test for the diagnosis of active alveolitis of sarcoidosis. Ga-67 may be markedly increased in the setting of a normal chest radiograph in early disease, and may be negative in the setting of an abnormal radiograph in inactive disease.

Pearl

Characteristic scintigraphic patterns of uptake of sarcoidosis are: 1) the "panda sign," due to uptake in the salivary glands, parotids, and nasopharyngeal region; and 2) the "lambda sign," due to paratracheal and hilar lymph node uptake.

Q: Which leukocytes are labeled with In-111 oxine and Tc-99m HMPAO?

A: In-111 binds to neutrophils, lymphocytes, monocytes, as well as erythrocytes and platelets. Tc-99m HMPAO preferentially binds to neutrophils.

Q: Which of the following statements is true regarding In-111 oxine leukocytes?

a. It is diagnostically useful for evaluating inflammatory lung disease.

b. It has a high sensitivity for detecting osteomyelitis of the spine.

c. It should not be used when the peripheral leukocyte count is less than 3,000/mm³.

d. It is the radiopharmaceutical of choice for intra-abdominal infection.

A: *c* and *d* are true. A minimal number of leukocytes are needed for adequate radiolabeling and sensitivity of the test. The lack of intra-abdominal clearance makes it ideal for detecting intra-abdominal infection. The false negative rate for osteomyelitis of the spine is high, in the range of 40%. It is insensitive and nonspecific for pulmonary inflammatory disease, although focal uptake noted should be pursued diagnostically.

Pearl

Tc-99m HMPAO is the preferred agent for localizing infection in pediatric patients because of In-111 leukocyte's high radiation dose to the spleen, in the range of 15–20 rads in the adult, but 30–50 rads in children.

Q: What is the optimal imaging time for In-111 labeled leukocytes and Tc-99m HMPAO leukocytes?

A: In-111 labeled leukocytes are routinely imaged at 24 hours. Imaging at 4–6 hours is less sensitive for detection of infection. The one exception is inflammatory bowel disease in which imaging should be done at 4 hours, because intraluminal shedding of inflamed cells may result in inaccurate localization at 24 hours. Tc-99m HMPAO leukocytes should be imaged at 1–2 hours for intra-abdominal infection because of biliary and renal clearance seen by 2 hours. Extra-abdominal infection can be imaged later, usually 4 hours, allowing more time for background clearance.

Pitfall

Leukocytes may accumulate at site of inflammation without infection, such as intravenous catheters, nasogastric, endogastric, and drainage tubes, tracheostomies, and colostomies. Leukocytes may accumulate at postoperative surgical sites for 2–3 weeks and low-grade uptake may be seen at healing fracture sites. Accessory spleens may be misinterpreted as infection and renal transplants accumulate leukocytes.

Pitfall

Intraluminal intestinal radioactivity can be the result of swallowed or shedding cells from pharyngitis, sinusitis, pneumonia or herpes esophagitis. Gastrointestinal bleeding is another cause for false-positive intraluminal leukocyte activity.

Pearl

Tc-99m fanolesomaba (NeutroSpec) is the newest approved radiopharmaceutical for infection imaging. It is a murine monoclonal antibody that binds to human neutrophils. It was initially approved for acute appendicitis; however, it will likely be used for osteomyelitis and other infectious etiologies. It is not excreted intra-abdominally. Its major advantage over In-111 oxine and Tc-99m HMPAO leukocytes is that no blood handling is required.

Pearl

F-18 FDG is expected to have a future role in infection and inflammation imaging.

Q: Which of the following statements is not true?
   a. A negative three-phase bone scan excludes osteomyelitis with a high degree of certainty.
   b. The specificity of the bone scan is poor in patients with underlying bone disease such as fractures, orthopedic hardware, and neuropathic joints.
   c. In-111 oxine and Tc-99m HMPAO leukocytes have poor specificity for the diagnosis of osteomyelitis in a patient with a hip prosthesis.
   d. Because the three-phase bone scan may be positive in a patient with a Charcot's joint, a radiolabeled leukocyte study should be performed.

A: *d* is not correct. A radiolabeled leukocyte study may also be a false positive. However, the combination of a bone marrow study with a leukocyte study can be diagnostic. Similarly hip and knee prostheses are best evaluated with a bone marrow study as well. In any clinical situation where the bone marrow distribution may not be normal, a Tc-99m SC study is indicated.

Pitfall

Although the three-phase bone scan has a high negative predictive value for osteomyelitis in general, false negatives have been reported in the neonate.

Q: Regarding osteomyelitis, which of these statements is false?
   a. The three-phase bone scan is a sensitive test for diagnosis.
   b. The three-phase positive scan is specific for osteomyelitis.
   c. A negative flow phase study almost always rules it out.
   d. In patients with prostheses, a bone marrow study can be useful to rule out a false positive In-111 leukocyte study.

A: *b.* The bone scan is the most sensitive test for osteomyelitis; however, it is not specific. For example, a three-phase bone scan can be seen with fracture, a Charcot joint, tumor, and so forth. Although false-negative bone scans are rare, ischemia due to arteriosclerotic vascular disease can result in a false-negative flow study. A bone marrow study in conjunction with a labeled leukocyte study is the most accurate method for diagnosing an infected prosthesis.

CENTRAL NERVOUS SYSTEM

Q: How is the diagnosis of brain death made?
A: The patient is in a deep coma with total absence of brainstem reflexes and spontaneous respiration. Reversible causes (e.g., drugs, hypothermia) must be excluded; the cause of the dysfunction must be diagnosed (e.g., trauma, stroke); and the clinical findings of brain death must be present for a defined period of observation (6–24 hours). Confirmatory tests such as electroencephalography (EEG) and radionuclide imaging may be used to increase diagnostic certainty, but the diagnosis is primarily clinical. The radionuclide study is more specific than EEG.

Q: Which radiopharmaceuticals are used to evaluate brain death, and what are the advantages of each?
A: Tc-99m DTPA is inexpensive but more technically demanding to use and interpret. Tc-99m HMPAO or Tc-99m ECD are often preferred because no flow study is required, just delayed images to visualize radiotracer fixed in cortex.

Pearl

A "hot nose" may be seen on the flow-phase images and delayed images as a result of shunting of blood from the internal to the external carotid system that supplies the face and nose in patients with severe carotid stenosis, brain death, psychoactive drug use, and use of other drugs that cause nasal congestion.

Q: What is the difference in mechanism of uptake between fluorine-18 fluorodeoxyglucose (F-18 FDG) and the Tc-99m cerebral perfusion agents?

A: F-18 FDG is a glucose analog, and its uptake represents regional glucose metabolism. It is metabolically trapped intracellularly. Tc-99m HMPAO and Tc-99m ECD are lipid-soluble cerebral perfusion agents taken up in proportion to regional cerebral blood flow. They fix intracellularly. In most cases, cerebral blood flow follows metabolism.

Pearl

An example of a decoupling of metabolism and blood flow is seen during the acute phase of a stroke. Blood flow may be normal or increased for the initial 1–10 days (luxury perfusion), but metabolism is decreased.

Q: How can single-photon emission computed tomography (SPECT) brain perfusion or positron emission tomography (PET) FDG imaging be useful in the differential diagnosis of dementia?

A: Multi-infarct dementia is characterized by multiple areas of past infarcts, recognized as areas of decreased uptake that correspond to the vascular distribution patterns as well as to changes in the deep structures such as the basal ganglia and thalamus. Alzheimer's disease exhibits a characteristic pattern of bitemporal and parietal hypoperfusion and hypometabolism. Pick's disease is associated with decreased frontal lobe uptake. AIDS-dementia complex is associated with a pattern of multifocal or patchy cortical regions of decreased uptake, seen particularly in the frontal, temporal, and parietal lobes and the basal ganglion.

Pearl

Although Alzheimer's disease has a characteristic bitemporal-parietal pattern on perfusion imaging, it is often *not* symmetrical. Decreased frontal lobe uptake may also be seen. This pattern often cannot be differentiated from the imaging pattern of Parkinson's disease and Lewey body disease, although they typically have very different clinical presentations.

Q: What is the purpose of cerebral perfusion imaging in patients with seizures? What is the expected PET or SPECT pattern?

A: F-18 FDG PET or SPECT cerebral perfusion studies can often localize the seizure focus in patients requiring surgery (typically temporal lobectomy) for seizure control. Interictally, a seizure focus shows decreased metabolism on FDG PET and decreased perfusion on SPECT; increased activity is seen during a seizure (ictal). Normally, perfusion follows metabolism. In many surgical seizure centers, depth electrodes are not required preoperatively if the clinical picture, EEG, and SPECT study are all consistent as to the location of the seizure focus.

Q: Which radiopharmaceuticals have been found useful in imaging brain tumors, and what is their clinical utility?

A: F-18 FDG PET imaging demonstrates increased uptake in tumors owing to increased glycolysis. Uptake of FDG is proportional to the malignant grade of glioblastomas. PET determines tumor viability after radiation therapy. SPECT with thallium-201 and Tc-99m sestamibi can be used in a similar manner. Both T1-201 and PET FDG can differentiate lymphoma from infection, most often toxoplasmosis, in AIDS patients. Uptake of T1-201 or FDG is indicative of lymphoma.

Q: Name the radiopharmaceutical used for cisternography and the most common clinical indication for this study.

A: In-111 DTPA. The most common use of this radiopharmaceutical in modern practice is to confirm the diagnosis of normal-pressure hydrocephalus, an obstructive communicating form of hydrocephalus. The next most common use is to localize cerebrospinal fluid (CSF) leaks.

Pearl

The symptoms of normal pressure hydrocephalus are incontinence, dementia, and gait disturbance.

Q: What is the characteristic pattern of normal pressure hydrocephalus on radionuclide cisternography?

A: Persistent ventricular filling and evidence of a convexity block.

CARDIAC

Pearl

Myocardial perfusion scintigraphy, whether performed with SPECT or PET, is a "map" of relative blood flow to viable myocardium. That is, for activity to be recorded in the image, it must be delivered (blood flow) and taken up by a myocardial cell (viable myocardium).

Q: How does the percent extraction of thallium-201 passing through the myocardial capillary bed compare with the extraction of Tc-99m sestamibi and Tc-99m teboroxime?

A: Tl-201 has a myocardial extraction fraction of approximately 0.85 in normal subjects at normal flow rates. The myocardial extraction of Tc-99m sestamibi and Tc-99m tetrofosmin is considerably lower, 0.50 and 0.60, respectively.

Q: What percentage of Tl-201, Tc-99m sestamibi, and Tc-99m tetrofosmin localizes in the heart?
A: For Tl-201, 3-4% of the administered dose localizes in the heart in normal subjects; for Tc-99, sestamibi, 1.5%, and for tetrofosmin, 1.2%.

Q: What are the advantages and disadvantages of Tl-201 as perfusion agent for stress and rest myocardial scintigraphy?
A: Advantages: Tl-201 requires only a single injection because of redistribution; imaging can be performed early after stress, within 10-15 minutes; it can be used to assess viability. Disadvantages: its low administered dose because of its high radiation dosimetry; its poor imaging characteristics with a low photopeak of 69 to 80 keV and high scatter fraction; and its susceptibility to the effects of attenuation.

Pitfall

Patient motion can cause image degradation, create a defect, or obscure a defect.

Q: What quality control should be routinely performed to detect patient motion?
A: Review raw data in cinematic display. Review of the sonogram can confirm the extent of the problem.

Pearl

The best method for correcting the problem of motion is to repeat the study. If this is not possible, motion correction programs should be used. However, this software only corrects for motion in the vertical axis. Motion in the horizontal or diagonal axes will not be corrected.

Pitfall

Attenuation of photons by soft tissue can result in decreased activity to the myocardium that might suggest myocardial infarction if seen on both rest and stress or as ischemia if only apparent on the stress study. With females, breast attenuation results in decreased activity of the anterior, septal, or lateral wall, depending on their size and shape. Males characteristically have attenuation of the inferior wall, so-called diaphragmatic attenuation.

Q: In what ways can the image interpreter determine if fixed decreased activity is indeed pathological (i.e., infarction) or merely due to attenuation?
A: Review the raw data in the cinematic display to look for soft attenuation. Review of the gated SPECT can help determine if there is wall motion and thickening that would indicate that it is not an infarct, but probably due to attenuation, not infarction. Attenuation correction programs can be helpful. Prone imaging has been used to differentiate attenuation from infarction in the inferior wall.

Pearl

To correct for attenuation, a transmission map must be acquired. This has commonly been done by acquiring transmission counts from a gamma source (e.g., gadolinium-153). With SPECT-CT systems, the acquired CT is used for attenuation correction.

Q: What is the significance of lung uptake on Tl-201 exercise studies?
A: Lung uptake on exercise stress images, but not the delayed images is consistent with exercise-induced cardiac dysfunction. This finding is usually associated with three-vessel coronary artery disease.

Pearl

Lung uptake on Tl-201 images is easily perceived on planar images, but may not be appreciated in SPECT reconstructed and reoriented images. Review of the cinematic display of the raw projection data (low count planar images at multiple angles around the patient) will nicely show the lung uptake.

Q: What other scintigraphic finding suggest three-vessel disease?
A: Exercise induced ischemic dilation. The normal heart dilates during stress but gated SPECT is acquired poststress when normal hearts have returned to baseline size.

Pitfall

Incomplete normalization on delayed Tl-201 imaging does not equate with a fixed perfusion defect. Insisting on complete normalization before accepting an abnormality as not "fixed" results in underdetection of ischemic areas versus scarred areas.

Q: What is the rationale for a second injection of Tl-201 versus simple delayed imaging to distinguish fixed from reversible defects?

A: Relying solely on delayed imaging overestimates the number of fixed myocardial defects. Redistribution may take longer than the usual 3- to 4-hour delay and may not even be complete by 24 hours. A low serum Tl-201 level may not allow for significant redistribution. Reinjection of Tl-201 increases the serum level, permitting further redistribution.

Pearl

Patients with left bundle branch block may have reversible stress-induced hypoperfusion of the septum. Patients with ischemia do not usually have isolated septal involvement, but also apical and anterior wall ischemia. This potential diagnostic problem can be avoided by performing pharmacologic stress with adenosine or dipyridamole.

Q: What is the relationship between the time after myocardial infarction and the sensitivity of perfusion imaging?

A: The sensitivity of perfusion imaging for detecting defects caused by acute myocardial infarction is greatest right after the infarct and diminishes with time. This is different from "hot spot" imaging with Tc-99m pyrophosphate, in which the greatest sensitivity does not occur for a day or two after infarction.

Pitfall

Although myocardial perfusion scintigrams are positive immediately after infarction, it is not possible to determine whether a given defect is new or old. A given cold area may be caused by myocardial scar or acute myocardial infarction.

Pearl

The primary cause of false negative exercise studies in the diagnosis of coronary artery disease is failure to achieve adequate exercise.

Pearl

After exercise, significant Tl-201 localization in the liver usually indicates a poor exercise level. At peak exercise, blood flow is diverted from the splanchnic circulation.

Pitfall

Quantitative analysis systems that rely on databases of "normals" may not reflect the patient population in a different nuclear medicine department. Care must be taken to not rely too heavily on these databases.

Q: What is the mechanism of action of dipyridamole?

A: Dipyridamole inhibits the action of adenosine deaminase. By augmenting the effects of endogenous adenosine, dipyridamole is a powerful vasodilator.

Q: What effect can a cup of coffee have on a dipyridamole or adenosine stress test?

A: Caffeine in coffee, tea, soft drinks, or foods such as chocolate are chemically related to dipyridamole and adenosine and can block the effect of dipyridamole pharmacological stress testing.

Q: What percentage of stenosis at rest is necessary in the coronary arteries for resting blood flow to be affected?

A: Coronary artery stenosis greater than 85–90% is required before flow is diminished at rest. Not all stenoses are created equal. Long irregular stenotic segments have more effect than discrete short-segment stenoses.

Q: Why is imaging delayed for 30–90 minutes after administration of Tc-99m sestamibi or Tc-99m tetrofosmin?

A: Although myocardial uptake is rapid with both Tc-99m sestamibi and Tc-99m tetrofosmin, lung and liver uptake are also significant. The lung and liver clear with time and the target-to-background ratio improves.

Q: What pharmaceutical is administered that allows the Tc-99m to bind to the red blood cell?

A: Stannous (tin) pyrophosphate is the usual agent. Stannous chloride has been used.

Q: To what part of the red blood cell does the Tc-99m label bind?

A: Tc-99m binds to the beta chain of hemoglobin when the patient is pretreated with stannous ion.

Pitfall

Injection of labeling materials through a heparinized intravenous line can significantly decrease the yield with in vivo and modified in vivo RBC labeling.

Pearl

The in vitro kit method (UltraTag) of radiolabeling red blood cells is the present day preferable methodology because it has the highest labeling efficiency, greater than 97%. This results in less background and higher accuracy.

Q: What are the considerations for selecting the number of frames in a gated blood pool study?

A: Selecting the number of frames to divide the cardiac cycle is a balance between having enough frames to capture the peaks and valleys of the ventricular time–activity curve versus the need to acquire a statistically valid number of counts in each frame. For gated ventriculography (MUGA), using 16 frames achieves this compromise. For gated SPECT myocardial perfusion imaging, 8 frames is the usual compromise. Too few frames will "average out" the peaks and valleys. Too many frames increases the imaging time required for a given number of counts per frame.

Pitfall

In calculation of the left ventricular ejection fraction, too high an estimate of the background counts per pixel will result in a falsely high ejection fraction. This can happen if the background area includes activity from the spleen.

Pearl

Variations in the length of the cardiac cycle can be recognized on gated perfusion or blood pool studies if the time–activity curve trails off or fails to approximate the height of the initial part of the curve. Significant asymmetry (>10%) of the height of the curve at the beginning and the end may indicate significant arrhythmia.

Q: What do amplitude and phase images portray?

A: Amplitude and phase images are parametric or derived images. The amplitude image portrays the maximum count difference at each pixel location during the cardiac cycle. High ejection fraction areas have high amplitude, and background areas have low amplitude. The phase image portrays the timing of cyclical activity with respect to a reference standard, usually the R wave.

Q: What is the hallmark of a ventricular apical aneurysm by phase analysis?

A: Aneurysms demonstrate paradoxical motion. Activity in the area of the aneurysm is typically 180 degrees out of phase with the rest of the ventricle.

PULMONARY

Q: What are the two most commonly used radiopharmaceuticals for ventilation imaging? What are their advantages and disadvantages?

A: Xenon-133 and Tc-99m DTPA aerosol. Xenon-133 demonstrates more clearly the physiology of respira-

tion and is very sensitive to detection of obstructive airway disease manifested by slow washout. The disadvantage is the rapid washout, limiting the views obtainable, its suboptimal image quality due to the low photopeak (81 keV) and poor count rate image. Tc-99m DTPA aerosol allows high count images in all projections; however, the images are comparable only to the inspiratory phase of xenon-133. With obstructive airway disease, particles impact in the proximal bronchi, potentially causing interpretation difficulties.

Pitfall

Xenon-133 will be taken up and cleared slowly from livers with fatty metamorphosis. This should not be confused with pulmonary delayed washout.

Q: What is the minimum number of particles recommended for pulmonary perfusion imaging?

A: Pulmonary perfusion scanning assumes a statistically even distribution of particles throughout the lung. This requires at least 100,000 particles in normal adults, and 200,000–500,000 particles are generally administered.

Q: How should the dose of technetium-99m macroaggregated albumin (MAA) be adjusted in pediatric patients?

A: Radiopharmaceutical doses are always adjusted with respect to patient size or age in the pediatric population. With Tc-99m MAA it is also necessary to reduce the number of particles.

Q: What is the size range of MAA particles?

A: In commercial preparations the majority of particles are 20–40 μm, with a range of 10–90 μm.

Pitfall

Withdrawing blood into a syringe with Tc-99m MAA particles may create a small radioactive embolus that shows up as a "hot spot" on subsequent images.

Pitfall

Failure to resuspend the Tc-99m MAA particles before administration may result in clumping of particles together and the presence of "hot spots" on subsequent imaging.

Q: What is the biological fate of MAA particles?

A: MAA particles are physically broken down in the lung. Delayed imaging performed several hours after pharmaceutical administration demonstrates activity in the reticuloendothelial system because of phagocytosis of the breakdown particles.

Pearl

One way to determine whether radioactivity outside of the lungs is caused by free Tc-99m or right to left shunting of Tc-99m MAA is to image the brain. Free pertechnetate should not localize in the brain, but rather in the thyroid, salivary glands, and stomach, whereas Tc-99m MAA particles that gain access to the systemic circulation will lodge in the first capillary bed that they encounter, including the capillary bed in the brain. If no brain uptake is seen, there is no significant right to left shunt.

Q: What is the preferred patient position during administration of Tc-99m MAA?

A: Administering Tc-99m MAA with the patient supine results in a more homogeneous distribution of particles in the lung than when the patient is sitting or standing. Gravitational effects result in more basilar distribution when injection is accomplished with the patient upright.

Pitfall

In lateral views of the lung obtained for a fixed number of counts, "shine-through" from the contralateral lung can give the false impression of activity arising from the side being imaged. This is most dramatically demonstrated in patients who after pneumonectomy show no activity on anterior or posterior views but a near-normal appearance can be seen because of the shine-through phenomenon.

Pitfall

In analysis of perfusion scintigrams, failure to recognize the significance of *decreased* versus *absent* activity is a potential pitfall. Not every clot is 100% occlusive of the circulation. Significantly diminished activity needs to be recognized as one of the patterns caused by pulmonary emboli.

Pitfall

In some patients with fatty liver, retained activity in the liver on Xe-133 scans can be confused with retained activity or delayed washout at the right base. Remember that xenon is fat soluble and will show significant accumulation in patients with fatty liver.

Pitfall

The pulmonary hili are photon-deficient structures caused by the displacement of lung parenchyma by large vascular and bronchial structures. Failure to remember this can result in false positive interpretations, especially for defects seen on posterior oblique images.

Pitfall

If the patient is placed supine for V/Q imaging but the chest radiograph was obtained with the patient upright, it can be difficult to correlate findings on the examinations. For example, free fluid may collect in a subpulmonic location or obscure the lung base in the upright position. With the patient supine, the fluid may layer out posteriorly or collect in the fissures. Also, the apparent height of the lungs may be different, as may the heart size. Ideally, imaging studies should be performed with the patient in the same position for all examinations. On the other hand, if there is significant pleural fluid, it may be desirable to image the patient in more than one position to prove that a defect is caused by mobile fluid.

Q: What is the stripe sign?

A: The *stripe sign* refers to a stripe or zone of activity seen between a perfusion defect and the closest pleural surface. Because pulmonary emboli are typically pleura based, the stripe sign suggests another diagnosis, often emphysema. Rarely, in the resolution of pulmonary emboli, a stripe sign develops as circulation is restored.

Q: What is the physiological basis for perfusion defects in areas of poor ventilation?

A: The classic response to hypoxia at the alveolar level is vasoconstriction. Shunting of blood away from the hypoxic lung zone maintains oxygen saturation.

Q: What is the shrunken lung sign?

A: The lungs may appear smaller than usual in patients sustaining multiple small emboli, such as fat emboli, that distribute uniformly around the lung periphery.

Q: What is the classic appearance of multiple pulmonary emboli on lung perfusion scintigraphy?

A: Multiple pleura-based, wedge-shaped areas of significantly diminished or absent perfusion. The size of the defects may vary from subsegmental to segmental or may involve an entire lobe or lung.

Q: What are the most common clinical signs and symptoms in patients with confirmed pulmonary embolism?

A: In the PIOPED study, the three most common presenting symptoms (and approximate percentage frequency) were dyspnea, 80%; pleuritic chest pain,

60%; and cough, 40%. Hemoptysis (15%) and leg pain (25–30%) were less common. On physical examination, lung crackles (60%) were encountered much more often than leg swelling (30%) or pleural friction rub (5%). Both the heart rate and the respiratory rate were elevated on average in the PIOPED study in patients with pulmonary embolism.

Q: What is the sensitivity of the high-probability scan category for detecting pulmonary embolism?

A: In the PIOPED study, 41% of patients with pulmonary embolism had a high-probability scintigraphic pattern. Thus the majority of patients with pulmonary emboli have intermediate or low-probability scans.

Index

Note: Page numbers followed by f refer to figures; page numbers followed by t refer to tables; page numbers followed by b refer to boxes.

A

Abdominal imaging
  for infections, 418
  for tumors, 272-273
Acalculous biliary disease. *See* Chronic acalculous cholecystitis
Accelerated acute graft rejection, 244
ACE. *See* Angiotensin converting enzyme
ACE inhibition renography, 230-234
  criteria for, 237b
  image interpretation of, 232-233
  imaging protocol for, 233, 235
  indications for, 230
  protocol for, 233b
  renogram pattern with, 237f
  reporting of, 233-234
Achalasia
  definition of, 557
  manifestation of, 347
  semisolid meal and, 351f-352f
Acquired immunodeficiency syndrome (AIDS), 431
Activity-induced enthesopathy, 139
Acute acalculous cholecystitis, 174-175
  cholescintigraphy for, 174-175, 174t
  conditions associated with, 174b
Acute cholecystitis, 168-174
  blood flow and, 548
  cholescintigraphy for, 170-174
    accuracy of, 170b, 171-172, 173t
    false positives in, 173b
    rim sign in, 173-174, 174f, 548
  clinical presentation of, 168
  pathophysiology of, 168, 169b
  ultrasonography for, 169-170, 170b
Acute epididymitis
  scrotal scintigraphy for, 260
  views of, 262f
Acute graft rejection
  dynamic renal scintigraphy for, 244, 251-252
  time course of, 249f-250f
  time-activity curves of, 248f, 250f
  views of, 247f-248f

Acute pyelonephritis, 255
Acute testicular torsion
  scrotal scintigraphy for, 260
  views of, 260f
Adenosine
  chemical structure of, 465f
  pharmacologic effect of, 461-462
  side effects of, 462-465, 465t
  stress test protocol with, 465b
Adrenocortical scintigraphy, 105-109
  androgen excess and, 108-109
  Cushing's syndrome and, 106-108, 108f
  hyperaldosteronism and, 108
  incidentalomas and, 109
  normal, 106
  protocol for, 106b
  radiopharmaceuticals for, 105-106
  suppression studies with, 106
Adrenomedullary scintigraphy, 109-112
  clinical applications of
    neuroblastoma and, 111-112
    pheochromocytoma and, 111
  drug interference with, 110, 110t
  normal, 111
  radiopharmaceuticals for, 110
  technique of, 110
Adult respiratory distress syndrome, 535-536
AIDS. *See* Acquired immunodeficiency syndrome
AIDS-dementia complex, 431
Akinesis, 486
Alcoholic liver disease, 197, 200
Alpha decay, 24-25
Alpha particles, 542
Alzheimer's disease
  imaging of, 428, 430-431
    bitemporal-parietal patterns and, 561
    PET, 429f, 430f
    SPECT, 429f-430f
  incidence of, 428
Angiotensin converting enzyme (ACE)
  physiology of, 232f
  renography with, 230-234
  renovascular hypertension and, 230

Angstroms, 21b
Anne Arbor staging system
  for HD, 270b
  for lymphomas, 336b
Antineutrino, 25
Antrum
  anatomy of, 356f
  gastric motility and, 355-356
Appendicitis, 412
Arterial stenosis, 246, 248
Arterial thrombosis, 246
Atomic mass unit
  formula for, 21b
  mathematic definition of, 23
Atoms
  Bohr model of, 21-22, 21f
  mass-energy equivalence of, 23
  structure of, 20-21
Auger electron
  definition of, 22b
  in radionuclide decay, 28
Avogadro's number, 21b

B

Background radiation, 40
Backscatter peak, 38
Barium esophagography, 351
Barium follow-through study, 382
Barrett's esophagus, 380
Basophils, 389
Becquerels, 28
Bell-clapper deformity, 259, 553
Bernstein acid infusion test, 351
Beta minus decay, 25
Beta particles, 30, 542
Biliary atresia, 180-182
  cholescintigraphy for, 550
  detection of, 549
Biliary diversion surgery, 186
Biliary duct obstruction, 177-180
  biliary-to-bowl transit and, 178, 179b, 180f
  clinical presentation of, 177t